Practical Clinical Medicine

# Practical Clinical Medicine

*Edited by*

John Davies, MRCP, FACC

*Consultant Physician, Royal Gwent Hospital and Clinical Teacher at the University Hospital of Wales;*
*Honorary Senior Lecturer, Cardiothoracic Unit, Royal Brompton National Heart and Lung Hospital, London*

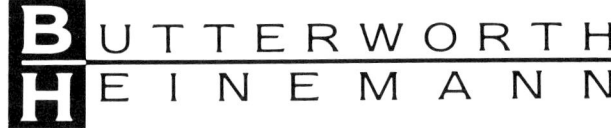

*For Wil and Nan*

Butterworth-Heinemann Ltd
Linacre House, Jordan Hill, Oxford OX2 8DP

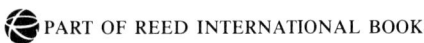 PART OF REED INTERNATIONAL BOOKS

OXFORD  LONDON  BOSTON
MUNICH  NEW DELHI  SINGAPORE  SYDNEY
TOKYO  TORONTO  WELLINGTON

First published 1992
Reprinted 1993

**British Library Cataloguing in Publication Data**
Practical clinical medicine
 I. Davies, John
 610

ISBN 0 7506 0026 8

**Library of Congress Cataloguing in Publication Data**
Practical clinical medicine/edited by John Davies.
 p. cm.
 Includes bibliographical references and index.
 ISBN 0 7506 0026 8
 1. Medicine.  I. Davies, John, Dr.
 [DNLM: 1. Clinical Medicine.  2. Physician–Patient Relations. WB
 100 P8951]
 R129.P68  1991
 616—dc20
 DNLM/DLC
 for Library of Congress
                                        91–29345
                                         CIP

Photoset by Wilmaset Ltd, Birkenhead, Wirral
Printed and bound in Great Britain by Bath Press Ltd, Bath, Avon

# Contents

# Contributors

LESZEK BORYSIEWICZ MRCP
Department of Medicine, University of Wales College of Medicine, Heath Park, Cardiff CF4 4XN

JOHN DAVIES MRCP FACC
Cardiology Department, Royal Gwent Hospital, Newport, Gwent

PAUL G. DAVIES MRCP
Department of Rheumatology, Chelmsford & Essex Hospital and Broomfield Hospital, Court Road, Broomfield, Chelmsford, Essex

PAUL FINUCANE MRCPI
Department of Geriatric Medicine, University Department of Geriatric Medicine, Cardiff Royal Infirmary, Newport Road, Cardiff, South Glamorgan CF2 1SZ

ANNE FREEMAN MRCP
Department of Geriatric Medicine, St Woolos Hospital, Newport, Gwent

HUMPHREY HODGSON DM FRCP
Department of Medicine, Royal Postgraduate Medical School, London W12 ONN

JOHN ISAACS MRCP
Immunology Division, Department of Pathology, University of Cambridge, Tennis Court Road, Cambridge CB12 1QP

IRENE LEIGH MRCP
Department of Dermatology, The London Hospital, Whitechapel, London E1 1BB

GLYN LEWIS, MRCPsych
Lecturer, Institute of Psychiatry, De Crespigny Park, Denmark Hill, London SE5 8AF

GARETH LLEWELLYN MRCP
Department of Neurological Science, Royal Free Hospital, London NW3 2PF

NEIL MCINTOSH FRCP
Department of Child Life and Health, University of Edinburgh, 17 Hatton Place, Edinburgh, EH9 1UW

KEITH PATTERSON MRCP MRCPath
Department of Haematology, University College Hospital, WC1E 6AU

IAN S. PETHERAM FRCP
Newport Chest Clinic, Postgraduate Organizer, Gwent Postgraduate Medicine Centre, Newport, Gwent

ANTHONY J. PINCHING FRCP
Department of Immunology, St Mary's Hospital Medical School, Norfolk Place, Paddington, London W2 1PG

NEIL SCOLDING MRCP (UK)
Department of Neurology, Addenbrooke's Hospital, Hills Road, Cambridge

DAVID J. SPALTON FRCS FRCP
Department of Ophthalmology, St Thomas' Hospital, London SE1 7EH

A. P. WEETMAN MRCP
Wellcome Senior Research Fellow, Royal Postgraduate Medical School, Hammersmith Hospital, London W12 0HS

# Section One

## Clinical Method

# 1

# APPROACH TO THE PATIENT

John Davies

## HISTORY

The best way to learn how to take a detailed, informative and useful history is by practice and experience. Every effort should be made to ensure that the patient is relaxed, comfortable and at ease. No leading questions should be asked and no suggested answers should be given. All questions should be neutral and the patient should be encouraged to give an account in his or her own words as to what exactly the trouble is.

Remember that there are many diseases that can be diagnosed on the basis of the history alone, for instance, angina pectoris, when the physical examination in most cases will be normal. Without a good rapport, based on mutual respect and sympathy, it will not be possible to obtain useful information concerning the patient's symptoms or to build up a comprehensive picture of the patient as an individual.

Each patient is unique. Even the most standard symptoms will manifest themselves in completely different ways from patient to patient. Circumstances at work or at home may be very relevant to symptoms. Most important of all, each patient will have an entirely individual response to a symptom. One patient may tolerate pain unflinchingly while others make much fuss over minor discomfort. Some are withdrawn while others are frankly theatrical.

The patient should never feel that the doctor is disapproving or a moralist. Because of the developing epidemic of AIDS it will probably become increasingly important to enquire delicately into each patient's usual sexual practice. Such information can only be obtained when a relationship of trust has developed.

A calm, gentle, kind but serious approach usually wins trust and cooperation, even when an elderly patient is interviewed by a young medical student. Outbursts of emotion by the patient during interviews are usually beneficial and the ability of the doctor to manage and not react to a period of anger scores many points in the patient's estimation of the doctor. It is always of benefit to a patient to be able to cry during an interview, in which case the doctor should not recoil or become worried but should gently touch and reassure the patient; the passing of a handkerchief or paper tissue to dry the eyes is usually appreciated.

As with any relationship, communication does not only take place via the spoken word. The physician needs to be perceptive of all types of unspoken communication—such as a nod of the head or roll of the eyes. Although the patient complains of headache, the real problem, such as marital difficulties, may be hinted at and, once the clue is given, the expert physician should home straight in and ask specifically: 'Is everything OK between you and your husband, Mrs Smith?'

Important clues about the patient's personality and therefore their reaction to presenting symptoms can be obtained from the type of dress, hairstyle and cleanliness, and by assessment of whether a patient is 'laid back' and relaxed or 'twitched' and anxious.

The patient's history should be taken in a quiet, relaxed and unhurried atmosphere. No matter how many people are waiting, or how much the doctor wants to dash off to a meeting, the patient should always be made to feel as though he or she has the doctor's undivided attention for as long as is required. It should be remembered that for many patients a visit to the doctor and especially attendance at the hospital outpatients can cause severe stress. For others, of course, frequent visits are highly enjoyable!

## The consultation

When the patient first enters the consulting room, the doctor should stand up, walk towards the patient and introduce himself or herself while shaking the patient's hand. The patient should then be taken towards a comfortable chair and asked if there are any accompanying relatives who would also like to be involved in the interview. If the patient is being seen in hospital, then it should be mentioned that the helpful letter or telephone call has already been received from the general practitioner. Rather than asking direct questions, general remarks should then be made, leaving the field entirely open to the patient—something like: 'Now tell me in your own words, Mrs Smith, what exactly the problem is that has brought you along today and when exactly did it start to bother you?'

## Direct questions

After the patient's own description some sort of order of questioning needs then to be introduced, starting with the presenting symptoms and the general questions regarding each particular system, followed by any past medical history. The patient should then be asked about personal habits, such as alcohol consumption, cigarette smoking (in younger patients to include possible drug addiction and unusual sexual habits), followed by the family history and some account of the patient's present social circumstances. The social history is obviously of considerable importance in an elderly patient.

Probably the best historian is a well-trained policeman who has always been disciplined to take careful notes and trained to give short and specific accounts. Most patients, of course, will be more vague and loquacious. Intelligent patients can sometimes be the most difficult to interview because they frequently have already put their own interpretation on their symptoms. On being asked what the problem is they may reply, 'Well actually I think it's probably angina, doctor.' Less intelligent patients should be guided but leading questions should always be avoided. For instance, when questioning a patient who may have angina it is better to ask: 'Tell me exactly where you get a pain or discomfort and what might bring it on?', rather than 'Do you get a pressure pain on exercise which goes away when you rest?'

If they cannot describe what exactly the matter is, then suggest gently, 'Well, is it a pain?' and then to go on slowly to ask where exactly it occurs and to where this pain may radiate. Premature interruption by questioning is to be avoided and specific questions should only be asked when the patient has completely finished his or her own description. The occasional nod may frequently be all that is required to show that the physician is still attentive and to encourage the patient to go on talking.

## Symptoms

Symptoms should then be characterized according to their type, severity, when they occur and whether there are any precipitating aggravating or relieving factors. It is sometimes common for a symptom to occur regularly as part of a group of symptoms. For instance, association of headache, flushing and palpitations in a hypertensive patient is very suggestive of a phaeochromocytoma. Any symptoms may be psychosomatic in origin. Indeed, most general practitioners complain that only a tiny minority of their patients turn out to have a definite organic cause for their symptoms. Symptoms simply serve as a means of communicating a need for help. The patient may be particularly worried about cancer or may have lost a close relative because of early ischaemic heart disease. It is often useful to ask the patient if he or she has any particular fears concerning a specific illness and it is frequently gratifying to see the enormous smile that appears at the end of a consultation when a patient is told that there are definitely no signs of any type of cancer.

If a particular symptom is present, it is worthwhile asking to what extent this symptom is limiting the patient's lifestyle. A man with angina may rarely get chest pain but this can sometimes be because he has turned into an invalid and is presently not exerting himself to any significant degree. The extent to which a particular symptom affects the patient's leisure activities and, in particular, sexual activity, should be specifically asked after.

## Previous medical history

After the presenting problem has been described in detail and specific direct questions asked about each system, then an account should be given of all previous medical events in the patient's life.

## Drug history

It is important to take a complete drug history. To avoid confusion it is always a good idea to suggest to the patient that when they visit the doctor they bring all their medication with them, in order that doses and frequency of administration can be carefully checked. A good example of drug-related disease is the extremely high incidence of gastrointestinal bleeding in elderly patients taking anti-inflammatory drugs. The administration of one drug frequently modifies the behaviour of another. Many drugs can potentiate the effect of warfarin. Any previous adverse reaction to drugs should be carefully enquired after and, in particular, whether or not the patient is allergic to penicillin, aspirin or any other drugs. Females should be specifically asked if they are, or have been, taking the contraceptive pill. Drug abuse should always be considered.

## Family history

Family history can be extremely important in many diseases. In some cases, for instance, Huntington's chorea, it may be diagnostic. Family history is one of the major risk factors for the development of early ischaemic heart disease. On the other hand, a symptom of atypical chest pain in a young man may be explained by the recent death of his father due to a myocardial infarction. A patient with headaches may have had a sister who developed a cerebral tumour.

## Social history

The patient's present and previous occupation is generally of interest and important in assessing their personality but may be of specific relevance if there is any possibility of industrial lung or other disease. In the presence of alcohol abuse, it may be difficult to find out from the patient how much is actually being consumed and this history may need to be obtained from relatives. Likewise, this may be the case regarding cigarette consumption. If the patient claims to be a non-smoker, the relevant question may be 'When did you stop?' He or she may now be a non-smoker having smoked 60 cigarettes a day for 20 years until the beginning of that week!

Specific questions regarding housing and diet may be relevant. Careful enquiry into the patient's social circumstances is particularly important in the elderly as it may well be possible to provide additional ancillary services. Living in a vandalized tenement block may well produce depression in a lonely, unmarried mother and this may be the cause of her symptoms of severe headaches.

Patients who are depressed and withdrawn will not volunteer much information and these patients need to be treated with patience and tolerance and generally require longer than the average period of time. On the other hand, the talkative, rambling patient needs to be treated with kind discipline.

If the patient is seen in Casualty confused or unconscious, then obviously a history is required from relatives, friends or neighbours. Remember that many deaf patients can lip read and that deaf and dumb patients are usually extremely good at communicating by short notes.

## Physical examination

The physical examination is very much secondary to a careful and complete history. Most disorders can be diagnosed on the history alone and in many conditions physical examination will be completely normal.

It is usually on the basis of the history that the decision is made as to whether the patient's symptoms are psychosomatic. A normal examination will go on to substantiate this suspicion. The history may strongly suggest a specific diagnosis, which can be confirmed on examination: for instance, a history of Raynaud's phenomenon with CREST (combination of calcinosis, Raynaud's Phenomenon, eosophageal dysmotility, sclerodactyly and telangiectasia) changes seen in the hands in systemic sclerosis.

Initial impressions on meeting the patient can give important clues and indeed may be diagnostic. The patient's gait on walking into the consulting room should be carefully observed. The characteristic short-stepped shuffling gait of Parkinson's disease will be easily recognized. When the patient walks into the consulting room there may be an immediate, striking abnormality such as jaundice, cyanosis or severe anaemia. Acromegaly should be obvious. It is frequently stated that the best clue to diagnosing hypothyroidism is that this is immediately thought of when the patient is first seen. Specific physical findings in this condition are frequently absent but the generalized myxoedematous state of a dull, lethargic patient with a gruff voice can be striking.

The patient should be comfortable when being examined. When female patients are being examined by male doctors, a nurse should be present as a chaperon and this may well make the patient feel more comfortable. All patients should be completely undressed apart from wearing underpants. A large blanket or sheet should, however, be available and whenever possible, the patient should be covered, this being particularly important in women. Any undue or unnecessary embarrassment should be carefully avoided; this thoughtfulness will help gain the patient's respect and avoid unnecessary tension.

The ideal position is lying on a couch with the patient's trunk at an angle of 45°, with the facility to lower the couch to the horizontal position, which is particularly important during palpation of the abdomen. Care should always be taken to make sure the patient is completely comfortable. In particular, patients with heart failure may feel dyspnoeic and therefore should *not* be put in a completely flat position.

The patient should be told at the beginning of the examination that the doctor would like to be told at any time if he or she is short of breath or uncomfortable for whatever reason. A physician who unnecessarily hurts a patient will immediately lose all chance of establishing a useful and satisfactory relationship with them.

The patient should then be examined in a systematic way, using a strictly adhered to routine. The examination should be performed thoroughly, using correct techniques for examination for each system. Through experience each physician needs to develop a method of examination that is comprehensive but also reasonably economical of time.

## A systematic approach

It matters not whether each system is examined separately or whether the patient is approached from the top of the head and then examined down to the toes, provided whichever system that is preferred by the physician is adhered to regularly and systematically. Right-handed physicians and also some left-handed ones find it best always to examine the patient by standing at the right-hand side of the couch. During undergraduate and postgraduate clinical examinations, candidates would always be expected to commence the examination from this position.

Most physicians start by holding and examining the patient's hands or feeling the pulse and then travel upwards to examine the face, neck and lymph glands. This can be done without the patient having to be uncovered and keeps the patient relaxed. The general technique of examination of each system or organ by inspection, palpation, percussion and auscultation should be used. Inspection should be done in a good light, natural sunlight being better than artificial light, and this is particularly important in the presence of mild jaundice. Palpation should always be gentle, and during palpation, particularly of the abdomen, talking to the patient can be useful in relaxing them and relieving tension in the abdominal muscles. Percussion is usually done by placing the third finger of the left hand firmly against the skin (for a right-handed physician) and then striking that finger with the third finger of the right hand with a free, pendular action of the right wrist. Although it is wise to listen to the noise produced, probably more information is obtained from the impression of the vibration produced, which is sensed by the left middle finger. Although most commonly employed in the examination of the chest, percussion is also useful in looking for ascites, estimating the actual size of the liver and also to confirm the absence of splenomegaly by finding resonance along the left ninth intercostal space.

The patient's height and weight should be recorded: the approximate ideal weight for a man of average height is about 70 kg, and for a woman about 68 kg. Apart from obtaining some objective assessment of obesity, regular weighing may be important to other conditions such as when assessing the response to diuretics in heart failure. Temperature should be recorded orally and should be 37°C. Urine should be looked at to see if it is cloudy or blood-stained and should be tested for albumin or glucose.

## Initial assessment

If the patient is acutely ill and, in particular, if shocked, then a quick general assessment, including measurement of vital signs such as the blood pressure, should be made and immediate resuscitation undertaken. Shocked patients look collapsed, weak and confused. Anaemic patients will be extremely pale and dehydrated patients will have sunken eyes, a dry tongue and the skin will have lost its normal elasticity.

If the patient is not acutely unwell, then a relaxed general assessment is made, looking for evidence of poor nutrition, rashes, lumps and abnormal pulsations. Gross features of acromegaly or Parkinson's disease will usually be obvious.

## The hands

Start with the nails. Their colour may suggest anaemia, which in severe iron deficiency may result in koilonychia where the nails are soft, brittle and 'spoon shaped'. The normal convexity is lost and replaced by concavity. White bands or ridges can be correlated with the length of the illness. Note should be taken of the presence of heavy staining in and around the nails by nicotine.

The presence of finger clubbing should be established. The main characteristic of clubbing is filling in and obliteration of the angle between the nail and nail bone. This area may actually appear convex instead of the usual, easily seen angle. The overlying skin may appear red and shiny and there may be increased curvature of the nail. The nail bed becomes thickened and soft, and it may be possible to elicit an increased fluctuation of the nail within the nail bed on palpation. It is important also to look for clubbing of the nails of the feet. Gross clubbing is usually found in association with severe, chronic cyanosis, as in congenital heart disease, and in association with chronic suppuration in the chest, which may occur in patients with long-standing bronchiectasis. Clubbing is a common feature of carcinoma of the lung and may rarely be seen in chronic abdominal conditions such as Crohn's disease and ulcerative colitis. If clubbing suddenly occurs in a patient with known heart disease, then infective endocarditis should be suspected. If this is present, there may be associated Osler's nodes and splinter haemorrhages of the nails.

A yellow discoloration of the palms is a feature of hypothyroidism and is seen in association with the elevated cholesterol found in that disorder.

In osteoarthritis the finger joints are often involved and there may be bony nodules, known as Heberden's nodes, usually above the distal interphalangeal joints. The swellings seen over the terminal joint in gout are different: these are yellow deposits (tophi) of uric acid in the skin, often over involved joints.

Trophic changes in the skin may be present in disorders affecting the peripheral circulation. In acromegaly the fingers will be thickened and the hands will have a broad, spade-like appearance.

Ulnar deviation is the hallmark of rheumatoid arthritis; arachnodactyly (long, spindly fingers) is seen in Marfan's syndrome. The small muscles of the hand may be wasted as part of a generalized cachexic state or due to some localized neurological disease or muscle disorder. Inspection of the palm may reveal contractures with flexion deformities of the fourth and fifth fingers known as Dupuytren's contracture. Palmar erythema is a mottled, red discoloration of the palm seen in liver disease but it may also occur in normal pregnant women.

After the examination of the hands, the patient should be asked to stretch out both hands. This gives a quick indication as to any definite weakness on one side, and a tremor may be noticed. A fine tremor is a common feature of thyrotoxicosis and a 'flapping' tremor occurs in liver disease. This 'flap' may be more marked if the patient is asked to extend both hands.

Both radial pulses should then be felt, and the character of the brachial pulse ascertained. If necessary the carotid also palpated to assess pulse character. The neck should be quickly looked at to see if there are any obvious swellings, such as a goitre, or enlarged cervical lymph nodes; then the head and face should be examined carefully.

## The head

During the interview there will have been ample opportunity to observe any obvious cranial and facial abnormalities. A large head in childhood may indicate hydrocephalus whereas in an elderly patient it may suggest Paget's disease. The actual colour of the face may have an unusual appearance, as with severe central cyanosis, or the slaty-grey appearance of a patient taking large doses of amiodarone. Facial pallor should be clearly distinguished from anaemia by careful examination of the conjunctivae, which are usually pale when the haemoglobin is less than 9 g/100 ml. Remember that cyanosis will not appear with low haemoglobin levels as the cyanotic colour is dependent on having an adequate concentration of reduced haemoglobin. Jaundice will be best detected on the conjunctivae, particularly with the patient in a good natural light, but actual yellow discoloration of the skin may also occur. The 'moon-face' appearance of a patient with Cushing's syndrome is very typical and the diagnosis can be confirmed by looking for a 'buffalo hump' over the thoracic vertebrae, the presence of striae and the characteristic and very unusual weight distribution found in this disease. A similar facial appearance may be found in patients taking high doses of steroids.

Severe weight loss and indrawing of the cheeks as occurs in cachexia due to cancer or advanced heart failure is usually a striking facial feature. The general demeanour of the patient is best observed by looking at the face—conditions such as myxoedema, thyrotoxicosis and Parkinson's disease are usually diagnosed during the interview.

## The neck

After examination of the head and face, the neck should next be inspected and palpated. Palpation of the neck is usually best performed with the patient sitting on a chair and the examiner standing behind.

An enlarged thyroid gland or goitre may be obvious and its movement with the larynx observed when the patient is asked to swallow. There may be an audible bruit on auscultation of an enlarged thyroid gland. It should be ascertained whether a goitre is uniform or nodular, hard or soft. Having felt the thyroid gland, the trachea should be gently palpated and any deviation carefully noted. This again is best palpated by standing behind the patient, and confirmation of a suspected tracheal shift may be obtained by feeling on both sides from behind to see if there is any difference in the gap between the clavicle and trachea. Any abnormal neck pulsation should be carefully noted. Forcible pulsations (Corrigan's pulses) are seen in aortic incompetence. A large right subclavian artery may be palpated, as may collateral vessels in coarctation of the aorta. The jugular veins may be distended and pulsatile in heart failure, whereas non-pulsatile distended veins are seen during superior mediastinal obstruction due to a goitre or a bronchial carcinoma. Enlarged lymphatic glands draining any infective focus are usually tender. Enlarged bilateral tender cervical glands are common in children with sore throats. Enlarged tuberculous cervical glands are rarely seen these days and the commonest causes of mobile rubbery glands in the neck are the lymphomas in young adults and secondary carcinoma in the elderly. It is important

to note whether enlarged glands are firm and distinct or fused together. Soft, rubbery glands may be suggestive of a lymphoma while hard, craggy and particularly immovable glands are always due to a carcinoma.

If the submandibular glands are enlarged, then these are usually swollen and tender, the most common cause being a salivary gland stone that has lodged within the salivary duct.

## The breasts

Breast cancer is treatable and therefore during any general examination of a woman a full, careful examination of the breasts is mandatory. The patient should be reclining and comfortable with arms to the side. Look initially for any abnormal swelling and note the symmetry of the breasts and nipples. Retraction of one nipple may suggest carcinoma underneath. Any discharge from the nipple should be carefully looked for. The breasts should then be palpated with the flat of the fingers, searching carefully for a lump. If a lump is discovered, its situation, size and shape, consistency and mobility should be ascertained. The axilla should then be examined for enlarged lymph nodes. Any swelling within the male breast is of equal importance. At some stage in puberty most normal boys will have a slight soft breast swelling; this will always be bilateral.

## The feet

Examination of the feet is important. The condition of the skin should be noted, particularly in diabetics. In peripheral vascular disease the skin may show cyanosis and be shiny, and there may be hair loss. It is important to feel for the dorsalis pedis and posterior tibial pulses. A sign of chronic ischaemia is the slow return of normal skin colour after compression and blanching. In most ambulant patients the feet and ankles are the best areas to look for pitting oedema. There may be trophic ulcers due to a peripheral neuropathy.

## Systemic review

Specific systems, e.g., cardiovascular, respiratory, should be carefully examined as outlined in later chapters.

## THE MENTAL AND EMOTIONAL STATE

An assessment of the patient's personality and intelligence is usually made early on in the initial interview. Mental retardation will be obvious. Simple tests of intelligence, such as by mental arithmetic and naming prominent public figures, may be necessary.

An anxious patient will be restless and fidgety. The lowered mood, slowness and depression of a myxoedematous patient may be clearly evident. Apparently severe disability without appropriate concern should suggest malingering or, more importantly, hysteria. Elderly patients can become quite clever at disguising considerable defects of memory and orientation.

Depression is often bound up with the patient's symptoms and may produce psychosomatic disorders. On the other hand, the patient's worry may stem quite reasonably from anxiety about new symptoms and fear of increasing disability.

### Psychiatric assessment

Remember that patients with psychiatric disorders can still present with very real somatic symptoms. Severe personality disorders, such as schizophrenia, are usually obvious at the onset of the interview. The organic psychoses, such as delirium or dementia, are usually easier to diagnose than the neuroses. An obsessive, persisting complaint, such as the sensation of a breast lump despite normal examination and a negative mammography, is a good example of masked depression manifesting itself as an obsessional neurosis. Many important organic disease states may form a large part of the development of a psychiatric disorder, e.g. toxic confusional states, cerebral vascular accidents and 'myxoedema madness'. If a psychiatric problem is suspected, then a detailed family history is essential and it may well be very informative to speak to a close family member. A family history of depression or attempted suicide may be contributory, whereas a family history of Huntington's chorea will be diagnostic. If family members are interviewed, care should be taken not to make the patient resentful or suspicious by giving the impression that he or she is thought to be a liar. Lastly, note that a complete physical examination is essential in every patient suffering from what is thought to be a psychiatric disorder. Special psychological tests of intellect, memory and personality, when available, can sometimes give valuable information.

## AFTER THE PHYSICAL EXAMINATION

When the examination has been completed, the patient is asked to dress and return to his or her seat. The doctor should explain slowly and carefully what initial impressions have been made and what further steps, usually in the way of a laboratory investigation, need to be undertaken. If at all possible, reassurance at this stage is of tremendous value because by now the patient has become increasingly worried about the diagnosis. Obviously, it would be wrong to reassure a suspected cancer patient in a banal and superficial way, but on the other hand, in such a case reassurance can take the form of explaining a course of action in order to reach a correct diagnosis, and to plan possible future treatment as early as possible. Even in the most serious cases, for the patient and the patient's family to know that they have a sympathetic friend who, with them, is making a plan for the future will produce tremendous relief and happiness, which sometimes a doctor can also feel and share. At all times the patient should be given the opportunity to ask questions, to which replies should be frank and explicit.

## MAKING THE DIAGNOSIS

Next try to make a differential diagnosis. This differential can be used as a basis for planning further investigations in order to reach a definitive diagnosis. Facts acquired from the history and examination should therefore be analysed; this becomes much easier and more rapid with clinical experience. Establish in your own mind what exactly has happened: for instance, exacerbations of bronchitis in a heavy cigarette smoker or the early development of ischaemic heart disease in a man with xanthelasma and hypercholesteraemia. On this basis a list of probabilities should be drawn up. (Generally the length of this list is inversely proportional to the physician's experience.) Obviously this differential diagnosis takes into account a patient's origin and geographical location. For instance, bloody diarrhoea in Africa would mean dysentery whereas the same in Yorkshire would probably be due to ulcerative colitis.

## DOCUMENTATION

With experience the traditional system of writing on a blank sheet of paper is probably the better and certainly quicker than using aids such as check lists and flow sheets. The history, physical findings, differential diagnosis, and investigations undertaken should be documented in a clear and logical way. All investigations should be recorded in the notes. If the patient is admitted, accurate and clear documentation of all decisions, investigations and the patient's progress is essential. The case records need to be readable, short and well ordered. They should include information on what the patient and/or the patient's relatives have been told. It is wise to include in a prominent position whether or not a 'crash team' should be called in the event of this patient's sudden collapse and this will be extremely useful to night nursing staff and covering doctors. This last point is controversial and not all physicians would agree.

On discharge from hospital the patient's general practitioner must be informed (sometimes by telephone) and details given of the final diagnosis and discharge treatment. This should be followed as soon as possible by a full discharge summary, which should be above all *succinct*.

## PRESENTING A CASE

Doctors have to present cases, frequently throughout their medical careers. For example, it needs to be done often and briefly by the houseman, senior houseman or registrar during post-intake ward rounds and in more detail at clinical meetings. The value of a physician's notes is much diminished if he or she is unable to communicate them in a concise form to other doctors. A short summary at the end of each history and examination is a useful way to practise and to start.

If a three sentence impression or summary is written at the end of each patient's notes throughout a doctor's medical career, it is possible to become expert at developing what is probably one of the most important skills. These summaries should emphasize both important positive and negative findings. Summaries should begin with the age, sex and occupation of the patient, the main symptom or symptom complex with its duration, and then the important positive physical findings. For instance.

> Mr A.G. is a 43-year-old accountant who presents with a 3-month history of pruritis and over the last week has noticed a painless, glandular swelling in his left axilla. The probable diagnosis is a lymphoma and he needs a lymph node biopsy as soon as this can be arranged.

When presenting a case, a physician should be concise and avoid irrelevances. Even with a long, involved and difficult case, it is usually possible to produce a short appraisal with a one- or two-sentence history and a further two sentences outlining the positive physical findings. There is nothing more tedious than listening to a long dissertation of irrelevant negative details or findings. Next describe the main positive symptoms and the main abnormality discovered in the main system affected. It is unusual to be able to reach a definitive diagnosis immediately; more commonly it is appropriate to give a short list of differential diagnoses. If specific questions are asked by colleagues, a short, concise answer is required.

# Section Two

## Emergencies and Special Settings

# 2

# EMERGENCIES AND ACUTE POISONING

## Neil Scolding

## MEDICAL EMERGENCIES

Common sense and a calm head are vital when dealing with acutely sick patients. Any amount of knowledge would be of small value without these qualities, and the information in this chapter would similarly be of little practical use. Thus each subsection contains broad outlines of management, which must then be tailored to suit the needs of each individual patient, and the stepwise approach, adopted in the interests of simplicity, brevity and clarity, is not intended to be inflexible and dogmatic.

Emergency medicine is now as rapidly changing a field as any other medical speciality and while the author has attempted to incorporate significant and well-substantiated recent advances into this chapter some omissions are unfortunately inevitable.

The management of some emergencies has been considered in other chapters and these will not be repeated here.

## Cardiac arrest

### Diagnosis

The patient is in a state of collapse, with no major arterial pulses and gasping or absent respiration.

### Management

(1) Feel for tracheal deviation to exclude tension pneumothorax. (This is obviously more relevant when a patient has just arrived in a state of collapse in the Casualty department than, for example, cardiac arrest in a previously admitted patient on the Coronary Care Unit [CCU].)

(2) Give a forcible blow to the sternum—this may (rarely) 'cure' asystole, complete heart block, ventricular fibrillation or ventricular tachycardia.

(3) If a defibrillator is instantly available, immediate defibrillation is occasionally rewarding (i.e., even without ECG monitoring).

*Basic resuscitation* ('**A-B-C**') follows:

(4) Clear the oropharynx (*Airway*) and insert an airway (e.g., Guedel).

(5) Start artificial ventilation (*Breathing*) giving oxygen via a mask, valve and Ambubag. These instruments are not easy to use, particularly for the inexperienced for whom mouth-to-mouth respiration is more effective. This may, however, carry the risk of acquired immune deficiency disease (AIDS) transmission.

(6) Commence *Cardiac massage*, one compression per second, using the heel of the left hand over the lower sternum, the right hand on top. Depress the sternum about two inches (5 cm) with the arms locked in hyperextension. Administer 15 cardiac compressions, pause to inflate the lungs twice, then continue this cycle.

*Advanced resuscitation* comprises consolidation of the above and treatment of the immediate cause:

(7) *Cannulate a large vein* (e.g., external jugular). Immediate bicarbonate administration is no longer recommended (in Britain), but intravenous drugs may be needed.

(8) *Endotracheal intubation* has advantages over an oropharyngeal airway, but for anyone other than a practising anaesthetist it is often time-consuming and yet unsuccessful. Furthermore, rapidly diagnosing a misplaced tube is far more difficult than is usually supposed. The time is better spent eliciting (electrocardiographically) and treating the cardiac rhythm. If no anaesthetist appears and

initial specific treatment has been attempted, *then* intubation may be attempted by the 'non-expert'.

(9) Attach an ECG monitor, and treat accordingly:

(a) *Ventricular fibrillation*. Defibrillate. Translucent conducting-gel pads are safer than electrode jelly. Place one over the left sternal edge and one over the apex. Apply the electrodes, disconnect other attendants from the patient and discharge the defibrillator. Follow Fig. 2.1.

If fibrillation persists despite all the manoeuvres outlined in Fig. 2.1 consider further lignocaine, intravenous bretylium (500 mg slowly), amiodarone (150–300 mg intravenously over 1–2 min) and/or shocking with one electrode over the left sternal edge and the other posteriorly. If, after success, infused lignocaine (2–4 mg/min) then fails to prevent recurrence, try

amiodarone (by central line, 5 mg/kg in 20 min if not preceded by a bolus, then up to 15 mg/kg in 24 h in 5 per cent dextrose; maximum 1.2g in 24hr).

Incidentally, this is not the best time to be discovering how the defibrillator works. Most are straightforward but always familiarize yourself with them when first starting a new job.

(b) *Asystole*. Check that there are no loose ECG monitor connections! Again, follow Fig. 2.1. Calcium gluconate has fallen from favour in Britain. Intracardiac adrenaline may be given (the subxiphisternal approach aiming toward the left scapula is best) and pacing (e.g., transthoracic or transoesophageal) is considered if there is evidence of mechanically useful electrical activity (implying a profound bradycardia).

(c) *Electromechanical dissociation*. No car-

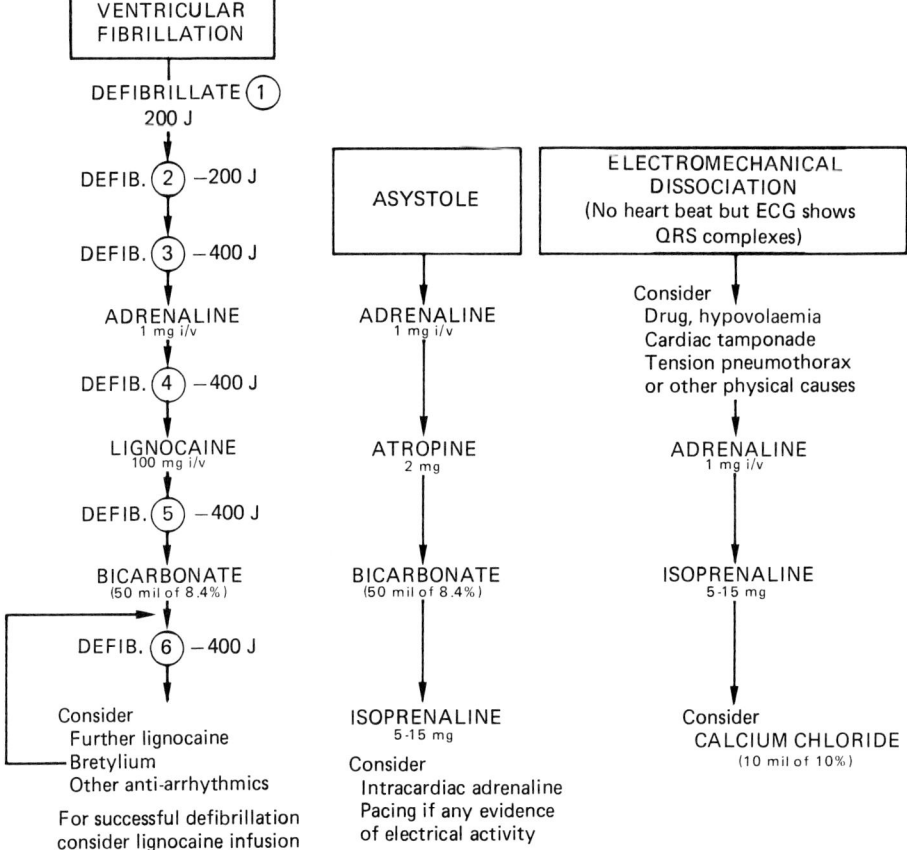

*Figure 2.1* 'Advanced' resuscitation (reproduced by kind permission of the Resuscitation Council [UK]).

diac output is detectable but QRS complexes continue. This may occur in massive pulmonary embolism, exsanguination, brain haemorrhage, myocardial rupture, drug poisoning, cardiac tamponade and tension pneumothorax. If the last two are excluded ('prospecting' by constantly aspirating in the region of the pericardial sac with a syringe and long needle may be necessary), try adrenaline then isoprenaline, then calcium gluconate or chloride (Fig. 2.1).

Some of the drugs mentioned above may usefully be given by injecting twice the dose down the endotracheal tube (e.g., adrenaline, atropine and lignocaine).

The decision to abandon resuscitation depends on a number of factors including the underlying condition, the duration of the attempt (survival after prolonged resuscitation may occur in drug-poisoning, near-drowning and hypothermia), and the exhaustion of therapeutic options. Fixed, dilated pupils do not necessarily imply irreparable brain damage. If resuscitation is successful, give intravenous dexamethasone to attempt prevention of cerebral oedema (and possibly adult respiratory distress syndrome) and check the electrolytes, arterial gases and chest X-ray.

Useful charts summarizing the above guidelines (Fig. 2.1) can be obtained from the Resuscitation Council (UK), Department of Anaesthetics, Royal Postgraduate Medical School, London, W12 0HS.

## Myocardial infarction

### Diagnosis

This is suggested by a history of severe central crushing chest pain radiating to the arms and jaw, with nausea and sweating. Unlike angina the pain often starts at rest, and is prolonged and unaffected by sublingual nitrates. There may be no abnormal signs but more often the patient is pale, sweaty, and distressed. Occasionally a fourth heart sound is audible. Alternatively, the general condition and signs may be dictated by the complications mentioned below. The ECG may be normal in the early stages but more commonly will show ST elevation followed by T-wave inversion and Q-wave formation.

### Management

(1) *An intravenous cannula* is inserted and intravenous diamorphine, 2.5 to 5.0 mg, or morphine, 5 to 10 mg, given if the patient is still in pain. Prophylactic antiemetics, e.g., prochlorperazine 12.5 mg, should also be given. The cannula is kept patent using 5 ml of heparinized saline 8- to 12-hourly.

(2) *Transfer to a CCU and commence ECG monitoring.* This should be done rapidly, even before detailed clerking if the diagnosis appears likely from the immediately performed ECG and brief history.

(3) *Oxygen* is not routinely given unless shock or pulmonary oedema is present.

(4) *Venesection* for cardiac enzymes (myocardial creatinine phosphokinase [CPK] isoenzyme is the most specific; most hospitals assay total CPK, aspartate transaminase and lactate dehydrogenase), electrolytes and haemoglobin. A *portable chest X-ray* is performed.

(5) *Low-dose subcutaneous heparin* (5000 u twice or thrice a day) reduces the incidence of thrombo-embolic complications, particularly if heart failure is present. Its value in uncomplicated infarction (with early mobilization) is not universally accepted, but as those patients destined to develop complications do not immediately announce themselves, it should be given in the early stages to all patients.

(6) *Aspirin* should be given unless specifically contra-indicated.

(7) *Limitation of infarct size*:

  (a) *Intravenous thrombolytic agents* appear to reduce both infarct size and mortality and streptokinally 1.5 million units over 60 minutes can now be recommended for all cases of myocardial infarction presenting within 6h without contraindications (see under 'Pulmonary embolism' for these). Isis 2 has convincingly demonstrated the use of streptokinase combined with aspirin, and Isis 3 has convincingly shown that there is no significant difference between the 3 major thrombolytic agents (streptokinase tPA and APSAC.)

  *Streptokinase* is antigentic and should not be re-administered in the period from 5 days to 6 months after first exposure. It should be avoided if there is significant hypotension and tissue plasminogen activator should be considered.

  *Tissue plasminogen activator (tPA)*

should be given when streptokinase cannot be repeated. The total dose of 100mg is divided into a 10mg bolus followed by 50mg over 1h then 40mg over 2h.

*Heparin* may be given for the 24h after tPA administration.

*Aspirin* 150–300 mg/day p.o. should be given to all patients without contraindications. The first dose should be given immediately on admission.

(b) *Intravenous β-blockers* (e.g., atenolol, 5 mg slowly, repeated once if the pulse remains above 60) have been shown to reduce infarct size, the incidence of ventricular tachycardia and overall mortality, at least in the short term.

Some recommend they be given to all patients except those with hypotension, cardiac failure, or bradycardia, though it seems it would be necessary to treat 100 to 150 patients to save one life.

(8) *Prophylactic lignocaine* remains controversial. It was formerly recommended for patients with 'warning arrhythmias', namely: (a) frequent ventricular extrasystoles (>5/min); (b) multifocal ventricular extrasystoles; (c) salvoes of two or more ventricular beats; or (d) early 'R-on-T' ventricular extrasystoles. However, the reliability of any of these as heralds of ventricular fibrillation is dubious, even the dreaded R-on-T phenomenon probably having no predictive value. It could therefore be argued either that prophylactic lignocaine should not be used at all, or that it be given to every patient. However, it is not a drug without side-effects, and its value in preventing ventricular fibrillation (in standard doses) has been questioned. There is as yet no consensus, though it appears that enthusiasm for prophylactic lignocaine is waning.

## Complications

Subsequent attention is directed towards seeking and treating complications as they arise. These are as follows.

## 1. Arrhythmias

See p. 17.

## 2. Heart failure

Causes include:

(1) *Loss of functioning muscle.* This is the commonest cause. In simplistic terms there are two aspects. Firstly, 'back pressure' causes pulmonary oedema with or without a raised jugular venous pressure, gallop rhythm and peripheral oedema. Secondly, 'pump failure' causes tachycardia with poor peripheral (and renal) perfusion, low urine output and hypotension (cardiogenic shock). Either or both may be present.

(a) *Pulmonary oedema.* See 'Acute heart failure', p. 00.

(b) *Cardiogenic shock.* These patients have a poor prognosis and there is little evidence that any therapy improves this, provided that surgically correctable, mechanical causes (see item [5] below) have been excluded. Nevertheless, most authorities still recommend invasive, haemodynamic monitoring with a Swan–Ganz catheter. This is, of course, uncomfortable for the patient and is anyway not often a practical proposition (few doctors have the necessary expertise), particularly in district general hospitals. Perhaps its most important role is in identifying that important, small subgroup of hypotensive patients, generally without pulmonary oedema, who are in fact hypovolaemic (often from previous diuretic treatment) and whose prognosis is better. However, these can probably equally well be identified by empirically giving all patients with hypotension but no clinical or radiographic evidence of pulmonary oedema an intravenous bolus (say 300 ml) of a plasma expander, closely monitoring the effect on the blood pressure, pulse rate and urine output.

If hypovolaemia is thus excluded *inotropic support* is usually attempted: a combination of dobutamine, 2 to 10 µg/kg/min, together with low-dose (i.e., renal vasodilating) dopamine, 0.5 to 2 µg/kg/min, has theoretical advantages. There is a growing and seemingly sensible tendency (albeit unsupported by firm evidence) to use inotropic support before shock develops, i.e., in patients who are pale, clammy and sweaty despite adequate analgesia, but not (yet) hypotensive.

Alternatively, *vasodilator therapy* with nitroprusside (starting at 10–15 µg/min and increasing in 10 µg increments every 5 to 10 min; range 10–200 µg/min) is often recommended, but this can exacerbate hypotension and should probably always be controlled in this situation with continuous monitoring of intra-arterial pressure.

*Chronotropic support* may also be necessary. Tachyarrhythmias should be treated but it should also be remembered that a rate of, say, 65–70 in a hypotensive, oliguric patient constitutes a functional bradycardia. If due to atrioventricular block, temporary artificial pacing at a rate of 90 to 100 should be undertaken. If the rhythm is sinus, then if the dobutamine/dopamine does not increase the rate, atrial pacing is used (as it preserves the atrial contribution to cardiac output).

*Balloon counterpulsation*—again there is often little expertise available for this in district general hospitals. ECG-controlled diastolic inflation and systolic collapse of the catheter-mounted balloon (positioned percutaneously in the aortic arch) does improve the outlook *providing* there is a correctable defect causing cardiogenic shock, e.g., acute ventricular septal defect. It should therefore only be considered for such patients.

(2) *Arrhythmias*—see p. 17.

(3) *Mechanical complications of infarction*—these occur two to ten days after infarction and include ventricular septal defect, ruptured papillary muscle or chordae tendinae, and cardiac rupture. The first three cause shock and/or a murmur. Echocardiography confirms the diagnosis. The traditional teaching is that surgical repair should be deferred, but for the septal defect early operation is now recommended. For acute mitral regurgitation, afterload reduction with nitroprusside (dose—see below) may help. Cardiac rupture causes shock and tamponade (see below) and is usually rapidly fatal.

(4) *Iatrogenic heart failure*—most anti-arrhythmic agents are negatively inotropic. Hypotensive crises after intravenous verapamil can probably be avoided by pre-administration of 10 ml 10 per cent calcium gluconate. Cardiac failure induced by β-blockers may respond to treatment with intravenous glucagon (as for β-blocker poisoning). Disopyramide and lignocaine are also negatively inotropic, digoxin and amiodarone are not.

Finally, particular mention should be made of *right ventricular infarction*. This may cause hypotension without pulmonary congestion, but accompanied by a raised jugular venous pressure, right ventricular gallop, and ECG signs of inferior infarction. Echocardiography shows a large, poorly functioning right ventricle. The high jugular venous pressure is a trap for the unwary, as diuretics can precipitate cardiogenic shock, cardiac output being dependent on higher venous pressure.

### 3. Peripheral embolus

This is uncommon but may affect the limbs, the gut, the kidneys or the cerebral circulation. Surgical embolectomy is the preferred approach, as medical management is unlikely to improve the outlook. Full anticoagulation should be started.

### 4. Pulmonary embolus

See p. 22.

### 5. Pericarditis

This is a common complication of Q-wave infarction, usually occurring around the second or third day. The patient complains of sharp chest pain, worse with movement, and a pericardial rub may be audible. A mild fever may be present. Indomethacin, 50 mg then 25 mg three times a day, is usually effective.

### Unstable angina

#### Diagnosis

The term can include: (a) angina rapidly increasing in severity and frequency (crescendo angina); (b) frequent angina developing at rest; and, (c) prolonged cardiac pain unrelieved by sublingual nitrates but without ECG or biochemical evidence of infarction. There is a 10 per cent risk of early myocardial infarction, increasing to 85 percent in 12 months if untreated.

#### Management

Standard quadruple therapy comprises:
(a) oral β-blockade—e.g., atenolol, to maintain a pulse rate below 60;

(b) calcium antagonists—e.g., nifedipine up to 20 mg four times a day;
(c) intravenous nitrates—e.g., isosorbide dinitrate, 2 to 5 mg/h;
(d) aspirin, 300 mg daily.
Bed rest is mandatory.

Transfer to a regional centre for angiography followed either by balloon angioplasty or bypass surgery is necessary for the (very) few patients unresponsive to this drug combination. Those who do respond may also need surgery, but this is better done electively after medical stabilization.

## Arrhythmias

In all arrhythmias, digoxin toxicity should be excluded, as should potassium imbalance and acid–base disturbance.

### Supraventricular tachyarrhythmias

#### Diagnosis

In *atrial fibrillation* the ECG shows small, patternless undulations between completely irregular ventricular complexes. The ventricular rate varies from normal (or even slow) up to perhaps 250 to 280 beats per min. In *atrial flutter* the ECG does show evidence of coordinated atrial contraction, with 'sawtooth' flutter waves (best seen in the inferior leads), 250 to 350/min. Again, the ventricular rate depends on the degree of resistance offered by the atrioventricular node. If there is 1:1 conduction, carotid sinus massage will temporarily increase the atrioventricular block, slowing the ventricular response and revealing the flutter waves (and also therefore the diagnosis). Other forms of *regular supraventricular tachycardia* result from various electrophysiological mechanisms, including enhanced atrial activity ('atrial tachycardia': atrial rate 130 to 250, often with a degree of atrioventricular block) and re-entry circuits (always with 1:1 conduction).

#### Management (Fig. 2.2).

(See [4], overleaf, for Wolff–Parkinson–White syndrome)
(1) *Carotid sinus massage.* Press the thumb over one carotid artery at the level of the upper border of the thyroid cartilage, rubbing an inch (2.5 cm) up and down. In all the above tachyarrhythmias this may temporarily slow the ventricular rate (allowing diagnosis), while in atrial and re-entry tachycardias, conversion to sinus rhythm occasionally occurs.

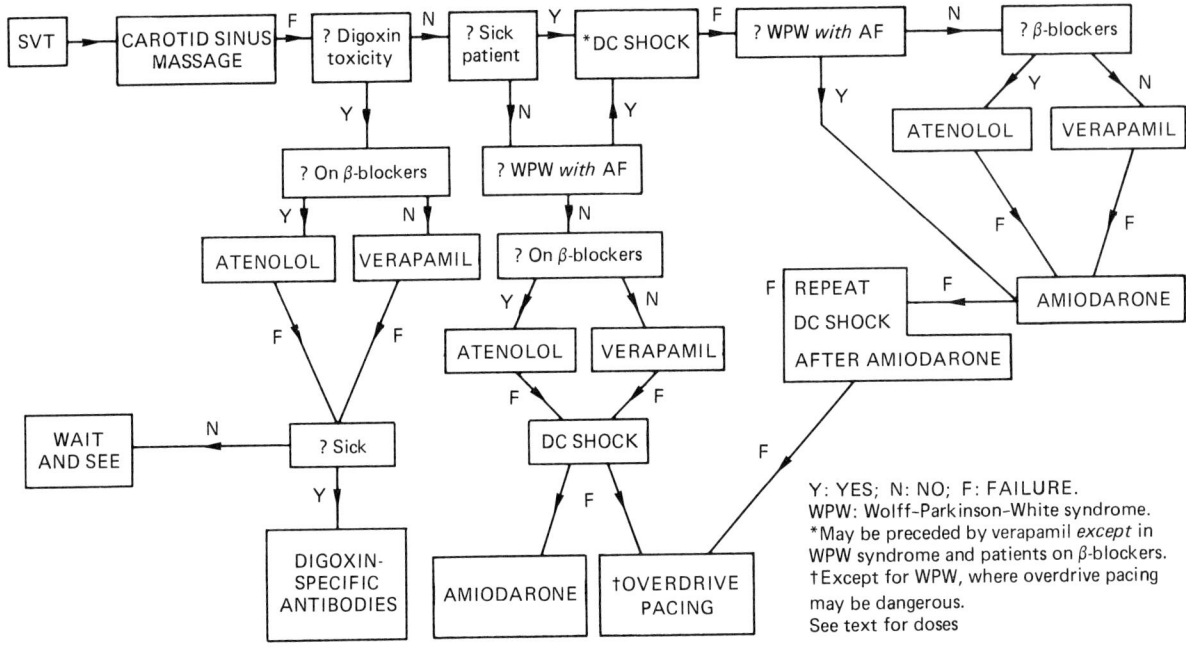

*Figure 2.2*  Management of supraventricular tachyarrhythmias (SVT).

If this fails the next step depends on the ventricular rate.

(2) (a) In all cases (*except where digoxin toxicity is suspected*—see (2[b]), when the ventricular response is fast enough significantly to reduce cardiac output (causing shock, collapse, etc.), the treatment of choice is *DC cardioversion*. If the patient is unconscious, this should be done immediately. If not, he or she should be rendered so by a short-acting agent delivered by an anaesthetist. (The seemingly increasing practice of shocking a patient who has merely been made drowsy by, for example, intravenous diazepam is barbaric and to be condemned.) Whilst waiting for the anaesthetist's arrival (or if DC shock is not possible for any reason) *intravenous verapamil* (as described below) should be given.

**Cardioversion.** A synchronized shock is used to reduce the possibility of inducing ventricular tachyarrhythmias. Electrode gel-pads are placed one at the left sternal edge and one over the apex and the electrode paddles applied to these. Start at 25 to 50 J for atrial flutter, 50 J for other supraventricular tachyarrhythmias, increasing the energy if unsuccessful. The efficacy will be reduced if the energy is shared with any hapless attendants in contact with the patient, and this is therefore best avoided.

If repeated shocks fail and verapamil is also ineffective, amiodarone 150 mg as a slow intravenous bolus, repeated once if necessary, should be considered.

(b) *Digoxin toxicity.* DC shock may be unsafe, but verapamil can still be used. If this fails and the patient is critically ill because of digoxin-induced arrhythmia, then intravenous digoxin-specific antibodies (e.g., Digibind) should be used.

(3) *If the patient is less compromised*, drug treatment may suffice. Verapamil, 5 to 10 mg intravenously as a rapid bolus (1–2 s), repeated after 10 to 15 min is the treatment of choice. Pretreatment with calcium gluconate (10 ml, 10 per cent) one minute before the verapamil is said to prevent the (rare) occurrence of hypotension or sinus arrest, without diminishing the efficacy of treatment. Verapamil will slow the ventricular response to atrial fibrillation and may convert flutter and other forms of supraventricular tachyarrhythmias to sinus rhythm.

*Verapamil should not be used if the patient is on oral β-blockers*; in this situation either an intravenous β-blocker may be used, e.g., atendot 2.5 mg over 2–3 minutes, repeated after 5 minutes or digoxin (orally, 1 mg in divided doses over 12–24 h, or intravenously, 0.75–1.25 mg in 50 ml saline over 30 min). Disopyramide has a negative inotropic effect and should probably be avoided in patients pretreated with either β-blockers or verapamil.

If this fails there are three alternatives:

(a) *'Semi'-elective DC cardioversion.* This is usually successful, particularly in the context of acutely arising tachycardias, and is probably the preferred next step.

(b) *Further drug treatment.* Digoxin can be added to verapamil either parenterally or orally. After this the next drug of choice is probably amiodarone given as an infusion through a central line (peripherally it causes severe thrombophlebitis and orally its onset of action is considerably delayed). Give 5 mg/kg over 20 min in 250 ml of 5 per cent dextrose, followed by 15 mg/kg over 24 h in 500 ml, adjusting the infusion rate according to the response. However, if the patient is not at all disturbed by the arrhythmia it might be more circumspect to wait until the verapamil and digoxin have been cleared and then try other more conventional therapy, e.g., β-blockers, disopyramide, etc.

(c) *'Overdrive pacing'.* A temporary pacing wire positioned in the right atrium is stimulated at a rate 20 to 30 per cent greater than the atrial rate. Pacing is then suddenly stopped. This may convert the tachycardia (particularly flutter) to sinus rhythm, but may also occasionally precipitate atrial fibrillation.

(4) *Wolff–Parkinson–White syndrome.* An extra conduction pathway from the atria to the ventricles results in a short PR interval together with a slurred upstroke on the QRS complex (a delta wave). The extra pathway predisposes both to atrial fibrillation and re-entry tachycardia. In fibrillation, delta waves are retained, exposing the diagnosis. A very fast ventricular response is possible, resulting in shock and occasionally ventricular fibrillation. Delta waves are lost in re-entry tachycardias, obscuring the diagnosis in the new patient.

In either case, tachycardias fast enough to

compromise cardiac output warrant emergency DC cardioversion.

Otherwise, in atrial fibrillation, elective cardioversion is the preferred treatment, as both *verapami and digoxin can increase the ventricular response*. Intravenous disopyramide, sotalol, flecainide or amiodarone are alternatives.

Regular, narrow-complex tachycardia (reentrant) is best treated as described in (3) above, with the exception that the digoxin is best avoided *in case* the patient should develop atrial fibrillation.

## Ventricular tachycardia

### Diagnosis

Distinguishing this from aberrantly conducted supraventricular tachyarrhythmia can be difficult. The rate, BP, and general condition of the patient provide *no* guidance, but:
(1) Capture beats, fusion beats, and differing QRS complexes (because of superimposed, independent P waves) all imply ventricular tachycardia.
(2) Pure QS in $S_1$ or $V_6$, chest lead concordance (i.e., all complexes positive or negative in $V_1$ to $V_6$), notched monophasic or biphasic QRS complexes and QRS complexes $>0.14$ s imply ventricular tachycardia.
(3) A normal or slight right axis, QRS complexes in $V_1$ or $V_6$ that are triphasic and $<0.14$ s, and preceding atrial events imply aberrantly conducted SVT.
(4) Completely irregular QRS complexes suggest aberrantly conducted atrial fibrillation.

## Management

Physical manoeuvres, such as a praecordial thump or a cough (patient not doctor) are occasionally successful and should be attempted. Otherwise *DC cardioversion* is necessary. As before, if the patient is not already unconscious, he or she should be rendered so before being electrified. Start at 100 J and work upwards.

If DC cardioversion fails, lignocaine should be tried (100 mg bolus, then an infusion of 4 mg/min, reducing to 1.5 mg/min). DC shock after pretreatment with lignocaine may be more successful. If not, the next drug of choice is probably amiodarone given as an intravenous bolus of 150 mg,

repeated if necessary, and followed by an infusion over 24 h (dose as for supraventricular tachyarrhythmia), if successful. Disopyramide, procainamide, flecainide, practolol and overdrive right ventricular pacing are all alternatives but all are said to carry the risk of converting the tachycardia to fibrillation (though the latter is not an unnatural progression anyway).

**Torsade de pointes** This is a ventricular tachycardia where the QRS complexes are of varying overall amplitude, forming a pattern or regularly waxing and waning size. It is often caused by antiarrhythmic agents and so does not take kindly to attempts at treatment with them. Overdrive pacing is the preferred approach, though an isoprenaline infusion (2–6 μg/min) may be effective.

## Bradyarrhythmias

If β-blockers are responsible, glucagon or prenalterol treatment may suffice. Sinus bradycardia in acute myocardial infarction may improve with analgesia. Otherwise, whatever the bradyarrhythmia, the treatment of choice if the patient is symptomatic is a bolus of atropine, 0.6 to 2.4 mg intravenously, perhaps followed by an isoprenaline infusion. Any effect is likely only to be short-lived and temporary pacing will probably be necessary. If the bradycardia is so slow as effectively to cause cardiac arrest, transoesophageal, transthoracic or even transcutaneous (electrodes on the skin surface) pacing may be attempted.

**Temporary cardiac pacing.** Access to a central vein is established as described on p. 24. Remember to check that the pacing wire fits through the cannula dilator before inserting the latter!

The pacing wire is passed through the dilator. If significant resistance is met, withdraw and start again. Under radiographic screening the wire is advanced to the right atrium. To traverse the tricuspid orifice, the wire is advanced and withdrawn repeatedly, perhaps applying a twist as well, until, often with a visible flick and a number of ventricular ectopic beats, the valve is crossed. The tip is then advanced to the apex of the ventricle, just above the left diaphragm. An inch (2.5 cm) more of wire is then inserted so that a slight curve of wire is left in the right atrium, improving stability.

Once stable and satisfactory, the poles of the wire are connected to the pacing box ('proximal' to 'positive'), and the threshold established, i.e., the lowest voltage at which the ventricle is 'caught' ('capture' being indicated by the presence of a pacing spike followed by a QRS shaped as in left bundle branch block). The target is anything below 1.0 V and the wire position should be adjusted to achieve this. Once done, the patient is asked to cough and to breathe deeply, an unchanging threshold confirming stability. The dilator can now be withdrawn, carefully holding the wire in constant position whilst this is done, and the wire is secured with a stitch, Opsite and Elastoplast. The pacing box is usually set on 'Demand' function, at a rate appropriate to the patient's general condition (usually 60–70) and at a voltage twice the threshold. The latter should be checked daily, but is expected to rise to 2–3 V in the first few days.

## Acute heart failure

### Diagnosis

Rapidly increasing breathlessness is accompanied by the production of pink, frothy sputum. The patient is often extremely breathless, cold and sweaty, with a normal or elevated BP. There is a tachycardia, raised venous pressure, a gallop rhythm and bilateral basal crackles, with or without wheezes. Signs of valvular or infective heart disease and of hypertension should also be sought. Otherwise, eliciting the cause rests on the history (chest pain, change in diuretic treatment, commencement of β-blockers, salt/water overload, etc.), and simple investigations (serial cardiac enzymes, blood count, electrolytes). The ECG may show signs of ischaemia, valve disease or hypertension. Alternatively, it may confirm the presence of an arrhythmia. If the latter is responsible for the heart failure (often hard to tell, but usually the rate must be either below 45 or over 150 to cause acute severe symptoms), then treatment of the heart failure obviously depends on that of the arrhythmia. The chest X-ray shows cardiomegaly, alveolar shadowing (classically a 'bat's wing' distribution), upper lobe venous diversion and Kerley 'B' lines.

Other common causes of acute dyspnoea, such as acute asthma, acute pulmonary embolus and pneumothorax, are relatively easily excluded by the story (particularly the mode of onset and type of sputum), signs and the X-ray. Other causes of pulmonary oedema, for example inhaled toxins and adult respiratory distress syndrome, are usually apparent from the clinical setting, and are not usually accompanied by cardiomegaly. An acute exacerbation of chronic airways obstruction is the commonest cause of confusion; much is often made of the value of various physical signs in differentiation (e.g., gallop rhythm), but if the patient is in extremis, their value is usually entirely lost. It is then acceptable to treat with intravenous diuretics, oxygen and nebulized bronchodilators, withholding opiates until the chest X-ray is available.

### Management

Oxygen is given (6 l/min) and the patient propped sitting forward. There is usually a dramatic response to intravenous opiates and diuretics (e.g., 40–80 mg frusemide; 2.5–5 mg diamorphine)—otherwise repeat after 30 min. If there is still no improvement, intravenous digoxin (of value, at least in the short term, even in patients in sinus rhythm, and no longer thought unsafe in acute myocardial infarction) may be considered, but unless there is a tachyarrhythmia, vasodilators are probably preferable. Intravenous nitrates (e.g., glyceryl trinitrate, 10 μg/min, increasing to a maximum of 200 μg/min) or nitroprusside (starting at 10 μg/min, increasing to 150–200 μg/min) may be used. Hypotension often limits the dose of the latter, headache the former. Swan–Ganz catheterization is helpful to monitor and control the wedge pressure (at about 18 mmHg) but this is often a counsel of perfection. An alternative to venodilation is venesection of 300 to 500 ml (provided the patient is normotensive with a raised jugular venous pressure), a very effective and rapid way of reducing the preload.

If despite these measures there is no response, positive-pressure mechanical ventilation should be considered. Balloon counterpulsation (if available) is another possibility *if* a potentially correctable cause has been identified.

Early echocardiography is essential to identify firmly those patients with mechanical defects (severe valvular stenosis, acute valvular regurgitation due to infarction or infection, etc.), who might benefit from transfer to a centre capable of corrective surgery.

## Cardiac tamponade

The fluid is usually a large effusion (e.g., malignant) or blood following a dissecting aneurysm, myocardial infarction, or chest injury.

### Diagnosis

The patient is often very ill, with hypotension, pulsus paradoxus (an inspiratory systolic pressure drop of more than 10 mmHg), tachycardia, raised jugular venous pressure with a further inspiratory rise and rapid 'Y' descent, absent apical beat, and muffled or inaudible heart sounds. A large area of cardiac dullness may be elicited on percussion. The ECG shows small complexes and the X-ray a large, globular heart unless the tamponade is particularly acute. Echocardiography confirms the diagnosis.

## Management

**Pericardial aspiration.** The patient sits at 45°, and the skin around the xiphisternum is cleaned with iodine.

After infiltration with lignocaine, a large bore needle is inserted 2 cm below the xiphisternum, 30 to 45° to the skin, advancing towards the left scapula, continuously aspirating. The butt of the needle should be attached using a crocodile clip to an ECG monitor. There is usually a 'give' as the pericardium is crossed and fluid enters the syringe. ST elevation occurs if myocardium is damaged by the needle and serves as a warning to withdraw. If the fluid is bloody, 3 to 4 ml should be placed in a tube: if it clots it is blood from within a cardiac chamber, implying rupture, otherwise it is simply a haemorrhagic effusion. As much fluid as possible is aspirated, providing rupture is excluded.

In a 'cardiac arrest' where tamponade is even suspected it is worth attempting aspiration; with the patient horizontal, a vertical approach at the left fourth intercostal space beside the sternum is best.

## Malignant hypertension

### Diagnosis

This is difficult to define. Symptoms are usually present (e.g., headache, drowsiness, blurred vision) and the diastolic blood pressure is usually over 130 mmHg. Fundal changes of grades III or IV are present (these grades, in fact, do not differ in prognosis). There is proteinuria, often with haematuria. Other features indicating 'malignancy' include secondary heart failure, myocardial ischaemia, renal failure and encephalopathy. Hypertensive emergencies may also be associated with aortic dissection, phaeochromocytoma and toxaemia of pregnancy.

### Management

In the past, immediate reduction with parenteral vasodilators was advocated, but after evidence that this treatment could actually precipitate (ischaemic) neurological deficits, it has fallen from grace. Bed rest is mandatory and the aim should be to reduce the pressure only to around 160/110 mmHg in the first 48 h. Sublingual nifedipine, 10

to 20 mg, will cause an adequately rapid fall whilst maintaining (or even increasing) cerebral flow. If ineffective, oral β-blockers (e.g., atenolol 100 mg) should be effective within an hour or two. If these drugs fail, if severe hypertensive heart failure is present (both drugs are negative inotropes), or if encephalopathic fits occur, intravenous nitroprusside is probably the drug of choice. It has a very short half-life, so that its effect can be very closely controlled and precipitous falls in blood pressure avoided. It should be started at a dose of 0.5 µg/kg/min (a freshly made up solution, protected from the light) and titrated according to response; 20 to 400 µg/min may be needed. It should not be continued for more than 48 h.

## Aortic dissection

### Diagnosis

This may cause severe ('tearing') pain in the chest and back, which may move as the dissection progresses. It is associated with shock, often with different blood pressures in the arm, or even absent pulses in the arms or legs, and tachycardia. Alternatively, the BP may be very high. Neurological signs may be related to carotid artery (hemiparesis) or spinal artery involvement (paraplegia), and the mesenteric and renal arteries may also be involved. Proximal (ascending aorta) dissection may result in tamponade, coronary occlusion and aortic incompetence. The chest X-ray may show aortic widening but the definitive method of diagnosis remains angiography. (CT scanning and digital subtraction angiography are gaining in popularity.)

### Management

(1) Pain relief with intravenous opiates (and antiemetics).
(2) Urgent control of BP if raised; a combination of intravenous nitroprusside (see above) and β-blockers is recommended.
(3) Relief of cardiac tamponade, if present (see p. 21).
(4) Cross-match blood (6–10 u).
(5) Aortography when stabilized.
(6) Consultation with the regional cardiothoracic team.

In proximal dissection, early surgery improves the prognosis and this is also advised for complicated distal dissection (e.g., occlusion of the renal or femoral artery). The prognosis for uncomplicated distal dissection is probably not affected by surgery.

## Pulmonary embolus

Pulmonary emboli that are silent, cause sudden death or chronic thrombo-embolic lung disease will not be considered here. The remainder, patients with acute symptomatic emboli, can be divided into: (a) those with minor (usually) peripheral emboli that do not cause cardiorespiratory embarrassment, and (b) those with larger, proximal emboli (usually obstructing over half the pulmonary vascular tree). In practice, of course, there is no strict dividing line. Furthermore, dislodgement or augmentation of embolus enables patients in either group to transfer themselves to the other. Nevertheless, it is useful, in terms of management, to distinguish the sick (and threatened) patient from the less compromised.

### Diagnosis

Patients in either group are likely to have pleurisy (though this is rather more common in those with minor embolism), dyspnoea, tachycardia and tachypnoea.

Features commoner in *minor pulmonary embolism* include haemoptysis, a pleural rub and a chest X-ray that is usually normal but may show wedge-shaped opacification.

In *massive pulmonary embolism* there may be a history of syncope. The patient may be cyanosed, shocked and sweaty, and with signs of right heart overload (raised jugular venous pressure with prominent 'a' wave, parasternal heave, loud $P_2$ and a right-sided gallop rhythm). Investigations confirm hypoxia and hypocarbia and the ECG may show the 'S1, Q3, T3' pattern (S wave in $S_1$, and a Q-wave and T-wave inversion in $S_3$) with right heart strain, right axis deviation and right bundle branch block. The chest X-ray may again be normal; alternatively it may show a 'black' lung, a dilated pulmonary artery with abrupt cut-off, or an elevated hemidiaphragm.

### Management

Chest X-ray, ECG and arterial gases are performed on all patients.

### Minor pulmonary embolism

(1) A perfusion lung scan, preferably done with a ventilation scan, is the investigation of choice.
(2) Confirmed cases, and those where there is reasonable suspicion but a delay in scanning, should be treated with intravenous heparin followed by oral warfarin as outlined in Tables 2.1 and 2.2. Heparin should be continued for five days, so there is no virtue in commencing warfarin until day 3. Patients without complications should continue on warfarin for six weeks.

### Massive pulmonary embolism

(1) Resuscitate!
   (a) Keep the patient lying flat.
   (b) Give oxygen (unlimited) via a face mask or nasal cannulae.
   (c) An intravenous bolus dose of heparin, 10 000 to 15 000 u, is given for its pulmonary vasodilating action (or rather its potential inhibitory effect on locally produced pulmonary vasoconstrictors).
   (d) Correct any acidosis with intravenous bicarbonate, 1.4 per cent.
   (e) Insert a central venous pressure line and infuse colloid to maintain a high–normal venous pressure.
   (f) Inotropic support (dobutamine and low-dose dopamine) if necessary.
   (g) If cardiac arrest occurs, cardiac massage may dislodge embolus distally.
   (h) If the patient remains critically ill, immediate thrombolytic therapy or even surgical embolectomy may be considered.
(2) If the patient responds to the above, the diagnosis should be confirmed either by perfusion/ventilation scanning or pulmonary angiography. The latter is the superior investigation but is probably only needed when the former is equivocal or if surgery is contemplated. Digital subtraction angiography carries less morbidity and is playing an increasing role.
(3) Having proved the diagnosis there are now three options.
   (a) *Heparinization.* This is inadequate for patients with massive emboli and shock.
   (b) *Thrombolytic agents.* Although there is still no evidence that these reduce mortality, they do clear the clot more rapidly

and are therefore recommended when there is persistent hypotension, oliguria or severe hypoxia. Contraindications include active or recent internal bleeding, and recent cerebrovascular accident (within two months), surgery or serious trauma (10 days). Pregnancy, puerperium, menstruation, hypertension and diabetic retinopathy are also contraindications. Heparin is stopped and when the kaolin–cephalin clotting time is within 10 s of the control, streptokinase is given

**Table 2.1 Flexible dose induction regime for warfarin—the Llandough scheme**

| | Kaolin–cephalin clotting time (KCCT)* (9–10 a.m.) | Heparin dose† | International Normalised Ratio (INR) (9–10 a.m.) | Warfarin dose‡ given at 5 p.m. (mg) |
|---|---|---|---|---|
| Day 1 | 1.5–2.5 × control | As per KCCT | – | 0.0 |
| Day 2 | | | – | 0.0 |
| Day 3 | | | <1.4 | 10.0 |
| Day 4 | | | <1.8 | 10.0 |
| | | | 1.8 | 1.0 |
| | | | >1.8 | 0.5 |
| Day 5 | | | <2.0 | 10.0 |
| | | | 2.0–2.1 | 5.0 |
| | | | 2.2–2.3 | 4.5 |
| | | | 2.4–2.5 | 4.0 |
| | | | 2.6–2.7 | 3.5 |
| | | | 2.8–2.9 | 3.0 |
| | | | 3.0–3.1 | 2.5 |
| | | | 3.2–3.3 | 2.0 |
| | | | 3.4 | 1.5 |
| | | | 3.5 | 1.0 |
| | | | 3.6–4.0 | 0.5 |
| | | | >4.0 | 0.0 |
| | | Stop heparin | | |
| Day 6§ | | | | Predicted maintenance dose (mg) |
| | | | <1.4 | 8.0 |
| | | | 1.4 | 8.0 |
| | | | 1.5 | 7.5 |
| | | | 1.6–1.7 | 7.0 |
| | | | 1.8 | 6.5 |
| | | | 1.9 | 6.0 |
| | | | 2.0–2.1 | 5.5 |
| | | | 2.2–2.3 | 5.0 |
| | | | 2.4–2.6 | 4.5 |
| | | | 2.7–3.0 | 4.0 |
| | | | 3.1–3.5 | 3.5 |
| | | | 3.6–4.0 | 3.0 |
| | | | 4.1–4.5 | Miss out next day's dose then give 2 mg |
| | | | >4.5 | Miss out next day's dose then give 1 mg |

  * The KCCT should be within or below therapeutic range (1.5–2.5 × control). If KCCT is above this range, the heparin effect of the INR is neutralized with protamine, 0.4 µg/ml plasma, added to the sample by the haematologist.
  † If heparin therapy is not being given, commence the schedule at day 3.
  ‡ Special care should be taken with patients with heart failure, liver disease or immediately postoperatively as their sensitivity to warfarin may vary with time.
  § If the INR on day 6 is less than 2.0, heparin can be recommended until the INR is within the therapeutic range.
Reproduced with kind permission from Fennerty A. *et al.* (1984). *B. Med. J.*, **288**, 1268–70.

**Table 2.2 Regimen for the use of heparin by intravenous infusion**

Loading dose—5000 u over 5 min

Infusion—*start* at 1400 u/h (e.g., 8400 u in 100 ml over 6 h)

Check the kaolin/cephalin clotting time (KCCT) after 6 h*

Adjust dose according to the ratio of KCCT to control (KCCT ratio) as follows:

| KCCT ratio | Change in heparin infusion rate (u/h) |
|---|---|
| >5.0 | Reduce 500 |
| 4.1–5.0 | Reduce 300 |
| 3.1–4.0 | Reduce 100 |
| 2.6–3.0 | Reduce 50 |
| 1.5–2.5 | No change |
| 1.2–1.4 | Increase 200 |
| <1.2 | Increase 400 |

Wait 10 h before next KCCT estimation, unless KCCT ratio is greater than 5.0, in which case more frequent estimation would be advisable

* If possible, measure the KCCT in the morning between 9 a.m. and 12 noon.

Reproduced with kind permission from Fennerty A. G. *et al.* (1985). *Br. J. Clin. Pharmacol.* **20**, p. 266 of the Proceedings supplement.

(250 000 u intravenously over 30 min, followed by 100 000 u/h, for 12–24 h). Concurrent administration of hydrocortisone and antihistamines may help prevent anaphylactic reactions. Control is complicated and target ranges unclear, so that some authorities do not consider even attempting it worthwhile. Tissue plasminogen activator may prove to be safer.

(c) *Surgical embolectomy.* This has an important role when hypotension or severe hypoxia persist after thrombolytic treatment, or when the latter is contraindicated. It should be preceded by angiography.

Filters or balloons placed (usually under local anaesthesia) in the inferior vena cava are superior to ligation or plication, and have a *preventative* role (in experienced hands) in patients with definite recurrence of embolism or when there is a further risk of embolism with a contraindication to anticoagulants.

**Central venous catheterization.** The main indications are severe hypotension or dehydration of any cause, and as a means of access for temporary cardiac pacing or for the administration of certain drugs (e.g., amiodarone) or parenteral feeding.

A number of anatomical approaches are possible. The infraclavicular route is associated with a higher risk of complications, including pneumothorax, but is often easier and quicker in an emergency. An approach to the internal jugular vein in the neck is usually safer, but more uncomfortable for the patient, particularly if the line is to be maintained for prolonged periods.

Whatever the approach the Seldinger technique, where a guidewire is inserted through a needle that is then withdrawn before the cannula is inserted over the guidewire, is to be recommended, as it avoids potentially dangerous conflict between the blade of the needle and the plastic cannula.

**Technique:** The bed is first tilted head down to engorge the veins and the patient's head turned to his or her left. Having chosen the site (see (4) below) the procedure is as follows:

(1) Sterility should be maintained. A gown and gloves should be worn, the chosen site swabbed with iodine and the surrounding area draped with green towels.

(2) Infiltrate with 0.5 or 1 per cent lignocaine (carefully aspirating before each injection to avoid intravascular administration).

(3) A nick is made in the skin with the point of a scalpel blade.

(4) Whatever site is chosen, first use a green needle to locate the vein (advancing while continuously aspirating) to help avoid damage to local structures from prospecting with the larger catheter needle. The latter is kept immediately to hand, so that as soon as the vein is located, the green needle is removed and the larger needle is inserted directly through the same hole at the same angle and to the same depth; the vein should be relocated with ease. The guidewire is inserted, floppy end first, through the needle (if any resistance is met, withdraw both and start again) and the cannula/dilator threaded over the guidewire after the needle has been withdrawn.

(a) *Internal jugular vein, high approach.* The right carotid artery is located and protected with the left finger tips at the level of the cricoid cartilage. The needle is inserted immediately lateral to the finger tips, directed caudally and slightly laterally at an angle of 30 to 40° to the skin. The internal jugular vein runs just deep to medial border of the sternomastoid at this point.

(b) *Internal jugular vein, lower approach.* The triangle formed by the sternal and clavicular heads of sternocleidomastoid with the clavicle as the base is identified. The needle is inserted, 30 to 40° to the skin, aiming caudally and toward the inner border of the anterior end of the first rib behind the clavicle.

(c) *Subclavian vein, infraclavicular approach.* The green needle is usually just long enough to locate the vein. It is inserted just below the lower border of the clavicle, slightly medial to the midpoint and directed medially and horizontally, 30 to 40° to the skin, aiming towards the suprasternal notch.

(5) If the purpose is to record central venous pressure, the cannula is connected (via a 3-way tip if it is to be used for other purposes as well) to a fluid column. Oscillation of the fluid level with respiration confirms an intrathoracic position. Chest radiography is performed; the preferred position of the tip of the catheter is 2 cm below a line joining the lower edges of the clavicles. The X-ray is also examined to exclude pneumothorax. The cannula is secured with a skin suture and then covered with, for example, an Opsite dressing. The cannula should also be secured further on with Elastoplast so that neither the stitch nor the dressing is required to 'take the strain' if the cannula should be pulled for any reason.

To measure the right atrial pressure a spirit level is used to set the 'zero' on the fluid column, level with the manubrosternal angle; the normal pressure is 3 to 10 cmH$_2$O.

## Gastrointestinal haemorrhage

Haematemesis and/or melaena are generally caused by a peptic ulcer, acute erosions or oesophageal varices. A minority are caused by Mallory–Weiss tears and a smaller number still by gastric neoplasm, haemangioma (e.g., Rendu–Osler–Weber disease) or general coagulation defects.

### Diagnosis and assessment

Unless the patient is collapsed and requires urgent resuscitation, a history of past peptic ulceration or dyspepsia, aspirin, other non-steroidal anti-inflammatory drug or steroid ingestion, and cigarette or alcohol abuse should be sought. Acute alcohol intake may cause gastric erosions, while chronic abuse increases the possibility of cirrhosis, portal hypertension and oesophageal varices (though only 50 per cent of patients with oesophageal varices and haematemesis are bleeding from the varices).

Pallor, sweating, anxiety or hyperventilation may immediately be obvious and shock may be confirmed by a low blood pressure and tachycardia. A well-looking patient may nevertheless have a significantly depleted intravascular volume: postural hypotension and postural tachycardia, together with an 'absent' (low) jugular venous pressure, are important clues and should *always* be sought. Other signs, including those of liver failure, or perhaps perioral telangiectasia, may be present; rectal examination is, of course, mandatory.

### Management

(1) Raise the foot of the bed if the patient is shocked!

(2) Blood should be taken for haemoglobin, urea and electrolytes, cross-matching (at least 6 u if there are signs of intravascular volume depletion), and prothrombin time. The haemoglobin is likely to be normal until haemodilution occurs; if less than 10.0 g/100 ml, transfusion is advised (even in the absence of shock).

(3) A significantly depleted intravascular volume must be replenished. If the patient is shocked, replacement should be commenced immediately with colloids, e.g., plasma protein fraction, or Haemaccel, until the blood is available.

(4) The urine output must be monitored.

(5) Fresh frozen plasma and vitamin K (10 mg intravenously) are given in those with disturbed coagulation.

(6) A central venous pressure line is advisable, especially in shocked patients, not only to manage the rate of fluid administration (maintain the central venous pressure in the upper normal range, i.e., 5–10 cmH$_2$O, measuring from the mid-axillary line with the patient supine), but more importantly to indicate early any further bleed.

(7) Some advise a nasogastric tube but, because this may conceivably irritate and cause further bleeding, the recommendation is far from universal.

(8) Similarly a 'nil by mouth' regimen is occasionally suggested on the grounds that emergency anaesthesia may later be required—if this should be the case, however, the stomach will obviously have already filled itself using its blood vessels, so this advice too is disputed.

(9) Oxygen may be needed, depending on the blood gases.

(10) Small doses of sedatives may help.

(11) The surgical team should always be asked to review the patient.

(12) (a) If resuscitation measures are failing, implying continued bleeding, then further management is complicated by

the absence at this stage of a diagnosis. Endoscopy is often unhelpful (nothing may be seen for the blood) but it should nevertheless be attempted (preferably in theatre) to exclude varices. Arteriography is then the investigation of choice. If the technique is available, it may also have an important therapeutic role in that bleeding of almost any cause can often be controlled either by local infusion of vasopressin, or by arterial embolization. Otherwise (occasionally anyway), urgent laparotomy is indicated.

(b) Rapid improvement implies that bleeding has stopped. The investigation of choice is now 'semi-elective' endoscopy (within 24 h, but immediately if varices seem likely). An urgent barium meal should be done if endoscopy is not available. Subsequent management depends on the diagnosis.

### Non-variceal bleeding

In *peptic ulceration*, intravenous $H_2$-blockers continue to be given despite the lack of any clear evidence of benefit. Antifibrinolytic agents or somatostatin are not routinely recommended and various methods of local treatment ('per endoscope'), such as laser photocoagulation and diathermy, are also currently being assessed. Indications for surgery include continued or rebleeding, particularly if the patient is over 50 years of age, and particularly if there is a history of chronic ulceration. A vessel visible on endoscopy at the ulcer base is also thought to imply a high risk of rebleeding. Surgery should be avoided if possible for *acute erosions*, as emergency gastrectomy, a hazardous procedure, usually proves necessary. Intravenous selective antihistamines and oral antacids should be given. The *Mallory–Weiss tear* also rarely requires surgery.

### Variceal bleeding

This carries a poorer prognosis. Immediate measures include vasopressin, 20 u intravenously in 50 to 100 ml of 5 per cent dextrose over 10 to 20 min, repeated 4-hourly if necessary. Alternatively, an infusion of 0.4 u/min may be used. Ischaemic heart disease is a contraindication. Triglycyl lysine vasopressin may be preferable and

is certainly more expensive. A Blakemore–Sengstaken tube can be used, either before vasopressin or if the drug is ineffective. The stomach balloon is inflated first to ensure corrected positioning and the oesophageal balloon, then inflated to tamponade the varices (pressure about 30 mmHg). The oesophagus is aspirated above the balloon, which should not be left inflated for more than 24 h (otherwise ischaemic necrosis may result). These measures will nearly always control bleeding. More definitive, subsequent measures include emergency endoscopic variceal injection (increasingly popular), or oesophageal transection with a stapling gun.

Neomycin and lactulose may be used to help prevent encephalopathy. Propranolol may reduce the incidence of rebleeding, but also prevents an adequate sympathetic response if bleeding does recur.

### Acute diarrhoea/colitis

#### Diagnosis

The diagnosis of a newly presenting patient with severe diarrhoea, with or without blood, can be extremely difficult—even sigmoidoscopy and biopsy may ultimately fail to distinguish various forms of colitis. Features such as arthritis or erythema nodosum should obviously be noted, but are not specific. A history of homosexual activity is important. Rectal examination may reveal blood, impacted stool (overflow diarrhoea) or carcinoma, though neither of the latter commonly cause severe diarrhoea of acute onset. Table 2.3 may be of some value and also gives some indication of the important initial investigations.

Fresh stool should be examined for ova, cysts, pus cells and organisms and then cultured. Blood should also be cultured and the electrolytes and urea, haemoglobin, white cell count and haematocrit checked. A low serum albumin and high ESR suggest severe disease. Serum calcium and magnesium may be low. Serology (*Campylobacter*, *Yersinia*, *Entamoeba*, *Giardia*, viruses, treponemes and human immunodeficiency virus [HIV]) should be checked (repeat specimens in 10 days). On a plain abdominal X-ray the extent of affected bowel can often be inferred from the amount of colon not filled with stool. Mucosal ulceration may be seen, as may the 'thumbprinting' of ischaemic bowel. A dilated colon (>6 cm)

**Table 2.3 Differential diagnosis of diarrhoea**

| Cause | Helpful features | Diagnosis |
|---|---|---|
| **Infections**—note the importance of contact and travel history | | |
| *Shigella* spp., enteroinvasive *E. coli* | IP*, 2–4 days—general malaise, headache, then high fever, bloody diarrhoea (acute onset) | Stool—red blood and pus cells and stool culture.—Rarely blood culture |
| *Salmonella* spp. | IP, 6–48 h—general symptoms then severe watery diarrhoea, often with blood; metastatic infection possible *typhi, paratyphi* A, B, C | Blood and stool culture—red blood and mononuclear cells in stool |
| *Campylobacter* | IP, 3–5 days—flu-like symptoms, high fever, abdomen pain (often severe), profuse, foul, watery diarrhoea, often bloody | Stool blood culture; serology |
| *Yersinia* | IP, 4–10 days—diarrhoea (rarely bloody), pain, usually right iliac fossa, fever; often erythema nodosum, arthritis | Stool, blood culture; serology |
| *Clostridium difficile* (pseudomembranous colitis) | Follows broad-spectrum antibacterials—low-grade fever, abdomen pain, watery or bloody diarrhoea; sigmoidoscopy—yellowish plaques | Stool, toxin assay and culture |
| *Entamoeba histolytica* | IP, 14–21 days—foul stool; ulcer on sigmoidoscopy | Stool microscopy (cysts); rectal biopsy; serology |
| *Giardia lamblia* | IP, 14 days—watery diarrhoea, prostration | Stool microscopy; jejunal biopsy or aspirate; serology |
| **The 'gay' bowel** | | |
| Anorectal syphilis | Acute bloody diarrhoea | Serology, stool culture, biopsy and microscopy |
| Cryptosporidiosis | Severe watery diarrhoea | Jejunal biopsy |
| *Gonococcus, Chlamydia trachomatis,* cytomegalovirus, herpesvirus | All can cause ulcerative proctitis | |
| **Viruses** | | |
| Rotavirus, Norwalk | Traveller's or institutional diarrhoea | Serology |
| **'Acute infective type colitis'** ('self-limited colitis') | Colitic symptoms | No infectious organism found; biopsy of value |
| **Non-infectious** | | |
| Acute inflammatory bowel disease | Acute bloody diarrhoea: possibly pyoderma gangrenosa, perianal sepsis, mouth ulcers, erythema nodosum; occasional severe systemic symptoms; may be past history | Sigmoidoscopy/biopsy; radiology |
| Ischaemic bowel disease | Acute onset of colitis: may be ischaemic heart disease, valvular disease, atrial fibrillation, etc. | Plain radiology ('thumbprinting') |
| Laxative abuse | History | History and biopsy |

* IP, incubation period.

suggests toxic megacolon, and gas under the diaphragm on the chest X-ray is of obvious importance. Sigmoidoscopy with careful biopsy forms the mainstay of diagnosis.

## Management

All patients should be barrier-nursed (even an exacerbation of known inflammatory bowel disease may prove to be due to infection).

(1) *The less sick patient* can be investigated as above at leisure and specific treatment started (if needed) when the diagnosis becomes clear, though dehydration and hypokalaemia may need swifter correction. Otherwise management is as follows.

(2) *The sick patient before diagnosis*

    (a) *General measures.* Features such as shock or tachycardia, high fever, confusion and/or prostration, sweating, peripheral vasodilation (or later, circulatory collapse with peripheral 'shut-down'), a low haemoglobin, neutrophilia, and low albumin suggest a toxic, ill patient with bacteraemia or septicaemia. Such patients require rapid correction of dehydration (using normal saline), electrolyte imbalance (hypokalaemia is common) and anaemia. A central venous pressure line is useful not only for monitoring fluid replacement but also because early parenteral feeding may be of benefit. Clear fluids only should be allowed orally. The urine output and stool frequency should be recorded. Abdominal girth and plain abdominal X-rays should be monitored to identify toxic megacolon, a complication of infectious as well as inflammatory colonic disease. Surgical referral and a joint approach to management are mandatory. The diagnosis will usually be made within a few days on the basis of biopsy and/or stool/blood cultures.

(b) *Drugs*. Intravenous antibacterials are given, e.g., ampicillin, gentamicin (beware renal failure—see Table 2.5 below) and metronidazole, later changed according to sensitivity. High-dose, intravenous steroids (e.g., hydrocortisone 100 mg 6 hourly) are also given immediately, despite the absence of an aetiological diagnosis—it is dangerous to delay them in ulcerative colitis and they are unlikely to be harmful to patients with septicaemic shock secondary to infectious colitis, providing they are not continued for more than the day or two needed to establish the diagnosis.

(3) *The sick patient—diagnosis known*
The general measures outlined in (2a) above are instituted. Specific treatment is as follows:

(a) *Inflammatory bowel disease*. A high frequency of liquid bloody stools (>6/24 h), in addition to the above features, suggests severe disease; liaison with surgeons is desirable from the onset. Parenteral steroids are given as above. Antibacterials, particularly metronidazole, are commonly used, though benefit remains unproven. Toxic megacolon or failure to improve on the above regimen are indications for surgery. Once improvement does occur, steroids orally and by enema, together with salazopyrine, can be commenced.

(b) *Infections*. Most are self-limiting; needlessly given antibacterials promote resistance and often prolong the period of infection. Nevertheless, severe infections with shock, high fever or severe colitis do need specific therapy—chloramphenicol, co-trimoxazole or amoxycillin for *Salmonella*, co-trimoxazole or ampicillin for *Shigella*, erythromycin for *Campylobacter*, tetracycline for *Yersinia*. All cases, trivial or otherwise, of amoebiasis or giardiasis require metronidazole.

(c) *The 'gay bowel'*. Specific treatment of *Candida*, herpes, *Neisseria*, syphilis and *Chlamydia* may be needed. Cryptosporidiosis (which may also occur in immunecompetent patients) *may* respond to spiramycin, if available. Diarrhoea is a common presentation of AIDS.

(d) *Pseudomembranous colitis*. If possible, current antibacterials are stopped. Vancomycin, 125 mg four times a day orally, was the initially recommended treatment, though metronidazole (400 mg three times a day) appears equally valuable.

(e) *Ischaemic bowel disease*. Most patients settle spontaneously with supportive therapy and antibacterials if necessary. Surgical liaison is again mandatory, as resection may prove necessary.

### Acute liver failure

#### Diagnosis

This condition occurs either acutely in patients with a previously normal liver (viral hepatitis, leptospirosis, hoalthane, paracetamol, etc.), or as a result of acute deterioration in cases of compensated chronic liver disease (e.g., cirrhosis). The latter may be precipitated by gastrointestinal bleeding, drugs (diuretics, causing potassium depletion, or opiates), infection, surgery, constipation, or alcohol, and these patients often have signs of chronic liver disease and portal hypertension in addition to the features of acute liver failure.

The latter include those of encephalopathy, ranging from mood change to confusion and coma (Table 2.4) together with a flapping tremor (asterixis) and constructional apraxia. Hepatic fetor is present. As coma progresses, pyramidal signs and then decorticate and decerebrate posturing with dilated pupils occur. Jaundice and ascites may be present. There is a predisposition to bleeding and to hypoglycaemia, and infection is common.

*Investigations* are directed towards finding the cause (electrolytes and urea; haemoglobin and white cell count; blood, spit and urine cultures; hepatitis and leptospirosis titre, and chest X-ray and liver ultrasound) and monitoring the effects and degree of liver failure (bilirubin, liver enzymes and albumin, glucose, prothrombin time, disseminated intravascular coagulation (DIC) screen, blood gases and possibly an EEG). Diagnostic paracentesis may be helpful if ascites is present (see below).

**Table 2.4 Grading of hepatic encephalopathy**

| Grade | Features |
|---|---|
| I | Euphoria or depression; disordered sleep, slurred speech, mild confusion |
| II | Lethargic, responding to command; moderate confusion |
| III | Sleeping but rousable; markedly confused, incoherent speech |
| IV | Coma, may or may not respond to pain |

*NB.* The EEG is abnormal in Grades II–IV.

## Management

Previously normal livers can acquire functional normality again if the patient survives the acute failure. Those with acute decompensation can do no more than return to their previous, precarious stability.

(1) Nursing care of the confused or comatose patient is of obvious importance, with attention to pressure areas, sphincters, etc. Barrier nursing is instituted if hepatitis B is not excluded.

(2) Treatment of the precipitating factor (electrolyte imbalance, infection, gastrointestinal bleed, etc.) or cause (if possible; e.g., leptospirosis) is also obviously important.

(3) Sedation is used only if absolutely necessary with *small* doses of diazepam or chlormethiazole.

(4) The above mentioned biochemical and haematological factors and the weight should be checked daily. Apraxia and, by implication,

encephalopathy itself can be monitored by daily recording the patient's attempts to copy a five-pointed star, or by a dot-to-dot 'apraxia chart'.

(5) Intravenous ranitidine, 50 mg three times a day, helps prevent stress ulceration and erosions.

(6) Other treatment is directed towards minimizing or reversing the effects of the failing liver:

(a) Hypoglycaemia—this may occur despite continuous 5 per cent dextrose and needs urgent correction.

(b) Bleeding tendency—vitamin K, 10 mg intravenously daily, is of some benefit. If bleeding becomes a problem, fresh frozen plasma or even clotting factor and/or platelet concentrates may be given.

(c) Jaundice—requires no treatment providing biliary obstruction has been excluded.

(d) Hypoxia—not uncommon and may necessitate assisted ventilation.

(e) Ascites is more common in chronic liver disease than acute. A diagnostic tap is necessary to exclude infection (fever and over 500 white blood cells/$mm^3$ fluid warrant antibacterial therapy) including TB, but therapeutic paracentesis is considered a bad idea. Strict restriction of sodium (30 mmol/day) and fluid (1.5 l daily except in hyponatraemia, when only 1 l is permitted *unless* postural hypotension indicates intravascular volume depletion) together with diuretics (spironolactone, up to 400 mg daily, to combat secondary hyperaldosteronism, with loop diuretics if necessary) may be effective—aim for a daily loss of ≤1 kg/day. Failure, or the development of intravascular volume depletion and a rising urea, indicate the need to consider either salt-poor albumin administration or ultrafiltration with intravenous re-infusion of ascitic fluid.

(f) Encephalopathy—oral protein should be restricted (20 g/day), the bowel emptied by neomycin, 1 g four times a day, and its remaining contents rendered acid (encouraging movement of ammonium into the bowel from the blood) by lactulose, 20 ml three times a day. Levodopa, bromocriptine and measures such as exchange transfusion are of unproven value. All patients with encephalopathy should be nursed head up, as this may help forestall the occurrence of cerebral oedema.

Cerebral oedema itself is probably the commonest cause of death, but is very difficult to diagnose on clinical grounds alone before it has caused decorticate or decerebrate posturing and fixed pupils, by which time the outlook is almost hopeless. The widely quoted advice to use mannitol for this complication is of little practical value unless the intracranial pressure is to be recorded.

(7) If transfer to a centre capable of considering charcoal haemoperfusion or liver transplant is thought worthwhile it should be done as early as possible. A considerably raised or persistently rising prothombin time, particularly if associated with encephalopathy of Grade II or more, indicates that the nearest liver unit should be contacted for advice regarding possible transfer. Hyponatraemia, declining renal function and metabolic acidosis are of similar significance.

## Hypercalcaemia

### Diagnosis

Symptoms include polyuria, polydipsia, abdominal pain, vomiting and behavioural changes. Acute renal failure and fatal arrhythmias may later occur. A short QT interval may be seen on the ECG. Symptoms commonly occur at levels over 3.5 mmol/l (remember to correct the serum albumin—add 0.02 to the calcium for every g/l by which the albumin is below 40 g/l), while levels over 4.0 mmol/l may be life-threatening. Such levels nearly always arise either from malignancy (including myeloma) or hyperparathyroidism. A low albumin and/or low chloride (<102 mmol/l) favour malignancy. Sarcoidosis, vitamin D intoxication, thyrotoxicosis, drugs and 'milk–alkali syndrome' very rarely cause extreme hypercalcaemia.

### Management

Dehydration is always present and up to 7–8 l/day of intravenous saline may be needed to correct it. Frusemide (100 mg intravenously every 3–4 h) facilitates a diuresis and causes hypercalciuria. A central venous pressure line is of obvious value; hypokalaemia should be sought and corrected. These measures alone usually lower the calcium to below 3.5 mmol/l. If not, other drugs are necessary. Steroids are ineffective in both hyperparathyroidism and malignancy (except myeloma). A combination of calcitonin (subcutaneous, 400 u 8-hourly for 48 h) and aminohydroxypropylidine (15 mg daily by intravenous infusion in 250 ml saline) has been shown to cause a rapid and sustained fall in calcium levels and is likely to become the treatment of choice. Plicamycin (1–1.5 mg infused over 4 h every three days) has a less sustained action and more side-effects. Dialysis or a single infusion of phosphate (50 mmol disodium phosphate over 8 h) can be used as a last resort. Further management naturally depends on the underlying cause.

## Acute fever

Most patients with an acute high fever have an infection. Malignancy, autoimmune disease, drug reactions, etc., more commonly cause the less acute 'pyrexia of unknown origin'.

### Diagnosis

Symptoms of cough and spit, dysuria, headache, arthralgia and myalgia, sore throat, diarrhoea and jaundice are clearly important. Equally important but less often ascertained are a history of travel, contact (with ill people, pets and other animals), occupation, recent surgery, sexual practice and menstruation (toxic shock syndrome). On examination, a flushed, hypotensive, sweaty and perhaps drowsy or confused patient suggests toxaemic or septicaemic shock. Examine the skin carefully (rash, jaundice, signs of endocarditis or needle marks), the fauces and the ears. Record the level of consciousness and seek meningism.

A provisional diagnosis can usually be made at this point and confirmatory investigations undertaken. A full blood count and film is essential. Blood cultures should be done even in apparently localized infections (e.g., pneumonia, meningitis), and throat-swab and stool samples should be taken in suspected viral infections (including meningitis). If no diagnosis is yet apparent, culture blood, urine, spit, stool and (if the patient is particularly sick) CSF, and send swabs from the throat, nares, ears, rectum, vagina and *any* skin lesion. Any ascitic and/or pleural fluid must be cultured. A chest X-ray should be done. Request a thick film if malaria is suspected. Send two clotted samples of blood, one for antibody titres (for viral illness), the other to be frozen and stored for any retrospective analysis.

## Isolation

Patients with a high fever, particularly if accompanied by diarrhoea or jaundice, should be barrier-nursed in a side ward. Exceptions are patients with abscesses, straightforward chest or urinary tract infections or malaria. HIV transmission is not common but febrile AIDS patients may harbour other more infective organisms and are therefore also best barrier-nursed.

*Viral haemorrhagic diseases* are a different matter. They include yellow fever (Central and West Africa and South America), dengue (as yellow fever plus South-East Asia), lassa fever (West Africa) and several others. Suspect them in febrile patients from these areas (especially rural regions) with systemic illness, conjunctival injection, haemorrhagic phenomena and possibly oropharyngeal signs (petechial ulceration or vesicles), a rash (maculopapular or petechial) or jaundice. If there is a low index of suspicion send a blood film to exclude malaria, but if this is negative or suspicion high, contact the regional 'high security' isolation hospital for advice and possibly direct transfer (i.e., without admitting or further investigating the patient locally). Advice can also be sought from either the London or Liverpool Schools of Tropical Medicine (telephone: 071 387 4411 or 051 708 9393, respectively).

## Management

In some cases immediate microbiological diagnosis is possible and specific treatment can be commenced (e.g., meningitis, malaria). In others (chest and urinary tract infections), treatment can reasonably be started as soon as specimens have been taken, based on prediction of the likely organisms. In most other cases it is best to withhold treatment until the causative organism is identified.

However, in *septicaemic shock* and other life-threatening infections, treatment cannot be withheld any longer than the few minutes needed to take the above specimens. Intravenous antibiotics are given, e.g., gentamicin, (dose depending on renal function; Table 2.5), ampicillin 500 mg four times a day (or even pipericillin or azlocillin), and metronidazole. The central venous pressure should be recorded and maintained at the upper

**Table 2.5 Gentamicin dosage in impaired renal function**

| Creatinine clearance (ml/min) | *Approx.* serum creatinine (μmol/l) (patient of 30 years) | | Gentamicin dose (mg/kg) | Dose interval (h) |
|---|---|---|---|---|
| | male | female | | |
| >80 | 100 | 95 | 1.5–2.0 | 8 |
| 60–80 | 140 | 125 | 1.5–2.0 | 12 |
| 40–60 | 200 | 170 | 1.0–1.5 | 12 |
| 20–40 | 340 | 290 | 1.5–2.0 | 24 |
| 5–20 | 800 | 700 | 0.5–1.0 | 24 |
| <5 | | | 0.2–0.5 | 24 |

This table is *not* a substitute for checking drug levels, but a guide to help achieve the targets of a peak level of 5.0–8.0 μg/ml (checked 15 min after intravenous dose), and a trough (immediately before administration) less than 2.0 μg/ml.

normal range with colloids and crystalloids. The bladder should be catheterized and urine output monitored. A combination of dobutamine with low-dose dopamine may help improve blood pressure and renal perfusion. Check the arterial gases and institute respiratory support if necessary. There is now good evidence that high-dose intravenous steroids (formerly given because of their occasional effect in elevating the blood pressure) confer no benefit at all and may even be harmful in uraemic patients. Recently, antibodies directed against endotoxin have been shown to be useful, whilst naloxone has been shown not to be.

## Malaria

All patients with a history of foreign travel should have blood films examined. A laboratory dealing infrequently with malaria cannot reasonably be expected confidently to identify malarial species, so advice should be sought from (and slides sent to) one of the Schools of Tropical Medicine. Broadly speaking, *P. falciparum* lives in Africa, South-East Asia and South America, while the other plasmodia abide in India, the Middle East and North Africa. (This is no basis for deciding on treatment! Your patient may have been bitten by an itinerant mosquito in the lounge at Heathrow Airport.)

Therefore for the first 24 (or at most 48) hours until expert advice is obtained I think it is probably most prudent to divide patients with malaria *not* into five or six groups depending on the area, severity and species but into just *two*:

(1) *Definite or probable malaria*—where the patient is not too sick—should be treated with oral quinine, 600 mg three times a day. Strictly speaking, of course, chloroquine should be used unless *P. falciparum* is suspected. The problem is that mild, chloroquine-resistant *falciparum* malaria can rapidly progress to malignant, so that serious consequences may arise from inappropriate attempts at treatment with chloroquine. Less harm, however, will come from treatment of chloroquine-sensitive *falciparum* or non-*falciparum* malaria with quinine. Therefore chloroquine (600 mg base orally, then 300 mg base 6 h later and 300 mg base daily for three days thereafter) should only be used when there is an unequivocal diagnosis of non-*falciparum* or chloroquine-sensitive *falciparum* malaria.

(2) *Severe malaria (i.e., malignant tertian)*. Alteration of conscious level (cerebral malaria), shock, acute anaemia (haemolysis), renal failure, DIC and adult respiratory distress syndrome only occur with *falciparum* infection. These patients need intravenous quinine, 16.7 mg base/kg over 4 h in 5 per cent dextrose (max. 1.4g), then 8.4 mg/kg over 4h, 8-hourly. Do not use these doeses if oral quinine has been given in the preceding 24h. Oral therapy should be commenced as soon as it can be tolerated. Cross-match 5 u of blood and consider exchange transfusion in very sick patients. Respiratory and/or renal support (i.e., ventilation or dialysis) may be needed. Fluid balance is monitored closely (preferably with a central venous pressure line), as are the electrolytes and haemoglobin. Control of convulsions and hyperpyrexia may be needed. All this is, of course, best done on an intensive care unit. Steroids and heparin should *not* be used.

## Status epilepticus

This is defined as repetitive fits without intervening return of consciousness. Complications include not only neuronal damage but also aspir-
ation, injury and anoxia. It may occur in known epileptic patients or be caused by metabolic disturbance (hypoglycaemia, hypocalcaemia, hyponatraemia, uraemia, hepatic failure, acute alcohol withdrawal, thiamine deficiency and drug poisoning), trauma, brain tumours, cerebrovascular disease and infection (meningo-encephalitis) in previously non-epileptic patients.

### *Management* (Fig. 2.3)

(1) Clear the airway (suction and a Guedel tube if necessary), and establish a semiprone position in bed with the cot sides up, padded if possible. Endotracheal intubation may be necessary, either now or later if drugs precipitate hypoventilation (i.e., monitor the arterial gases!). All cases not rapidly responsive to first line treatment should be managed on an intensive care unit.

(2) Establish and *secure* an intravenous line. Check the electrolytes, urea, glucose, calcium, full blood count and (if appropriate) anticonvulsant drug levels.

(3) If you are unable *immediately* to exclude hypoglycaemia, give 50 ml 50 per cent dextrose. Similarly it is worth giving thiamine, 100 mg intramuscularly or intravenously, if alcoholism appears a possibility.*

(4) *Diazepam* should be used first (10 mg intravenously, repeated if necessary at 5-minute intervals to 30–40 mg):

  (a) *If the diazepam treatment is successful* its effect is likely to be short-lived (e.g., 20–30 min). Intravenous phenytoin (18 mg/kg at less than 50 mg/min, monitoring the blood pressure and the ECG) should therefore be given *unless* the patient is already on this. As the diazepam wears off, so the phenytoin is becoming active. It has the advantage of not being hypnotic.

  If the patient is already on phenytoin a diazepam infusion (e.g., 100 mg Diazemuls in 500 ml dextrose, around 40 ml/h according to response and respiratory effect) may be needed.

*The CSM has recently recommended that parental thiamine should only be administered with caution where *essential*; i/v injections should be given over 10 minutes with observation in case of anaphylaxix.

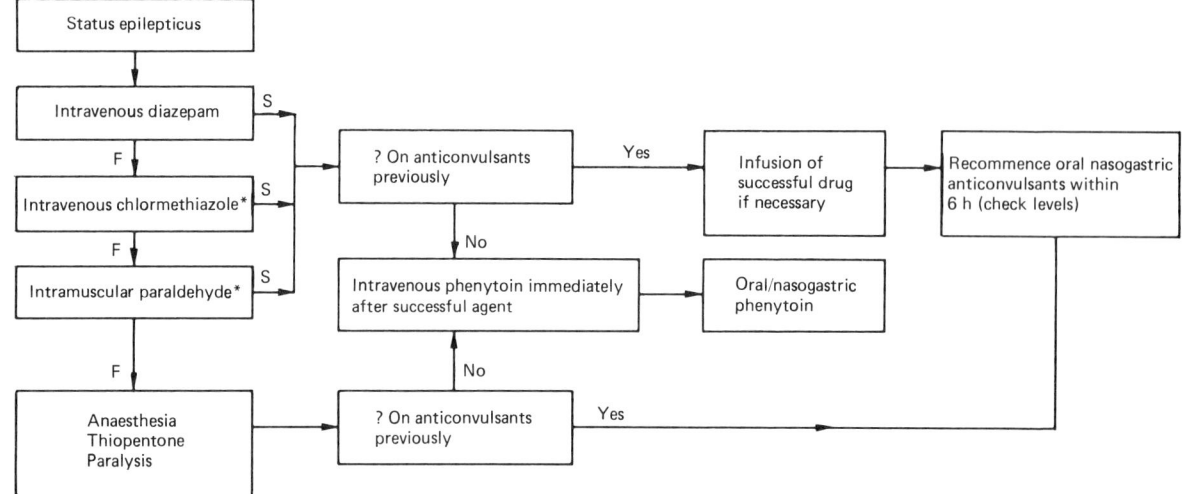

F: Failure; S: Success.
Doses as given in text.
*Paraldehyde may be tried before chlormethiazole depending on availability.
If respiratory depression occurs at any time consider mechanical ventilation.

*Figure 2.3* Management of status epilepticus.

(b) *If the diazepam fails*, try chlormethiazole, 0.8 per cent infusion (40–100 ml over 5–10 min then 10–15 drops/min), which has a short half-life, causes little respiratory depression but can cause prolonged sedation.

An alternative is paraldehyde, 5 ml intramuscularly to each buttock, or as a 6 per cent infusion (30 ml in 500 ml dextrose—remember it dissolves plastic syringes).

(c) *If the diazepam, chlormethiazole and paraldehyde all fail* (or succeed but cause unacceptable respiratory depression), enlist the aid of an anaesthetist, as intravenous thiopentone with mechanical ventilation are necessary. If paralysis is used, continuous EEG monitoring is mandatory to assess epileptic activity.

(5) It is vital to start definitive, longer-term treatment at the earliest possible stage, administering (if necessary via nasogastric tube) either the patient's previous treatment or (usually) phenytoin in the new patient.

Once fits are controlled, consider further investigations, e.g. CT head scan, if necessary.

**Meningitis**

*Diagnosis*

This is suggested by the presence of a headache and vomiting, with fever and a rigid neck. Impaired consciousness may be present. If this has progressed to coma, meningism may be absent. A maculopapular rash and story of 'flu-like' illness suggest a viral aetiology while a petechial, haemorrhagic rash suggests meningococcal disease (and a poor prognosis). A more protracted history with systemic illness and focal neurological deficit raises the possibility of tuberculous meningitis (look for choroidal tubercles in the fundi). Focal signs, including personality change, seizures, dysphasia and cranial nerve deficits, may be present in herpes encephalitis. Localized infection, such as an abscess or subdural empyema, may also cause fever, headache, meningism and focal signs, often accompanied by raised intracranial pressure.

*Management*

(1) *Check* the full blood count, glucose, electrolytes and blood cultures, together with throat swabs and stool specimen or rectal swabs (to help identify viruses).

(2) If the patient has a *petechial/haemorrhagic rash* give 2.4 g benzylpenicillin intravenously immediately, *before* the lumbar puncture. If the patient is allergic to penicillin give chloramphenicol, 1 g intravenous.

(3) **Lumbar puncture** If focal neurological signs, coma, papilloedema, or other evidence of raised intracranial pressure (e.g., falling pulse rate and rising BP) are present, defer lumbar puncture until a CT scan has been done, *but start antibacterial chemotherapy anyway* if the suspicion of meningitis is high and/or the patient is deteriorating (see 4 [d]).

**Procedure**: Turn the patient to his or her left side, hips maximally flexed, head and thoracic spine moderately flexed. The lumbar area is swabbed with iodine and draped with green towels. Wear gloves and maintain a sterile technique. The anterior superior iliac spine is vertically above the L3–4 interspace. This, L2–3, or L4–5 can be used—the spinal cord ends at L1–2. The chosen site is infiltrated with 1 per cent lignocaine and a minute or two is allowed for this to work. The spinal needle (size 18–20) is then advanced; a slightly cranial direction may be best, and the needle should be perpendicular to the actual plane of the back, i.e., not necessarily horizontal. There is a palpable 'give' as the interspinous ligament is crossed, then a second at the ligamentum flavum. Withdraw the stylet and CSF should drip out. If no fluid is seen, simple rotation of the needle may produce results. Otherwise withdraw and start again, possibly in another space.

Check the pressure of the CSF, remembering that the fluid in the manometer can form the first specimen. Five to ten millilitres in total are collected and sent for microscopy (including Gram and Ziehl–Nielsen stains), protein, glucose and culture. **Results**: (Table 2.6). The CSF pressure may be elevated in all types of meningitis. In *bacterial meningitis*, identifiable organisms are usually seen on Gram stain, but may be absent in, for example, cases treated with antibacterials before admission. In these circumstances (if available), countercurrent immune electophoretic identification of specific bacterial antigens (i.e., meningococcus, pneumococcus and *Haemophilus influenzae*) in the CSF may allow rapid diagnosis. In *tuberculous meningitis*, acid-fast bacilli *may* be seen in the sediment. C-reactive protein levels in CSF can be useful in equivocal cases, being grossly elevated in bacterial meningitis and normal in viral disease.

(4) *Treatment* is with intravenous antibacterials, intrathecal administration no longer being recommended (apart for Gram-negative meningitis). It is continued for 10 to 14 days in the commoner forms of the disease.

(a) *Meningococcal meningitis*. Intravenous benzyl penicillin, 2.4 g 4-hourly, is given. Chloramphenicol, 1 g four times a day, is the alternative in penicillin allergy.

(b) *Pneumococcal meningitis*—may be secondary to otitis media, sinusitis or pneumonia and is more common in patients with sickle cell anaemia, a past splenectomy, alcoholism or lymphoreticular malignancy. Benzyl penicillin in the above doses is used, chloramphenicol is again the alternative.

(c) *H. influenzae* is uncommon in adults. Chloramphenicol (25 mg/kg four times a day in children) intravenously is used; ampicillin, 250 mg 4-hourly, may be added.

(d) *Pyogenic meningitis, unknown organism*. Benzyl penicillin plus chloramphenicol is usually recommended but the newer cephalosporins, such as cefotaxime, have been shown to be effective used alone. Cefotaxime plus ampicillin may be preferable in immune-compromised patients.

(e) *Listeria monocytogenes* is the fourth commonest cause of bacterial meningitis (usually elderly or immune-compromised patients). The CSF may be reported either as showing no organisms or 'diphtheroid' contaminants. Intravenous ampicillin, 1 g four times a day, is the drug of choice.

(f) *Gram-negative meningitis* is uncommon except in immune incompetence. Ampicillin plus cefotaxime (up to 12 g daily in six divided doses) are used. Piper-

**Table 2.6 Cerebrospinal fluid in meningitis**

| Cause | Appearance | Protein | Glucose | Cells/mm |
|---|---|---|---|---|
| Pyogenic | Cloudy | 1.5–5.0 g/l | Low (<40% blood glucose) | >1000, mostly neutrophils |
| TB | 'Cobweb' pattern on standing | 1–4 g/l | Low | 20–500, mostly lymphocytes |
| Viral | Clear | <1.5 g/l | Normal* | <1000, mostly lymphocytes |

* May be low in herpes zoster and mumps.

acillin or azlocillin with tobramycin or possibly intrathecal gentamicin are used for *Pseudomonas*.

(g) *Tuberculous meningitis*. Isoniazid (10 mg/kg once daily), rifampicin (10 mg/kg once daily, maximum 600 mg/day), pyrazinamide, 30 mg/kg/day, and ethambutol, 15 mg/kg/day orally (or via nasogastric tube), are used, with pyridoxine, 10 mg daily. Some advocate adding streptomycin (intramuscular, 0.5 g twice daily), some also steroids, particularly after the first two to three days of treatment.

(h) *Herpes simplex encephalitis*. Acyclovir, 800mg five times daily for 7 days, is effective and should be used whenever this is suspected, e.g., lymphocytic meningitis with focal signs and/or diminished consciousness. Brain biopsy is unnecessary.

## Subarachnoid haemorrhage

### Diagnosis

This is suggested by a story of extremely severe, often occipital headache of very sudden onset, with vomiting and variable depression of conscious level or syncope (occasionally deep coma). Neck stiffness is usually present. In the fundi, subhyaloid haemorrhages may be seen and confirm the diagnosis. (Changes of hypertension should also be noted.) Focal neurological signs may be detected as may an intracranial bruit. A high fever should arouse suspicion of meningitis rather than subarachnoid haemorrhage.

### Investigation

The diagnosis may be confirmed by lumbar puncture, which is vital not only as a means of urgently excluding meningitis, but also because normal CSF will properly intensify the search for other diagnoses (metabolic disturbance, drug poisoning, etc.) in the confused or comatose patient. However *if there are focal neurological signs, coma or any evidence of raised intracranial pressure, an urgent CT scan should be done before (or more often instead of) lumbar puncture*. (If there is serious suspicion of infection, antibacterials for meningitis should be started without awaiting the result.)

Spinal fluid in subarachnoid haemorrhage is blood-stained from six to eight hours onwards and xanthochromia may be seen in the supernatant. Blood may also be seen in the traumatic lumbar puncture, in which case the staining is in streaks rather than uniform, red cell counts in sequential CSF specimens show a serial decline, and xanthochromia is absent.

### Management

(1) 'Standard' nursing care of the unconscious patient is instituted if necessary. This includes clearing and protection of the airway, nursing in a semiprone position with frequent turning, neurological nursing observations and care of the 'pressure areas' and sphincters. Urethral catheterization may be necessary, though in men condom drainage is preferable. Fluid balance is carefully controlled. Nasogastric fluids and feeding may be needed—if the cough and gag reflexes are absent the tube should be inserted under direct vision using a laryngoscope (or a drip is needed).

(2) The electrolytes and glucose are monitored and controlled.

(3) Fits are treated, as described elsewhere.

(4) Headaches are treated with mild analgesics, avoiding opiates if possible.

(5) Subcutaneous low-dose heparin is commenced.

(6) *Hypertension* usually settles with bed rest. If the blood pressure remains grossly elevated (e.g., diastolic >120 mmHg) after 6 to 12 hours, oral treatment is commenced (e.g., nifedipine). In the unconscious patient, intravenous nitroprusside is used because of its very short half-life and the consequent sensitivity of control it affords, with frequent recording of BP and aiming only for a modest and slow reduction. Remember that if accompanied by a low pulse rate, the hypertension may indicate raised intracranial pressure (see below) rather than a cardiovascular problem.

(7) Contact the regional neurosurgical centre. Most are keen to investigate (angiography) patients with little neurological disturbance and a normal conscious level—this group is likely to benefit from surgery to prevent rebleeds.

(8) Current evidence suggests antifibrinolytic agents offer no overall advantage, any

reduction in rebleeding being offset by an increase in the occurrence of ischaemia.

(9) Nimodipine 60 mg 4-hourly is, however, thought to help prevent ischaemic neurological complications.

(10) Deterioration after an early period of stability may have a number of causes:

(a) *Cerebral ischaemia*—probably caused by arterial spasm, this causes depression of conscious level with the development of focal signs and no fresh CSF blood. A CT scan may show an area of infarction. There is some evidence that manipulating the central venous pressure to a level at or slightly higher than the normal upper limit by infusing fluids is beneficial if undertaken early; nimodipine 1 mg/h i/v for 2h then 2 mg/h for 5 days (less if <70 kg) may help.

(b) *Rebleeding*. A repeat lumbar puncture may show fresh blood. Acute surgical intervention is too hazardous and conservative management is advised.

(c) *Acute hydrocephalus*—signs of increased intracranial pressure may be present, including increasing headache, papilloedema, and bradycardia with hypertension; new focal neurological signs may appear, and the patient may become drowsy. The diagnosis is confirmed by CT scanning. If the deterioration is particularly acute, give intravenous mannitol, 20 per cent (1–2 g/kg over 20 min), which may help temporarily, and contact the neurosurgeons as a shunt may be needed.

## Stroke

This is due to infarction or haemorrhage and causes an acute neurological defect, with or without impairment of consciousness. A number of clinical pictures are possible depending on the arterial territory affected (Table 2.7). If the neurological defect resolves completely within 24 h, the diagnosis becomes one of transient ischaemic attack, the implication being that a now dispersed embolus was responsible.

### *Diagnosis*

A large number of other causes of acute neurological deficits, ranging from the unlikely to the very

**Table 2.7  The commoner clinical pictures of stroke**

| Artery/territory | Clinical features |
| --- | --- |
| Middle cerebral artery | Contralateral hemiplegia and hemianaesthesia (mostly face and arm); dysphasia if dominant hemisphere affected |
| Anterior cerebral artery | Contralateral weakness and anaesthesia, mostly leg |
| Posterior cerebral artery | Contralateral homonymous hemianopia |
| Posterior inferior cerebellar artery | Ipsilateral: Horner's syndrome, cerebellar ataxia, Vth nerve sensory loss, palatal and pharyngeal weakness, diminished gag reflex<br>Contralateral pain and temperature impairment in the limbs<br>Vomiting, hiccough and vertigo |
| Central pontine stroke (basilar artery) | Coma and/or quadriplegia, pinpoint pupils, depression (or grossly disturbed pattern) of respiration<br>*or*<br>'Locked in' syndrome—consciousness and sensory pathways preserved, no voluntary movement except eyes (occasionally limited to vertical movement only) |
| Cerebellar haemorrhage | Rapid onset of headache, nausea, vomiting and impaired consciousness; cerebellar signs minimal or absent |

rare, must be excluded (Table 2.8). This process of exclusion must be particularly active in the younger patient and in those with an atypical history.

If the diagnosis does appear to be a stroke, then evidence of predisposing factors must be sought, for example, sources of emboli (past myocardial infarction, arrhythmias, valvular disease, cardiomyopathy, arterial myxoma, endocarditis, carotid artery stenosis), hypertension, diabetes, use of the oral contraceptive pill, polycythaemia (and other causes of hyperviscosity) and, in the case of suspected cerebral haemorrhage, coagulation disorders. It is therefore obvious that a complete and thorough history (if necessary from the family and general practitioner) and examination (always including fundoscopy and auriscopy) are mandatory.

**Table 2.8 Differential diagnosis of 'cerebrovascular accident'**

Subdural haematoma (particularly suggested by unequal pupils, variable depression of conscious level and progressive neurological signs)
Extradural haematoma
Cerebral abscess
Cerebral tumour
Epilepsy (postictal or Todd's paresis)
Meningitis (particularly TB, herpes meningo-encephalitis)
Vasculitis (e.g., SLE, polyarteritis, temporal arteritis, syphilis)
Diabetes (hypoglycaemia)
Migraine (e.g., migrainous hemiplegia)
Demyelination (particularly suspected brainstem strokes)

The *investigations* can largely be predicted from the above, and include a blood count and ESR, serum glucose, urea and electrolytes, syphilis serology, chest X-ray and ECG. Skull X-ray and echocardiography may be helpful. The need for a CT scan is hard to define but a history that is atypical (e.g., a slowly progressive disability) or includes severe headaches or trauma, the presence of papilloedema or fever, or the suspicion of malignancy, are reasonable indications. If a source of possible emboli is identified, CT scanning is useful to confirm that the stroke is not haemorrhagic, so permitting possible anticoagulation. Similarly, patients suffering a stroke whilst on anticoagulants need a scan to help decide whether this treatment should be stopped. CSF examination (if thought necessary) in these circumstances should never precede a CT scan.

*Management*

Steps (1) to (6) of the management of subarachnoid haemorrhage (above) (itself, of course, a form of stroke) are followed. Remember simple rules such as always approaching the patient from his or her 'good' side.

(7) Full doses of heparin may be indicated in those patients with a source of non-septic emboli, after a CT scan has excluded haemorrhage (or tumour, etc.). Some authorities prefer just using warfarin, yet others withhold all anticoagulants for several days for fear of precipitating haemorrhage into the infarct. There is no consensus.

(8) A wide variety of manoeuvres aimed at reduc-

ing oedema or improving perfusion of the ischaemic area has been proposed, including barbiturates, low molecular-weight dextran, vasodilators, steroids, anaesthesia and hypothermia, but none has proved useful. Recent evidence suggests that glycerol may be of value.

**Acute paraparesis**

*Diagnosis*

Acute paraparesis with a sensory level and (possibly) localized spinal pain may have a variety of causes including transverse myelitis, spinal artery occlusion, or compression from abscess, tumour, vertebral body collapse, or prolapsed disc. If compression is responsible, only urgent relief may prevent permanent neurological damage.

As well as assessing the level of neurological disturbance from the distribution of the motor and sensory impairment, remember also to look for sphincter disturbance and for evidence elsewhere of any neoplastic, neurological, vascular or infective disease. Investigations are directed towards looking for malignancy, together with plain radiography of the spine, looking for vertebral collapse, erosion, metastatic deposits and paravertebral masses. The nearest neurosurgical centre should be contacted and *immediate full length myelography* (preferably accompanied by spinal CT scanning) must be arranged. In suspected or proven compression, intravenous dexamethasone, 10 mg four times a day, may be helpful pending immediate decompressive surgery. In malignant disease, radiotherapy is indicated.

**Acute inflammatory polyneuropathy (Guillain–Barré syndrome)**

*Diagnosis*

The classical story is of weakness, often with paraesthesia, starting in the legs and spreading proximally over a course of days to weeks. There is commonly a history of a (usually) mild, self-limiting illness one to two weeks earlier. The neuropathy may involve any of the cranial nerves and the respiratory muscles may also be affected. The tendon jerks are absent and sensory signs may be present. A probable variant, the Miller–Fisher syndrome, comprises cerebellar ataxia, areflexia and external ophthalmoplegia. The CSF has a high protein content (occasionally normal early on) with normal cell counts. The differential diagnosis may include acute myelitis, lyme disease, diphtheria and other causes of neuropathy (toxins, connective tissue disorders, porphyria, etc.).

## Management

Most patients recover spontaneously and completely over a period of weeks to months. The assessment of any specific treatment is therefore difficult but it is generally now considered that steroids are not useful while plasma exchange may well be. Management is largely supportive but if necessary the utmost vigour in treating complications is completely justified by the potential for recovery. Possible causes of avoidable death include:

(1) *Respiratory insufficiency.* The vital capacity and arterial gases must frequently be monitored. Vital capacities around the 1 l mark indicate that ventilation may well be necessary. The decline in respiratory ability can sometimes be quite precipitous so that even in apparently uncompromised patients diligence is vital.
(2) *Bulbar paralysis.* Difficulty in swallowing and nasal regurgitation may necessitate endotracheal intubation, followed by tracheostomy to protect the airway. Nasogastric feeding is then required.
(3) *Autonomic instability.* Sudden tachycardias or hypertension may respond to β-blockers. Cardiovascular collapse can also occur; bradyarrhythmias may necessitate cardiac pacing.
(4) *Pulmonary embolism.* As with all bedridden patients, prophylactic, subcutaneous low-dose heparin should be administered.

If paralysis is prolonged, expert nursing care and physiotherapy are vital to prevent pressure sores, contractures, foot and wrist drop. Constant encouragement is needed to help maintain morale.

*Acknowledgements.*

My thanks to Dr M. J. Ward and Professor D. A. S. Compston for their kindness and help in reading and commenting on the manuscript.

## Further reading

### General

Kennedy H. J., ed. (1985). *Medical Emergencies.* Oxford: Blackwell Scientific.

*Med. Clin. N. Am.*, **70**, No. 4, July 1986 and No. 5, Sept. 1986 (Reviews a wide spectrum of medical emergencies)

### Specific

Anon. (1986). Central venous catheterisation. *Lancet*, **ii**, 669–70.
Anon. (1986). Herpes simplex encephalitis. *Lancet*, **ii**, 535–6.
Bayer A. J., Patny M. S. J., Newcombe R. (1987). Double-blind randomised trial of glycerol in acute stroke. *Lancet*, **i**, 405–7.
Bone C. R., Fisher C. J., Clemmer T. P., *et al.* (1984). A controlled clinical trial of high dose methyl prednisone in the treatment of severe sepsis and shock. *N. Engl. J. Med.*, **311**, 1137–43.
Cairns J. A. *et al.* (1985). Aspirin, sulfinpyrazone or both in unstable angina. *N. Engl. J. Med.*, **313**, 1369–75.
De Sanctis R. W., Doroghazi R. M., Austen W. G., Buckley M. J. (1987). Aortic dissection. *N. Engl. J. Med.*, **317**, 1060–6.
Ferner R., Barnett M., Hughes R. A. C. (1987). Management of Guillain-Barré syndrome. *Br. J. Hosp. Med.*, **38**, 525–30.
Fraser C. L., Arieff A. J., (1985). Hepatic encephalopathy. *N. Engl. J. Med.*, **313**, 865–73.
GISSI (1987). Long term effects of intravenous thrombolysis in acute myocardial infarction: final report on the GISSI study. *Lancet*, **ii**, 871–4.
Gorbach S. L. (1987). Bacterial diarrhoea and its treatment. *Lancet*, **ii**, 1378–83.
Heim C. R., Des Prez R. M (1986). Pulmonary embolus: A review. In *Year Book of Medicine*. Chicago: Year Book Medical Publishers, pp. 187–212.
Kertes P., Hunt D. (1984). Prophylaxis of primary ventricular fibrillation in acute myocardial infarction. *Br. Heart J.*, **52**, 241–7.
Pitt A. *et al.* (1980). Low dose heparim in acute myocardial infarction. *Am. Heart J.*, **99**, 574–8.
Ralston S. H., Aizaid A. A., Gardner M. D., Boyle I. T. (1986). Treatment of cancer-associated hypercalcaemia with combined aminohydoxypropylidine diphosphonate and calcitonin. *Br. Med. J.*, **292**, 1549–53.
Sandercock P., Molyneux A., Warlow C. (1985). Value of computerised tomography in patients with stroke. *Br. Med. J.*, 193–7.
Scot D. B. (1986). Endotracheal intubation: friend or foe? *Br. Med. J.*, **292**, 157–8.
Solomon R. A., Fink M. E. (1987). Current strategies for the management of aneurysmal subarachnoid haemorrhage. *Arch Neurol.*, **44**, 769–74.
Wirth M. A. *et al.* (1984). Intravenous amiodarone: UK clinical experience. *J. Int. Biomed-Information and Data*, **5**, 3–9.
Zuckerman G. (1984). A controlled trial of medical

therapy for upper gastrointestinal bleeding and prevention of rebleeding. *Am. J. Med.*, **76**, 361–6.

Randomised trial of intravenous atenolol among 16 027 cases of suspected acute myocardial infarction ISIS-1. *Lancet* (1986) **ii**, 257–66.

## SELF POISONING

Patients presenting after self poisoning form a significant proportion of most acute general medical intakes. Most are medically trivial and need only observation, but this and the low overall mortality cannot justify the cursory way in which medical staff at all levels often deal with these patients. The responsibility for ensuring that the minority of patients who are both seriously poisoned and potentially treatable do receive prompt and appropriate management usually rests with the house physician.

It is also important to remember that once the necessary medical treatment has been carried out, management remains incomplete without a psychosocial assessment of the patient's reason for self poisoning and risk of repeat. It is no longer recommended that all patients necessarily be reviewed by a psychiatrist before discharge. This increases the responsibility of physicians, particularly to predict future risks. Serious pointers are a history of depression, a middle-aged or elderly patient, and signs that suicide was really intended—a suicide note, an attempt to prevent discovery, or simply a subsequent admission of intent. Such patients do need expert psychiatric review.

### Assessment and resuscitation of the patient

A brief evaluation of vital functions involves examination of:
(1) *Respiratory function.* The first priority is to clear and then maintain the airway. If the cough reflex is suppressed, a cuffed endotracheal tube must be inserted to prevent aspiration. Subsequently respiratory function can be assessed. The Wright spirometer can be used as a screening method; patients with a minute volume less than 4 l need further investigation by blood gas analysis. If the $pCO_2$ exceeds 6.5 kPa ($\sim$50 mmHg) or if the $pO_2$ is below 10 kPa ($\sim$75 mmHg) and falling, then ventilation should be assisted. Localized crackles in the chest may suggest aspiration of vomitus or other fluids; generalized crackles may indicate pulmonary oedema. Radiography is then mandatory. Respiratory function should subsequently be assessed at regular intervals.
(2) *The level of consciousness.* The Glasgow Coma Scale (p. 87–8) should be used to assess, record, and follow the progress of the patient with depressed consciousness. The activity of the brainstem reflexes (pupillary, gag, corneal and oculocephalic) and tendon jerks should also be noted. General nursing care of the unconscious patient is instituted as necessary, including nursing in a semiprone ('coma') position and care of the airway, eyes and sphincters.
(3) *Cardiovascular function.* If the systolic blood pressure is below 90 mmHg in patients over the age of 50 years, or below 80 mmHg in younger patients, action is needed. The traditional (and often neglected) expedient of simply raising the foot of the bed may be all that is required, together with the correction of hypoxia. If not, then providing the jugular venous pressure is not markedly elevated, plasma expanders should be infused (e.g., plasma protein fraction or Haemaccel, 0.5–1 l). If the blood pressure is not readily restored, a central venous catheter should be inserted to ensure that there is no gross deficit in venous pressure, and subsequent fluid balance adjusted to maintain a central venous pressure of 0 to +5 cmH$_2$O (measured from the angle of Louis with the patient supine and horizontal). If the blood pressure remains low despite correction of hypovolaemia, then an infusion of dobutamine (2–20 µg/kg/min) together with dopamine (2.5 µg/kg/min) is necessary. A urinary catheter to monitor renal function is mandatory at this stage.

Other important aspects of immediate management include the correction of hypothermia (which may be missed unless a low-reading thermometer is used) and cardiac arrhythmias (if the latter have not responded to the correction of hypoxia and/or acidosis), and the control of convulsions by conventional methods.

### Urgent antidotes

It is important rapidly to exclude or treat two specific poisons where immediate antidotes are vital.

### Cyanide poisoning

The smell of bitter almonds is not necessarily present. The patient may be deeply unconscious and profoundly hypotensive with dilated pupils. If the diagnosis is certain, give dicobalt edetate, 600 mg intravenously over one minute, followed by a further 300 mg if there is no response after another minute. Oxygen should be administered. Dicobalt edetate can cause hypotension and vomiting and so should not be used indiscriminately. If it is not available, sodium nitrite (10 ml of a 3 per cent solution intravenously over 2–4 min) followed by sodium thiosulphate (25 ml of 50 per cent solution over 10 min) is used.

### Opiate poisoning

This causes pinpoint pupils, depression of respiration and conscious level and hypothermia. Rapid and effective reversal is achieved with intravenous naloxone, 0.8 to 1.2 mg repeated at 2-minute intervals if needed, or given as a continuous infusion at a rate of up to 5 mg/h, often for prolonged periods (especially with long-acting opiates such as methadone). The dramatic success of naloxone treatment can often obscure the need in these patients *to seek and treat paracetamol or aspirin poisoning*, many widely prescribed analgesics containing mixtures of opiates and these drugs.

### Diagnosis

This is usually volunteered by the patient, but anyone of serious suicidal intent may attempt deception, so it is still necessary to attempt to substantiate the story and exclude additional poisons. Third-party evidence may be obtained from attending relatives, ambulance staff or the police.

On examination, attention is directed to the smell of the patient's breath (alcohol, organic solvents, cyanide), the presence of blisters (most commonly occurring between two opposed skin surfaces in barbiturate poisoning), burns around the mouth (corrosives, including paraquat) and needlemarks (indicating 'recreational' drug abuse—remember to mark all specimens with 'BIOHAZARD' labels and take the usual precautions when in contact with the patient until he or she is proven to have negative serology for both hepatitis B and HIV). In single-agent poisoning the diagnosis may be aided by the pattern of physical signs (Table 2.9).

Blood or urine should be sent for paracetamol and salicylate identification in *all* cases. Both poisons are commonly taken, potentially fatal and usually treatable. This is particularly important in poisoning with mild analgesic–opiate combinations, and in the (sleeping) benzodiazepine patient, where the temptation is simply to observe overnight. The only other poisons where urgent serum levels may sometimes justifiably be requested (i.e., have therapeutic and/or prognostic implication) are digoxin, ethanol, ethylene glycol, iron, lithium, methanol, paraquat and theophylline. (Do not use lithium heparin bottles for lithium levels!) Not all of these poisons always need measuring (ethanol rarely). Paraquat is easily screened for by a simple urine test. Samples of urine and gastric aspirate or vomitus should be retained, as should a further sample of blood for any later analysis that might prove necessary.

In cases where the trade name of the ingested substance is known, but not its contents, particularly household, agricultural or industrial substances, help can be sought from any of the regional Poisons Information Services (see list). Alternatively, the manufacturer can be contacted by telephone and will often be able to identify toxic elements and advise on management and complications. When tablets arrive with the patient, 'Pill Charts' kept in the Accident and Emergency Department may be useful. Laboratory analysis of the pills can be used as a last resort, though this facility is very rarely available locally or on an emergency basis, nor is it very often required.

*Poisons centres (phone numbers)*

| | |
|---|---|
| Belfast | 0232 240503 |
| Birmingham | 021 554 3801 |
| Cardiff | 0222 709901 |
| Dublin | 0001 379964/6 |
| Edinburgh | 031 229 2477 |
| Leeds | 0532 432799 |
| London | 071 955 5095 |

### Elimination of poison from the body

### Emptying the stomach

Either lavage or induced emesis (with syrup of ipecacuanha, 30 ml in adults, 15 ml in children, followed by 200 ml water) should be carried out in all but the most trivial of cases presenting within

**Table 2.9 Some of the features of single-agent poisoning**

| | Salicylates | Neuroleptics | Tricyclic antidepressants | Benzodiazepines | Barbiturates | Opiates | LSD | Volatile solvents | 'Magic' mushrooms | Amphetamines | Organo-phosphorus compounds |
|---|---|---|---|---|---|---|---|---|---|---|---|
| Temperature | N* to ↑ | → | N, ↑ or → | N | → | → | N – ↑ | N | N | N to ↑ | N |
| Skin | Sweaty | Cold, dry | Warm, dry | N | Cold, dry | Cold, moist | Cold, moist | N | Clammy | N to clammy | Sweaty |
| Mouth | N | Dry | Dry | N | — | Dry | N | — | Dry | — | Salivation |
| Conscious level | N or confused | Impaired—coma | N, confused or coma | Drowsy—coma | Coma | Coma | Confusion | Confusion | Confusion | Confusion | N to coma |
| Convulsions | 0 to + | Lower threshold | ++ | 0 | 0 | 0 to ++ | ↓ + ↑ | + | + | 0 to +++ | ++ |
| Motor activity | Restless | Extrapyramidal movements Restlessness | Ataxia | → | → | → | → or ↑ | N to ↑ | N to ↑ | ↑ | Ataxia Twitching Weakness |
| Pupils | N | Constricted Sluggish reaction | Dilated | N | N to small | Pinpoint | Dilated | Dilated | Dilated | Dilated, sluggish or absent reflex | Pinpoint |
| Plantar reflexes | → | → | → or ↑ | N to absent | ↑ or → | → | → | N to absent | → | ↓ or ↑ | N |
| Tendon jerks | N | N | N or ↑ | → to absent | → or N | N or → | N or ↑ | → to absent | ↑ | ↑ | N |
| Respiration | ↑ rate | N to → rate | ↑ rate | → | ↓ rate; respiratory failure | ↓ rate; respiratory failure | N | → to absent; ↑ rate | Occasional wheezing | ↑ rate | Wheezing; respiratory failure |
| Pulmonary oedema | Rare | 0 | ++ | 0 | Rare | +++ | 0 | 0 | 0 | 0 to + | +++ |
| Heart rate | N to → | N, ↑ or → N to → | ↑ | N | N to → | → or ↑ N to → | N to ↑ | N to ↑ | ↑ | N to ↑ | → to ↑ |
| Blood pressure | N to → | N to → | ↓, N or ↑ | N to → | → | N to → | N to ↑ | → | →← N | N to + | +++ |
| ECG changes | 0 | 0 to +++ | +++ | 0 | 0 to + | 0 to + | + | ++ | | | Arrhythmias Prolonged QT |

\* N, normal.

Adapted and modified from the *British Journal of Hospital Medicine* (1978) (with kind permission from the editor).

four hours *except* those of petroleum distillate or corrosive ingestion, where such procedures are dangerous. In poisoning with salicylates, oral opiates, antispasmodics, tricyclic antidepressants or sustained-release theophylline preparations, stomach emptying may help up to 12 h after ingestion (possibly 24 or even 48 h for salicylates). If the patient is unconscious, a cuffed endotracheal tube must be inserted before lavage to prevent pulmonary aspiration. Emesis is preferable to lavage in children.

### Activated charcoal

This has two distinct though related roles. Given early (ideally within an hour) and in a dose of approximately 10 times the suspected dose of drug (e.g., up to 50–100 g in water), it will bind to and significantly reduce the absorption of most drugs, including aspirin, paracetamol, theophylline, tricyclic antidepressants and digoxin. It should therefore be given routinely after lavage or ipecacuanha. (Some authorities advocate its use instead of emesis or lavage.)

There is also good evidence that if given later in repeated doses it will accelerate clearance of the drug. This may be by interrupting the enterohepatic cycle, or possibly by 'gastrointestinal dialysis', whereby the charcoal binds within the gut lumen that amount of drug which has diffused across the gut wall from the blood. As long as the activated charcoal is replaced by further doses, continued clearance occurs. Repeated doses (50 g 4-hourly) should be given orally or by nasogastric tube in poisoning with aspirin, theophylline (though persistent vomiting may limit its value here), barbiturates, digoxin, carbamazepine and phenytoin, bearing in mind that this augments rather than replaces other established therapeutic manoeuvres.

### 'Forced' diuresis

This is most commonly used in the management of salicylate poisoning, for which complicated regimens of 'forced alkaline diuresis' continue to be recommended. Their apparent success may be due in good part simply to rehydration. The administration of excess fluid is fraught with dangers and these regimens should no longer be encouraged. It is more reasonable to (a) correct dehydration (a central venous pressure line should be inserted and the pressure maintained at the upper limit of normal), and (b) correct any metabolic acidosis and then maintain a urine pH >7.5 (preferably closer to 8.5) using 1.4 per cent sodium bicarbonate infused as necessary. Urinary catheterization is necessary to allow urine pH monitoring. Urine alkalinization is also useful for phenobarbitone poisoning. Acidification of urine (to pH <7.0, achieved by infusing either ammonium chloride, 1.5 g in 500 ml of 5 per cent dextrose, or lysine hydrochloride, 10 g in 500 ml dextrose, both over 30 min) may be of value in amphetamine poisoning.

In all cases, strict fluid balance charts should be kept and the central venous pressure regularly checked. The serum electrolytes should be monitored frequently (2-hourly) and potassium imbalance corrected promptly. No attempt should be made to maintain a high–normal central venous pressure in patients with impaired renal or cardiac function.

Other methods of active elimination include *peritoneal dialysis*, useful in lithium, ethylene glycol, methanol and ethanol poisoning and in those cases of salicylate poisoning where alkalinization of urine is thought inappropriate (e.g., patients with renal failure). *Haemodialysis* is probably more appropriate in the latter situation and is generally more effective than peritoneal dialysis. *Haemoperfusion* involves passing blood through columns of either resin or activated charcoal, which adsorb the poison. Transfer to a unit with this facility should be considered in severe cases of poisoning with barbiturates, meprobamate or theophylline.

### Specific poisons

#### Anticoagulants (e.g., warfarin, phenindione)

Patients with a high INR (International Normalized Ratio) and haemorrhage should be given 5 to 10 mg phytomenadione, intravenously and slowly, and fresh frozen plasma. Major bleeding necessitates intravenous vitamin K together with infusion of vitamin K-dependent clotting factor concentrates (II, IX, X). Oral cholestyramine speeds the removal of warfarin.

#### Antidepressants

*Tricyclic antidepressant poisoning* (e.g., amitryptyline, nortryptyline) causes anticholinergic effects (dry mouth, blurred vision, urinary retention) together with fits, coma (which may resemble 'brainstem death'), and cardiac arrhythmias. Serious poisoning is suggested by any of the last three features, by prolongation of the QRS complex ($>0.11$ s), arterial acidosis, or by a dose of over 1 g. Management is essentially with lavage followed by a single dose of activated charcoal and, importantly, ECG monitoring and correction of any acidosis, hypoxia or potassium imbalance. Dialysis is ineffective, and haemoperfusion is suggested only by a few authorities. Physostigmine is no longer recommended and arrhythmias are best managed conventionally.

*Monoamine oxidase inhibitor overdose* (e.g., phenelzine, tranylcypromine) is less common. If shock is present, sympathomimetic support is not used; hydrocortisone may be tried. Alternatively, hypertensive crisis may occur, which should be treated with phentolamine (5–60 mg intravenously over 20 min) or phenoxybenzamine (1 mg/kg in 250 ml of 5 per cent dextrose over 60 min). Hyperthermia may respond to chlorpromazine (25–50 mg intramuscularly).

### Barbiturates (e.g., phenobarbitone)

This form of poisoning is now uncommon. Other than 'routine' supportive management, urine alkalinization may help with serious poisoning with phenobarbitone and barbitone. Haemoperfusion is indicated for very severe poisoning (dense coma, respiratory or circulatory failure).

### Benzodiazepines (e.g., diazepam, nitrazepam, etc.)

Poisoning is extremely common but even massive doses require only supportive management. Mechanical ventilation is rarely needed.

### β-adrenergic blockers (e.g., propranolol, atenolol, etc.)

These (predictably) may cause severe bradycardia, hypotension and occasionally coma. Atropine, 0.6 mg intravenously, should be given before lavage to prevent vasovagal collapse. Glucagon, 5 to 10 mg intravenously then 3 mg/h as an infusion, is often effective in severe hypotension; prenalterol, 2.5 to 15 mg intravenously (slowly) is an alternative. An isoprenaline infusion may be used if prenalterol is not available—occasionally very large doses are necessary. Temporary cardiac

pacing may be needed, and bronchospasm may necessitate nebulized salbutamol.

### Bleach, other household products and corrosives

Household bleaches contain around 5 per cent sodium hypochlorite, toxic as a corrosive and through inhalation of chlorine gas liberated in the stomach. The foul taste usually prevents severe poisoning. Cautious lavage is not contraindicated, but the instillation of sodium thiosulphate is no longer considered helpful. Milk or 'milk of magnesia' have been used.

*Disinfectants* may contain isopropanol, which is toxic. *Detergents* rarely lead to problems, but *drain cleaners* can be serious because of their corrosive effects. The management of *strong alkali* or *acid* poisoning is similar. The risk of perforation contraindicates lavage or emesis. Large volumes of milk or water should be given. Cautious endoscopy should be performed within 24 h. Hydrocortisone, intravenous 200 mg 6-hourly, may reduce the chances of oesophageal stricture.

### Carbon monoxide

The hypoxia does not cause cyanosis (carboxyhaemoglobin maintains in the skin and mucosae a deceptive pink colour) but does cause tachyarrhythmias, myocardial ischaemia, pulmonary oedema, hyperpyrexia, confusion and a spectrum of neurological deficits, including hemi- and monoplegia, cerebellar signs, parkinsonism, akinetic mutism and coma. Pure oxygen and 20 per cent mannitol (1–1.5 g/kg over 15 min) and dexamethasone (4 mg 8-hourly, intravenous) to reduce cerebral oedema are indicated. Hyperbaric oxygen, the preferred treatment, is almost never available in the critical first half-hour or so of poisoning; but may still be useful even after several hours.

### Cyanide

See above ('Urgent antidotes').

### Digoxin

Acute overdose is uncommon but can be fatal. The normal therapeutic range is 1 to 2 ng/ml. Toxic effects include visual disturbance, vomiting, diarrhoea, hyper- or hypokalaemia, and almost any cardiac arrhythmia. Supportive therapy with lavage and immediate and repeated doses of activated charcoal is instituted. Haemoperfusion may be effective in digitoxin poisoning, but neither dialysis nor haemoperfusion is useful in digoxin poisoning. Serum potassium levels should be kept within the normal range. Magnesium sulphate is said to counter the toxic effects of digoxin (2 ml of 50 per cent solution in 50 ml saline over one hour intravenously).

Bradyarrhythmias (including sinus arrest) usually respond to intravenous atropine (0.6–2.4 mg); if not a temporary pacemaker is necessary. Supraventricular arrhythmias usually respond to β-blockade, ventricular arrhythmias to lignocaine (50–100 mg intravenously, followed by an infusion). Intravenous amiodarone may be more effective. *DC cardioversion may be dangerous.*

Digoxin-specific antibody fragments (e.g., Digibind) are now commercially available and appear to be of very great value in life-threatening cases.

### Ethanol

This is common both alone and with tablets, causing inebriation followed by ataxia, blurred vision, stupor, coma, hyporeflexia, respiratory depression, vasodilation contributing to hypothermia and hypotension, and hypoglycaemia. It may cause lactic acidosis and alcoholic ketoacidosis. Blood levels of 150 mg/100 ml indicate moderate poisoning and 300 mg/100 ml severe, but clinical assessment is of paramount importance because of the variability due to tolerance. Treatment is supportive, including the correction of hypoglycaemia. In life-threatening poisoning (concentrations usually over 500 mg/100 ml), especially if complicated by metabolic acidosis, haemodialysis should be considered. Alcoholic ketoacidosis responds to glucose with fluid replacement, and insulin is not usually required.

### Ethylene glycol

The fatal dose of this antifreeze agent is around 100 g. Clinical features resemble those of ethanol poisoning, but later include vomiting and haematemesis, coma, fits, papilloedema and optic atrophy, hypotension, hypocalcaemia, bradycardia, pulmonary oedema and acute tubular necrosis. Supportive treatment includes the correction of acidosis and hypocalcaemia. Ethanol may be effective (competing for alcohol dehydrogenase

delays conversion of ethylene glycol to toxic metabolites) and is given in a dose of 1 g/kg in 5 per cent dextrose orally, then as an intravenous infusion at around 10 g/h, maintaining serum ethanol levels of 100 mg/100 ml. Pyridoxine (100 mg intravenously) and thiamine (100 mg intravenously) may also help prevent toxic metabolite production. Severely symptomatic patients and those with plasma levels over 500 mg/l should be treated with peritoneal or haemodialysis.

### Iron

Clinical features include epigastric pain, vomiting and haematemesis, then after an apparent recovery of up to 24 h, acute encephalopathy and circulatory collapse. Acute hepatic failure may occur up to three days later. Levels over 90 μmol/l at four hours indicate severe poisoning, particularly in children. Treatment should be commenced urgently. Desferrioxamine chelates iron and should be given immediately, 2 g in 10 ml of sterile water intramuscularly (for an adult). After gastric lavage using a solution of 2 g desferrioxamine in 1 l warm water, 5 to 10 g in 50 ml of water is left in the stomach. An intravenous desferrioxamine infusion is commenced at a rate of 15 mg/kg/h, giving up to 80 mg/kg/day. The haemoglobin and serum iron should be monitored and the infusion discontinued when the latter falls below 90 μmol/l. If oliguria or anuria occur, intravenous desferrioxamine becomes unsafe and dialysis is required.

### Lithium

Poisoning may cause polydipsia, polyuria, vomiting, diarrhoea, drowsiness, tremor and muscular hypotonia. Fits, electrolyte imbalance, bradyarrhythmias and shock are occasionally seen. Toxicity may occur at levels over 1.5 mmol/l (therapeutic range: 0.7–1.3 mmol/l) and is serious if over 3.5 mmol/l, although clinical features may correlate poorly with blood levels. Supportive therapy includes lavage and close monitoring of electro¹/te levels. A diuresis should be encouraged and alkalinization of urine is advised by some authorities. Caution should be exercised as lithium can lead to resistance to antidiuretic hormone, resulting in hyperosmolality, which may be dangerously exacerbated by sodium infusion (chlorthiazide treatment may be helpful). In severe cases (including those with hyperosmolality), dialysis is necessary.

## Metals

A variety of antidotes is available. *Lead* poisoning can cause severe abdominal colic, vomiting, diarrhoea, fits, coma, encephalopathy and circulatory, renal and liver failure. Supportive treatment includes lavage, mannitol for encephalopathy and dialysis for renal failure. Sodium calcium edetate, 25 to 35 mg/kg intravenously over an hour, should be given twice daily for five days. The addition of intramuscular dimercaprol, 3 mg/kg 4-hourly for 48 h may help, while oral penicillamine, 20 to 40 mg/kg/day after the acute phase helps prevent chronic toxicity. Dimercaprol is also effective in poisoning with *arsenic*, *gold* and *mercury*, penicillamine in *mercury*, *copper*, and *zinc* poisoning. *Radioactive plutonium*, *thorium*, *uranium* and *yttrium* are chelated by sodium calcium edetate, though one hopes the need might not too frequently arise.

## Methanol

Doses over 30 g can be fatal. Features include abdominal pain and vomiting, papillitis (progressing to optic atrophy and permanent blindness), ataxia, confusion, and metabolic acidosis, correction of which is an important part of supportive management. Ethanol (given as for 'Ethylene glycol' above) inhibits metabolism to formic acid and formate. Serious poisoning, indicated by levels over 50 mg/100 ml, mental, visual or fundoscopic changes, or severe metabolic acidosis, warrants haemodialysis—peritoneal dialysis is less effective. Folinic acid, 30 mg intravenous 6-hourly, may help protect against ocular toxicity.

## Mushrooms

'Magic mushrooms', *Psilocybe semilanceata*, contain the hallucinogen psylocybin, which produces euphoria, hallucinations (especially flashing coloured lights) and sympathomimetic effects including brisk tendon jerks, mydriasis, tachycardia, dry mouth and apprehension. Lavage is indicated. Convulsions rarely occur and require standard treatment, and sedation may be needed. Nearly all patients recover spontaneously and completely within 12 h.

Other species are less commonly encountered. Identification is paramount and standard texts should be consulted.

## Opiates

(E.g., morphine, dihydrocodeine, etc.)—see above ('Urgent antidotes'.)

## Organophosphorus compounds

These insecticides inhibit cholinesterase, causing both muscarinic effects (bronchospasm, sweating, hypersalivation) and nicotinic (muscular twitching, fasciculation and weakness, vomiting, colic and diarrhoea, blurred vision and miosis). Coma, fits, bradycardia, hypotension, pulmonary oedema and respiratory failure may also occur. Supportive management includes lavage followed by charcoal, removal of contaminated clothing and washing the skin. Plasma cholinesterase activity below 30 per cent indicates significant poisoning. Atropine is given, but only after correction of hypoxia as ventricular fibrillation may otherwise result; large doses (e.g., 50 mg in 24 h) may be needed. Pralidoxime (often only available from the nearest Poisons Centre), 30 mg/kg intravenously (at less than 500 mg/min) repeated 4-hourly in the first 24 h, specifically reactivates cholinesterase. Intravenous diazepam, 10 mg, helps sedate the patient, prevents fits and decreases muscle twitching.

## Paracetamol

This is common both alone and in analgesic combinations. In adults, doses over 10 g can cause serious toxicity. This results from a metabolite, inactivation of which is facilitated by the antidote. Features include nausea and vomiting then, after an apparent recovery of several days, tenderness over the liver and acute hepatic failure with encephalopathy. Hypoglycaemia, acute tubular necrosis and hypotension may occur.

Lavage should be performed and specific treatment immediately commenced if there is any suspicion of serious poisoning, avoiding the delay of waiting for plasma-level findings. This is because both acetyl cysteine and its cheaper, oral alternative methionine, less often used because of the possibility of vomiting preventing its absorption, are only effective in the first 8 to 10 h (though still *probably* worth giving up to 16 h after ingestion). The decision to continue treatment can later be taken according to the plasma levels (Fig. 2.4). The latter are not estimated before four hours after ingestion, when they reach their peak.

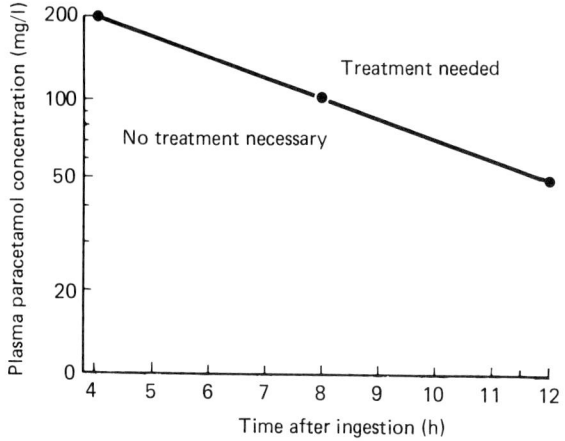

*Figure 2.4* Paracetamol poisoning: need for treatment.

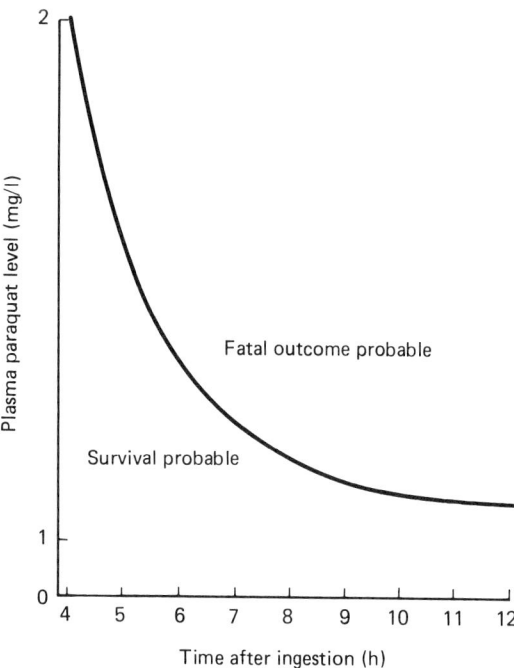

*Figure 2.5* Outcome of paraquat poisoning.

Acetyl cysteine is given as an intravenous infusion of 150 mg/kg in 200 ml of 5 per cent dextrose over 15 min, followed by 50 mg/kg in 500 ml of dextrose over 4 h, then 100 mg/kg in 1 l of dextrose over 16 h.

Hepatic failure is assessed by clinical features, dramatic elevation of aminotransferase levels, and a prolonged prothrombin time, and managed as described elsewhere (p. 29). Those livers that do recover usually do so completely.

### Paraquat

This herbicide may cause early pulmonary oedema, metabolic acidosis and cardiovascular collapse. Severely painful ulceration of the mouth is often seen. Later on (three to four days), renal failure may occur. In those yet surviving, pulmonary fibrosis with respiratory failure may cause death in three days to two weeks. Urine testing confirms the diagnosis, and plasma paraquat concentrations can be used to predict the outcome (Fig. 2.5). A dose of 2 to 3 g (e.g., 10–15 ml undiluted Gramoxone) is likely to be fatal. Gastric emptying is followed by instillation into the stomach of Fuller's earth or activated charcoal. Repeated doses of Fuller's earth and purgatives should be given 4-hourly. Copious irrigation of exposed mucosal surfaces may help prevent ulceration. Adequate hydration should be ensured. Haemodialysis and haemoperfusion both help lower paraquat levels but neither appears to affect prognosis. Cyclophosphamide may be considered.

### Petroleum products (e.g., paraffin)

Symptoms include apparent inebriation followed by nausea, vomiting and diarrhoea, blurred vision, coma and convulsions. If inhaled, chemical pneumonitis may occur. Emesis or lavage must be avoided, although in severe poisoning lavage after insertion of an endotracheal tube is worthwhile. Corticosteroids do not seem to prevent the development of pneumonitis if aspiration does occur.

### Salicylates

Features are summarized in Table 2.9 but also include deafness and tinnitus, dehydration, cardiac arrest, renal failure and the adult respiratory distress syndrome. Laboratory findings may include respiratory alkalosis (from the hyperventilation) or metabolic acidosis, hypo- or hyperglycaemia, hypokalaemia and a prolonged prothrombin time. General measures include lavage, even if presentation is delayed up to 24 h, instillation of activated charcoal in repeated doses, and close monitoring and correction of biochemical abnormalities (including vitamin K, 10 mg intravenously if necessary). Dehydration should also be corrected (preferably with the aid of central venous pressure measurements because of the risk of pulmonary and cerebral oedema) and the urine alkalinized (see 'Forced diuresis') if salicylate levels are over 3.1 mmol/l (approximately 50 mg/ 100 ml). In severe poisoning (levels over 50 mmol/l or 80 mg/100 ml), haemodialysis should be considered.

**Solvents** (e.g., glue, cleaning fluids, nail varnish remover, etc.)

Features resemble alcoholic intoxication, although hallucinations may also occur. Coma, convulsions and respiratory depression are uncommon. A rash around the mouth and nose, together with the characteristic odour, may be present. Treatment may include sedation or respiratory support. Hepatorenal damage and encephalopathy rarely occur.

**Xanthine bronchodilators** (e.g., theophylline, aminophylline, etc.)

These may cause vomiting and haematemesis, abdominal pain, supraventricular and ventricular tachycardias, restlessness, tremor, fits, coma and hypotension. Hypokalaemia is common. Measures include early and repeated doses of charcoal (if vomiting can be controlled), correction of hypokalaemia and acidosis, control of fits, and prophylactic ranitidine. Haemoperfusion is advised in severe poisoning.

*Acknowledgement.*

I am very grateful to Dr P. A. Routledge for his helpful comments, criticism and advice.

## Further reading

### *General*

Mathews H., Lawson A. A. H. (1979). *Treatment of Common Acute Poisonings*, 4th edn. Edinburgh: Churchill Livingstone.
Polson C. J., Green M. A., Lee M. R. (1983). *Clinical Toxicology*, 3rd edn. London: Pitman.
Proudfoot A. T. (1982). *Diagnosis and Management of Acute Poisoning*. Oxford: Basil Blackwell.

### *Specific*

Farmer R. (1986). Deliberate self-poisoning. *Br. J. Hosp. Med.*, **36**, 437–41.
Hanrahan J. P., Gordon M. A. (1984). Mushroom poisoning. *J.A.M.A.*, **251**, 1057–61.
Lewy J. (1982). Gastrointestinal clearance of drugs with charcoal. *N. Engl. J. Med.*, **307**, 676–8.
Litowitz T. L. (1986). Emesis versus lavage for poisoning victims. *Am. J. Emerg. Med.*, **4**, 294–5.
Pond S. M. (1984). Diuresis, dialysis and haemoperfusion: indications and benefits. *Emerg. Med. Clin. N. Am.*, **2**, 29–45.
Prescott L. F., Balali-Mood M., Critchley J. A. J. H. *et al.* (1982). Diuresis or urinary alkalinisation for salicylate poisoning? *Br. Med. J.*, **285**, 1383–6.
Proudfoot A. T. (1986). A star treatment of digoxin overdose. *Br. Med. J.*, **293**, 642–3.

# 3

# APPROACH TO THE PATIENT SUSPECTED OF HAVING AIDS

Anthony J. Pinching

## INTRODUCTION

Since their first recognition in 1981, the acquired immune deficiency syndrome (AIDS) and the range of clinical disorders caused by the human immunodeficiency virus (HIV) have presented many challenges to clinical medicine. First, HIV-related disorders have had to be included in virtually every list of differential diagnosis; secondly, in order to determine whether a patient is likely to have HIV infection, basic history taking has had to include more specific, though no less sensitive, enquiries about sexual and drug-taking behaviour than have been usual hitherto; thirdly, these disorders have re-emphasized the importance of maintaining a high standard of clinical technique for control of blood-borne viral infection, notably in the use and disposal of 'sharps'; finally, they have highlighted some of the most difficult aspects of clinical practice, including communication, confidentiality and consent.

Many of these themes are thoroughly discussed elsewhere and it is inappropriate to explore them in detail here. Nevertheless, it is vital for clinicians to acknowledge the complexity of the issues raised and to respond positively to the challenges, rather then denying or minimizing their importance. As with any other area of clinical medicine, good practice emerges from the application of sound knowledge, substantial practical experience and a willingness to learn. In this chapter, I will concentrate on issues relevant to the practical clinical management of HIV-related disease.

### The nature of HIV

HIV is an enveloped RNA virus that has an enzyme for reverse transcriptase, which allows a DNA copy of the genome to be made in infected cells. This copy can then be inserted into the host's DNA to act as a template for further viral replication—in other words, establishing latency. The principal AIDS virus is HIV-1, found in Central and East Africa, North and South America, Europe, South-East Asia and Australasia. However, a related but distinct virus, HIV-2, has recently been found in West Africa. It has similar biological properties but may be less rapidly pathogenic; it is not detected by most assays for HIV-1. HIV has a particular tropism for the CD4 (T4) molecule on cells of the immune system; it has cytopathic effects, direct or indirect, as well as causing changes in the function of cells in the immune and nervous systems. Although the main specific target is the CD4 (helper) lymphocyte, macrophages and other accessory cells can serve as a reservoir of virus, as infection appears less liable to lead to their elimination. Activation of latently infected cells appears to increase viral replication; this may be the way that intercurrent events (infection, pregnancy) act as cofactors for progression and infectivity.

### The origins of the HIV pandemic

While the origin of HIV is still uncertain, it seems likely that it represents the shift of a virus of non-human primates into a human population in recent decades, its subsequent adaptation to our species and the acquisition of uniquely human pathogenicity. Wherever it originated, it has spread rapidly in a manner that reflects its mode of transmission and the prevalent social and sexual anthropology of diverse (sub-)communities.

## HIV TRANSMISSION

HIV is transmitted sexually by either homosexual or heterosexual contact, through the inoculation of infected material into blood or tissues (especially by the use of contaminated 'works' by intravenous drug users and by transfusion of unscreened blood) and transplacentally from mother to fetus. The fact of these routes has been established through extensive epidemiological study and is covered in detail elsewhere; the possibility of casual transmission by other means has been investigated and found not to occur, or to occur with such rarity as to be undetectable. This is despite a pandemic of HIV infection that has emerged rapidly over the last 10 to 15 years and is already thought to affect several million people.

### Infection control

Studies on health care staff after needlestick accidents or exposure of broken skin or mucous membranes have shown that infection can occur by these routes, albeit rarely. HIV infection is thought to ensue after about 0.3 per cent of such incidents, from prospective study and identification of cases that may have arisen under similar circumstances. In most, the exposure was substantial and the circumstances unusual, standard practices for control of infection not having been followed. This low rate of infection contrasts with the incidence of 20 to 35 per cent for hepatitis B infection after inoculation through injury, suggesting that the necessary inoculum for HIV infection is much larger.

As would be expected from the epidemiology, the main objective in control of infection among health care workers is to avoid percutaneous inoculation of blood or other material from HIV-infected patients. In practice this means the avoidance of 'needlestick' injury and exposure of broken skin or mucous membranes to HIV-infected material. This can be achieved by applying simple, basic standards of care with all patients, regardless of HIV status. For example, the great majority of needlestick incidents would have been avoided if needles had not been re-sheathed and if all 'sharps' had been immediately disposed of in penetration-proof containers.

## HIV ANTIBODY AND ANTIGEN TESTING

As with other organisms, infection with HIV is followed by the development of an antibody response. These antibodies are usually detected by enzyme-linked immunosorbent assays, either anti-globulin or competitive, and should be confirmed by at least one other method, including Western blot. Newer assays use recombinant viral antigens and offer greater specificity. Antibodies are usually detectable from four weeks to four months after infection, but persist thereafter. With some assays, antibody titres may fall in late disease. Antibodies against core proteins of HIV (anti-*gag*) fall in those HIV-infected patients who subsequently go on to develop AIDS or the AIDS-related complex (ARC).

It is now possible to assay serum for HIV antigen. This may be detectable before the emergence of antibodies, usually for only a few days or weeks. If antigen persists or reappears in asymptomatic, HIV-infected individuals, it seems to indicate a greater likelihood of progression. It generally reappears in patients progressing to AIDS. It is likely that antigenaemia indicates a higher rate of viral replication, and hence more effects on cells of the immune and nervous systems, and also probably the level of 'infectiousness'. Antigen assays are important in studies of the natural history of AIDS and in the monitoring of antiviral treatment because they offer direct evidence of *in vivo* viral replication. This is in contrast to isolation of virus, which depends on detecting cells with latent viral genome and which cannot reliably determine the extent of viral replication.

### Use of HIV antibody testing

Because HIV infection is persistent and productive, leading to a state of lifelong infectiousness, antibody testing has offered a simple, technical means for identifying the vast majority of HIV-infected persons. This has been, for example, critical to safeguarding blood transfusion supplies, together with self-exclusion of high risk persons from the donor population. Outside this and analogous settings of voluntary donation, the use of HIV antibody testing has been controversial.

### Personal implications of testing and consent

Knowledge of one's HIV status has major psychological, social and practical implications that go far beyond those resulting from many other tests; testing for HIV antibody is not 'just another test', a view usually promulgated by those with the least clinical experience of HIV. The implications include the permanent threat of disease, the threat to social and sexual relationships, and the effects of discriminatory policies still adopted by some sectors of society, commerce and even medicine. While these problems may be minimized or averted by adequate counselling before and after the test(s), a person should have the opportunity to choose whether or not they are tested in the light of their particular circumstances. This is especially true if testing is being used for non-clinical purposes. Even where testing is thought helpful for clinical diagnosis, although there may be no legal obligation to inform and obtain consent before testing, experience has indicated that it is wise and good clinical practice to do so. The worst casualties are often those who consider themselves to be at low risk and are therefore least prepared.

### Limitations of testing

Is the test able to answer the question being addressed? The possibility of false negatives must be considered, especially those resulting from the delay between infection and the antibody response. False positives can largely be obviated by confirmatory testing and this must be done, especially where positivity is unexpected. Another consideration is whether the result uniquely enables change, for example in behaviour or clinical policy, or whether there are better and/or less harmful means of achieving the same end. This applies where testing may be proposed for control of infection and where it is generally possible to effect policy without an obligation for testing. It also applies where testing is being considered as a motivation for behavioural change, to reduce spread in the community. It should be determined whether knowledge of the result of the test can in itself and uniquely effect the necessary change.

Although HIV testing may sometimes clarify clinical diagnosis, this is surprisingly infrequent. It is most likely to be relevant to a clinical presentation if the patient is at low risk for HIV, because finding HIV antibodies in a person from a population at high risk (with high prevalence) does not necessarily signify a causal relationship. On the other hand, a negative test may be helpful where genuine doubt exists. If negative in the face of an

obvious clinical diagnosis of AIDS or other HIV-related disorder, it may need to be ignored.

### Counselling

It is inescapable that a person must be told the result of testing, not least because he or she may otherwise find out indirectly and without benefit of counselling. Counselling is essential because the result has so many implications to the individual and as a means of guiding them through the crisis that inevitably follows. It must be given or at least started at the same time as the result is divulged, and by the same person. This should be the person who initiated the test, who obtained consent and who counselled before it. It should continue as needed, if appropriate using specialist counsellors. Information given must not only include detail about what the result does and does not signify, but should also clarify what is going to be done with the information, who will and who will not be informed and by whom. It should be made clear that it is the duty of the patient to inform those whom he or she may have inadvertently put at risk. It is unwise and unreasonable (if consent for testing has been obtained) for health care professionals to have to shoulder responsibility for all the social consequences of people's behaviour, although they must be able to offer guidance and practical help.

### THE CLINICAL SPECTRUM OF HIV INFECTION

Clinical responses to HIV infection encompass the following:

(a) acute viral infection, sometimes with evidence of immune complex disease (acute HIV infection; Center for Disease Control classification—Group I);

(b) chronic persistent virus infection (asymptomatic infection, Group II; and persistent generalized lymphadenopathy [PGL; Group III]);

(c) chronic active viral infection with constitutional symptoms (ARC, Group IVA);

(d) mild or moderate immunodeficiency disease leading to opportunistic infections and/or tumours from the effects of HIV on cells of the immune system (ARC, Group $IVC_2$; or AIDS, Groups $IVC_1$ and D);

(e) chronic encephalopathy and/or neuropathy

from the effects of HIV on the cells of the nervous system (Group IVB);

(f) chronic active viral infection in other tissues, immune complex disease (e.g., lymphocytic pneumonitis, thrombocytopenic purpura—Group IVE).

Because HIV establishes latent and persistent productive infection in all those infected, it must be assumed that people in all these categories are potentially infectious to others. There is now evidence that risk of transmission is greater at two stages, the early viraemia before antibodies are formed and the later stages of chronic active infection, for example in patients with late ARC and AIDS.

## HIV-RELATED DISORDERS

### Acute retrovirus infection

Some weeks after exposure, 10 to 15 per cent of patients suffer a glandular fever-like illness with malaise, fever, lymphadenopathy, sometimes with rash, arthropathy and headaches, occasionally complicated by an acute encephalopathy. Some of these features may be due to immune complexes and some to direct effects of viral replication. Most cases resolve spontaneously. HIV antibodies are negative or equivocal at onset and become positive in convalescence.

### Asymptomatic HIV infection and persistent generalized lymphadenopathy

Whether or not they have an acute illness with seroconversion, all patients then pass through a phase lasting many months or several years when they are symptomless. Amongst these are people in whom infection is being contained and those in whom sufficient time has yet to elapse before pathogenicity is evident. In a proportion of symptomless persons, persistent, symmetrical enlargement of lymph nodes in all peripheral sites may be palpable, but is rarely gross. In the absence of constitutional symptoms or signs of minor opportunist infection, such as thrush or shingles, PGL appears to be relatively benign; its rate of progression to AIDS seems no greater than that of asymptomatic infection without lymphadenopathy. PGL due to HIV must be distinguished from lymphadenopathy due to other causes; lymph node biopsy is only rarely necessary in PGL, unless another diagnosis is strongly suspected. Where HIV infection is present, care must be taken to seek clues that may suggest infection, Kaposi's sarcoma or associated lymphoma such as asymmetrical enlargement, marked splenomegaly or hepatomegaly, haematological abnormalities and symptoms. In asymptomatic HIV infection and PGL, antigenaemia and absent anti-*gag* antibodies are adverse prognostic markers, as is constitutional a falling CD4 cell count.

### Thrombocytopenic purpura

Some otherwise symptomless patients may develop severe thrombocytopenia, which appears to be immune-complex mediated. Bleeding is rarely life-threatening and the condition may resolve spontaneously after months or years. Treatment with steroids and splenectomy, though temporarily resolving the haematological defect, may increase the risk of progression to AIDS. Transient elevation of platelets to cover bleeding episodes or surgery may be usefully achieved by intravenous gamma globulin. Zidovudine (AZT) has been shown to benefit such patients.

### AIDS-related complex

This term has been used to encompass a wide variety of disorders, sometimes including PGL, but with the increasing recognition of the latter's distinctive natural history, it is now restricted to patients with severe HIV infection having constitutional symptoms (unexplained fevers, marked weight loss, persistent diarrhoea—Group IVA) or with minor opportunistic infection (oral candidiasis, shingles, hairy oral leukoplakia, salmonellosis or tuberculosis—Group IVB). Lymphadenopathy, if present, is generally less than that found in PGL and patients progressing from PGL to ARC or to AIDS may notice a marked reduction in the size of the nodes.

ARC patients may be severely ill—for example, more so than most AIDS patients with Kaposi's sarcoma; many will progress to AIDS itself over a few months. Such patients usually require investigation to exclude other causes for their symptoms and, if HIV-infected, AIDS itself will need to be excluded—for example, oesophageal candidiasis, gastrointestinal opportunist infection and lymphoma.

## AIDS

### Pathogenesis

The immunodeficiency of AIDS is due largely to loss of CD4 T-helper cells, both numerically and functionally. Cell damage is by direct viral cytotoxicity, lysis or syncytium formation, or immune elimination by cytotoxic lymphocytes or antibody-dependent cytotoxicity; the functional defects may result from selective loss of cell subpopulations or latent retroviral infection. Associated defects in macrophage and natural killer cell function are largely due to reduced secretion of lymphokines by CD4 cells; polyclonal activation of B cells is promoted by HIV proteins.

### Characteristics of the immune deficiency

The biological defect is thus one of cell-mediated immunity, leading to increased susceptibility to infection by intracellular pathogens and other organisms normally eliminated by similar mechanisms; most of the organisms are ones that remain latent from prior infection and cause disease when immune defence becomes impaired. Because of the profound immune defect, many of the presenting symptoms, the signs and the chest radiographic features may be subtle and the rate of progression insidious. This is an important background to clinical assessment of AIDS patients. The dysgammaglobulinaemia may lead to an additional susceptibility to infection with capsulated bacteria, such as pneumococcus and haemophilus, and sometimes staphylococcus. It also makes serology of secondary infections unreliable for clinical diagnosis. Opportunistic tumours arise and are generally thought to be virally associated. Kaposi's sarcoma is commonest amongst the sexually active and, if it presents without infection, may have a relatively benign course, apparently indicating less severe immunodeficiency; lymphomas are also seen.

AIDS patients become ill during episodes of infection, many of which will respond to early treatment with appropriate antimicrobials. Between infections, they may be relatively well and able to return to normal life and work, especially during the early months or year following diagnosis. Patients with Kaposi's sarcoma affecting skin and lymph nodes, and those with limited mucosal disease, may feel quite well and have no systemic symptoms. The best index of the severity of immunodeficiency is the type of infection or tumour; immunological tests may be quite misleading in both directions. AIDS patients characteristically have low CD4-positive cell counts, absent delayed-type hypersensitivity skin reactions, reduced *in vitro* mitogen and antigen responses, hypergammaglobulinaemia and reduced natural killer cell function.

### Respiratory presentations

The commonest presentations of pulmonary disease in AIDS include dry cough, gradually increasing dyspnoea on exertion and fever. By far the commonest cause in developed countries is *Pneumocystis carinii* pneumonia. Symptoms may develop insidiously over several weeks and some patients present with a pyrexia of unknown origin (PUO). The physiological disturbance may initially be quite modest, but increased respiratory rate, reduced diffusing capacity for carbon monoxide and reduced arterial oxygen are valuable indicators. Chest X-ray may be normal until quite late but when abnormal usually shows diffuse interstitial mid-zone shadowing, often bilaterally, but not always symmetrical; gallium scanning has been advocated, but in most hands the sensitivity is low.

The other common respiratory pathogens found in AIDS are *Mycobacterium tuberculosis* or atypical mycobacteria (*avium-intracellulare*, *kansasii* and *xenopi*). Infection by *M. tuberculosis* tends to occur early in the course; it is also the most common respiratory complication in developing countries. Mycobacterial infection may present with miliary disease and/or pleural effusion, which is rare in *Pneumocystis* infection; cavitation and fibrosis are rare. Patients are not often sputum-positive initially. Cytomegalovirus pneumonitis may present like *Pneumocystis* infection, but is surprisingly uncommon. Reticular shadowing on X-ray is typical and may extend to the periphery, unlike *Pneumocystis* infection. Associated retinitis or colitis from cytomegalovirus may give important clues to differential diagnosis. Cryptococcal infection of the lung may resemble that of *Pneumocystis* but is less severe and may present with effusion. Bacterial pneumonia is generally accompanied by purulent secretions and the radiological appearances are more typical because neutrophil function is well maintained; bronchoscopy is only needed with such presentations if other infections are suspected.

Patients with Kaposi's sarcoma of the lung usually have skin or mucosal disease and the latter may be apparent at bronchoscopy. Bronchial lesions may cause obstruction with secondary infection; pleural plaques may cause largish effusions. Parenchymal infiltration may develop gradually, with increasing dyspnoea, slight cough and patchy interstitial shadowing on X-ray. Tuberculosis or Kaposi's sarcoma or lymphoma may cause mediastinal or hilar adenopathy.

Where an opportunistic infection or Kaposi's sarcoma of the lung is suspected, confirmation is essential. Sputum rarely yields diagnostic material, but when induced by inhalation of nebulized hypertonic saline may give enough material for diagnostic cytology; this procedure is rather uncomfortable and has a relatively low yield. The optimal procedure to establish diagnosis is fibreoptic bronchoscopy with bronchoalveolar lavage transbronchial biopsy. Good communication with histopathology, cytology and microbiology laboratories is vital to make best use of the material obtained. If the appearances are typical of *Pneumocystis* infection, patients can be started on empirical, high-dose co-trimoxazole, pending a result or bronchoscopy if this has to be delayed for a few days.

There are three main reasons for using this approach to investigation. First, it allows substantive identification of an infection on which AIDS itself can be diagnosed and the resulting certainty helps in counselling and further management. Secondly, although infection with *Pneumocystis* is the most common, several other important pathogens must be distinguished to enable prompt and appropriate therapy, and there may be dual infection. Thirdly, should the patient fail to respond to adequate treatment for all pathogens known to be present, rational decisions can be made concerning assisted ventilation.

Treatment of *Pneumocystis* infection is with high-dose co-trimoxazole for three weeks, initially intravenously. In the event of the notably common allergic or other intolerance to sulphonamides, dapsone/trimethoprim is equally effective. Pentamidine isethionate may be given intravenously (slowly) but is more toxic and no more effective. Recent studies have suggested that, at least in milder cases, inhaled pentamidine may be effective. For patients with rapid deterioration, a short course of methylprednisolone (40 mg thrice daily for three days) may be a valuable adjunct. The risk/benefit ratio of prophylaxis is not clear, but

weekly Fansidar, or daily co-trimoxazole or dapsone, have been effective in several studies. Adverse reactions, usually allergic, may limit the role of prophylaxis and could reduce the options available when treatment is required. Inhaled pentamidine prophylaxis has been widely used and seems effective; extra pulmonary pneumocystis can occur however.

Triple therapy for tuberculosis is effective but may be needed for long periods, with at least isoniazid maintenance for life; atypical mycobacteria are more resistant to treatment but some palliation may be achieved with standard antituberculous agents, or with rifabutin substituted for rifampicin. Cryptococcal infection is treated with at least one month of amphotericin and flucytosine but fluconazole and itraconazole are proving valuable alternatives with much lesser toxicity. Cytomegalovirus responds to intravenous ganciclovir and possibly phosphonoformate. Standard antibacterials are used for bacterial pneumonia but, if this is recurrent, gamma globulin replacement has been of value. Pulmonary or severe bronchial Kaposi's sarcoma are indications for chemotherapy (see below), and recurrent pleural effusion can be satisfactorily treated by instillation of bleomycin.

### Gastrointestinal presentations

Oral candidiasis should always be sought in such patients and is a common and early marker of immunodeficiency; it may or may not be symptomatic and the accompanying oesophagitis, which can be picked up on barium swallow or oesophagoscopy, only sometimes leads to dysphagia. Ketoconazole or the newer fluconazole or itraconazole are effective but topical agents rarely control it. Maintenance therapy is needed and is well tolerated, though malabsorption may necessitate increasing doses. Ketoconazole cannot be used with rifampicin.

Hairy oral leukoplakia, typically whitish corrugated lesions on the lateral border and underside of the tongue, should be distinguished from thrush. No therapy is needed, but in ARC it is a marker for progression. Gingivitis is common, for which metronidazole with oral rinses is helpful. Other causes of oesophagitis include herpes simplex and cytomegalovirus. Herpes simplex stomatitis may occur and chronic mucocutaneous ulceration may necessitate long-term, low-dose acyclovir.

Perianal or genital lesions of herpes simplex are more common and present with progressive, low-grade ulceration. Acyclovir treatment leads to healing to be followed by maintenance at low dose to prevent relapse.

Diarrhoea, abdominal pain and distension, weight loss and fever are common symptoms of bowel disease in patients with AIDS but several characteristic patterns may be seen. Cryptosporidiosis causes severe, watery diarrhoea and colicky pain with associated malabsorption; stool microscopy or biopsy shows the typical oocysts. This is physically one of the most unpleasant infections in AIDS and there is no definitive treatment; symptom control and dietary supplementation are possible and some patients have benefited from treatment with interleukin 2.

Abdominal pain and distension, with fever and rebound tenderness in the left iliac fossa, are typical of cytomegalovirus or adenovirus colitis. Plain abdominal X-ray shows distended loops of bowel with some thickening of the wall. Characteristic inclusions may be seen on sigmoidoscopic biopsy and culture should be attempted; both infections respond well to ganciclovir and phosphonoformate. Salmonellosis may present with fever alone, or with mild diarrhoea and abdominal pain; the organisms can be cultured from stool; bacteraemia is usual. Antibacterial therapy is given according to the sensitivity, but maintenance treatment (usually trimethoprim) is almost always needed.

Mycobacterial infection, which is usually caused by atypical organisms, may cause no symptoms and be found incidentally on biopsy; granulomas are absent. Sometimes a Whipple's-like appearance is seen with malabsorption. Abdominal masses, usually mesenteric nodes, may be palpable though painless and may be seen on CT scanning. Percutaneous biopsy can yield diagnostic material. Mild, intermittent diarrhoea and some degree of malabsorption are not uncommon in AIDS and ARC; they appear to result from partial villous atrophy, perhaps due to direct effects of HIV; symptomatic relief is readily achieved.

Kaposi's sarcoma is commonly seen as flat or raised plaques on the palate and around the gums. Oesophageal or gastric lesions are less common but may cause dysphagia, nausea, vomiting, obstruction or bleeding; diffuse or extensive gastric or bowel lesions may present as a protein-losing enteropathy or diarrhoea. Severe or symptomatic disease may necessitate chemotherapy, but flat plaques or small sessile symptomless lesions may be best left alone. The gut is also one of the commoner extranodal sites of lymphoma in AIDS.

## Nervous system presentations

The two most common opportunistic pathogens in the central nervous system are *Toxoplasma gondii* and *Cryptococcus*.

### *Cryptococcus*

Cryptococcal meningitis may present as a PUO; symptoms and signs of meningitis are minimal or absent unless diagnosis is long delayed. There may be central ataxia and, rarely, focal signs; sometimes the diagnosis is first made from peripheral evidence of cryptococcosis, such as skin lesions or pulmonary disease. Lumbar puncture should only be undertaken after CT scanning, because toxoplasma abscesses, especially those in the posterior fossa, may have similar presentations. The CSF has few or no white cells, raised protein and low sugar; cryptococci may be seen microscopically and prolonged culture is advised as some grow very slowly. Assay of serum and CSF cryptococcal antigen is sometimes helpful in diagnosis, but more so in monitoring for relapse after treatment. This consists of intravenous amphotericin (0.6 mg/kg daily) with flucytosine for four to six weeks. Fluconazole offers a valuable and better tolerated alternative with apparently good efficacy. Without maintenance, relapse tends to occur within a few months but the optimal regimen is not clear. Amphotericin given intermittently seems effective but oral fluconazole or intraconazole may give equally good results with lesser toxicity. Some patients may develop secondary hydrocephalus after recurrent attacks.

### *Toxoplasma*

Cerebral abscesses are common, occurring in about a third of AIDS patients who are seropositive for *Toxoplasma* (indicating latent infection). They may present with focal signs, ataxia, fits or abnormal higher function developing subacutely over several weeks; headache, if present, is rarely severe. CT scanning usually shows multiple, low-density lesions, usually with irregular, central ring enhancement; magnetic resonance imaging may be more sensitive. The differential diagnosis in AIDS is cerebral lymphoma and tuberculoma (rare).

It is usual in patients who are seropositive for *Toxoplasma* to try two weeks of sulphadiazine and pyrimethamine at high dose (with folinic acid). If there is no clinical or radiological improvement, which usually is evident by the second week, brain biopsy is advisable. Earlier biopsy may be indicated where appearances suggest lymphoma or in seronegative patients, but some centres have reported a high complication rate on biopsy of acute lesions. Dapsone or clindamycin may be used in the event of sulpha allergy. After four weeks of treatment at full dose, it may be reduced and tapered over several weeks to daily or thrice weekly Fansidar (sulphadoxine/pyrimethamine) or dapsone/pyrimethamine, but long-term maintenance is required. Isolated cerebral lymphoma may be treated with radiotherapy but the results are relatively poor.

### Other neurological changes

Progressive, multifocal leucoencephalopathy is occasionally found and presents with diffuse changes in mental and physical function. Patchy, low-density change in the white matter on CT scan is characteristic; there is no effective treatment. Subacute encephalitis due to cytomegalovirus is seen but appears not to be as common as initially suspected. There are few specific clinical or radiological features but the virus may be cultured from the CSF, or retinitis may accompany the central signs. Ganciclovir appears effective.

In retinitis from cytomegalovirus, the characteristic, irregular white areas of choroiditis are accompanied by flame haemorrhages and there may be associated cottonwool spots, but these alone are not a basis for diagnosing cytomegalovirus infection. Retinal lesions are only symptomatic if central vision or large areas are affected, so fundoscopic examination at each visit is essential for early detection. Retinal detachment may occur as a result of damage by the virus. Prompt treatment with ganciclovir or phosphonoformate will stem spread, but there will be little recovery of vision. Maintenance with ganciclovir three or five times weekly is necessary as without it early relapse with further loss of vision is apparently inevitable. Ganciclovir may cause myelosuppression, especially when used with zidovudine.

HIV itself causes encephalopathy with gradual loss of higher function, starting with short-term memory and concentration, progressing over many months to more overt dementia with mood or personality change, pyramidal, extrapyramidal or (pseudo-)cerebellar signs, incontinence and extreme withdrawal. It is clinically evident in about 25 per cent of AIDS cases at the end of their course and may sometimes dominate the clinical picture; it can sometimes occur in the absence of immunodeficiency. Early there are no changes on CT scan and the CSF has only elevated protein; magnetic resonance imaging is believed to show earlier changes. Later there is diffuse cerebral atrophy. However, HIV encephalopathy is a diagnosis of exclusion, so CT scan and examination of the CSF are mandatory in a patient with unexplained cerebral deterioration. Myelopathy due to HIV has been seen. Peripheral neuropathy may present not uncommonly with glove-and-stocking sensory loss and dysaesthesia, amyotrophy or mononeuritis multiplex; autonomic neuropathy, myopathy and a disorder clinically resembling amyotrophic lateral sclerosis have been described.

### Kaposi's sarcoma

The main cutaneous manifestation of AIDS is Kaposi's sarcoma, a tumour of probable endothelial origin. It is most common in patients with sexually acquired infection, especially amongst homosexual men. It has been suggested that the tumour is due to an as yet unidentified oncogenic virus that is sexually transmitted; early evidence suggested that it might be cytomegalovirus but this is disputed.

There are flat or usually slightly raised skin plaques that typically are purplish, but may appear erythematous in the early stages. The coloration is due to the entrapment of red cells; a surrounding, yellowish discoloration is sometimes seen in larger lesions, indicating extravasation. Lesions may appear anywhere but may tend to follow Langer's lines or veins. Many patients present with one or two solitary lesions; others develop rapid cropping of lesions, suggestive of more advanced disease. Some early lesions may recede spontaneously but larger lesions (> 0.5 cm) do not. Induration and redness are the best markers of lesional activity. Rates of change may vary between lesions and over time in individual patients; different patients show different patterns. The tumour is multifocal and does not metastasize. Lesions may preferentially arise at sites of trauma or inflammation.

Although the developed lesion is very characteristic, early ones can be hard to distinguish from several other conditions, so biopsy is mandatory; this may be a punch or excision depending on site. Early histological changes may be hard to interpret, but the typical lesions have spindle cells separated by slits in which free red cells are seen.

Several lesions of Kaposi's sarcoma may occur together on mucosal surfaces, especially on the palate, and there may be lymph node involvement and splenomegaly. Diffuse subcutaneous disease may be seen around regional lymph nodes, especially in the groin, and may also follow the course of veins or lymphatics, notably in the upper thighs; lymphoedema may be seen in association with such involvement. Visceral disease has been described above; it occasionally occurs in the absence of skin lesions.

Treatment options require an overall assessment, including cosmetic and psychological effects, rate of progression and extent of lesions, and the presence of symptomatic, visceral disease. Cutaneous lesions may either be left or given local radiotherapy (facial lesions are best treated this way) or intralesional vinblastine. These treatments leave some residual skin pigmentation but this is less than that of the original lesion. Radiotherapy is with low doses in four fractions over a few days. More extensive or rapidly progressive disease affecting the skin has been treated by α-interferon or chemotherapy.

Alpha-interferon certainly has considerable efficacy for cutaneous disease but has a minimal effect on visceral disease and in patients with more severe immunodeficiency, especially those with opportunistic infections. Its main drawbacks are its side-effects, not only the 'flu-like symptoms, which may occur on starting treatment and which gradually diminish, but also the more insidiously severe malaise, anorexia, weight loss and mental changes, including severe depression. The quoted incidence of these varies, but they can be dose limiting. Given that patients most likely to benefit from α-interferon are those without any constitutional symptoms, a treatment that causes these may not be ideal, even if the tumour resolves, given that there are other ways of achieving this. For this reason many centres prefer to use local therapy.

For more aggressive disease, including rapidly developing skin lesions, lymphatic disease causing oedema and symptomatic visceral involvement, especially of lung and gut, one of the chemotherapeutic agents is the preferred treatment. A variety of chemotherapies has been advocated but the need is for those with minimal myelo- or immunosupresion. Vinblastine, etoposide and bleomycin/vincristine have been used to good effect; our current preference is for the latter combination, which is more rapidly efficacious and is also better tolerated than the former two. Treatment is given at monthly or 3-weekly intervals for six to seven courses, after which it may be discontinued or reduced to vincristine alone. If peripheral neuropathy develops, vinblastine is substituted. In the event of tumour escape, other agents may be needed, albeit at the expense of greater toxicity. Irradiation of regional lymph nodes may also have a limited place where there is local lymphoedema, but mucosal radiation is very poorly tolerated.

## Lymphoma

Both non-Hodgkin's and Hodgkin's lymphoma occur in HIV infection, and may present atypically. The former especially tends to present with extranodal disease although some lymphadenopathy is usual. The lymphoma is relatively aggressive in character in many cases. Aside from lymphoid sites, lymphoma of the central nervous system is the most common presentation, but involvement of gut and skin is not uncommon; haematological abnormalities and type B symptoms are common. Diagnosis is usually made by biopsy of a lymph node, cerebral mass lesion or other site. The histological appearances are of the diffuse, lymphocyte-depleted type. Various regimens have had some limited success in treatment but the optimal regimen is as yet unclear as many of the agents normally used would seem inadvisable because they are immunosuppressive. Combination regimens without prednisolone have been used to some effect. The ultimate prognosis is relatively poor, especially perhaps in non-Hodgkin's lymphoma.

## Skin disorders

The skin is rarely unaffected in symptomatic HIV infection. It is typically dry and scaly and may benefit from emulsifying agents; pruritus can be marked. Seborrhoeic dermatitis, folliculitis and molluscum contagiosum are very common. Topical antifungals with or without low-dose steroids may be helpful for the dermatitis and folliculitis; topical phenol may cause the molluscs to abate temporarily. Vasculitic or herpetiform lesions over the trunk, limbs and face are often troublesome and respond poorly to topical treatment; they may become secondarily infected. Treatment is largely symptomatic or directed at the infection.

### Other problems

In AIDS, lymph node or splenic enlargement may be due to lymphoma, Kaposi's sarcoma or the related angiofollicular hyperplasia. However, an increase in node size may also occur in mycobacterial infections, typical and atypical, and in disseminated fungal infections like histoplasmosis (not endemic to the UK but found in patients who have lived in, for example, the American mid-west or the Caribbean). Marked systemic symptoms, disease at other sites, lymphadenopathy that is asymmetrical or also involves internal node systems (e.g., hilar, para-aortic) and haematological abnormalities are indications for biopsy or aspiration.

An important, additional diagnosis that is easily missed and is not uncommon is Addison's disease due to cytomegalovirus or occasionally to tuberculous infection of the adrenals. It may occur without disease at other sites. Affected patients often have systemic symptoms, such as fatigue, malaise or weight loss, which both they and their physicians readily ascribe to nonspecific effects of HIV or other intercurrent illness. Important clues to diagnosis are symptoms and signs of postural hypotension (although autonomic neuropathy is another possible cause) and, notably, reduced skin turgor in the absence of sites of loss and recurring despite repletion. Replacement therapy with fludrocortisone (150–200 µg daily) and hydrocortisone (20 mg, twice a day) produces a swift and gratifying response.

## TREATMENT

There are four broad approaches to the treatment of AIDS and other HIV-associated disease: (a) treatment or prophylaxis of specific opportunistic infections or tumours; (b) general management; (c) antiretroviral agents; (d) immunorestorative therapy.

### Opportunistic infection

Hitherto, the main focus of medical management, as outlined above, has been the treatment of opportunistic events as they arise, supplemented by maintenance therapy for some infections. Prompt diagnosis and appropriate treatment of many of the opportunistic infections can restore patients, albeit temporarily, to a state of good or reasonable health. Many patients remain well between episodes of infection, even though their susceptibility may be gradually increasing with time. Antimicrobial prophylaxis for specific pathogens has done much to reduce the incidence of some opportunistic infections; however, drug hypersensitivity and reduced absorption due to enteropathy have limited their value. The development of new drugs for secondary diseases still has considerable potential for reducing morbidity and improving survival in AIDS.

Patients with solely cutaneous Kaposi's sarcoma have relatively less severe immunodeficiency and, in addition, may feel quite well—apart from the not inconsiderable psychological effects of the skin blemishes. Thus the therapeutic approach to such tumours must take account of the fact that over-zealous treatment may exacerbate the immunodeficiency as well as making the patient feel more ill. Similar principles underlie the management of thrombocytopenic purpura in HIV infection. In both settings, no treatment may be in the patient's best interests.

### General measures

In addition to specific therapies, general measures to reduce risk of progression and to make the best of the patient's remaining immune defence are important. These include avoidance of cofactors, such as intercurrent infection, and attention to good nutrition. Advice about the avoidance of the relatively few opportunistic organisms that are newly acquired rather than already latent (e.g., salmonella) should be simple and practical. Access to prompt diagnosis and treatment of secondary complications, counselling and education about AIDS and HIV, and strong hospital and community support, are essential adjuncts to management. A positive approach by patients towards their disease, whether or not it has any effect on the immune system, is critical to the quality of life of people with AIDS.

Much can be achieved by establishing good lines

of communication between the patient and health care staff, and by outlining a philosophy of management that involves the patient in maintenance of health and in decision making. The patient must be assured that he or she retains control over information about their disease and that staff will be frank and open with them, whether the news is good or bad. The issue of death and dying must be addressed and anxieties about them resolved so that the patient can, thereafter, get on with the business of living with AIDS. This is best discussed at the time of diagnosis and an adequate investment of time and thought at this stage can greatly enhance further delivery of care; it serves as a foundation of knowledge and principles that enable the patient to cope with the many anxieties and conflicting advice that will inevitably follow.

## Antiretroviral therapy

Given the fact that AIDS results from the effects of active, chronic viral infection, strategies to reduce viral proliferation are clearly likely to be of benefit. In principle, this is especially so if they are used early in HIV infection, before much damage has been done to target cells and tissues; later on, in AIDS and ARC, they may be able to reduce the rate of progression or even allow some limited regeneration of function; alternatively they could be used in combination with immunorestorative approaches. The latter alone, although theoretically attractive for the treatment of immunodeficient patients, have hitherto been of rather limited benefit, presumably because of continued viral replication.

The only drug to have emerged from the very many clinical trials done with these objectives in mind has been zidovudine (AZT). This is a reverse transcriptase inhibitor that interferes with the means whereby HIV establishes latent infection in newly infected target cells. After encouraging phase I studies, a phase II, placebo-controlled clinical trial among patients with ARC or AIDS (presenting with *Pneumocystis* pneumonia) showed that those receiving the drug had substantially lower short-term mortality and fewer and less severe opportunistic infections than those receiving the placebo. These differences became apparent after the first six weeks of treatment. Benefit was also seen in placebo patients when crossed over to the active drug. In addition to this and some indication of modestly improved, cell-mediated immune function, viral antigen titres

fell during treatment, a marker of reduced viral replication. There are also reports of improvement in cognitive, neuropsychological function in the treated group and this is borne out by clinical experience; this suggests that there is a significant and useful degree of reversibility in HIV encephalopathy and neuropathy.

Widespread clinical use has confirmed and extended these findings, including a possible preventive effect on HIV encephalopathy. Wider experience indicates that patients with AIDS and ARC show less frequent and less severe opportunistic infections, especially in the first 6 to 12 months of treatment. Even in patients able to continue taking full doses, the effects in the second year are less striking. Overall, the impression is that the drug prolongs the period over which such patients remain well but does not prevent the eventual progression to more severe disease. Most clinicians feel that all patients with AIDS and those with ARC features should be offered zidovudine. There is evidence that lower doses may be effective and better tolerated. There are early encouraging data on its use in symptomless or PGL patients, but longer-term trials remain under way.

Initial regimens of 4-hourly dosing were recommended on the basis of pharmacokinetic studies, but 6-hourly or even 12-hourly schedules are now being tried, as are lower doses, apparently with equal efficacy. Patients commonly develop systemic side-effects, notably in the first few weeks; these include malaise, headache, nausea, myalgia, rash and insomnia; they generally settle with continued treatment. After prolonged treatment some patients complain of fatigue and lassitude, which resolve on discontinuing the drug.

The toxicity of zidovudine is substantial at high doses in symptomatic disease. The major effect is on bone marrow and in particular on the red cell series: severe anaemia arises in 20 to 30 per cent of patients, necessitating transfusion in most of these, as often as 4- to 6-weekly; lesser degrees of anaemia may be found in some other patients. Macrocytosis occurs in virtually all patients and is not linked to the development of anaemia. Neutropenia tends to occur later, and can give rise to serious infective complications (staphylococcal, Gram-negative and systemic fungal infections). Platelet counts tend to rise initially in patients with lower baseline counts; this may be due to an effect on HIV-associated thrombocytopenia and severe thrombocytopenia may itself be an indication for zidovudine. However, after prolonged treatment, platelet counts tend to fall due to marrow suppression.

The myelotoxicity of zidovudine appears to be exacerbated by some other agents used for opportunistic infection, notably ganciclovir and dapsone (daily or alternate daily treatment), but other agents have little observable effect. Although anaemia is commoner in patients who are already anaemic, or who have low CD4 counts and low levels of vitamin $B_{12}$, toxicity cannot be entirely predicted from the patient's prior state; some patients with AIDS may tolerate zidovudine without myelotoxicity yet others with only mild ARC may have severe problems. Reducing the dose of zidovudine or stopping it entirely allows reversal of the myelotoxicity, although recovery may take some weeks. However, the efficacy of the drug appears to be less at lower dosage.

A new form of toxicity, seen in patients being treated in the longer term, is a necrotizing myopathy, which tends to affect the proximal parts of the lower limbs. There may be associated pain and tenderness and CPK (creatine phosphokinase) levels are typically raised. Symptoms and enzyme changes resolve slowly after stopping zidovudine. Its pathogenesis appears to be due to mitochondrial dysfunction.

In some patients, reducing or stopping zidovudine may be followed in the succeeding days or weeks by an acute meningoencephalitic illness causing headache, fever, neck stiffness, confusion or a depressed level of consciousness. In others there may be an acute transverse myelitis. This apparent 'rebound' phenomenon seems only to occur in some patients and to be self-limiting over several days or weeks in most. It may be avoided by more gradual reduction in dosage where this is possible. Although this illness has not been temporally associated with a rise in serum or CSF antigen, such a rise does occur in many patients after the treatment is stopped or reduced.

The effects of zidovudine offer considerable hope that this and future antiretroviral agents may be able to contain the progression of the disease in the longer term and possibly to prevent disease if used in early infection. It is to be hoped that infectiousness to others may also be reduced by such treatment. However, the substantial toxicity of zidovudine means that agents with similar effects on HIV but which are better tolerated will need to be developed. Drug combinations could also improve the therapeutic ratio. It is also vital that further, licensed use of zidovudine be properly monitored so that more information on its value, its role and its toxicity can be gained without delay. Other drugs under development are being watched with interest, but despite the relatively high profile of many, none has yet reached a stage where usage can be considered outside the context of the clinical trial. Combinations of antiretrovirals or of such drugs with immunorestorative therapy may offer additional benefits, but further trials are necessary.

## CONCLUSIONS

AIDS and HIV have posed considerable challenges to the medical profession. These have included a need to understand a wide range of new or unfamiliar clinical conditions, the social milieu in which the infection is contracted, the basic principles of infection control, the wider implications of AIDS and the tests that are used to identify HIV infection, the nature of the contract between physician and patient, and the constantly changing therapeutic opportunities. Many of these issues are not so much new ones as old problems that have been thrown into rather sharp relief. If we are able to develop understanding and to respond to the needs of our patients, we will be better physicians for it.

### Further reading

Dournon E., Matheron S., Rozenbaum W. *et al.* (1988). Effects of zidovudine in 365 consecutive patients with AIDS or AIDS-related complex. *Lancet*, **ii**, 1297–1302.

Fischl M. A., Richman D. D., Grieco M. H. *et al.* (1987). The efficacy of azidothymidine (AZT) in the treatment of patients with AIDS and AIDS-related complex: A double blind, placebo-controlled trial. *New Engl. J. Med.*, **317**, 185–91.

Glatt A. E., Chirgwin K., Landesman S. H. (1988). Treatment of infections associated with human immunodeficiency virus. *New Engl. J. Med.*, **318**, 1439–48.

Gold J. W. M. (1988). Infectious complications in patients with human innumodeficiency virus infection. *AIDS*, **2**, 327–34.

Gottlieb M., Jeffries D. J., Mildvan D., Pinching A. J., Quinn T. C., Weiss R. A., eds. (1987). *Topics in AIDS* vol. 1. Chichester: John Wiley.

Gottlieb M., Jeffries D. J., Mildvan D., Pinching A. J., Quinn T., Weiss R. A., eds. (1989). *Topics in AIDS* vol. 2. Chichester: John Wiley.

Krown S. E. (1988). AIDS-associated Kaposi's sarcoma. *AIDS*, **2**, 71–80.

Miller D., Weber J., Green J., eds. (1985). *The management of AIDS patients*. Basingstoke: Macmillan.

Pinching A. J., ed. (1986). *AIDS and HIV infection.* Clinics in Immunology and Allergy 6, pp. 441–687. London: WB Saunders.

Pinching A. J. (1989). Zidovudine in asymptomatic HIV infection: knowledge and uncertainty. *Int. J. STD & AIDS*, **2**, 157–61.

Pinching A. J. (1988). Prophylaxis and maintenance therapy in patients with AIDS and ARC. *AIDS*, **2**, 335–43.

Pinching A. J., Helbert M., Peddle B. *et al.* (1988). Clinical experience with zidovudine in the treatment of patients with AIDS and ARC. *J. Infect.* (in press).

Richman D. D., Fischl M. A., Grieco M. H. *et al.* (1987). The toxicity of axidothymidine (AZT) in the treatment of patients with AIDS and AIDS-related complex; a double blind, placebo-controlled trial. *New Engl. J. Med.*, **317**, 192–7.

# Section Three

**Clinical Specialities**

# 4

# CARDIOLOGY

John Davies

## APPROACH TO THE PATIENT

When taking a cardiac history the patient should be encouraged to give spontaneously a full account of the symptoms and only then cross-examined on specific points. In general, cardiac symptoms are caused by myocardial ischaemia, a decrease in efficiency of left ventricular contraction or by a disturbance of cardiac rate or rhythm. Exercise may induce cardiac symptoms but remember that there will be enormous differences in exercise capacity between, for example, young, fit labourers and middle-aged, sedentary office workers. The most important point to establish is whether there has been a *change* in the patient's exercise capacity.

After the detailed history, it is important to make a careful examination, and in most cases to proceed to some baseline investigations such as an ECG and chest X-ray. Further investigations, such as echocardiography and radionuclear studies, are rarely needed; invasive studies, such as cardiac catheterization, are only necessary for a few patients.

Non-invasive tests are only an aid to diagnosis and must not replace a good history and examination. Invasive investigations involve a risk, are time consuming, costly and should only be done to answer a carefully thought out question and when the answer to this question will change the management of the patient.

The general public is well informed about the extent and severity of cardiac problems, particularly ischaemic heart disease, and patients with a strong family history of this condition frequently present complaining of atypical and nonspecific symptoms. The correct approach to such a patient should be to take a careful history, make a thorough examination and ECG, which, if normal, can be followed by assertive yet sympathetic reassurance.

Among the many medicaments which doctors carry in their bags, there can be none more precious than Reassurance, precious in that it is the 'Pill' he has to dispense most frequently and so often does most good.

*William Evans*

## SYMPTOMS

### Chest pain

Chest pain is probably the most challenging symptom in clinical medicine. The correct diagnosis of angina pectoris is in most cases based entirely on the careful interpretation of a well-taken history. It is one of the most difficult but most important diagnoses to get right. Misdiagnosis of ischaemic chest pain in a young, fit man under 40 years of age with heavy family commitments can produce dire professional and medicolegal consequences. Unfortunately, despite a careful history, normal examination, normal ECG, and even a negative stress test, a patient can still leave a medical outpatients department reassured, run to catch a bus and drop down dead of an acute myocardial infarction! For a careful and elegantly written description of angina pectoris, it is difficult to improve on William Heberden's classical description made in 1768 (see Suggested Reading).

Disorders that cause chest pain are manifold because so many structures in the thorax share afferent pain fibres. For example, the pain due to a hiatus hernia is frequently confused with angina.

The most important feature of anginal pain is its close relationship to *exercise*. Angina is often first experienced when walking quickly or uphill against the wind, often exacerbated by very cold weather. However, emotion, stress, worry or excitement can also induce typical ischaemic chest pain and the relief of this pain by rest or by sublingual nitroglycerine is also suggestive of an ischaemic origin.

The nature of the pain, especially if spontaneously described by the patient as crushing, heavy or pressing, is helpful in making a diagnosis as is the spontaneous application of a pressing fist on the front of the sternum by the patient.

Anginal chest pain is most commonly experienced in the mid-sternal region of the chest, often spreading to one or both arms and sometimes up into the neck, jaw, epigastrium or through to the back.

The diffuse distribution of anginal pain helps diagnosis. If a patient can localize the exact site of the chest pain with a finger tip it is probably not ischaemic. If the chest pain is brought on by exercise, and disappears following a few seconds of rest, it is less likely to be ischaemic chest pain than if it persists for two or three minutes.

Patients rarely refer to true anginal chest pain as 'pain'. They more frequently refer to the sensation as one of extreme discomfort and if they reply 'It's not really a pain, doctor', it is unlikely to be ischaemic in origin, particularly if accompanied by dyspnoea.

The pain of myocardial infarction is exactly the same as angina. The duration is much longer and it may occur at rest. It is often accompanied by other symptoms, such as sweating, faintness, dyspnoea, and the signs of shock.

### Other forms of cardiovascular pain

The pain of pericarditis is sharp, continuous and uncomfortable with a pleuritic element, sometimes referred to the tip of the left shoulder, particularly when there is involvement of the diaphragmatic pericardium. Many patients obtain relief by sitting forward.

The pain of a dissecting aortic aneurysm is similar to that of myocardial infarction. It is usually severe and often radiates through to the back. It may be accompanied by obliteration or inequality of peripheral pulses.

A massive pulmonary embolus may cause severe retrosternal pain. This is often associated with sudden collapse, shock, dyspnoea and cyanosis.

### Dyspnoea

Shortness of breath in cardiac disease is produced most commonly by pulmonary congestion causing increased lung stiffness. This may occur early in certain conditions such as mitral stenosis and late in others such as aortic stenosis. In pulmonary hypertension, dyspnoea is probably due to the failure of enough blood to get to the lungs because of the massive increase in pulmonary vascular resistance. The sensation of dyspnoea is subjective; objective assessment, either by questioning or by testing to see how many stairs the patient can manage, is useful. There are many causes other than cardiac for dyspnoea; cardiac dyspnoea can be exacerbated by additional problems such as anaemia and chronic bronchitis.

### Paroxysmal nocturnal dyspnoea

Sudden attacks of severe shortness of breath occurring at night may be the first manifestation of left ventricular failure or mitral stenosis. Typically the patient awakes from sleep gasping for breath with a feeling of being suffocated and describes this attack as 'asthma'. Indeed, this condition is sometimes referred to as 'cardiac asthma'. Pulmonary oedema is a potent cause of bronchospasm, sometimes making cardiac asthma difficult to distinguish from true asthma—the late onset of which is rare and not usually accompanied by heart murmurs.

### Orthopnoea

Orthopnoea is defined as breathlessness at rest and is exacerbated by lying flat. This is probably because gravity no longer helps the usual descent of the diaphragm. To be comfortable the patient props him- or herself up with pillows and the number of pillows used gives an indication of the severity of the orthopnoea. When assessing severity it is helpful to ask such questions as, 'What are you now unable to do that you used to do and would still like to do?' Gradual increase in severity of exertional dyspnoea is a good guide to the increasing severity of a valvular gradient, as in mitral stenosis, or gradually decreasing left ventricular function, as in congestive cardio-myopathy.

## Palpitation

Palpitation is the awareness of one's heart beat. It is important to establish whether the sensation is of a fast or a slow heart beat and whether it is regular. It is often helpful to ask the patient to tap out the actual rate and rhythm of the palpitation. The sensation of a normal, regular heart beat, especially on going to bed at night, is perfectly normal.

Most palpitations are fast but occasionally, as in complete heart block, the increased stroke volume may cause awareness of the heart's slow action. Short episodes of fast, irregular beating are often due to atrial fibrillation. Atrial flutter manifests itself as longer episodes of slightly slower palpitation, either regular or irregular.

Remember to consider other causes such as thyrotoxicosis when a patient complains of palpitation. The most common cause is anxiety, often potentiated by stress and overwork. Extrasystoles are common and the patient may complain of a 'missed' beat. In the absence of myocardial or valvular disease, atrial extrasystoles are benign. Ventricular extrasystoles are also often normal, even long episodes of *bigeminy* (i.e., regularly alternating normal sinus beats and unifocal ventricular extrasystoles) can occur in the normal heart. In the case of ventricular extrasystoles, however, underlying cardiac disease should be carefully excluded.

## Oedema

Mild, bilateral oedema of the ankles occasionally occurs in a normal person. This is simple dependent gravitational oedema, noticed after long episodes of inactivity such as an air flight—where the knees are bent with no active muscle tone contributing to venous return.

Heart failure causes fluid to accumulate in the tissue spaces causing swelling, most frequently of feet and ankles. As well as ankles other dependent areas such as buttocks and scrotum may accumulate fluid as congestive heart failure develops. Remember that heart failure is not the only cause of oedema, which also occurs in liver and/or kidney failure and in hypoproteinaemic states.

If only one leg is swollen, the most likely cause is a deep venous thrombosis. This can sometimes occur without the usual symptoms of inflammation and pain.

## Syncope

A characteristic feature of cardiac syncope as opposed to other causes of sudden loss of consciousness is that there is usually no warning and the fall frequently results in a head injury. An elderly patient who complains of 'drop attacks' in whom a head injury is noticed should be taken very seriously. This symptom is almost pathognomonic of intermittent heart block and is treatable by permanent pacing.

In addition to arrhythmias, other cardiac causes of syncope include sudden, low-output states, which can occur in conditions such as Fallot's tetralogy, hypertrophic cardiomyopathy and tight stenosis of the aortic valve.

## Other symptoms

### Tiredness

Although fatigue is common in any illness, excessive tiredness is the symptom that most patients with severe heart failure complain of bitterly.

### Cough

Pulmonary oedema frequently presents as a cough, which may be dry and non-productive but more commonly results in pink, frothy sputum. Bright red blood may be coughed up by patients with heart disease and this is common in young people with tight mitral stenosis, and also in advanced pulmonary hypertension from any cause. Acute haemoptysis, especially if associated with pleuritic chest pain, is most frequently due to an acute pulmonary embolus.

### Cachexia

Patients with severe and longstanding heart failure may look thin, ill and wasted; this has been described as 'cardiac cachexia'. It is due to longstanding underperfusion of tissues and results in loss of facial tissue and muscle wasting, particularly of the cheeks.

## GENERAL EXAMINATION

There is no more difficult art to acquire than the art of observation

*Sir William Ossler*

The cardiovascular system should be examined systematically. It does not matter which system you use so long as an exact format is repeated regularly.

A suggested method is to start with both radial pulses, followed by the right brachial to assess pulse character.

The blood pressure should be carefully measured.

The head, face, mouth and eyes should be looked at and the presence and height of an elevated jugular venous pressure measured. Other signs of heart failure include hepatosplenomegaly, ascites and ankle oedema. Any abnormal thoracic pulsations should be noted and the heart apex accurately located. Lastly, the heart should be auscultated with the patient and the stethoscope in several different positions.

*Remember that most cardiac diagnoses can be made without a stethoscope.*

Examination of the cardiovascular system does not simply mean cardiac auscultation, which indeed may be much less informative than assessing the character of the pulse. An important abnormal physical finding should spark off in your mind a list of other clinical signs, which should be sought. For instance, if coarctation is suspected on the basis of absent femoral pulses, then hypertension in the arms and rib notching on the chest X-ray should be looked for. Likewise, if a young person presents with a sudden attack of atrial fibrillation the neck should be examined because there may be a goitre.

### The hands

Finger clubbing (remember that the toes may also be clubbed) has several cardiac and other causes. The actual temperature of the fingers and all extremities can be a useful guide to left ventricular output. In a warm room, the finding of cold fingers and toes in a patient after myocardial infarction is a poor prognostic sign and suggests cardiogenic shock. Excessive sweating may be due to anxiety or thyrotoxicosis. If the fingers are blue, the presence of absence of central cyanosis should be established. If the tongue is pink, the blue fingers are due to peripheral cyanosis. Splinter haemorrhages, which occur in both finger *and* toe nails, may be an important clue. If bacterial endocarditis is suspected, a daily check of finger and toe nails is important because the appearance of new splinter haemorrhages would be of diagnostic importance. Anaemia exacerbates heart failure and this diagnosis may be suspected by looking at the hands and confirmed by inspection of the conjunctiva.

### The head and face

A shimmering iris caused by lens dislocation is characteristic of Marfan's syndrome; a high arched palate should also be looked for. The cornea should be inspected for an arcus, the presence of which is only a relevant finding under the age of 50 years. The characteristic 'malar flush' of dilated venules in the cyanosed skin in both cheeks is almost pathognomonic of mitral stenosis.

### The chest

Any chest deformity may be relevant because conditions such as pectus excavatum almost invariably result in innocent systolic murmurs. Obvious thoracic pulsations should be noted and the left ventricular apex localized. Other pulsations may include a right ventricular heave, or a diffuse, and sometimes paradoxically moving impulse covering a large area around the left ventricular apex, which is suggestive of a left ventricular aneurysm. The shape of the thorax may be due to longstanding heart disease as in the 'pigeon breast' deformity resulting from longstanding right ventricular hypertrophy, often due to congenital heart disease. If coarctation is present, arterial pulsations can often be seen over the posterior intercostal spaces in enlarged collateral vessels. The best method of detecting these arterial pulsations is to place the patient in a good light, bent forward over the upright of a chair. The lung bases should be auscultated, listening for fine, late crackles, which do not clear on coughing and which are due to pulmonary oedema. Pleural effusions may be present and these can be detected by percussion and auscultation (detailed in Chapter 5). In severe heart failure, 'pitting' oedema may be present, particularly over the lower part of the back.

## CARDIAC PHYSICAL SIGNS

### The pulse

It is just as easy to palpate both radial pulses as it is one. Delay or absence of one pulse suggests a previous or ongoing aortic dissection, particularly in a patient with severe chest pain. Having felt both radial pulses, the femoral and carotid pulses should be palpated on both sides and bruits listened for.

The rate, rhythm, character and volume of one peripheral pulse should be determined; Paul Wood (see Suggested Reading) taught that placing the examiner's thumb over the patient's right brachial pulse was the method of choice. Count the rate over 15 s to ascertain the rhythm. The rhythm is either regular, regularly irregular as with regular ventricular extrasystoles, or irregularly irregular as in atrial fibrillation. The brachial pulse should be only lightly palpated because too firm a pressure, particularly in an elderly, atherosclerotic patient, may simulate a bisferian's pulse (see next subsection).

The pulse volume is either normal and strong, or weak and low. A pulse of weak volume is due to impaired left ventricular function and is a poor prognostic sign. Ventricular bigeminy, or coupling, results from a normal beat being regularly followed by an ectopic beat. It may be that the stroke volume from the second and smaller beat will fail to produce a pulse wave that reaches the wrist and, in this case, the pulse rate felt at the wrist is half that heard over the heart. It is important to search for a pulse 'deficit' because it is more relevant to control the heart rate than the pulse rate.

### Abnormal pulses

Experience is required to tell by palpation the different types of pulse character. Special varieties of pulse form are as follows.

A *plateau pulse* is found in aortic stenosis because the systole of the heart is more sustained than usual. A *collapsing pulse* is of a short duration with a very rapid upstroke and an equally swift descent. It is this rapid fall in pulse pressure that gives the characteristic 'collapsing' quality. This particular pulse character can be exaggerated by palpating the radial pulse, preferably with the whole of the examiner's hand when the patient's arm is lifted well up above the head. This is found most commonly in aortic regurgitation but can also be felt in the presence of an arteriovenous fistula such as a patent ductus arteriosus. A *bisferian pulse* of combined aortic regurgitation and stenosis has a rapid rise, a double peak, and a fall not quite so dramatic as a true collapsing pulse. Hypertrophic cardiomyopathy produces an abnormal and characteristic *jerky pulse* with an initial sharp rise followed by prolongation as in aortic stenosis. Volume alterations of the pulse may occur from beat to beat. Two variations of the force of the pulse may occur, as follows.

*Pulsus paradoxus* occurs during inspiration. The thorax sucks in blood from the periphery as the pulmonary vascular bed expands, which results in a reduction in the flow of blood from the lungs to the left ventricle during inspiration. Normally this is hardly descernible but it becomes more marked in the presence of severe asthma or if the heart is surrounded by fluid and is unable to expand as usual. The diminished output at the height of inspiration that is detected in these conditions is termed 'pulsus paradoxus'. In *pulsus alternans* there is an alternate variation in the size of the pulse wave, always due to severely impaired left ventricular function.

### Blood pressure

Although the measurement of blood pressure is the most frequently performed ancillary investigation, it is one of the least standardized. Blood pressure is variable and an isolated reading can be misleading. Grossly elevated levels may be found when patients are anxious, and in obese patients care should be taken to use a larger cuff. Good technique in measuring blood pressure is essential. The brachial artery should be carefully palpated and the area of maximum impulse located. The diaphragm of the stethoscope is placed over the brachial artery with the arm extended fully. The armlet of the sphygmomanometer should be pumped up until all sounds disappear. It is then gently released until a soft, thin noise is first heard, which represents the systolic pressure. Pressure within the armlet is slowly reduced until a loud knocking noise is heard, which increases in intensity and then passes suddenly into a softer sound, the sharp transition from the loud knocking to the soft, flowing sound is taken as the diastolic pressure.

### The jugular venous pressure

Estimation of the jugular venous pressure and description of the various wave forms causes much diagnostic difficulty. The patient should be properly positioned at about 45° in a good light and, most importantly of all, feeling relaxed and not tensing the neck muscles. The jugular venous pressure is measured in centimetres above the sternal angle. If difficulty is encountered in seeing this on one side of the neck, try looking at the other side. The internal jugular vein lies between the two heads of the sternomastoid angle. If there is any doubt as to whether a particular pulsation is arterial or venous, try obstructing the venous return as this will obviously have no effect on arterial pulsation. Another useful trick is to press gently but quite hard over the abdomen as this will raise an elevated jugular venous pulsation, and indeed may even bring a normal jugular venous pressure into view. Abdominal compression (called the 'hepatojugular reflux') may also be helpful in making an elevated pressure clearer and thus establishing its wave form. The jugular venous pressure is said to be raised when it is easily visible in the 45° position, the normal being 2 cm above or below the sternal angle. The normal pressure has a physiological 'a' wave resulting from atrial contraction and a physiological 'v' wave resulting from ventricular contraction.

Help in differentiating the 'a' from the 'v' wave on inspection of the jugular venous pressure may be obtained by palpating the radial pulse. The 'v' wave should occur in time with systolic contraction, i.e., at the same time as the pulse, whereas 'a' wave occurs before (Fig. 4.1a).

Giant 'a' waves (Fig. 4.1b) are produced by atrial contraction against an increased resistance. This will occur in any situation where there is raised right ventricular end-diastolic pressure. Because of the raised pressure, the right atrium is contracting by Starling's law to try and augment right ventricular filling and therefore improve cardiac output, usually in the failing right ventricle. Obviously this cannot occur in the presence of atrial fibrillation. The commonest clinical condition giving rise to giant 'a' waves is

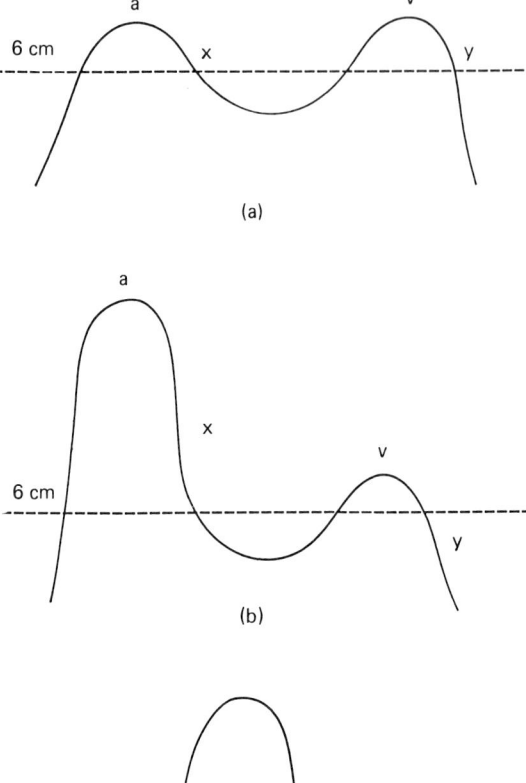

*Figure 4.1* (a) The normal jugular venous pressure. (b) A giant 'a' wave. (c) A cannon wave.

pulmonary hypertension. Pulmonary and triscuspid valve stenosis will also give rise to a giant 'a' wave. The only cause of a large 'v' wave is tricuspid incompetence.

Cannon waves (Fig. 4.1c) occur regularly in atrial tachycardias when the atrium is depolarized after ventricular contraction and therefore the right atrium contracts against a closed tricuspid valve. They occur irregularly in the presence of ventricular extrasystoles and in complete heart block. In these last two conditions the right atrium may contract by chance when the tricuspid valve is closed, producing irregular cannon waves.

## The apex beat

After careful observation and any relevant palpation over the chest, locate the heart apex beat, i.e., the most lateral and inferior part at which the left ventricle can be palpated, normally in the fifth interspace in the mid-clavicular line. Cardiac enlargement, particularly of the left ventricle, will result in lateral and downward displacement of the apex beat.

It is important to palpate the apex beat carefully and determine its character. The apex beat may be *thrusting* when there is left ventricular volume overload such as occurs in mitral or aortic incompetence, or *sustained* due to left ventricular hypertrophy, as occurs in severe aortic stenosis. It was once thought that a *tapping* apex was due to right ventricular hypertrophy but it has now been established that the tapping single apex beat is caused by vibrations associated with a loud first heart sound, typically due to severe mitral stenosis. The main outward pulsation felt at the apex is caused by ventricular systole but is preceded by a smaller pulsation due to atrial contraction. When there is atrial hypertrophy, this atrial impulse may be felt as a bifid beat. This extra-atrial impulse is particularly impressive in hypertrophic cardiomyopathy. A *double impulse* is occasionally felt over a diffuse area and is always due to a left ventricular aneurysm.

## The right ventricle

The right ventricle is only palpated when there is considerable right ventricular hypertrophy, most commonly due to pulmonary hypertension. A right ventricular 'heave' may be palpated at the left sternal edge and is best felt by placing the hand completely flat over this area. Rarely, when the pulmonary artery is grossly enlarged, its pulsation may be felt by pressing two fingers firmly into the second or third left intercostal space.

## Auscultation

After palpation, the heart should be auscultated over the four important areas (see Figs. 4.2 to 4.8 below). Although these areas do not accurately reflect surface markings of heart valves or other structures, they are useful for their uniformity of description.

### Heart sounds

The first heart sound, usually heard as a single sound, is produced by the closure of the mitral and tricuspid valves. Increased intensity is virtually always due to mitral stenosis.

The second sound is caused by the audible closure of the aortic and pulmonary valves. The right ventricle ejects blood into the pulmonary artery a little more slowly than does the left ventricle into the aorta and therefore the aortic component of the second sound occurs before the pulmonary component. On inspiration, more blood is drawn into the thorax and into the right ventricle. Thus normal splitting is exaggerated and more easily audible.

On expiration, likewise, the right ventricular ejection time is shortened and splitting may not be discernible at all. Reverse or paradoxical splitting occurs in aortic stenosis, and left bundle branch block. For either mechanical or electrical reasons closure of the aortic valve is delayed and therefore it will now close after the pulmonary valve. A full inspiration will therefore reduce the splitting, whereas in expiration this 'reversed' splitting will be more easily discernible.

For the same physiological reasons, wide splitting of the second heart sound will occur where there is an increase in the right ventricular ejection time such as with an atrial septal defect or right bundle branch block.

The third and fourth heart sounds are heard in diastole. The third sound is heard when there is rapid left ventricular filling, often in conditions where the left ventricle is dilated. As the blood suddenly enters from the atrium, it causes a shudder of the left ventricular wall in early to mid-diastole (sometimes well discerned on two-dimensional echocardiography), giving rise to a filling sound. This is often very loud in mitral incompetence and when left ventricular function is impaired. A third heart sound is normal up to the age of 35 years but if it is easily discerned after this age, it is probably pathological.

The fourth heart sound occurs in late diastole just before the first and represents atrial contraction. It can occur in the healthy heart but more commonly is a sign of an attempt by the atrium to augment a failing of left ventricular filling at the end of diastole. If loud and easily palpable it may indicate hypertrophic cardiomyopathy. Both the third and fourth heart sounds are low pitched and are therefore best auscultated with the bell of the stethoscope.

As with the overall cardiac examination, the heart should be auscultated using a regular routine. Lie the patient flat and probably start with the aortic area and carotids, moving down through the tricuspid and pulmonary areas to the apex.

Auscultation should also be done with the patient turned over to the left (listening with the bell for a mitral rumble) and with the patient leaning forward (listening with the diaphragm for an early diastolic murmur). The specific timing of heart murmurs and extra sounds can be facilitated by feeling the carotid artery to see if these murmurs or sounds occur during systole or in diastole.

### Additional heart sounds

Loud, high-frequency, early systolic ejection clicks may occur before the systolic ejection murmur in bicuspid aortic valves or in pulmonary valve stenosis. They are best heard in the aortic or pulmonary areas but may also radiate to the mitral area. Clicks that occur later in systole are usually due to mitral leaflet prolapse. These are generally mid to late systolic clicks, frequently followed by a crescendo late systolic murmur, varying in intensity according to the patient's position and usually loudest in the mitral area. The opening snap of the stenosed mitral valve, if present, occurs early in diastole and is followed by the low-frequency, rumbling, diastolic mitral stenotic murmur. All clicks are high-frequency noises and are therefore better appreciated with the diaphragm than the bell of the stethoscope.

Additional sounds may occur in pericardial disease, when a loud pericardial 'knock' may be auscultated or even palpated in severe calcific constrictive pericarditis.

### Signs of heart failure

Careful auscultation of the lung bases may reveal early crepitations that do not clear on coughing, or there may be evidence of pleural effusions. Fluid may accumulate on one side of the chest more than the other, this results because the patient frequently feels better in one particular position, usually leaning forward and to the left. Right heart failure causes an enlarged, tender liver, and if tricuspid incompetence is present, it will pulsate.

Fluid retention developing in heart failure will swell the ankles, and perhaps the scrotum or the sacral area, especially when the patient is confined to bed.

### Heart murmurs

#### Innocent murmurs

These are common in children, young adults and pregnant women. The most common cause is a pulmonary flow murmur, best heard at the left sternal edge. A venous hum is a continuous murmur, common in children, and is usually reduced by neck vein compression or by turning the head laterally. These are always loudest in the neck and around the clavicles and are entirely benign. The following features characterize innocent as opposed to pathological murmurs:
(1) Innocent murmurs are always ejection systolic murmurs. Pansystolic murmurs are more likely to be pathological, commonly due to mitral regurgitation or ventricular septal defects. Diastolic murmurs are always pathological.
(2) There should be no palpable thrill. The aortic and pulmonary components of the second heart sound should be present, equal in intensity and heard to split physiologically on inspiration.
(3) The character of the pulse should be normal.
(4) There should be no systolic ejection click.
(5) There should be no signs of cardiomegaly.
If in doubt it may be necessary to proceed to an ECG, chest X-ray (beware of the pregnant patient) and echocardiography.

#### Pathological murmurs

These are organic, due to valve abnormalities.

The grading of pathological cardiac murmurs is rather a subjective exercise but can be useful, particularly if the patient with a progressive valve lesion is being followed by the same auscultator on a yearly basis. Overall they should be graded as being just audible, soft, moderate or loud. Figures 4.2 to 4.8 illustrate the characteristics of common pathological murmurs.

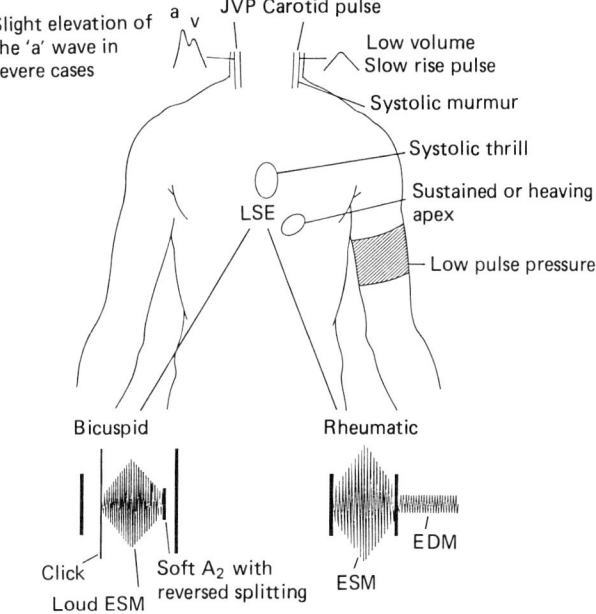

Figure 4.2 Physical signs of aortic stenosis. JVP—jugular venous pressure; LSE—left sternal edge; ESM—ejection systolic murmur; EDM—early diastolic murmur.

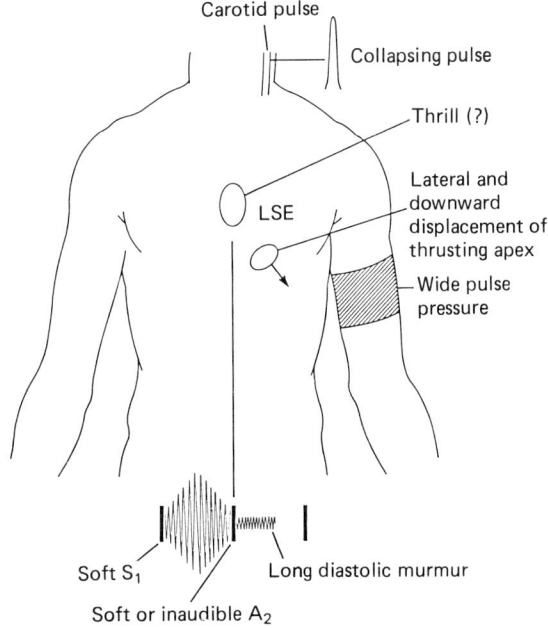

Figure 4.3 Physical signs of aortic regurgitation. LSE—left sternal edge.

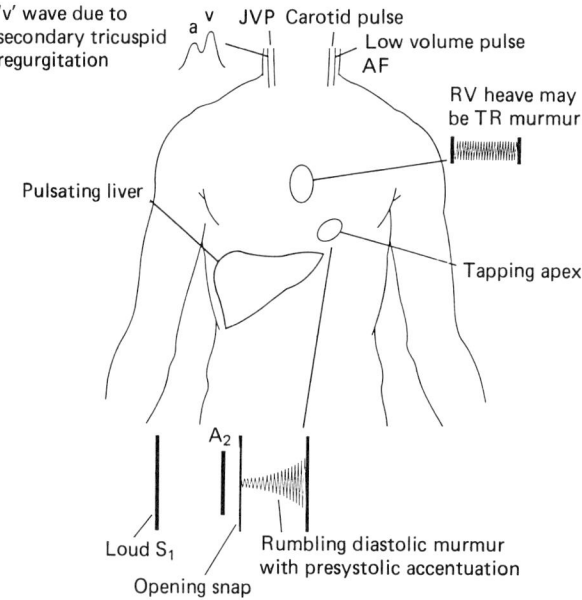

*Figure 4.4* Physical signs of mitral stenosis. JVP—jugular venous pressure; AF—atrial fibrillation; RV—right ventricle; TR—tricuspid. NB. Remember to listen laterally with the bell of the stethoscope as the mitral diastolic murmur may be loudest in the mid-axillary line.

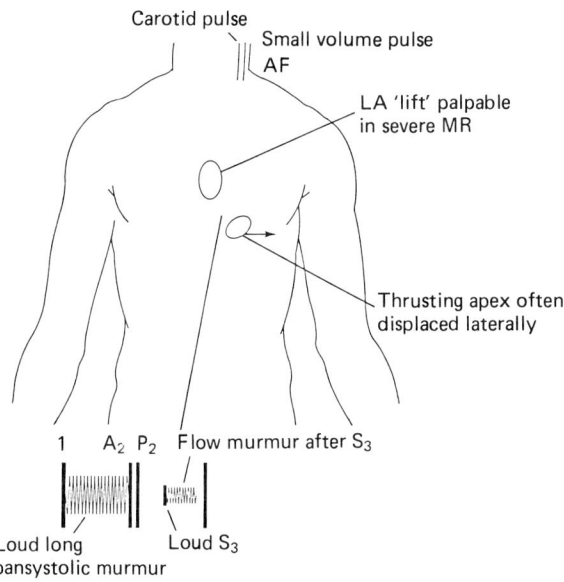

*Figure 4.5* Physical signs of mitral regurgitation (MR). AF—atrial fibrillation; LA—left atrium.

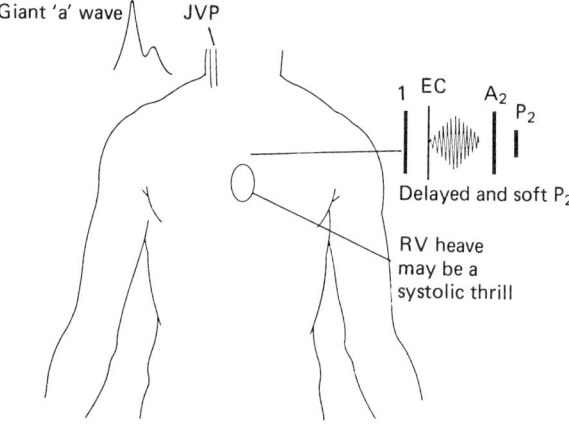

*Figure 4.6*  Physical signs of pulmonary stenosis. JVP—jugular venous pressure; RV—right ventricle. NB. In children the systolic murmur of pulmonary stenosis is often well heard over the back.

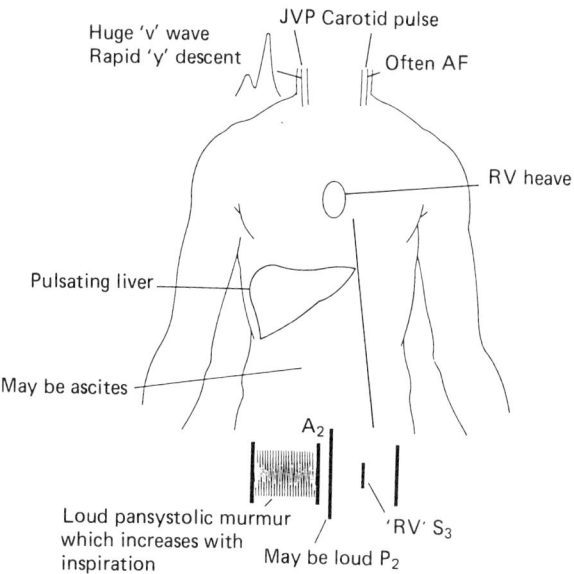

*Figure 4.7*  Physical signs of tricuspid regurgitation. JVP—jugular venous pressure; AF—atrial fibrillation; RV—right ventricle. NB. Tricuspid stenosis is very rare; tricuspid regurgitation is mostly functional or secondary to pulmonary hypertension or severe mitral regurgitation.

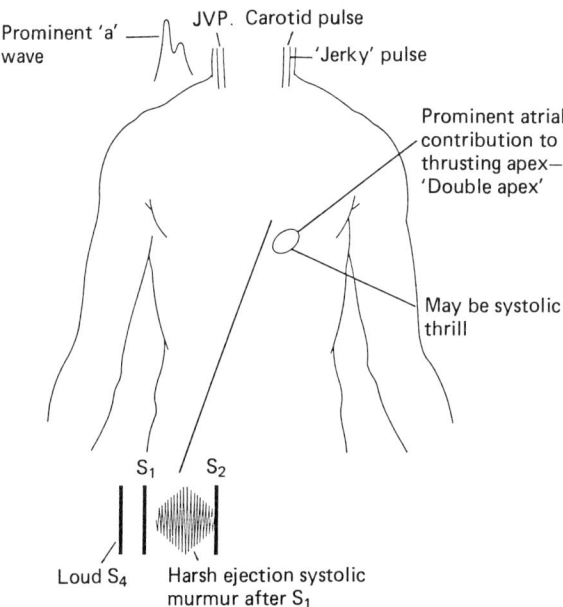

*Figure 4.8* Physical signs of hypertrophic cardiomyopathy. JVP—jugular venous pressure.

## SPECIFIC CARDIAC CONDITIONS

### Angina

There are many causes of chest pain and the specific diagnosis of angina pectoris ('strangulation of the breast') can be difficult.

Typically angina presents as chest tightness or heaviness *brought on by effort* and relieved by rest. The sensation of discomfort rather than actual pain usually starts in the retrosternal region and radiates across the chest, often associated with a heavy feeling in both arms, more commonly the left than the right. It may present in more unusual sites such as the epigastrium or jaw. Angina is often exacerbated by heavy meals, cold air and emotional upset. It may be brought on by stress at work or at home, such as watching a lively football match on television.

#### Aspects of differential diagnosis

##### Non-cardiac pain

Retrosternal pain can be caused by gastrointestinal problems especially hiatus hernia. This pain is often described as a fullness in the chest associated with 'heartburn', an acid feeling in the mouth, and may be precipitated by bending, or by particular foods such as spices or onions. Remember, how-ever, that angina can be brought on by a heavy meal through redistribution of blood from the heart to the intestine.

Spondylosis over the upper spine can also produce retrosternal pain but usually there is a history of arthritis, perhaps tenderness over the thoracic spine and the pain may be exacerbated by twisting movements. Arthritic changes may be seen on a lateral chest X-ray.

A massive pulmonary embolus may cause severe retrosternal pain associated with collapse, dyspnoea and severe cyanosis.

#### Cardiac anxiety

Many patients are worried that they may have premature heart disease, often because of family history or bereavement of a friend. They present with a chest pain that is usually quite easy to differentiate from cardiac ischaemic pain. It is often localized to a small area and described as a 'knife sticking in the chest'. The pain occurs at any time, even at rest. It may be a continuous, dull ache. On examination it may be possible to simulate the pain by palpation of the muscles of the intercostal spaces. This type of pain in the chest wall is very common and naturally causes anxiety. The resting ECG is normal. It is probably better to reassure these patients rather than to perform further tests, such as exercise testing, which usually do more harm than good. Such patients should be discharged with the reassurance that they can always come back if the pain continues or gets worse.

### Clinical examination

In patients complaining of angina pectoris, examination of the cardiovascular system and other systems may be completely unremarkable. However, an aortic ejection murmur suggestive of aortic valve stenosis should be carefully looked for and the physical signs of hypertrophic cardiomyopathy should be obvious. Both may present with a history of angina pectoris. If either condition is suspected, an echocardiogram should be done at an early stage. All peripheral pulses should be carefully palpated. Look for evidence of associated peripheral vascular disease, with or without femoral and carotid artery bruits. Examine the patient for signs of heart failure. If the pulse is irregular it is important to establish what sort (if any) of arrhythmia is present. The blood pressure should be taken lying and standing.

### Investigations

It should be emphasized that the clinical description of typical chest pain and its relation to effort is the most important single aspect in the correct diagnosis of angina pectoris. An ECG may help by showing old ischaemia but more frequently the resting ECG is entirely normal.

If angina is suspected in the presence of a normal ECG, an exercise stress test should be performed (Fig. 4.9). This is important for prognosis but also because if strongly positive (particularly if associated with hypotension) then early coronary angiography is indicated.

Careful monitoring and observation are essential during an exercise stress test to ensure the patient's safety and to clarify the diagnosis. It should not be done simply for an analysis of ST segment changes, but also to assess further the site, severity and character of pain and to look for concomitant haemodynamic changes such as a fall in blood pressure.

Thallium scanning can be used instead of, or in addition to, exercise testing in the diagnosis of angina pectoris. Its sensitivity and value are similar to treadmill testing and the choice depends on the available facilities. In most hospitals, treadmill

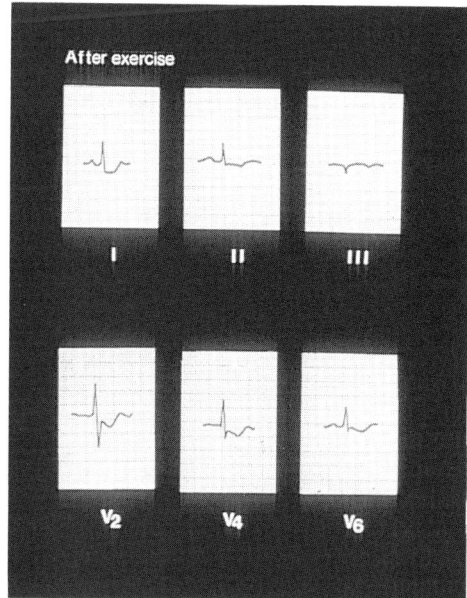

*Figure 4.9* A positive exercise test with ST segment depression best seen in standard lead I and chest lead $V_2$.

exercise testing is easier where a large number of patients may require this assessment. A thallium scan is particularly useful when the standard exercise test is equivocal because, in combination, the two tests have increased sensitivity. If the exercise test is equivocal and the thallium test definitely negative, the patient can be reassured and coronary angiography avoided.

The chest X-ray is usually normal in patients with angina. However, if there are signs of heart failure, an exercise stress test should be avoided.

### When should a patient be referred for coronary angiography?

This is a controversial question. However, because of the poor correlation between the severity of symptoms and the extent of coronary disease found on investigation, some cardiologists argue that all patients with angina should have coronary angiography. Because bypass surgery is now well established as an effective treatment for angina pectoris where medical treatment has failed, in the absence of other severe medical problems, any patient with disabling angina despite maximum medical treatment should be referred for further investigation with a view to surgery. Patients under 40 years (and some would say under 50 years of age) with angina should always be further investigated. Patients with a strongly positive exercise test at an early stage should also be investigated because it is likely that they have left main-stem disease.

Another reason to embark on coronary angiography is an absolute need for a diagnosis of puzzling chest pain and, indeed, it may be less expensive than repeated hospital admissions for an anxious patient.

### Other investigations

If a hiatus hernia or peptic ulceration is suspected, the preferred investigation is outpatient endoscopy but, should this not be available, a barium swallow and meal should be done. Ambulatory monitoring—although not routinely used in the investigation of angina pectoris—may be helpful in looking for symptomatic or asymptomatic arrhythmias accompanying chest pain. Also, if calibrated carefully, it may be useful in ascertaining the number and severity of changes in the ST segment that occur with or *without* angina.

### Management of angina pectoris

Management of the patient with angina is directed towards improvement in the quality of life by relief of symptoms. It may be that prognosis can also be improved, although this has not been clearly established. Initial steps to be taken are the relief of pain and the control of risk factors, especially cigarette smoking, hypertension and hypercholesterolaemia.

### Mild angina

When mild, angina can sometimes be wholly managed by careful explanation and slight modification of the patient's activities. Avoiding the activities known to bring on angina, such as lifting heavy weights, may be the only treatment needed. The patient should be strongly advised to stop smoking as it has now been well established that this is the main risk factor in the progression of early ischaemic heart disease. Emotional stress and anxiety can be treated with tranquillizers, but careful counselling and explanation may be more effective. Although obesity is not an established risk factor it increases the workload of the heart, and weight reduction should be advised.

Glyceryl trinitrate is effective in relieving angina if taken correctly. Nitrates remain a mainstay in the management of angina pectoris. Glyceryl trinitrate can be used in a sublingual, buccal or spray preparation and it is probably advisable to allow the patient to try each method and choose the most suitable. It takes about two minutes to work so a preparation should be taken at the onset of an attack of angina or even before if an activity such as sexual intercourse is known to bring on pain. Glyceryl trinitrate is a profound vasodilator and its main side-effects are therefore flushing and headaches, which can be quite severe. It is quite safe and patients can be reassured that they can take more than two or three tablets daily, provided that headaches are not troublesome. However, should they need much larger quantities of trinitrate, further treatment is indicated.

### Moderate angina

Management includes the same principles as for mild angina but the following further therapies should be considered.
(1) *Long-acting nitrates.* The action of glyceryl trinitrate lasts between 30 and 45 minutes. Longer acting oral nitrates have been developed and used with efficacy and safety for many years. The newer preparations of isosorbide mononitrate are now supplanting the older isosorbide dinitrates, their advantage being that they do not need to undergo first-pass metabolism in the liver and their bioavailability is thus greater. Nitrate preparations have been successfully developed where the drug is administered from a small plaster with a rate-limiting membrane that controls its release over a 24-h period. The plasters are waterproof. Oral and transdermal nitrates are useful in the long-term control of angina but intolerance does occur in some patients. The main side-effect is headache.
(2) *β-blockers.* These work by reducing heart rate and cardiac output by blocking sympathetic drive and lowering the oxygen consumption of the myocardium. There are over 20 β-blockers to choose from in the UK and, as for hypertension, it is wise to use only one or two preparations and get to know their actions and side-effects well. The patient's heart rate will usually drop to around 60/min and, more importantly, it will fail to accelerate rapidly on moderate exercise. Ancillary properties, such as a membrane stabilizing effect and the

presence of intrinsic sympathomimetic activity, which are often stressed by pharmaceutical companies, are of relatively little importance clinically. The only important ancillary effect is cardioselectivity (which means that these β-blockers affect the cardiac $\beta_1$-receptors more than the respiratory $\beta_2$-receptors) and are therefore more suitable in patients with bronchospasm, although they should always be used with care. They may also be better tolerated in patients with peripheral vascular disease. Side-effects, such as airways resistance, cold extremities and fatigue, can occur; other effects, such as depression and impotence, may not be volunteered by the patient and therefore should be sought by the physician.

(3) *Calcium antagonists.* Calcium blockers reduce the transmembrane transport of calcium ions on which vascular tissue depends for contraction and impulse formation, playing an important part in the degree of contraction and tone of coronary and other arteries. These drugs are particularly useful when 'coronary artery spasm' is thought to contribute to anginal symptoms. This may be a particular syndrome in young smokers with highly vasoactive coronary arteries, or may play a part in development of pain in patients with occlusive atheroma. Calcium antagonists may be useful alone or combined with β-blockers in the treatment of angina.

### Severe angina

The first step is to ensure that the management procedures of mild and moderate angina are being followed. Is the patient still smoking? Is he or she adequately β-blocked? The latter question can be answered by taking the patient's heart rate at rest and again after a short walk around the outpatients department. Only if the heart rate barely alters is the patient fully β-blocked and therefore deriving maximum benefit.

When medical treatment is failing to enable the patient to lead a happy and full life, a coronary artery bypass graft should be considered. This procedure involves taking a length of saphenous vein from the patient's leg, reversing the vein and sewing it on to the aorta and into the coronary artery distal to the coronary artery stenosis. There are three main coronary arteries (Fig. 4.10) and

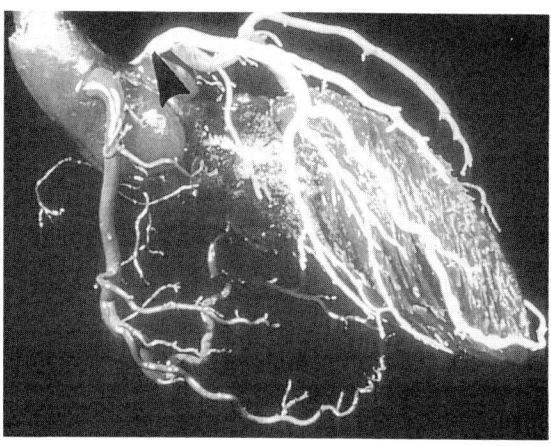

Figure 4.10   Illustration of a normal coronary arterial tree. The arrow is pointing to the 'left main stem'.

grafts can be placed on all of these and even on some of the larger branches. Proximal, single occlusions are more easily treated than distal, diffuse lesions.

When the most important part of the coronary tree, i.e., the left main stem (see arrow on Fig. 4.10), is involved, and also when all three major arteries are involved and grafted, it has been shown that surgically treated patients live longer than medically treated patients. On the other hand, if only one or even two of the larger vessels are involved (and the left main stem is clear of disease), there is no statistical proof that surgery improves prognosis.

Whatever the severity or extent of anatomical disease, this operation can be dramatically successful in the relief of disabling angina.

The important questions to ask when contemplating surgical treatment are:
(1) Is medical treatment producing side-effects, and how bad are they?
(2) Although medical treatment may have relieved pain, is this because the patient is now severely limiting his or her physical activity?
(3) More specifically, ask the patient, 'Is there anything presently you are not doing because of your angina (or its medical treatment)?'

If a young patient is unable to work because of severe side-effects, he or she is probably better off with surgery. On the other hand, if an elderly patient is well managed with only occasional pain on moderate doses of anti-anginal therapy, then it is meddlesome to interfere.

### Unstable angina

Many of these patients will be known to have angina. A sudden change in crescendo, 'pre-infarction' or unstable angina should therefore be taken seriously. It is defined as increasing frequency and severity of angina and is particularly worrying if it is associated with rest or nocturnal pain. Investigation and surgery carry an increased risk, so it is now well established that these patients should be managed medically until the symptoms settle and then they should be investigated early with a view to elective surgery.

Patients with unstable angina should be admitted to hospital and put on complete bed rest. It is wise to restrict visitors. Light sedation should be employed if necessary. The patient should be assessed clinically and by ECG monitoring. The role of analgesia is controversial because some feel this masks ongoing symptoms and is therefore detrimental to management. Most clinicians, however, would give diamorphine when required.

Patients should be on a combination of nitrates (in any form that they find most tolerable), a β-blocker and also a calcium antagonist. Provided that there are no gastrointestinal contraindications, daily aspirin should be started. If symptoms do not settle on this regimen, then intravenous nitrates are very useful, increasing the dose until the pain and the change in the ST segment have settled or side-effects, including severe headaches and/or hypotension, supervene. If the blood pressure is normal, the pain is ongoing and the patient is not experiencing headaches, he or she is probably *not* getting enough intravenous nitrates. If the pain persists and, in particular, if the ST segments continue to fluctuate after 48 h, coronary angiography should be considered. Subsequent management depends on the catheter findings. If a critical proximal lesion in one artery is found, angioplasty should be considered, whereas diffuse three-vessel disease will need surgery.

All procedures carry an increased risk in the patient with unstable angina and are better done on an elective basis. However, emergency invasive therapy may be mandatory.

There is no evidence yet that thrombolysis is effective in the management of unstable angina, but much useful research is currently being done in this area.

## Heart failure

### Symptoms

The most common presentation of a patient with heart failure is with dyspnoea. However, it is important to ascertain that the dyspnoea is due to heart failure as opposed to one of the other common causes of shortness of breath, which are:

Respiratory disease
Anaemia
Diabetic ketoacidosis
Uraemia
Anxiety

Remember that acute pulmonary oedema can present with a wheeze very similar to asthma. The patient's age is the best clue. Although asthma does occur in middle-aged or elderly people, acute pulmonary oedema is a more common cause of acute dyspnoea.

Shortness of breath is subjective, defined as a feeling of suffocation, the need to take an extra breath, or having to breathe more deeply to feel comfortable. In heart failure this is produced by increased lung stiffness caused by pulmonary oedema. Although there are many ways of assessing severity of dyspnoea, such as the commonly used New York Heart Association grading system, the severity is probably best described by the patient in terms of distance walked, or number of stairs climbed without having to stop. It may be helpful to watch the patient undressing, or to walk a short distance with him or her to see how quickly dyspnoea develops.

Orthopnoea is the feeling of shortness of breath when lying flat, produced by fluid accumulating at the bottom of the lungs. It usually occurs as the heart failure and dyspnoea get worse.

Paroxysmal nocturnal dyspnoea is manifested as feelings of suffocation when going to sleep, or having to sleep upright, or waking breathless and having to climb out of bed to open a window. Wheezing is common and a cough productive of pink, frothy sputum often accompanies the breathlessness.

Fatigue is a common and disabling symptom of heart failure.

## Clinical examination

The patient should be assessed in a relaxed atmosphere. Note if the patient is dyspnoeic at rest and if he or she gets short of breath doing simple things like undressing or climbing onto the examination couch. Signs of left and right heart failure should be sought. The general examination includes looking for the other causes of dyspnoea, such as anaemia. The blood pressure should be measured.

The pulse should be examined for regularity, volume and character. Arrhythmias may be contributing to the heart failure. A low-volume pulse may be due to aortic stenosis or simply a sign of severe left ventricular dysfunction. It is a bad prognostic sign. The character of the pulse may help to make a specific diagnosis, such as aortic regurgitation or hypertrophic cardiomyopathy. Auscultation of the heart is mandatory. The sudden onset of severe failure in association with a new systolic murmur may be due to a myocardial infarction and the patient may need to be referred to a cardiothoracic centre for either closure of a ventricular septal defect or repair of a ruptured mitral valve. The typical murmurs of aortic and mitral valve disease have already been illustrated and it should be emphasized that these murmurs will not always be easy to hear in the presence of loud crackles due to pulmonary oedema. It is important to auscultate the patient daily as important physical signs may be easier to elicit once the patient is more comfortable, relaxed and has a slower respiratory rate.

## Investigations

The chest X-ray is important and often shows signs, even in mild heart failure. The first abnormality to occur is cardiomegaly followed by signs of pulmonary oedema with upper lobe blood diversion, pleural effusions (which may be bigger on one side than the other) and Kerley's 'B' lines (Fig. 4.11).

There are many methods of assessing left ventricular function but echocardiography is safe, simple, cheap and probably as effective as the others. Ejection fractions worked out by this method are not very accurate but it is usually easy to ascertain if the reduction in left ventricular function is mild, moderate or severe.

An ECG may show ischaemic changes or hypertrophy due to valvular heart disease. In the presence of an irregular pulse, a long rhythm strip will ascertain what type of arrhythmia is present.

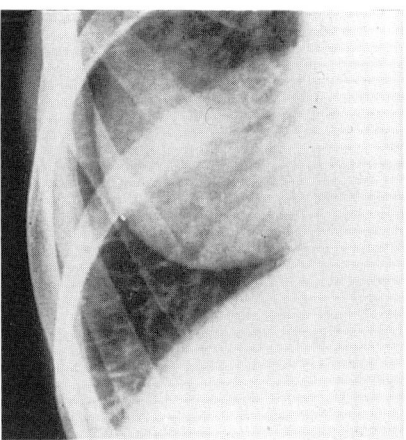

*Figure 4.11*  Kerley's 'B' lines.

Exercise testing is not usually necessary in the diagnosis of heart failure and can indeed be dangerous. Graded exercise tests, however, may be useful in mild to moderate heart failure in the analysis of various drug therapies.

### Cardiac catheterization

Most of the important information regarding valvular dysfunction and left ventricular performance can be obtained non-invasively by echocardiography. Cardiac ultrasonography combined with Doppler techniques can now easily diagnose aortic and mitral valve regurgitation. It can also measure valve gradients.

The main use of cardiac catheterization is therefore in the assessment of the presence and/or severity of coronary artery disease. Left ventricular angiography is also necessary if there is a suspicion of a left ventricular aneurysm; here removal of the aneurysm, usually combined with coronary artery bypass grafting, may dramatically improve left ventricular function.

Most surgeons prefer to know the anatomy of the coronary arteries before replacement of an aortic valve, even in relatively young patients. If necessary, coronary artery bypass grafting can then be done at the same time as valve replacement.

Invasive tests are also required before heart transplantation.

### Management of heart failure

First look for and treat any precipitating cause of heart failure such as thyrotoxicosis or anaemia.

Patients with chronic heart failure may also be helped by treatment of specific arrhythmias, most commonly with digoxin if the patient is in atrial fibrillation with a fast ventricular response. Next, any surgically correctable cause such as aortic stenosis should be excluded.

In advanced disease of the coronary arteries there is no convincing evidence that bypass surgery improves left ventricular function, but it may still be necessary to consider this in patients with heart failure if they suffer from severe concomitant angina. Reducing risk factors, such as smoking and hypertension, may prevent worsening of coronary artery disease but will not improve existing dysfunction. Although there is doubt as to whether there is a specific entity called 'alcoholic cardiomyopathy', it is certainly true that alcohol depresses myocardial function and should be avoided in patients with left ventricular failure.

## Mild heart failure

Many patients are able to lead a normal life if taking oral diuretics and digoxin. Digoxin is particularly important in controlling the ventricular response to atrial fibrillation but also has a small positive inotropic effect in some patients, although of short duration. Watch for side-effects, however, particularly in elderly patients and those with impaired kidney function, as 80 per cent of this drug is excreted by the kidneys. Side-effects include gastrointestinal symptoms, anorexia, nausea and, occasionally, diarrhoea. Too much digoxin can potentiate arrhythmias, e.g., paroxysmal atrial tachycardia with a varying block, and also ventricular ectopics (especially bigeminal rhythm). Serum digoxin levels can be estimated (the therapeutic range being taken as 1.5–3 ng/l).

Frusemide is still the most popular diuretic in heart failure. Any aldosterone antagonist can be used in combination with frusemide and will potentiate a diuresis. Both drugs can also be combined with a thiazide with further beneficial action as all three drugs have a separate mode of action. The main side-effects of diuresis are those associated with hypokalaemia. Potassium depletion is very common in patients taking thiazides. Serum potassium levels should be regularly checked in all patients who are on any sort of diuretic.

A concomitant rise in serum urea can also be detrimental and may give rise to confusion in the elderly. Thiazides can precipitate gout.

## Moderate heart failure

These patients need larger doses of frusemide and spironolactone. Vasodilators have probably been supplanted by angiotensin-converting enzyme (ACE) inhibitors such as captopril or enalapril. These drugs are effective and have fewer side-effects. There is inceasing evidence that patients in heart failure have a longer life expectancy and better quality of life on regular ACE inhibition.

ACE inhibitors are vasodilators and also lower aldosterone levels, thus reducing sodium and hence water retention. As with other vasodilators, their main side-effect is hypotension, and therefore they need to be used with care in moderate to severe heart failue, where blood pressure is frequently low.

## Severe heart failure

Digoxin, diuretics and ACE inhibitors in optimum doses should be used as a first step; metolazone potentiates the effect of diuretics. If no improvement is noted, more drastic treatment has to be considered, such as reducing fluid and salt intake. Regular daily bed rest is often beneficial and it may be helpful to hospitalize the patient for a week or 10 days of complete bed rest.

Heart transplantation should be considered in young patients. Results continue to improve each year. The present prognosis for the transplanted heart (not the patient, who can be given two or even three transplants) is about 50 per cent success at five years. If transplantation is to be considered, the patient should be assessed in a specialist unit. Consideration is given to the patient's general systemic health, age and psychological ability to tolerate the rigors of transplantation, including immunosuppression, long-term follow-up, and regular endomyocardial biopsy. If successful, however, cardiac transplantation can produce dramatic improvement in health and quality of life.

## ARRHYTHMIAS

Palpitation is the sensation of the heart beating. This may be fast or slow, regular or irregular. When a patient complains of palpitations he or she should be encouraged to keep a diary of these events, to ascertain their length and frequency, whether they are daily or nocturnal and, also to discover any precipitating factor such as alcohol.

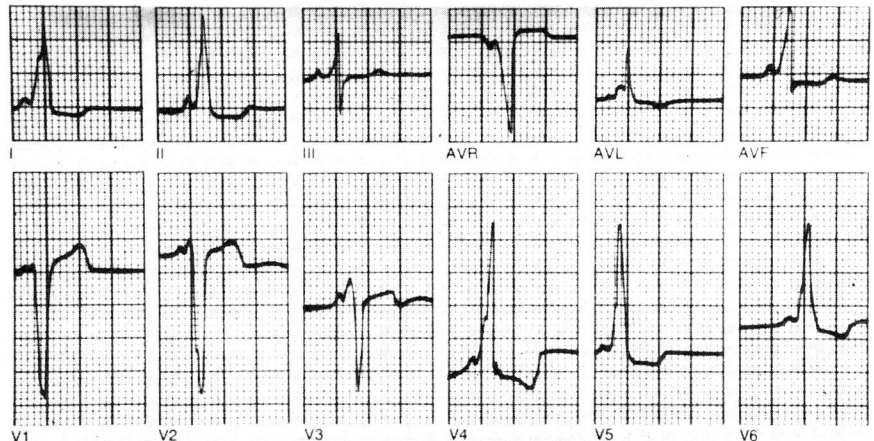

*Figure 4.12* The Wolff–Parkinson–White syndrome showing a short PR interval, a slurred upstroke delta wave and a broadened QRS complex.

Possible systemic disease such as thyrotoxicosis should be carefully sought. Palpitations may also accompany angina, or dyspnoea due to heart failure.

Lastly, and most importantly, when interviewing a patient complaining of palpitations, an assessment of their personality, mood, family and financial worries should be made. The most frequent cause of palpitations is mild anxiety. Patients, more often women than men, with domestic problems suffer palpitations and this symptom can be real and very distressing. There may also be an element of cardiac neurosis, especially if there is a concomitant family history of heart disease—this is more common in men. Patients with anxiety-related palpitations most commonly notice their symptom on going to bed. Alcohol is a potent precipitator of palpitations, particularly in men with lone or idiopathic atrial fibrillation.

A systemic examination should be made and, in particular, signs of thyrotoxicosis sought. Examination of the cardiovascular system may reveal a definite organic cause, such as mild mitral stenosis, hypertrophic cardiomyopathy or heart failure. The blood pressure should be taken, although hypertension is not a common cause of palpitations.

### Investigations

#### The ECG

If during the interview or examination, the patient begins to have an attack of palpitations, a rhythm strip should be performed immediately. The resting ECG may be diagnostic as in Wolff–Parkinson–White syndrome (Fig. 4.12).

#### Echocardiography

If there is clinical or electrocardiographic suspicion of hypertrophic cardiomyopathy, an echocardiogram will be diagnostic. It also helps in the presence of a diastolic murmur (or even in the absence of such a murmur) in the patient with intermittent episodes of atrial fibrillation, when it may reveal 'silent' mitral stenosis.

#### Chest X-ray

In the absence of abnormal auscultatory findings or signs of heart failure, the chest X-ray is likely to be normal.

#### Ambulatory monitoring

Ambulatory monitoring may be useful in the detection of symptomatic and asymptomatic tachy- and bradyarrhythmias. Continuous monitoring is by far the more useful investigation if bradyarrhythmias are suspected, but can also be useful in detecting tachyarrhythmias. The main use of the 'cardiac memo' seems to be in reassuring young people of the benign nature of attacks of sinus arrhythmia or sinus tachycardia.

Continuous ambulatory monitoring is useful in assessing the efficacy of various anti-arrhythmic drugs. This investigation should always be done in patients with hypertrophic cardiomyopathy because these may have long episodes of asymptomatic ventricular tachycardia, which if treated with amiodarone will result in an improved overall prognosis.

### Electrophysiological studies

Measurement of the conduction time interval and programmed atrial and/or ventricular stimulation are not required in most patients complaining of palpitations, but may be useful in the following situations:

(1) To confirm the presence of and investigate the site of aberrant pathways when conditions such as Wolff–Parkinson–White syndrome are suspected—particularly if surgical transection of this pathway is contemplated.

(2) To investigate refractory supraventricular tachycardias and therefore to outline the best treatment. Once treatment has begun, provocative electrophysiological studies may be undertaken later to ensure it has been effective.

(3) To delineate the site of an ectopic ventricular focus of electrical instability (for example, myocardial scars following myocarditis or small aneurysms following myocardial infarction).

(4) It may be necessary to assess conduction times within different parts of the conducting tissue of the heart before the insertion of a permanent pacemaker. This is unusual, however, and the decision to insert a pacemaker can almost always be made on clinical grounds supplemented by ambulatory monitoring.

## Treatment of specific arrhythmias

Arrhythmias are common. They may occur in people with normal hearts or they may represent a clinical manifestation of serious cardiac disease.

There are two groups of arrhythmias—fast and slow. In some clinical situations, particularly the 'sick sinus syndrome', both may occur.

### Bradyarrhythmias

#### Sinus bradycardia

Sinus bradycardia may be a normal rhythm particularly in a fit athlete. Other causes include β-blocking agents, which are the commonest cause of a sinus bradycardia, so a careful drug history is essential. A slow heart rate may also be due to sinoatrial disease, especially in elderly patients, and its context always has to be judged with reference to the patient's age, other cardiac problems and general health.

#### Sinus node disease

Any part of the heart can work as its own intrinsic pacemaker, but the specialized conducting tissue is especially geared for pacemaking activity. The further down the heart, from the sinus node through the atrioventricular node to the ventricle, the slower the intrinsic activity of each area, i.e., the idioventricular pacemaker activity is about 20 to 30/min, the atrioventricular node is 40 to 50, and the sinoatrial node normally fires at 60 to 70. What happens within a heart is that the impulse from above 'captures' the pacemaker below and stops it from firing. However, if this impulse from above does not occur then the pacemaker below (which will be the atrioventricular node in the case of sinoatrial node arrest) will 'escape'. An example of sinoatrial arrest is shown in Fig. 4.13. This shows an episode of sinus node arrest followed by a pause and then a normal atrioventricular node escape beat (note the normal QRS complex that occurs in this situation).

Sinus node arrest may occur in normal people with high vagal tone, but more commonly it reflects a diseased node often exacerbated by drugs, electrolyte disturbances or ischaemia.

*Figure 4.13* Sinus node arrest.

## Heart block

Heart block occurs as a congenital variant but more often results from pathological processes affecting the conducting tissue, such as idiopathic fibrosis or ischaemia. Drugs like digoxin and β-blocking agents frequently cause varying degrees of heart block. Calcification associated with aortic valve stenosis may extend into the conducting tissue and cause heart block. Heart block is also a common postoperative complication of aortic valve replacement or repair of a ventriculoseptal defect.

It is important to know whether heart block is the precise cause of the presenting symptoms. It may be a coincidental finding in a patient who has syncopal episodes due to epilepsy. Ambulatory monitoring or careful observation on stress testing may help to correlate symptoms with intermittent episodes of heart block.

**First degree atrioventricular block.** This is an ECG finding diagnosed by a prolonged PR interval (Fig. 4.14). It may be normal in young athletes with high vagal tone. More commonly it is a manifestation of disease, such as inferior myocardial infarction, or of electrolyte disturbances or hypothermia. Many drugs, especially digoxin, prolong the PR interval.

**Second degree atrioventricular block.** There are two forms of second degree atrioventricular block.

*Mobitz type I*—is also known as the Wenckebach phenomenon. This is shown in Fig. 4.15. Here the PR interval progressively lengthens with each succeeding beat until finally an atrial complex is not followed by a QRS complex and a 'dropped' beat therefore occurs.

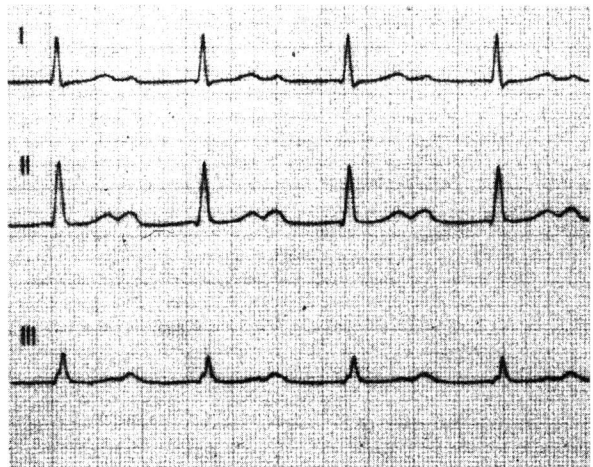

*Figure 4.14* An ECG showing first-degree atrioventricular block with an extremely long PR interval seen in all three leads.

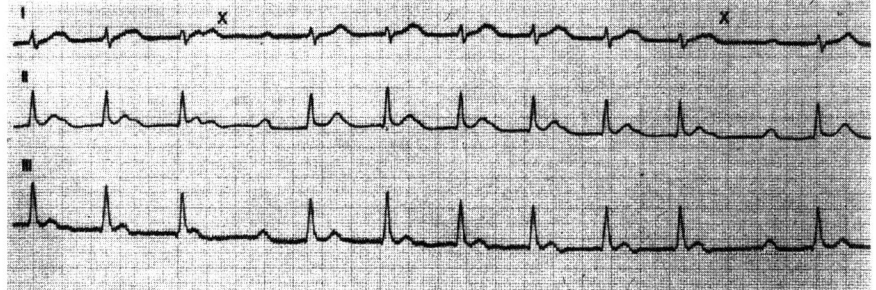

*Figure 4.15* An ECG showing a sinus tachycardia complicated by second-degree (type I) atrioventricular block (the Wenckebach phenomenon). There is a progressive increase in the PR interval with the sequence terminating in a blocked sinus impulse: a P wave (x) that is not followed by a QRS complex.

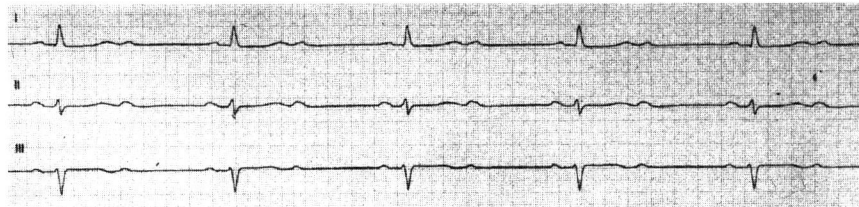

*Figure 4.16* An ECG showing sinus bradycardia with second-degree (type 2) atrioventricular block. There are two P waves before each QRS complex.

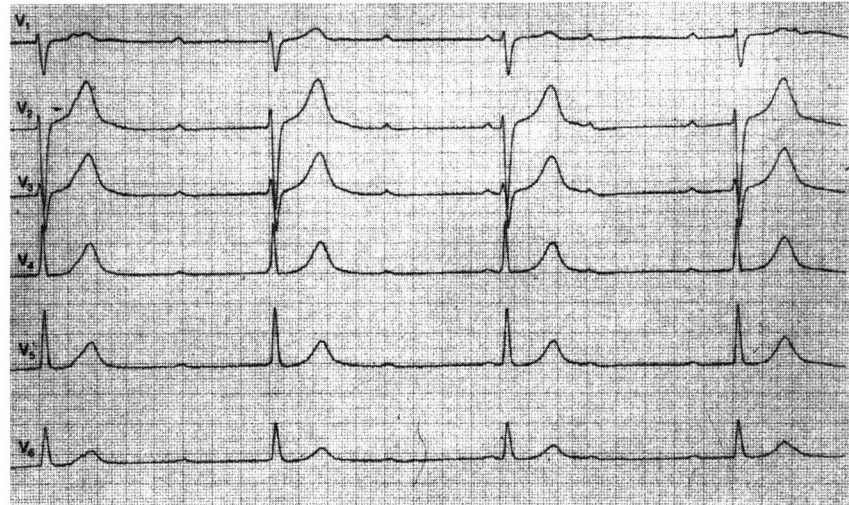

*Figure 4.17* An ECG showing third-degree heart block with complete disassociation between P wave and QRS activity.

*Mobitz type II*—occurs when not all the atrial complexes are conducted and usually there is a consistent, unvarying degree to this block where there may be two preceding P waves before each complex (2 to 1) (Fig. 4.16). The PR interval in this case does not vary.

**Third degree atrioventricular block.** In this degree block P waves occur independently of the QRS complexes (Fig. 4.17). This can be associated with a slow ventricular rate that provides an inadequate blood supply to the brain; this results in syncope (the Stokes–Adams attack). This slow ventricular rate may also give rise to heart failure, particularly where there is associated reduced left ventricular function. Dramatic symptomatic improvement will occur after the insertion of a pacemaker. When complete heart block occurs with a narrow QRS complex the impulse to depolarization is coming from the atrioventricular node or the bundle of His, but when associated with an idio-ventricular rhythm this type of complete heart block is considered more sinister and more frequently associated with symptoms of syncope and heart failure.

**Treatment of heart block.** It is important to treat the patient rather than the patient's ECG. First degree atrioventricular block almost never requires any treatment and frequently reverts to normal. This is particularly true if it is associated with resolving myocardial oedema after recent infarction. Second and third degree block may well be associated with symptoms that should be treated, with a permanent pacemaker. Complete heart block usually, but not always, is associated with symptoms that can be easily relieved by permanent pacing. Because of the improved technology associated with permanent systems and the extremely low morbidity and negligible mortality associated with this operation, permanent systems are now being inserted on the basis of 'softer' clinical evidence. It is also argued that the arrhythmia, from whatever cause, is unlikely to improve and may well deteriorate, so symptoms can be averted by the 'prophylactic' presence of a pacemaker. Nevertheless, implantation rates in the UK are much lower than in Europe and the USA.

If a patient with Stokes–Adams attacks is admitted via casualty, a temporary pacemaker is usually inserted before a permanent system is provided. However, if theatre space and technical staff are available it is better to insert a permanent system immediately the conduction defect is diagnosed.

### Tachyarrhythmias

These are arrhythmias associated with fast beating of the heart. First exclude a normal sinus tachycardia or a mild sinus arrhythmia due to anxiety exacerbated by caffeine, cigarettes or alcohol. Then the more significant tachyarrhythmias should be considered and differentiated as follows.

Paroxysmal atrial tachycardia (PAT)
Paroxysmal atrial tachycardia (PAT) with block
Atrial flutter
Atrial fibrillation
Pre-excitation syndrome (usually Wolff–Parkinson–White syndrome)
Ventricular extrasystoles
Ventricular tachycardia (VT)
Ventricular fibrillation (VF)

Clinical examination is important to exclude diseases that can produce disorders of cardiac rhythm such as thyrotoxicosis or mitral stenosis. A drug history is essential. Often electrocardiography is unhelpful because the record is taken over a short, limited period. Ambulatory monitoring and/or transtelephone monitoring systems can be used for the transmission of arrhythmic events.

### Supraventricular extrasystoles

Isolated supraventricular ectopic beats—arising from within the atrium but outside the sinoatrial node—are common and almost always benign. Typically the P waves will have a slightly different size and shape and the PR interval will be different and usually shorter than the normal PR interval.

### Paroxysmal atrial tachycardia

Atrial tachycardia occurs with a sudden onset and equally sudden termination. The rate is 170 to 220 beats/min and there is usually normal atrioventricular conduction, particularly with atrial rates of less than 200 beats/min. Most episodes therefore produce a QRS complex of normal shape and size, although so-called conduction with aberration may occur, producing the patterns of left or right bundle branch block. When this occurs the differential diagnosis between an atrial tachycardia with aberrant conduction and actual ventricular tachycardia is difficult.

Tips that help distinguish ventricular tachycardia from supraventricular tachycardia (SVT) with aberration are as follows.

(1) SVT is *usually* faster than VT.
(2) A wider, bizarre-shaped QRS complex is much more in favour of VT.
(3) There should be evidence of atrioventricular dissociation with discernible P waves in a VT:
   (a) in VT the complexes will not be *exactly* the same because of the concealed independent P-wave activity;
   (b) in VT a therapeutic trial of a short-acting β-blocker (e.g., pindolol) may exaggerate atrioventricular dissociation and produce a PR interval.
(4) The QRS morphology may be helpful:
   (a) if the primary R wave in $V_1$ is more positive than the second R wave then this is strongly in favour of SVT;
   (b) deep S waves in $V_6$ suggest VT.

*Remember*:
(1) The patient's haemodynamic response is a poor guide. The patient may walk into casualty smiling and still be in VT.
(2) There is a bias amongst doctors to favour SVT. Look at the tracings carefully and do not be afraid to diagnose VT.
(3) If in doubt it is safer to assume the patient has VT and to treat accordingly.

PATs are benign and occur in the healthy heart. They may be produced by an abnormal ectopic focus within the atria but are more commonly due to a re-entry phenomenon, and are often terminated by vagal manoeuvres. Attacks may be stopped by a Valsalva manoeuvre, carotid sinus massage (one side may be more effective than the other and both sides should *not* be massaged at the same time), a cold drink or by rebreathing into a paper bag.

If these manoeuvres are not successful, pharmacological treatment is aimed at slowing or blocking conduction at some point within the re-entry circuit. The various options have already been discussed in Chapter 2. The attacks may be asymptomatic and short, or be long and quite distressing. If the latter, both patient and physician need to decide if long-term therapy is justified, given that side-effects may be encountered in a relatively benign condition that is not life threatening.

### Paroxysmal atrial tachycardia with block

Most cases of PAT with block are caused by digoxin toxicity. When PAT occurs with varying degrees of atrioventricular block, an irregular pulse is produced and a misdiagnosis easily made that the patient is in atrial fibrillation and not receiving enough digoxin. Careful analysis of the ECG, however, will show that the patient is receiving too much digoxin. Digoxin should immediately be stopped and, if necessary, potassium supplements given.

### Atrial flutter

In this arrhythmia (Fig. 4.18), the rhythm strip of atrial flutter is characterized by close coarse atrial flutter waves that occur at a frequency of about 280 to 320 per min. They give a 'saw tooth' appearance to the isoelectric line of the ECG and are usually best seen in standard lead II or in lead $V_1$. Atrial flutter is characterized by regular, repetitive wide atrial deflections of identical size, shape and timing. The rate of atrial discharge may be related to atrial size, slow rates being associated with large atria. Atrioventricular conduction shows variable degrees of block. Although one-to-one conduction may occur with slow rates of flutter, this is very uncommon and more usual two-to-one or four-to-one are seen. The number of P waves is always one more than that apparently seen, as one of the P waves is 'concealed' within the QRS complex. Therefore note that in Fig. 4.18 the amount of block is four-to-one and not three-to-one as might initially be thought.

There may also be transient episodes of atrial fibrillation alternating with flutter. The causes and treatment of atrial fibrillation and flutter are more or less identical. Frequently the block varies rather than being regular and this produces a completely irregular pulse.

Digoxin is still the treatment of choice, but amiodarone is being increasingly used, particularly for elderly patients. Quinine may be useful in suppressing paroxysms of atrial flutter. It is

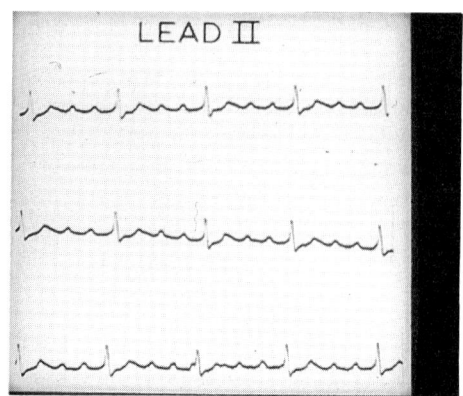

*Figure 4.18* Atrial flutter with a fixed 4:1 atrioventricular block.

important to differentiate atrial flutter from paroxysmal tachycardia because verapamil is not very useful in the treatment of atrial flutter.

### Atrial fibrillation

Although there is a small group of patients who have what is called 'lone atrial fibrillation', most cases of atrial fibrillation are due to underlying heart disease (Fig. 4.19). This is a common arrhythmia in patients with mitral valve disease or heart failure. It is identified on the ECG, as is shown in Fig. 4.19, as low-voltage, irregular atrial activity occurring at a frequency of over 300/min. It is usually coarser and more irregular than flutter but the two can be confused. The pulse is irregularly irregular. It is important to emphasize that the pulse rate may give an erroneous representation of what is happening in the heart and in a patient with atrial fibrillation *both* the pulse and apex rates should be measured and any 'pulse deficit' should be calculated.

Atrial fibrillation can profoundly reduce cardiac output because atrial contraction contributes to about 20 per cent of the total cardiac output. This may make young people with healthy hearts feel unwell and uneasy, or put patients with compromised ventricles into pulmonary oedema.

Digoxin is still the drug of choice in the treatment of atrial fibrillation because it is effective in slowing the ventricular response to the fibrillatory waves by profoundly slowing conduction through the atrioventricular node. β-blocking agents can sometimes be useful added to digoxin. Usually small doses (e.g., propranolol 10–20 mg, twice a day) are sufficient to help slow the ventricular

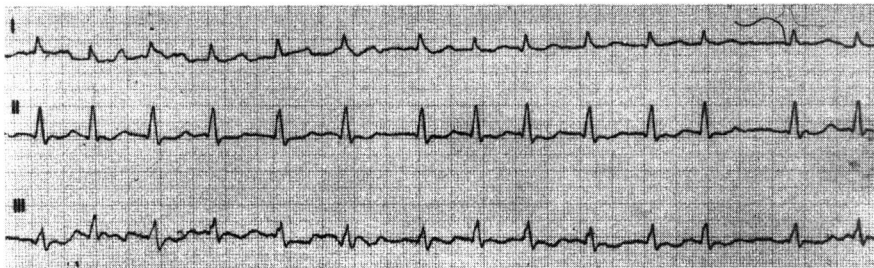

*Figure 4.19*  Atrial fibrillation.

response. Cardioversion can sometimes be successful but usually the atrial fibrillation will recur while the cause of the fibrillation, for instance an enlarged left atrium, remains unchanged.

It is generally accepted that all patients with evidence of mitral valve disease *should be* anticoagulated. If the atrial fibrillation is due to another cause, such as disease of conducting tissue, the use of anticoagulation is controversial.

### Pre-excitation syndromes

The most common condition associated with pre-excitation is the Wolff–Parkinson–White syndrome. This is due to an aberrant pathway called the 'bundle of Kent', which connects the sinoatrial node via a high-speed conduction pathway to the bundle of His just below the atrioventricular node. This results in a short PR interval and a broad QRS complex with a slurred upstroke or delta wave (see Fig. 4.12). There are often abnormalities of repolarization in that there are changes in the ST segment in association with T-wave abnormalities. These are simply the effects of the syndrome and should not be confused with concomitant ischaemia or drug effects.

Although the pre-excitation syndrome can occur as an asymptomatic, incidental finding in otherwise normal individuals, it can produce symptomatic tachyarrhythmias. Particularly in symptomatic patients, it is important not to use drugs that profoundly depress conduction at the atrioventricular node (e.g., digoxin) because this simply encourages the use of the aberrant pathway and exacerbates the symptoms.

Physical examination of patients with pre-excitation syndrome is usually normal.

For the suppression of troublesome symptoms associated with tachyarrhythmia, the most effective drugs are disopyramide and amiodarone. If symptoms are mild, no treatment is required. If

the patient is experiencing syncopal attacks, electrophysiological studies should be done. The purpose is to ensure the patient will not conduct one-to-one down the aberrant pathway during an episode of atrial fibrillation, thereby producing ventricular fibrillation that results in death. Under carefully controlled conditions, the atrium is put into atrial fibrillation via a catheter placed in the right atrial chamber. Conduction studies are then done in the presence of facilities for urgent DC conversion should ventricular fibrillation ensue. If this does not happen, the patient can be reassured. If it does, aggressive therapy, either in the form of amiodarone in suitable doses or surgery should be considered.

### Ventricular extrasystoles

Ventricular extrasystoles are common and usually benign. They often occur in young people and, in the absence of demonstrable myocardial or valvular heart disease, the patient should be reassured. Even ventricular bigeminy can be a completely benign arrhythmia and is often noticed by an anaesthetist in a preoperative assessment. Benign ventricular extrasystoles are often associated with a slow heart rate and will disappear on exercise. They are unifocal with the same shape and configuration. Multifocal extrasystoles, those occurring in pairs or longer runs and the so-called 'R' on 'T' extrasystoles are thought to be pathological and may require treatment. If rapid treatment is required in the short term, intravenous lignocaine is effective. If oral therapy is required for longer term suppression, disopyramide, mexiletine or amiodarone are all effective.

### Parasystole

Parasystole is due to an ectopic ventricular pacemaker that discharges independently of the sinus pacemaker and bears no relation to the rate or rhythm of the sinus pacemaker. Parasystole is thus a form of dual rhythm wherein two pacemakers can currently and independently govern the rhythm of the heart. It is a relatively uncommon arrhythmia and although it occurs with myocardial disease and may be associated with digoxin overdose, it is also found in normal individuals. The treatment is that of the underlying condition if it exists.

Parasystolic ventricular extrasystoles are characterized by the fact that there is no regular coupling interval between the ectopic beat and the preceding sinus beat, whereas there is with the more usual ventricular extrasystoles previously described. Another helpful distinguishing feature is that when both pacemakers discharge in synchrony, the resulting QRS configuration is intermediate between the sinus beat and the ventricular parasystole beat and is known as a 'fusion beat'.

*Ventricular tachycardia and ventricular fibrillation* are extremely important tachyarrhythmias, always associated with severe cardiac pathology, and require urgent treatment, as outlined in Chapter 2.

## VALVULAR HEART DISEASE

The aortic and mitral valves are the main heart valves to become stenosed or incompetent. Currently the most common cause of aortic valve replacement is a bicuspid, calcified aortic valve. Although rheumatic fever has virtually disappeared from Western countries, mainly due to improvement in social and economic circumstances, its sequelae are still found in elderly and late middle-aged populations. Rheumatic fever is still common in the Third world.

### Rheumatic fever

Rheumatic fever is primarily a disease of adolescence and begins with a β-haemolytic streptococcal sore throat. Three weeks later the signs and symptoms of rheumatic fever begin with malaise, fleeting joint pains, erythema marginatum, subcutaneous nodules, pyrexia and most important of all, evidence of carditis. An antibody is produced

to the streptococcus, which has a similar antigenic property to the joints and heart valves. The basic pathological lesion in these tissues is a granulomatous vasculitis. A positive diagnosis can be made if there is a raised antistreptolysin O (ASO) titre (greater than 250) and if two of the major and one minor or two minor and one major of the modified 'Ducket–Jones' criteria exist (Table 4.1).

**Table 4.1 Criteria for the diagnosis of rheumatic fever**

| Major | Minor |
|---|---|
| Polyarthritis | Fever |
| Carditis | Raised ASO titre |
| Chorea | Abdominal pain |
| Subcutaneous nodules | Malaise |
| Erythema marginatum | Raised white cell count or ESR |
| | Prolonged PR interval seen on the ECG |

Although the patient's main complaint in acute episodes is of joint pains, the major long-term effect follows from carditis. It has been said that rheumatic fever 'licks the joints and bites the heart'. The heart can be affected in various ways. Pericarditis and myocarditis are common but the long-term problems are produced by endocarditis affecting the heart valves. Initial swelling of these valves may cause transitory murmurs but later cordal thickening, fibrosis and rupture may seriously damage the valves. In the acute episode, bed rest, aspirin and prednisolone are effective. The most important treatment, however, is the prevention of further attacks by long-term penicillin. The specific β-haemolytic streptococcus has never been shown to be resistant to penicillin, which is still the recommended prophylactic.

The severity of subsequent chronic lesions of the heart valves in rheumatic fever is not dependent on the initial attack, however severe, but upon the number of recurrent attacks. The length of prophylactic treatment is controversial but probably needs to continue until the age of 21 years or possibly 25 years. The valves involved in rheumatic fever are the mitral, aortic and tricuspid (MAT), in that order and the pulmonary valve is rarely, if ever, involved. The commonest cardiac lesion after rheumatic fever is mixed mitral valve disease.

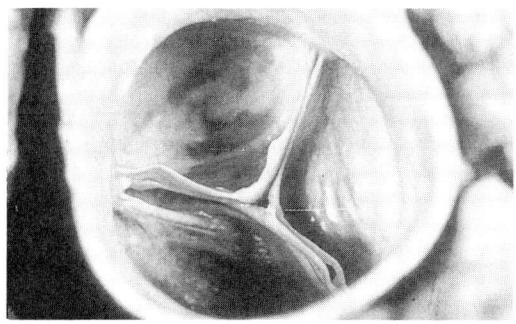 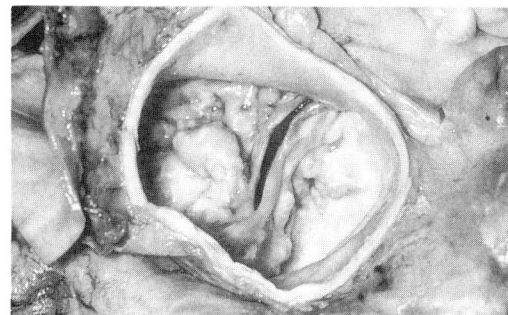

*Figure 4.20*   (a) A normal tricuspid aortic valve. (b) A severely calcified biscuspid aortic valve.

TO PREVENT BACTERIAL ENDOCARDITIS

Antibiotic cover is required under the following circumstances

1.  Dental procedure other than simple fillings:
    amoxycillin 3 g single oral dose 1 hour before dental work (1.5 g for childeren under 10)
    \*For patients allergic to penicillin, erythromycin 2 g should be given instead (1 g for children under 10)

YOU SHOULD VISIT YOUR DENTIST REGULARLY

2.  Other sepsis
    Tonsillitis (oral penicillin for one week)

3.  Minor surgical procedures
    Any potentially septic operation, particularly instrumentation of the bladder or rectum:
    amoxycillin 1 g and gentamicin 30 mg half an hour before

4.  No antibiotics needed for normal childbirth

YOU SHOULD REPORT ANY UNEXPLAINED FEVER TO YOUR DOCTOR

*Figure 4.21*   The 'antibiotic card'.

### Bicuspid aortic valve stenosis

A comparison of a normal tricuspid aortic valve with a bicuspid calcified stenosed valve is shown in Fig. 4.20. Bicuspid aortic valves are common in the general population (an estimated 4 per cent), but the progression to calcific aortic stenosis is obviously rare. The most common presentation of this condition is that of a systolic ejection murmur on a routine insurance or other examination. In some patients the additional turbulence caused by movement of blood through these variant valve cusps gives rise to a mild thickening, followed by fibrosis and calcification. The rate of progression is not predictable but it is known that a major exacerbating factor is an attack of acute infective endocarditis. Therefore the most important action when such a murmur is discovered and a bicuspid valve is confirmed by echocardiography is to give the patient an antibiotic card. This needs to be shown to the dentist or during any hospital admission when appropriate antibiotic cover is advised. Details of the card are shown in Fig. 4.21.

The usual clinical findings of a bicuspid aortic valve are an ejection aortic systolic click heard in early systole (frequently heard best at the mitral area) followed by an ejection systolic murmur, often with a short gap between this murmur and the second heart sound. The aortic component of the second heart sound is preserved and normal.

### Idiopathic billowing mitral valve leaflet syndrome

This common syndrome is usually a mild valvular abnormality, affecting about 10 per cent of females. A cusp or part of a cusp may 'prolapse' into the left atrium, and this is often associated with a non-ejection systolic click and a late crescendo systolic murmur. With varying end diastolic volumes these murmurs and clicks may become louder or disappear. They therefore may become audible or get louder when the patient changes position by leaning to the left or by squatting.

Usually this congenital valvular variation is of no significance but occasionally cordal rupture may occur, giving rise to significant valvular regurgitation. Also, for reasons ill understood, the benign billowing leaflet syndrome may be associated with arrhythmias, particularly recurrent supraventricular tachycardias, and with atypical chest pain. Many of these symptoms are improved by β-blockers. It is important to make the diagnosis clinically and if possible confirm it with an echocardiogram as all of these patients should have prophylactic antibiotic cover for dental procedures.

## Marfan's syndrome

Marfan's syndrome is a dominantly inherited congenital abnormality. It results in fibrous dysplasia of connective tissue affecting the aortic media, eyes and skeleton. It is recognized clinically in patients who have spindly digits, a high-arched palate and in whom there is a tendency to lens dislocation. The main cardiac complications are aortic dilatation, aortic root dissection and aortic valve regurgitation. The mitral valve is frequently affected, giving rise to mild or severe prolapse. A striking echocardiographic example of this condition is shown in Fig. 4.22.

### Other causes

Aortic incompetence may be associated with a dissecting aortic aneurysm. An acute attack of bacterial endocarditis can cause sudden and severe haemodynamic incompetence. Rheumatoid disease can affect the aortic valve and necessitate its replacement. This is particularly important in juvenile rheumatoid arthritis (Still's disease) where acute aortic regurgitation may produce life-threatening pulmonary oedema. Libman–Sacks condition, a complication of systemic lupus erythematosus, may produce acute aortic and/or mitral valve disease.

Very mild and haemodynamically insignificant mitral regurgitation is frequently heard as a functional complication of left ventricular dilatation. A soft, systolic mitral murmur is a common finding in patients with advanced left ventricular dysfunction due to ischaemic heart disease or congestive cardiomyopathy.

### Aortic stenosis

#### Symptoms

Patients with aortic stenosis usually present late in the pathology of their disease. The most important symptoms are syncope and angina, although arrhythmia and heart failure can occur. Symptoms in patients with aortic valve stenosis are significant and should often be considered an acute medical emergency. The average survival time following the onset of symptoms without treatment is about

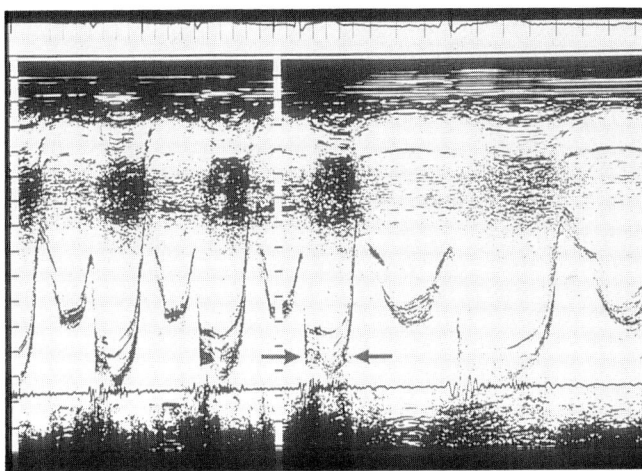

*Figure 4.22* An echocardiogram showing a severe case of mitral valve prolapse in a young man with Marfan's syndrome.

two years, and patients with heart failure have the worst prognosis.

## Signs

The characteristic findings have already been described (p. 73). In severe aortic stenosis there is usually a loud and long ejection aortic systolic murmur and there may be a thrill. There is often reversed splitting of the second heart sound with a soft $A_2$. An aortic ejection click (best heard in the mitral area) is a frequent finding with a bicuspid aortic valve and mild aortic stenosis, but tends to disappear with the onset of significant valvular calcification. It is important to remember that severe chronic stenosis of the valve may present as a profound state of low output in the *absence* of *any* normal auscultatory findings.

## Investigations

The ECG usually shows left ventricular hypertrophy with or without a 'strain pattern'. The atrioventricular node can be involved by the calcific process, producing varying degrees of heart block. The chest X-ray rarely shows cardiomegaly unless left ventricular failure has developed, in which case there may be signs of pulmonary oedema. Post-stenotic dilatation of the aorta can occur. A well-penetrated lateral X-ray often shows calcification around the aortic valve ring. Echocardiography gives a characteristic appearance with mul-

tiple dense shadows within the aortic route as opposed to the usual 'box opening and closing' appearance of the normal aortic valve (Fig. 4.23). An accurate aortic valve gradient can be measured non-invasively by Doppler ultrasonography. Cardiac catheterization is only necessary to delineate the coronary arteries. Coronary angiography is necessary to look for coronary artery disease, which may be dealt with at the same time as aortic valve replacement.

### Aortic incompetence

### Symptoms

Unlike aortic stenosis, symptoms of heart failure develop gradually in incompetence of the aortic valve. Patients experience gradually worsening exertional dyspnoea, but can go on for many years without marked deterioration. Occasionally, however, an acutely damaged, often infected aortic valve can present with sudden and life-threatening pulmonary oedema. The timing of surgical intervention is controversial, but most commonly is advised because of significantly increasing symptoms. More objective signs, such as increasing cardiac size on chest X-ray and an increasing end-diastolic left ventricular diameter measured by echocardiography (some take an upper limit of 7 cm), can be used as objective criteria for aortic valve replacement. However, these criteria are not accepted by all cardiologists; possible benefits

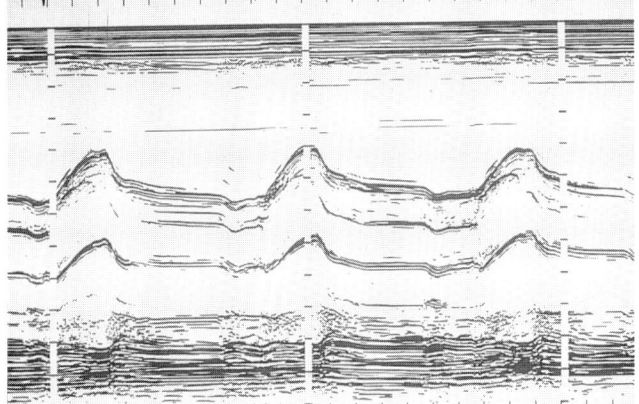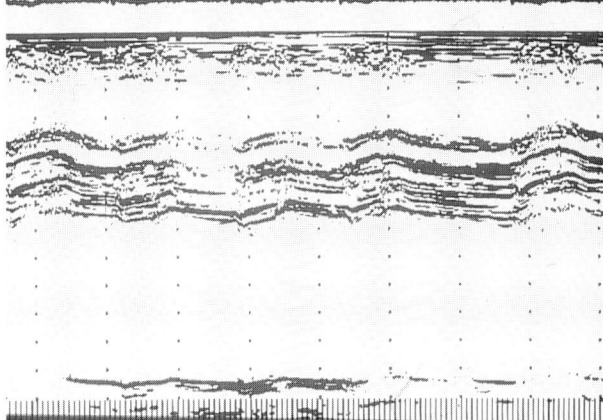

*Figure 4.23* (a) Normal aortic root with normal aortic valve opening. (b) A heavily calcified aortic valve with multiple echoes seen within the aortic root during systole and diastole. Note also that there is an enlarged left atrium.

have to be measured against the risks of surgery, particularly in asymptomatic young patients.

### Signs

The usual physical signs have already been illustrated (p. 73). An ejection systolic murmur is almost invariable, particularly with moderate or severe aortic regurgitation, due to the large systolic volume of blood giving rise to a flow murmur. However, the combination of aortic valve stenosis and regurgitation is not uncommon and the presence or absence of organic stenosis should be determined.

It is important to appreciate that as the degree of incompetence increases, the early diastolic regurgitant murmur generally becomes longer and louder. This continues up to the point when left ventricular failure sets in, and then because of the rising left ventricular end-diastolic pressure, the degree of regurgitation lessens and the murmur becomes less impressive. *This represents severe aortic incompetence.*

### Investigations

In moderate or severe cases the ECG shows a pattern of diastolic overload with left ventricular hypertrophy and T-wave inversion over the lateral chest leads. A chest X-ray will usually show cardiomegaly, a dilated aorta and sometimes pulmonary oedema. There are no specific signs of aortic valve regurgitation on echocardiography but indirect signs include a large left ventricular end-diastolic volume and flutter of the anterior mitral valve leaflet. Doppler ultrasonography will confirm the presence and assess the severity of the regurgitant flow. Doppler studies can also confirm the presence and measure the gradient of concomitant aortic valve stenosis. Cardiac catheterization was once used extensively to assess the severity of regurgitation by studying the amount of flow back into the ventricle during the aortogram. However, as for aortic valve stenosis, catheterization is now only needed to assess the presence and severity of concomitant disease of the coronary arteries.

### Mitral stenosis

Ninety-nine per cent of cases of mitral stenosis are due to chronic rheumatic valvular disease. Rarely, membranous lesions occur above or below a 'normal' mitral valve.

### Symptoms

The commonest symptom is breathlessness. This may occur acutely, precipitated by a sudden onset of atrial fibrillation, or be due to chronic pulmonary venous congestion. Pulmonary hypertension gradually worsens and this brings on associated right heart failure, symptoms of fatigue and more breathlessness. Because of the chronic vascular congestion, respiratory symptoms—such as haemoptysis, either acute or chronic, and symptoms resembling bronchitis with a dry, hacking cough—may also supervene. A large left atrium causes atrial fibrillation. The first symptom of mitral stenosis may be a systemic embolus.

### Signs

The 'malar' flush, a plethoric colour over the cheeks, often combined with central cyanosis, is a classical sign of mitral valve disease, although it tends to occur late. The 'tapping' apex beat, the right ventricular heave, and the characteristic loud first heart sound, opening snap and rumbling diastolic murmur have already been described (p. 73). Note that once the cusps become rigid and calcified, some of these auscultatory signs may disappear. A loud, pulmonary-component second sound indicates the presence of pulmonary hypertension. The presystolic accentuation of the late diastolic murmur is said to be due to atrial contraction and indeed usually does disappear in the presence of atrial fibrillation. It should always be remembered that this is also a sign of pliable mitral valve cusps and therefore should always be present in patients who are considered for closed mitral valvotomy. A pliable valve gives a loud first heart sound, a crisp opening snap and an easily audible, presystolic accentuation to the diastolic murmur.

### Investigations

The ECG usually shows atrial fibrillation, with or without signs of pulmonary hypertension. The typical chest X-ray appearance is shown in Fig. 4.24. Pulmonary oedema frequently occurs, following which pulmonary hypertension gradually develops. Calcification of the mitral valve may be seen, particularly on a well-penetrated lateral

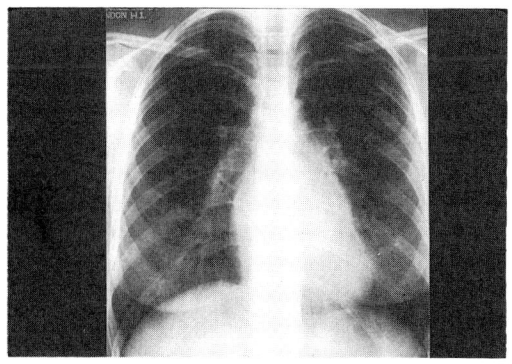

*Figure 4.24* A chest X-ray of a patient with mitral stenosis showing a markedly enlarged left atrial cavity. Note the upward displacement of the left bronchus produced by the enlarged left atrium.

chest X-ray. Echocardiography gives a clear and specific picture in mitral stenosis, as shown in Fig. 4.25. Coronary angiography may be indicated in late middle-aged patients, particularly male smokers in whom mitral valve replacement is contemplated.

### Mitral incompetence

Still the most common cause of significant mitral regurgitation is chronic rheumatic valvular heart disease. Acute chordal rupture, often producing dramatic signs of pulmonary oedema, may occur after acute myocardial infarction. It should be particularly considered in postinfarct patients who have suddenly developed heart failure. Floppy mitral valves are common in Marfan's syndrome, and may become haemodynamically significant, particularly should they become infected.

The idiopathic, billowing mitral valve leaflet syndrome is a common and usually incidental finding. It is generally of no haemodynamic significance.

### Symptoms

Palpitations and atypical chest pain are common in patients with the billowing mitral leaflet syndrome. Otherwise, symptoms are generally related to pulmonary venous congestion. The severity of symptoms correlates closely to the severity of regurgitation. Concomitant with left atrial enlargement, supraventricular arrhythmias, particularly atrial fibrillation, are common.

### Signs

The left ventricle is dilated and the apex beat is usually thrusting. A right ventricular heave due to pulmonary hypertension is common and, in severe mitral incompetence, a left atrial 'lift' may be palpable at the left sternal edge. The classical long and loud pansystolic mitral murmur has already been described. Because of the sudden and severe back rush of blood from the left atrium into the left ventricle in mid-diastole, a loud third heart sound is commonly heard. A short diastolic rumble may also be present following the third heart sound and this is more common in rheumatic disease of the mitral valve.

It is important to remember that in severe mitral regurgitation, there may be *no* systolic murmur because the left ventricle and left atrium have become a continuum.

### Investigations

The ECG shows left ventricular hypertrophy with a pattern of diastolic overload similar to that seen in aortic incompetence. The chest X-ray shows cardiomegaly with left atrial enlargement. There may be signs of pulmonary oedema and/or signs of pulmonary hypertension. Calcification of the mitral valve is not as common as in mitral stenosis. An unusual X-ray appearance, typically seen in longstanding severe rheumatic mitral regurgitation, is calcification over the posterior aspect of the left atrial wall (Fig. 4.26). This is probably due to chronic regurgitation and turbulence of blood at the back of the left atrial wall, causing thrombosis, fibrosis and later calcification. Mitral incompetence cannot be specifically diagnosed by echocardiography although occasionally prolapsing leaflets can be visualized. There will be enlargement of the left atrium, which will usually correlate with the severity of the regurgitation. Left ventricular function is usually normal and indeed often vigorous. Doppler ultrasonography is extremely useful in assessing the severity of mitral regurgitation, especially in difficult cases when there is no systolic murmur, or in assessing the competence of a prosthetic mitral valve. Cardiac catheterization can be used to assess the

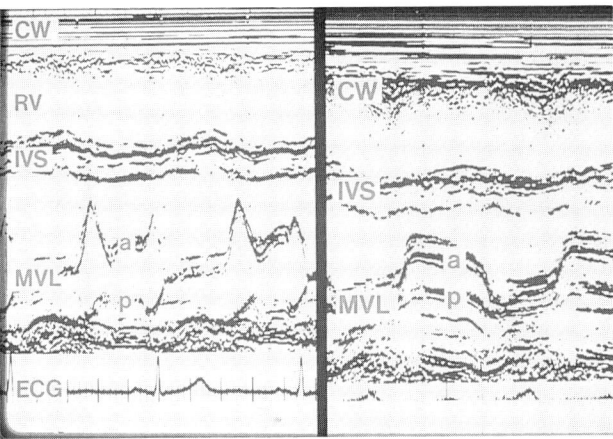

*Figure 4.25* Two echocardiograms showing a normal mitral valve on the left and severe mitral stenosis on the right. Note the considerable thickening of the anterior mitral valve leaflet (a) and the posterior mitral valve (p).

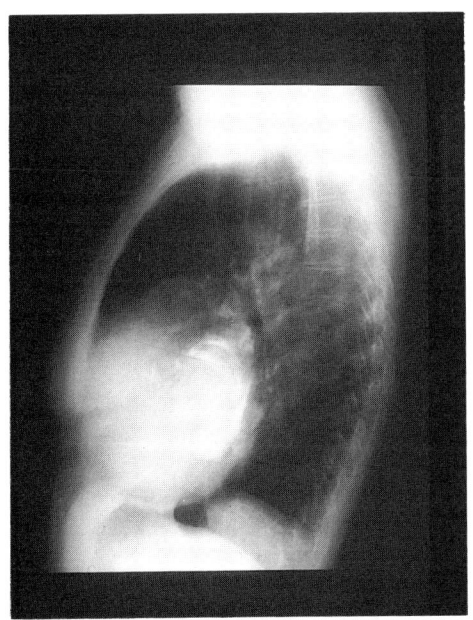

*Figure 4.26* Lateral chest X-ray showing gross calcification over posterial wall of left atrium.

severity of mitral regurgitation by calculating the amount of dye going into the left atrium after left ventricular angiography, but this is usually not necessary. Again, catheterization is generally reserved for assessing the state of a patient's coronary arteries before mitral valve replacement.

### Tricuspid stenosis

Tricuspid stenosis is rare, occurring in a few patients with chronic rheumatic valvular heart disease.

#### Symptoms

The complications of right-sided heart failure predominate, particularly liver congestion and peripheral oedema.

#### Signs

A high jugular venous pressure is commonly found, usually with a giant 'a' wave. There is ankle or sacral oedema with a large and often painful liver. The murmur is similar to mitral stenosis but is heard in the tricuspid area. There may be an opening snap.

#### Investigations

The ECG characteristically shows 'P' pulmonale due to right atrial enlargement. The chest X-ray shows cardiomegaly due to right atrial enlargement—calcification of the tricuspid valve is rarely seen. The diagnosis can be specifically made by echocardiography: stenosis of the tricuspid valve has a similar shape, pattern and delay of opening and closing to that of mitral stenosis. Tricuspid stenosis very rarely occurs on its own: there is commonly evidence of concomitant disease of the mitral and aortic valves.

### Tricuspid incompetence

Tricuspid incompetence is common and is usually functional due to dilatation of the tricuspid valve. The tricuspid valve is large and easily stretched and therefore any condition that causes considerable enlargement of the right ventricle is likely to give rise to stretching of the tricuspid valve and functional tricuspid incompetence.

### Symptoms and signs

Symptoms are predominantly right-sided with distension of the neck veins, liver and ankles.

There will be an elevated jugular venous pressure with a large 'v' wave. This venous pressure may be so elevated as to be best visualized with the patient *standing up*. The liver is enlarged, tender, and pulsatile. There is usually peripheral oedema. The murmur has already been described (p. 73) and is similar to that of mitral incompetence but is heard best over the tricuspid area and its intensity is increased by inspiration.

### Investigations

The ECG will show evidence of right ventricular and right atrial enlargement. There is usually considerable cardiomegaly on the chest X-ray. Echocardiography is not specific but Doppler ultrasonography can be diagnostic. Cardiac catheterization is usually unnecessary.

### Treatment of valvular heart disease

### Medical therapy

The treatment of peripheral and pulmonary venous congestion has already been outlined. Arrhythmias, most commonly atrial fibrillation, need to be treated with digoxin and/or any other anti-arrhythmics. Particularly in the presence of atrial fibrillation, anticoagulation with warfarin is mandatory. Infective endocarditis on previously damaged valves carries a high mortality and adequate antibiotic cover is essential when the patient is at risk (e.g., during dental extractions).

### Surgical treatment

Mitral valvotomy, a common operation 20 years ago, is rarely done today. The stenosed mitral valve is dilated with the surgeon's finger, the fused leaflets being 'split', often with considerable relief of pulmonary venous congestion. The advantage of this procedure is that it does not require facilities for complete open heart surgery, but the disadvantage is that it is only effective for tight, pliable mitral stenosis, and in older valves, particularly those which are heavily calcified, secondary mitral regurgitation is common. This operation has become obsolete in the Western world where young patients with tight, pliable mitral stenosis are rare, but is still of paramount importance in those countries where virulent rheumatic fever persists.

As a general principle it is better to repair a valve than replace it. Reattaching ruptured chordae and/or reducing the size of the valve ring (annuloplasty) can bring considerable symptomatic relief. Sometimes these operations need to be repeated and, if a repair fails, then the valve is replaced. Valve replacement can be with homografts (human grafts or valves constructed from the patient's own tissue), xenografts (heart valves from other animals such as pigs) or artificial valves such as the Starr–Edwards ball-and-cage valve. The advantage of homografts over synthetic valves is that anticoagulation is not needed, but the disadvantage is that in time they disintegrate.

Synthetic valves require permanent anticoagulation but may last a lifetime. Homografts are usually reserved for where the valve is only needed for five or six years, in elderly patients, or where patients cannot be anticoagulated, such as women planning further pregnancies. In this latter situation the homograft valve is usually replaced by a prosthetic valve several years later.

The outcome of aortic valve replacement is generally better than that of mitral valve replacement, probably because the round prosthetic valve fits better in the round aortic root than does the mitral replacement in the elliptical mitral valve area. Arrhythmias and reduced left ventricular function are common complications after mitral valve replacement.

The timing of valve replacement will depend on the patient's symptoms. Other criteria, such as signs of 'strain' on the ECG or increasing cardiomegaly, can also be used as a guide to the timing of surgery. A middle-aged man with tight aortic stenosis, angina and syncopal attacks should be considered a surgical emergency.

### Infective endocarditis

Infective endocarditis may develop on *normal heart valves*. Much more commonly, however, infective vegetations develop on congenital or acquired cardiac lesions. Due to turbulence and pressure phenomena, the mitral and aortic valves are much more commonly infected than pulmonary or tricuspid valves although recently lesions on tricuspid valves are becoming more common due to intravenous drug abuse.

Clinical presentation may be acute or subacute.

### Acute bacterial endocarditis

Acute bacterial endocarditis is a severe form of endocarditis that is much less common than the subacute variety. It often develops on normal valves and is usually associated with a very severe infection. It is most common among immunosuppressed patients and drug addicts. *Staphylococcus aureus* is the most common organism involved; the mortality is high. The usual clinical features of subacute endocarditis are not seen because they do not have time to develop. However, there is usually a very high fever and often a new and loud heart murmur. Rapidly developing heart failure is common. Abscesses may occur, which can result in heart block or arrhythmias. These latter complications may further exacerbate heart failure and are a bad prognostic sign. Patients require immediate hospitalization, early intravenous antibiotic therapy, and should be immediately considered for replacement of the infected valve.

### Subacute bacterial endocarditis

The presenting features of subacute bacterial endocarditis are often vague and nonspecific, causing late diagnosis. Weight loss is common. General symptoms are vague ill-health, pyrexia, nausea and lack of energy. The following physical findings are strongly suggestive of this condition.
(1) Splinter haemorrhages in finger and toe nails.
(2) Osler's nodes—these are painful nodules, usually occurring on the finger tips.
(3) Anaemia.
(4) Finger clubbing.
(5) Splenomegaly.
(6) Arteritic lesions, called Roth's spots, may be seen on fundoscopy.
(7) Haematuria due to microemboli in the kidneys.
(8) A heart murmur will be present in most patients but it is possible to have infective endocarditis *without* a heart murmur.
(9) Signs of heart failure.

The complications of infective endocarditis may be subdivided into cardiac and extracardiac.
*Cardiac*:
(a) heart failure due to valve damage;
(b) myocardial infarction due to an infected embolus of a coronary artery;
(c) myocardial abscesses may develop, which can produce conduction abnormalities, particularly heart block.
*Extracardiac*:
(a) systemic or pulmonary emboli;
(b) mycotic aneurysms;
(c) glomerulonephritis;
(d) a cerebrovascular accident due to an infected embolus;
(e) Osler's nodes;
(f) anaemia.

*Blood cultures are vital*—if adequate blood cultures are taken, usually at least six over a 24-h period before starting intravenous antibiotics, it is possible to isolate the relevant organism in most cases. (Therapy should not, however, be inordinately delayed in order to take blood cultures.) The importance cannot be overemphasized of taking multiple cultures from both arms because once treatment has begun, it is virtually useless to try again.

### Diagnosis of infective endocarditis

An anaemia occurs, which is most frequently normochromic and normocytic, and the ESR is usually very high. Urine abnormalities such as microscopic haematuria are frequent. Echocardiography is helpful and may demonstrate valvular vegetations, which are particularly dramatic in fungal endocarditis. Remember that a normal echocardiogram does *not* exclude the diagnosis of infective endocarditis.

### Organisms

Although any organism can cause infective endocarditis, most cases are still due to streptococcal and staphylococcal infections. Overall, the main culprit is *Strep. viridans* (about 40 per cent). Other streptococci, *Staph. aureus* and *Staph. epidermidis* are the next most common causative organisms. Gram-negative bacilli account for about 10 per cent of infections and other rarer causes include fungi, *Coxiella* and even *Chlamydia* (in which case serology may be more useful than blood culture). *Strep. epidermidis* and fungi are the most important organisms to infect prosthetic valves. About 5 per cent of cases of infective endocarditis remain culture negative.

### Drug therapy

The antibiotic chosen should be bactericidal because bacteriostasis alone is inadequate. Penicillin remains the most useful drug but it must be given in adequate doses for an adequate period of time, usually at least four weeks. Penicillin and gentamicin act synergistically against *Strep. viridans* and the combination has been shown to be effective clinically. So, following blood cultures, treatment should be started with large doses of penicillin intravenously combined with gentamicin. Subsequent therapy depends on the result of the blood cultures. Adequate doses of penicillin are too high to be given intramuscularly, therefore regular intravenous therapy is mandatory. The patient will probably find a central subclavian or internal jugular venous line more comfortable than frequent resited peripheral cannulae. 'Cidal' levels of the antibiotic in the patient's serum can be tested against the stored organism in culture to ensure that therapy is adequate. After about four weeks the intravenous route is usually exchanged for the oral route for a further two weeks.

### Penicillin sensitivity

The patient may be known to be sensitive to pencillin before treatment is started or it may develop during treatment. If known previously, erythromycin or vancomycin should be used instead, erythromycin being the easier and safer. If the history of penicillin sensitivity is vague or inconclusive, it is reasonable to start with penicillin and await developments, monitoring the patient carefully. This is usually quite safe and treatment should certainly never be delayed because of worries about sensitivity.

### Culture negative endocarditis

Cultures are negative in about 5 per cent of cases of endocarditis. The most common cause is previous antibiotic therapy. Frequently the patient has visited his or her general practitioner over the preceding few days and been given a broad-spectrum antibiotic to treat the general ''flu-like'' symptoms.

If not, non-bacterial organisms including *Cox-*

*iella*, fungi and *Chlamydia* should be suspected, and appropriate serological tests performed. The presence of fungi should be particularly suspected in the presence of prosthetic valves. Treatment includes a combination of penicillin, flucloxacillin and gentamicin.

### Prophylaxis for infective endocarditis

Prophylaxis should be done before dental work, tonsillectomy, bronchoscopy, genito-urinary and gynaecological procedures; some clinicians include radiological investigations, such as barium enemas, in this lists. It should certainly be given before cystoscopies. *If in doubt give antibiotic prophylaxis.* The purpose of prophylaxis is to kill bacteria released by such procedures so the aim is to obtain an adequate bactericidal blood level of antibiotic for one hour following the procedure. (For further information see the antibiotic card in Fig. 4.21.)

### Pericardial disease

### Acute pericarditis

Acite pericarditis is acute inflammation of the pericardium and is usually viral in origin. The chest pain produced is sharp, pleuritic and often worse when lying in a particular position. Other causes include uraemia and drugs, such as hydralazine. Pericarditis is common after myocardial infarction, occurring acutely due to pericardial rupture, or more commonly about a week later due to anticardiac antibodies—Dressler's syndrome. This condition is also known as the 'post-cardiotomy syndrome' and can follow any cause of direct cardiac muscle injury such as trauma or, rarely, pacemaker insertion.

On examination, a characteristic pericardial rub is frequently heard in both systole and diastole. This is a superficial 'scratchy', high-pitched sound. High-pitched noises are best heard with the diaphragm of the stethoscope and further accentuation of this noise can be obtained by pressing hard on the stethoscope, which removes extraneous low-frequency sounds.

### Investigations

The ECG is characteristic (Fig. 4.27). It can easily be distinguished from acute ischaemic changes because the elevation of the ST segment is wide-

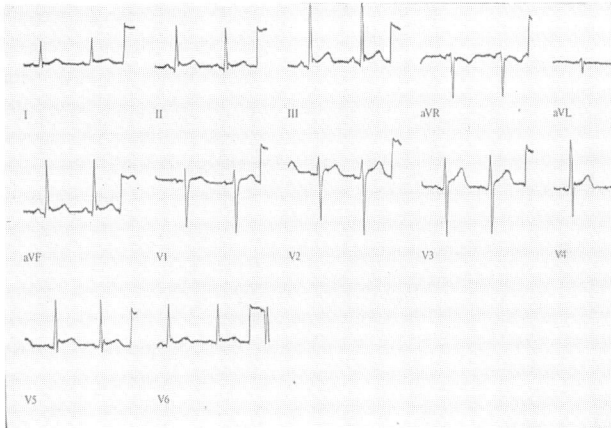

*Figure 4.27* An ECG in acute pericarditis with widespread, saddle-shaped, concave upwards elevation of the ST segment.

spread and there is no reciprocal depression of the ST segment. The chest X-ray is normal, as is the echocardiogram, because there is rarely enough fluid to produce a pericardial effusion.

### Treatment

The pain can be frightening because it is sharp and understandably causes patients to become worried about more serious cardiac pathology. It responds well to aspirin but occasionally steroids are needed. It usually settles down without any long-term sequelae, but sometimes it can take a long time to resolve. Reassurance, analgesics and anti-inflammatory drugs are all that is required.

### Pericardial effusion

Following the advent of echocardiography, small pericardial effusions have been discovered in many conditions, such as heart failure and hypoproteinaemic states. Large pericardial effusions occur in the collagen diseases and are common in malignancy, when metastatic 'pericardial seedlings' can sometimes be demonstrated by echocardiography.

### Tamponade

Initially the pericardium will stretch in response to the effusion but a point is reached when this can no longer occur and the heart becomes compressed. This is a dangerous situation and is called pericardial tamponade.

Pulsus paradoxus occurs and this is usually a sign that the cardiac tamponade is severe. The heart sounds are soft and distant and may be difficult to hear when the effusion is large. A pericardial rub may or may not be present. The jugular venous pressure is high and tends to rise further with inspiration (Griesinger–Kussmaul sign). This sign is also seen in constrictive pericarditis. Hepatomegaly, ascites and peripheral oedema may develop but tend to be more marked when the accumulation of fluid is chronic. The chest X-ray shows an enlarged globular heart. The ECG is characteristic with low voltage complexes throughout. Echocardiography is extremely useful and always diagnostic in this condition.

Sometimes it is difficult to ascertain whether the sudden accumulation of fluid in a patient and newly apparent severe 'heart failure' is due to tamponade or primary myocardial disease. As the former is so amenable to treatment it is important to make this diagnosis as quickly as possible. A typical pericardial effusion is shown in Fig. 4.28, where the heart can be seen swinging due to respiratory fluctuations within the bag of pericardial fluid. In this case the pericardial effusion is large enough to be shown both posteriorly and anteriorly. Pericardiocentesis can be life saving in such a situation.

Echocardiography is also useful in assessing the success of pericardiocentesis and in searching for recurrence.

Most pericardial effusions will resolve spontaneously and only a minority require pericardiocentesis. Tamponade is unusual. Occasionally

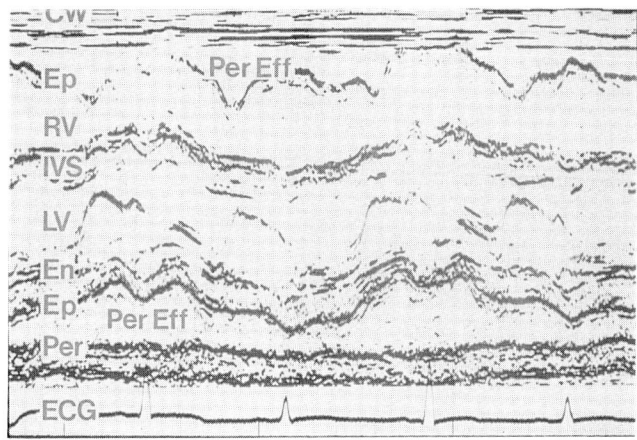

*Figure 4.28* An echocardiogram showing anterior and posterior pericardial effusions. Note that the heart is swinging within the bag of pericardial fluid.

pericardial effusions need to be 'tapped' for diagnostic reasons, a protein content can be measured and cytological examination made for neoplastic cells. The fluid can be cultured if infection is suspected. Blood-stained pericardial effusions are almost always malignant. Repeated pericardiocentesis, possibly even with the insertion of a permanent pericardial drain, can be useful in the relief of symptoms due to large, chronic, malignant pericardial effusions.

### Constrictive pericarditis

Constrictive pericarditis results from longstanding inflammation of the pericardium, which becomes fibrosed, thickened and may even calcify (Fig. 4.29). Calcification is best demonstrated on a well penetrated lateral chest X-ray and can often be difficult to see clearly on echocardiography or even cardiac catheterization. Because the heart is small and unable to expand, there are signs of back pressure or 'heart failure' with a high jugular venous pressure, a large liver and chronic peripheral oedema resulting more in ascites than in leg oedema for reasons that are not well understood.

The physical signs are similar to those seen in cardiac tamponade but tend to be more profound because of the chronic nature of this condition. The elevated jugular venous pressure is sometimes so dramatic that it can only be properly seen when the patient is standing.

The Griesinger–Kussmaul sign is frequently positive. A loud, early, third heart sound occurs due to the heart filling quickly and tapping against the calcified pericardium; this is known as a pericardial 'knock' and may even be palpable. The ECG shows a widespread, low voltage pattern. The echocardiogram is usually nonspecific and is not diagnostic. The chest X-ray shows a normal or small heart and calcification may be seen on the lateral film. On cardiac catheterization the diastolic pressures are equal in all four chambers and there is a characteristic early and sudden plateau of pressure in both ventricles.

Worldwide, the commonest cause of constrictive pericarditis is chronic tuberculous disease but, in the UK, the cause is usually unknown or sometimes termed 'postviral' although no viruses have ever been isolated.

Treatment involves diuretics for the relief of symptoms, particularly spironolactone, as there is often secondary hyperaldosteronism. Great care, however, has to be taken not to overuse diuretics in these patients because a sudden reduction in stroke volume may result. These patients are dependent on a high end-diastolic pressure to maintain cardiac output. *Dehydration, therefore, is to be avoided at all costs.* Arrhythmias should be treated in the usual way and digoxin started if there is atrial fibrillation.

Pericardial resection can be performed when symptoms are disabling, with a satisfactory symptomatic result. Resection may need to be repeated at a later date, particularly in young patients. Prognosis is dependent upon the availability of surgical intervention, as myocardial structure and function are normal. Unfortunately,

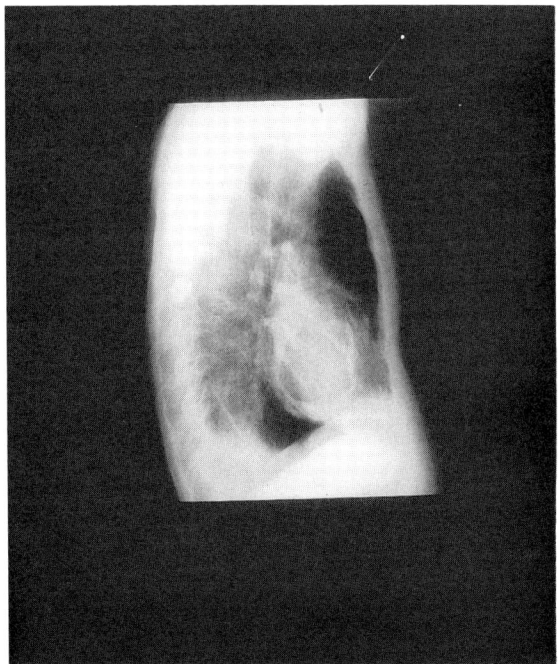

*Figure 4.29* A well-penetrated lateral chest X-ray showing severe calcific constrictive pericarditis.

in areas where tuberculous pericardial disease is common, such facilities are often not available.

### Acute myocarditis

Acute myocarditis is defined as any inflammatory process involving the myocardium. It may result from parasites or fungi but by far the commonest cause in temperate regions is viral. Although it has long been known to occur in acute rheumatic fever, it is now also thought to play a part in the heart failure that may develop in chronic collagen disorders such as chronic rheumatoid disease or ankylosing spondylitis.

Acute myocarditis occurs throughout the world and in all age groups. Specific infecting organisms, however, have a distinct geographic distribution. Chagas' disease (caused by *Trypanosoma cruzi*) is common in South America (estimated to affect over 10 million people), and is probably the most common cause of acute myocarditis in the world. Indeed, in these areas, any patient with heart failure or arrhythmia, particularly in combination with right bundle branch block, has Chagas' disease until proven otherwise.

In Europe and the USA, probably the most common cause of acute myocarditis is the Coxsackie B enterovirus. Electrocardiographic abnormalities are often seen in patients with acute infection. After a ''flu-like' illness, many patients describe palpitations, which then resolve spontaneously. In all of these cases, the myocardium has been involved and, had these patients been subjected to specific tests, acute myocarditis would have been discovered. Such diagnoses are not of clinical importance, except in those who develop chronic heart failure because this is probably the cause of congestive cardiomyopathy. Treatment is largely symptomatic with bed rest and appropriate treatment of heart failure. Steroids, if given early in acute cases, may be beneficial but there is no clinical information available concerning the efficacy of steroids because it is almost impossible to conduct controlled clinical trials in these circumstances. It would seem logical, however, that acute reduction of severe inflammation can only be beneficial. The patient should be carefully followed up and assessed for the development of chronic heart failure. Most patients recover spontaneously with no sequelae. A few develop 'congestive cardiomyopathy' for reasons not fully understood.

### Cardiomyopathies

Cardiomyopathies have been defined by John Goodwin as 'heart muscle disease of unknown cause and unknown association'. This definition particularly excludes unusual conditions associated with heart disease such as sarcoidosis, amyloid and acromegaly. The three main subgroups of cardiomyopathies are:
(a) hypertrophic cardiomyopathy;
(b) congestive cardiomyopathy;
(c) restrictive cardiomyopathy.

#### Hypertrophic cardiomyopathy

Hypertrophic cardiomyopathy can be described as a type of 'congenital muscular dystrophy' affecting only the heart muscle. In this condition the heart is hypertrophied and its muscle bulk is considerably increased but this hypertrophy is abnormal and does not give the heart any increased power. The myofibrils are abnormal in size, shape and distribution. The characteristic pathology is a thickened left ventricle encroaching upon a small left ventricular cavity. The septum, in particular, is thick and immobile and although this condition has been described as 'asymmetric septal hypertrophy' (ASH), there is usually additional hypertrophy of the posterior left ventricular wall. Pressure gradients can occur within the ventricular cavity and may produce syncopal attacks. Heart failure and arrhythmias are common. There is a marked spectrum of disease severity in that the condition may present at birth with severe heart failure or may be found as an incidental finding in an asymptomatic patient. This condition runs in families and has an autosomal-dominant pattern of inheritance.

## Symptoms

Syncope is the most worrying and dangerous symptom. This may be due to either cavity obliteration or arrhythmia. Other symptoms include chest pain, dyspnoea, and palpitations.

## Signs

There is usually a 'jerky' pulse. The blood pressure is normal. Palpation of the apex beat may be helpful because there may be a characteristic double impulse to this beat. The apex beat will also have a forceful and sustained character. There may be an audible fourth heart sound and there is usually a long, pansystolic murmur.

## Investigations

The ECG usually shows left ventricular hypertrophy with a marked pattern of left ventricular strain. There may be cardiomegaly on the chest X-ray. Echocardiography is diagnostic and shows specific changes of septal hypertrophy and systolic anterior movement of the mitral valve (Fig. 4.30). It is thought that this systolic movement of the mitral valve produces the frequently heard, concomitant flow murmur of mitral regurgitation.

These patients are prone to a variety of arrhythmias, most alarmingly ventricular tachycardia, which can be present in totally asymptomatic cases.

## Treatment

Patients with hypertrophic cardiomyopathy die suddenly from symptomatic or 'silent' ventricular tachycardia. The most effective prophylaxis is amiodarone. The dose needed is usually small, 200 to 300 mg daily; the lowest required dose can usually be discovered by repeated ambulatory monitoring in patients on treatment. Surgery to remove discrete areas of hypertrophied muscle has proved to be moderately successful, and mitral valve replacement may be life saving.

Having made the diagnosis, it is sensible to look for other patients within the family that may have subclinical hypertrophic cardiomyopathy. This can easily be done non-invasively and an echocardiogram is usually all that is needed. In the absence of demonstrable arrhythmias these patients will require no treatment.

### Congestive cardiomyopathy

Congestive cardiomyopathy is also known as 'dilated cardiomyopathy'. The probable cause of these dilated and poorly contracting hearts is a

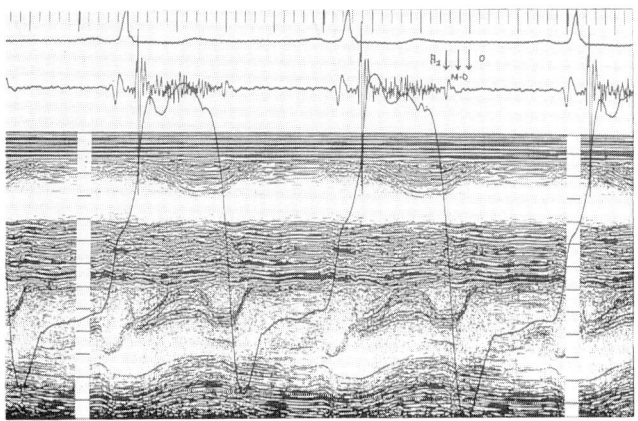

*Figure 4.30* Hypertrophic cardiomyopathy with marked septal and posterior left ventricular wall thickening.

previous myocarditis. Viruses and viral inclusion bodies have been isolated within these hearts. Raised viral antibody titres are uncommon, probably because by the time the patient presents with heart failure, the infective agent has long gone. At one time this condition was also described as 'alcoholic heart disease' but generally patients with other alcohol-related problems such as liver cirrhosis have normal hearts. It is certainly true, however, that if myocardial function is depressed then alcohol will make it worse. A past history of severe hypertension may be relevant, in which case the residual, poor pump function may be termed 'burnt out hypertensive heart disease'. This is probably a different entity to most dilated cardiomyopathy cases where there is no cause or association.

The most common cause of reduced left ventricular function in the UK is ischaemic heart disease and this must be ruled out before the patient can be defined as having true cardiomyopathy.

### Symptoms

One or both ventricles may be affected. A very large, dilated and poorly contracting right ventricle may be discovered with virtually normal left ventricular function (Uuhl's syndrome). The symptoms and signs are those of heart failure.

### Investigations

The ECG shows nonspecific ST- and T-wave changes without definite evidence of myocardial infarction. Ventricular arrhythmias are common. The chest X-ray shows cardiomegaly, with or without signs of pulmonary oedema. The echocardiogram shows a dilated left ventricle with posterior displacement of the mitral valve. The ejection fraction is always very low.

### Treatment

Treatment is similar to that for heart failure using diuretics, nitrates, vasodilators and ACE inhibitors. Beware of severe cases in whom the blood pressure is low. Atrial fibrillation should be treated with digoxin. Hypokalaemia should be carefully sought and treated because patients with this condition are particularly prone to arrhythmias.

Young patients with this condition are probably the best candidates for heart transplantation.

### Restrictive cardiomyopathy

Restrictive cardiomyopathy is a rare condition consisting of endomyocardial fibrosis, often with superadded thrombus, which results in reduction and eventual obliteration of both ventricular cavities. It occurs both in tropical and temperate climates and the pathology in either is indistinguishable. In the tropics it occurs with or without eosinophilia and is suspected to be associated with filariasis. Outside tropical areas it is virtually always associated with a profound eosinophilia and has also been described as Loeffler's of eosinophilic endocardial disease. Treatment includes cytotoxic drugs to lower the eosinophil count when this is markedly raised and conventional treatment of 'heart failure'. Anticoagulation is essential because many of the peripheral complications of this condition are due to embolization from the abnormal left ventricle. Surgery has recently produced encouraging results and consists of mitral and/or tricuspid valve replacement, with or without endocardectomy.

### Pregnancy and heart disease

### Hypertension in pregnancy

Uncontrolled or poorly controlled hypertension in pregnancy used to cause substantial fetal and neonatal mortality. Although bed rest and sedation are effective, it is often not practical in mothers with other young children. Thiazide diuretics have adverse fetal side-effects and calcium channel-blocking agents have not yet been shown to be completely safe. The most widely used drugs are β-blockers.

Adequate antihypertensive therapy has been shown to reduce the incidence of mid-trimester abortions in women with idiopathic hypertension but it does not influence the onset of pre-eclampsia or eclampsia. The most commonly used β-blocker in pregnancy is labetalol, which has been shown to be safe. Methyldopa is also used but causes more side-effects in the mother.

### Anticoagulation in pregnancy

Anticoagulation is most commonly needed in young women with prosthetic heart valves. For this reason, homograft valves are sometimes preferred because they do not require long-term anticoagulation. Warfarin does carry a risk of teratogenicity in the fetus in early pregnancy but if the mother has a metallic valve this risk is generally thought to be acceptable because the consequence of no anticoagulation might be disastrous. If it is decided to continue warfarin throughout the pregnancy, low-dose subcutaneous heparin is introduced during the two weeks before delivery because of the increased risk of fetal haemorrhage induced by warfarin combined with birth trauma. The advantage of heparin is that it does not cross the placenta and therefore has no adverse effects on the fetus. However, continuous long-term subcutaneous or intravenous heparin therapy throughout pregnancy is thought not to be practical, and can cause osteoporosis. A compromise regimen is to administer heparin subcutaneously (the mother can usually be taught to administer this herself) for the first trimester, reverting to warfarin for the rest of the pregnancy and then subcutaneous heparin two weeks before delivery. Full anticoagulation should be commenced post-delivery as soon as is thought to be safe.

Vitamin K supplements can be given to the baby if there are any possibilities that warfarin may have crossed the placenta to the child. Warfarin appears in breast milk and therefore babies of these mothers should always be bottle fed.

If warfarin is continued through the pregnancy, the risk of spontaneous abortion is increased and the chances of having a live, deformed baby are probably in the region of 8 per cent. The clinical decision is always a difficult one.

### Mitral stenosis in pregnancy

Mitral stenosis is now much less of a problem in pregnancy because of the dramatic decrease in the incidence of acute rheumatic fever in the Western world. The increased cardiac output, tachycardia, fluid and sodium retention of pregnancy may cause haemodynamic deterioration. Symptoms usually become apparent by the twentieth week of pregnancy and may be aggravated at the time of labour due to the associated increases in cardiac output. This is a serious problem because maternal and fetal death can occur.

When severe mitral stenosis is identified before pregnancy, mitral valve surgery (preferably a mitral valve repair) should be undertaken before conception. When an asymptomatic woman with mitral stenosis becomes pregnant no special treatment is required. If symptoms are severe during late pregnancy despite medical treatment, closed mitral valvotomy is the safest operative procedure because it does not involve putting the mother and hence the child on a cardiopulmonary bypass machine. If open heart surgery is required, fetal mortality is usually about 40 per cent. If thromboembolic complications occur, anticoagulation is advised, irrespective of the risks to the child.

### Cardiac tumours

Cardiac tumours are rare. The most common and most pleasing to diagnose is a left atrial myxoma.

A myxoma may occur in the right as well as the left atrium and bilateral atrial myxomas have been described. Frequently there are systemic symptoms, such as fatigue, tiredness and intermittent pyrexia. A high ESR is common. Clinical manifestations include arrhythmia, intermittent pulmonary oedema and a murmur suggestive of mitral stenosis. In particular, this murmur may be intermittent or only audible when the patient is put in a particular position. There may be evidence of present or past embolic problems.

The investigation of choice is an echocardiogram, when a specific diagnosis can be made quickly and easily (Fig. 4.31). Cardiac catheterization can be dangerous. After echocardiographic confirmation the patient should go straight to surgery.

The result of surgery is immediate and gratifying but unfortunately 10 per cent of these tumours are malignant. For such tumours, radiotherapy and chemotherapy can be helpful and may prolong life. Sometimes atrial tumours grow into the pulmonary veins where complete resection may be impossible.

Primary cardiac tumours, such as fibromas or rhabdomyomas, or rhabdomyosarcomas, are extremely rare but the latter may occur in association with tuberosclerosis. Malignant tumours, particularly secondary deposits (often from lung primary sites), are common, but are rarely associated with any clinical problems and most often are discovered as incidental post mortem findings.

Primary myocardial tumours often present with palpitations as these abnormal areas give rise to abnormal electrical activity. Resection may be possible, depending upon the anatomical site of the tumour. If the tumour is resectable, sequelae are uncommon and secondary deposits rare.

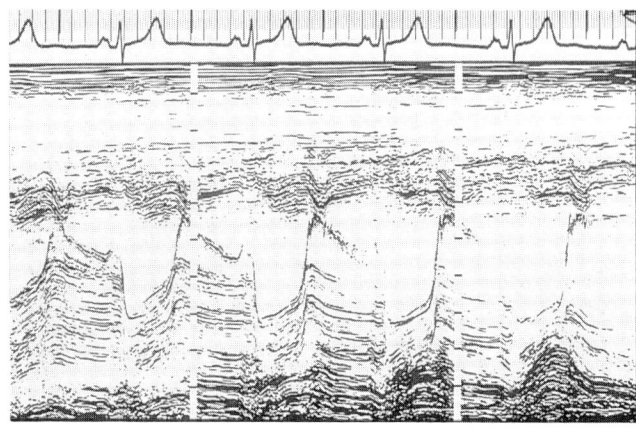

*Figure 4.31* An echocardiogram showing a left atrial myxoma better seen on the left of the diagram than the right because of variation in the position of the transducer during the patient's inspiration.

## PREVENTION OF HEART DISEASE

Much work is now being done in an attempt to reverse the present epidemic of early ischaemic heart disease in the UK. By far the most significant type of heart disease, which affects 'young' people and produces a high mortality within young, wage-earning men, is acute myocardial infarction due to ischaemic heart disease.

Although it is true that about half of acute myocardial infarctions are *not* associated with any known risk factors, it is still worthwhile to try and educate the public in an attempt to reverse the known preventable factors. The most important risk factors—age, male sex and a family history of ischaemic heart disease—cannot be reversed. Other exacerbating factors, however, in particular cigarette smoking, are well worth concentrating on. The other known risk factors include hypertension, poor control of diabetes, hypercholesterolaemia, excessive stress, and high-oestrogen contraceptive pills. Although not a specific risk factor, obesity, especially when associated with a low level of physical activity, should be discouraged.

Much attention is currently directed toward stopping children from starting smoking. Seminars are organized in schools for children and teachers. The general public is presently encouraged to stop smoking, eat a healthier diet (to grill rather than fry foods and to avoid fatty animal and dairy products) and to get their blood pressure checked by general practitioners. In South Wales, which has an extremely high incidence of early ischaemic heart disease, an epidemiological experiment is currently taking place, under the auspices of 'Heartbeat Wales' to see if general persuasion and advertising using the mass media can change people's habits and actually reduce the incidence of ischaemic heart disease.

### Suggested reading

Feigenbaum H. (1986). *Echocardiography*, 4th edn. Lea and Seibiger.

Hurst J. W. (1989). *The Heart*, 5th edn. McGraw Hill.

Major R. H. (1978). *Classic descriptions of disease*. Charles C. Thomas.

Opie L. (1986). *Drugs for the Heart*, 2nd edn. Grune and Stratton.

Schamroth L. (1989). *An Introduction to Electrocardiography*, 6th edn. Blackwell Scientific.

Swanton (1989). *Cardiology*. Blackwell Scientific.

Van Jones J., Blackwood R. (1983) *Outline of Cardiology*. Wright.

Wood P. (1988). *Diseases of the Heart and Circulation*, 3rd edn. Eyre and Spottiswoode.

# 5

# RESPIRATORY MEDICINE

Ian S. Petheram

## INTRODUCTION

Respiratory disease is a major cause of ill health and death in the community and accounts for about 29 million days of lost work per year and up to 20 per cent of all general practitioner consultations. Many of these illnesses are smoking-related and, therefore, theoretically preventable. There seems a disappointing lack of will by political leaders to tackle this widespread environmental hazard at a time when atmospheric pollution is socially and politically topical.

Other causes of respiratory disease are becoming increasingly recognized. There is much evidence that there is a true increase in the incidence and prevalence of asthma. Modern treatment controls symptoms in the majority of asthmatic sufferers but attacks of acute, severe asthma remain a significant risk to life in all age groups. Occupational inhalation of organic or non-organic substances is becoming recognized as an increasingly significant cause of some respiratory diseases and the physician needs to become aware of the diversity of industrial processes that might be causing respiratory symptoms. Pulmonary complications of the acquired immune deficiency syndrome (AIDS) are now well recognized and are likely to become an increasing problem for respiratory physicians. This disease is dealt with separately in Chapter 3.

## PRESENTING FEATURES

There are six principal symptoms of respiratory disease—breathlessness, cough, sputum, haemoptysis, wheeze and chest pain.

### Breathlessness

The speed of onset of breathlessness is the most useful information leading to diagnosis. The following non-pulmonary disorders can present with breathlessness:

Cardiac disease
Anaemia
Uraemia
Diabetic ketoacidosis
Hysterical hyperventilation

A practical guide to the causes of breathlessness depending on rate of onset is given in Table 5.1.

### Cough

Cough may be due to stimulation of irritant receptors anywhere in the upper or lower respiratory tract or may be a nervous habit. Special features in the history pointing to the cause of cough are shown in Table 5.2.

### Sputum

Production of sputum is always abnormal and attention should be paid to quantity, colour, presence of blood and whether changes of posture increase production. Infected sputum is yellow or green (purulent), though asthmatic sputum may appear yellow due to the eosinophil content. Regular, morning production of clear (mucoid) sputum suggests chronic bronchitis, daily production of purulent sputum despite antibiotics suggests bronchiectasis and the sudden production of purulent, sometimes 'fetid', sputum may be due to a lung abscess. Unusually viscid sputum occurs in asthmatic patients, when it is usually mucoid, and in cystic fibrosis, when it is usually purulent.

**Table 5.1 Practical classification of causes of breathlessness according to speed of onset**

|  | Sudden (hours) | Day(s) or weeks | Months or years |
|---|---|---|---|
| Respiratory | Laryngeal oedema | Exacerbation of bronchitis/ emphysema | Chronic bronchitis/emphysema |
|  | Major airway obstruction | Pneumonia | Pulmonary fibrosis |
|  | Acute severe asthma | Left ventricular failure | Pulmonary hypertension: |
|  | Pneumothorax | Pleural effusion | Primary |
|  | Pulmonary embolism | Severe asthma | Thromboembolic |
|  | Pulmonary oedema | Progressive bronchial obstruction | Mitral valve disease |
|  | Toxic fumes |  |  |
|  | Pneumonia |  |  |
|  | Allergic alveolitis |  |  |
| Non-respiratory | Septicaemia | Anaemia | Pregnancy |
|  | Haemorrhage | Uraemia | Obesity |
|  | Poisoning | Diabetic ketoacidosis |  |
|  | Diabetic ketoacidosis | Pregnancy |  |

**Table 5.2 Diagnostic aspects of cough**

|  | Features | Likely significance |
|---|---|---|
| Unproductive | Harsh, painful | Laryngitis (croup), tracheitis |
|  |  | Early acute bronchitis or pneumonia |
|  | Sudden, short, repeated | Inhaled foreign particle |
|  | Repeated with swallowing | Aspiration |
|  | Harsh with inspiratory 'whoop' | Pertussis |
|  | Continuous, short | Early left ventricular failure, nervous habit, lymphangitis |
|  | Weak, ineffective | Vocal cord paralysis, abdominal/thoracic pain, myasthenia gravis, polyneuritis |
|  | Nocturnal | Left ventricular failure, asthma |
|  | Repeated followed by 'collapse' | Cough syncope |
|  | Becoming productive | Acute bronchitis/pneumonia |
| Productive | Daily, especially mornings | Chronic bronchitis |
|  | Daily, affected by posture | Bronchiectasis, cystic fibrosis |
|  | Sudden, purulent sputum | Lung abscess, bronchopleural fistula |
|  | Sudden, affected by posture | Pharyngeal pouch, achalasia |
|  | Containing blood | See under 'Haemoptysis' in text |

## Haemoptysis

Blood in the sputum is common in acute bronchitis and pneumonia but its presence should always raise suspicion of serious underlying disease. Pink, frothy sputum is characteristic of pulmonary oedema; recurrent haemoptysis for a few days at a time over years occurs in bronchiectasis but recent onset of daily production of blood-streaked sputum is suspicious of bronchial carcinoma or tuberculosis. Haemoptysis with breathlessness and pleurisy suggests pulmonary infarction. Massive haemoptysis (more than 600 ml of blood in 24

h) is a medical emergency and is discussed in Chapter 2.

## Wheeze

If patients complain of breathlessness they should be asked if they wheeze, because this is characteristic of airways obstruction. Daily, wheezy breathlessness with little day to day variation suggests chronic bronchitis and emphysema but, if intermittent, suggests asthma. Nocturnal wheeze or wheeze early in the morning is highly suggestive of asthma. Occasionally wheeze can be localized to one side of the chest and may indicate a localized bronchial obstruction, such as carcinoma.

## Chest pain

Pain in the chest may be due to cardiac, respiratory, gastrointestinal, musculoskeletal or neurological disease. Respiratory diseases cause chest pains of the pleuritic, central or lateral types.

### Pleuritic pain

This is stabbing or lancinating in character, worsened by coughing or deep inspiration, and is usually localized to one side. It is caused by pneumothorax, pneumonia or pulmonary infarction. A similar but more persistent and 'dragging' pain may be the first symptom of pleural mesothelioma.

### Central chest pain

This chest pain, which is worse on coughing and deep breathing, may be due to tracheal inflammation.

### Lateral chest pain

This may be due to pressure on or infiltration of a rib due to tumour. Herpes zoster of a thoracic dermatome may mimic pleural pain or rib infiltration and can be confusing until the typical vesicular rash appears.

## OTHER HISTORY

Important diagnostic information can be obtained from the familial, social and occupational history.

## Familial

A history of pulmonary disease may be obtained from patients with cystic fibrosis (1 in 4 chance of sibling affected), emphysema ($\alpha_1$-antitrypsin deficiency) and immune deficiency states (recurrent infections).

## Social

Cigarette smoking is a major cause of respiratory disability in the UK. Patients should be asked more about smoking habits over their whole life-time rather than their current consumption of tobacco. The increased risk of bronchial carcinoma in a one-time smoker falls to that of a non-smoker only after about 15 years of abstinence. Ex-smokers may have subclinical airways obstruction, which might become relevant if they develop other conditions such as late-onset asthma or heart failure. Passive inhalation of cigarette smoke can exacerbate asthma, cause an increased incidence of respiratory infections in children and statistically has been claimed to increase the likelihood of bronchial carcinoma in non-smokers.

Damp or dusty housing, certain types of central heating, bedding, carpets and curtains may be relevant to asthma sufferers. Hobbies such as keeping pigeons (not necessarily the patient's!), budgerigars or other pets are relevant to patients with alveolitis or asthma.

## Occupational

Lung disease related to occupation has been recognized since the beginning of the century. Occupational lung diseases can be classified simply, as follows.
(1) *Mineral dusts* that cause fibrosis—such as silica, asbestos, talc (severe), tin, iron and barium (mild) inhalation.
(2) *Chemical fumes*—isocyanates, hardening agents, platinum salts causing asthma. Metal fumes produce a variety of respiratory illnesses. Ammonia, chlorine and the nitrogen oxides may cause acute or chronic inflammation of airways or acute pulmonary oedema.
(3) *Organic materials* may cause asthma, acute alveolitis or chronic fibrosis (often upper lobe). Examples are farmer's lung (mouldy hay), cotton (byssinosis), proteolytic enzymes (asthma), laboratory animals or insects (asthma) and cereal dusts (asthma).
(4) *Malignancy*. Pulmonary and pleural malignancy have been attributed to industrial inhalation. The best-known example is asbestos exposure (pleural mesothelioma, bronchial carcinoma).

Many of these conditions are recognized by law as compensatable. Readers are advised to consult reference works for more detailed descriptions of occupationally related lung diseases (see Further Reading).

## EXAMINATION

### Physical signs

Certain external signs may give clues to underlying respiratory disease. The rate and difficulty of breathing should be noted and the sternomastoid and trapezius muscles should be inspected for overuse or hypertrophy. Cyanosis or anaemia may be obvious but even experienced clinicians can make subjective errors. Fingers may be nicotine stained or clubbed. Although clubbing is a well-known external marker of serious intrathoracic disease it is not always present, e.g., it is not seen in small cell carcinoma of the lung. Patients seldom notice the onset of clubbing but if it is present enquiries about arthralgia should be made because hypertrophic pulmonary osteoarthropathy may coexist. The thoracic diseases that cause clubbing are:

*Neoplasms*
Benign
Malignant
*Sepsis*
Bronchiectasis
Cystic fibrosis
Lung abscess
Empyema
*Fibrosis*
Fibrosing alveolitis
Asbestosis

Raised jugular venous pressure with predominant 'v' waves due to tricuspid regurgitation, peripheral oedema and a tender, pulsatile liver are signs of right ventricular failure (cor pulmonale) secondary to lung disease.

### *Respiratory signs*

#### Inspection

The chest should be inspected for scars of previous surgery or trauma and the shape should be assessed for kyphoscoliosis, pectus excavatum and Harrison's sulci. Longstanding airways obstruction may be suspected from the following signs:

Increased anteroposterior diameter
Hypertrophy of sternomastoid muscles
Supraclavicular and intercostal insuction
Immobile lower half of chest
Elevation of clavicles and shoulders during inspiration
Unilateral reduction in chest wall movement or a contracted hemithorax is best seen in the infra-clavicular region.

#### *Palpation*

Deviation of the trachea towards a poorly moving or contracted hemithorax suggests underlying collapse or fibrosis of that lung. The trachea often remains central in pleural effusion or pneumothorax unless there is raised intrapleural pressure (i.e., under tension). Chest expansion is measured objectively, using a tape at nipple level, and normally there is a 4 to 5 cm difference between maximum inspiration and expiration. Comparison of the movement of either side can be estimated anteriorly or posteriorly by apposing the thumbs in the midline with the fingers fanned out symmetrically on either side and comparing movement during deep inspiration. The scalene lymph node is often felt behind the medial end of the clavicle when mediastinal nodes are infiltrated by malignancy; nodes in the axillae and groins may be enlarged in sarcoidosis, Hodgkin's disease or lymphoma. Tactile vocal fremitus is a useful sign when it is reduced or absent over a pleural effusion. Other more reliable signs will be present.

#### *Percussion*

Production of a resonant note is relatively easy over normal lungs with a thin chest wall but difficulties can arise in obese or muscular patients. A dull clavicular percussion note is a good sign of collapse, consolidation or fibrosis of the upper lobe. The chest should be percussed at approximately 10-cm intervals anteriorly and posteriorly and the note compared on the two sides. Unilateral loss of resonance may be due to:

Pleural fluid
Pleural thickening
Collapse/consolidation
Pulmonary fibrosis

#### *Auscultation*

This should be done with the stethoscope diaphragm at about 10-cm intervals, starting at the top of the chest both anteriorly and posteriorly, comparing the two sides. At each site the following should be assessed:

*Breath sounds*
Loudness
Quality (bronchial breathing)

Vocal resonance (whispering pectriloquy)
*Added sounds*
Crackles
Wheezes

Breath sounds vary depending on the amount of tissue between their source and the stethoscope. Thus over the trachea relatively more high-pitched frequencies are heard whereas over the scapulae and shoulder muscles these are attenuated. Over areas of underlying consolidation, collapse and fibrosis, and at the upper level of a pleural effusion, fewer low-frequency sounds penetrate, giving rise to bronchial breathing (similar to normal sounds heard over the trachea). Vocal resonance may be increased due to the same mechanism but this is not an easy sign and a more reliable and striking sign is whispering pectriloquy.

Much unjustified importance has been attributed to the quality of crackles in lung disease. Of more use is their timing in the respiratory cycle. Crackles heard early in inspiration are typical of pulmonary oedema but in fibrosing alveolitis they are late and high pitched. In both disorders the crackles are bilateral. Unilateral crackles may be heard over an area of pneumonia. Early or mid-inspiratory crackles may be heard in obstructive chronic bronchitis or bronchiectasis. Recent research suggests that crackles are caused by sudden opening of small, gas-conducting airways due to high transmural and intrabronchial pressure gradients.

Wheezes (formally called rhonchi) are thought to be caused by vibrations in the walls of bronchi on the point of closure and are the hallmark of airflow limitation. The wheeze of an asthmatic patient may be higher in pitch than in obstructive bronchitis and emphysema but this is not reliable diagnostically because some patients with emphysema may have little wheeze. Monophonic wheeze confined to one side of the chest should suggest bronchial stenosis, most commonly due to carcinoma.

## RESPIRATORY DISEASES PRESENTING AS SUDDEN, LIFE-THREATENING EMERGENCIES

Relatively few respiratory conditions present as sudden life-threatening emergencies (see also Chapter 2) but in all there will be severe circulatory upset. Thus breathlessness, sweating, pallor,

confusion, exhaustion, cyanosis, pulsus paradoxus and hypotension are common to all. There may be little or no history available or time to obtain assistance from chest radiography, arterial blood gases or measurement of central venous pressure. Priorities are to support circulatory and respiratory function by ensuring an adequate airway and obtaining access to the circulation.

### Acute airway obstruction

Common causes are inhaled, foreign bodies, such as dentures or food debris in adults, and sweets, peanuts or small toys in children. Occasionally tracheal stenosis due to carcinoma or following previous tracheal surgery can present acutely. The patient develops sudden breathlessness and cyanosis. If the obstruction is likely to be a food bolus impacted in the larynx or trachea, then the Heimlich manoeuvre can be life saving. This is performed by encircling the arms around the patient's upper abdomen and producing an explosive exhalation by sudden pressure. Intratracheal intubation or rigid bronchoscopy under general anaesthesia would be necessary to remove other foreign bodies and restore the airway.

### Tension pneumothorax

Sudden, unilateral chest pain and breathlessness should suggest a pneumothorax. If the site of the air leak acts as a one-way valve, increase in intrapleural pressure causes mediastinal shift and impairment of venous return with cyanosis and hypotension. There may not be time for a chest X-ray to be taken; intercostal drainage needs to be established immediately using a sharp, hollow instrument, e.g., a Medicut. Recovery from the circulatory abnormality is usually rapid. Underlying diseases that particularly predispose to pneumothorax are asthma, emphysema, cystic fibrosis and any cause of 'honeycomb lung'.

### Pulmonary oedema

(See Chapter 4.)

### Acute severe asthma

Life-threatening attacks of asthma may develop suddenly over minutes in a previously asymptomatic patient or as a sudden worsening in a patient with chronic, persistent asthma. The following physical signs should alert the doctor that cardiovascular collapse is imminent:

Inability to speak
Pulse rate greater than 120 (do not assume this is due to medication)
Pulsus paradoxus (often palpable at the brachial artery but best measured by a sphygmomanometer)
Respiratory distress and exhaustion

In the presence of these signs it is better to intubate electively with the assistance of an anaesthetist rather than delay and allow cardiorespiratory arrest to occur.

If cardiorespiratory collapse is not imminent the following basic information should be obtained:

Chest radiograph (to exclude pneumothorax)
Arterial blood gas analysis
Peak expiratory flow rate (PEFR; this should be documented even if it is zero)

All patients with acute severe asthma are hypoxic and should be prescribed oxygen in high concentrations. Only very few patients with severe asthma (usually the elderly) will develop carbon dioxide narcosis. The following medication should be prescribed:

Nebulized bronchodilator, e.g., salbutamol or terbutaline (5 mg 4-hourly)
Intravenous hydrocortisone, 200 mg 6-hourly
Oral prednisolone, 30 to 60 mg in divided doses
Oral antibiotics if infection is present

Provided that patients do not delay in seeking medical attention, most will improve on this regimen. Improvement can be monitored by PEFR at 4-hourly intervals and by observing a fall in tachycardia and pulsus paradoxus. If little improvement is observed in four hours, then an intravenous infusion of bronchodilator, either $\beta_2$-stimulants, such as salbutamol or terbutaline, or aminophylline should be started. Before prescribing the latter it is important to note whether long-acting or a slow-release theophylline has been prescribed before admission. An improving PEFR reassures that the attack is subsiding but if there is little clinical improvement despite these measures, then respiratory effort may be dulled by exhaustion and serious consideration should be given to elective intubation with the help of an anaesthetist. Mechanical ventilatory assistance can then be provided until the airways obstruction has been adequately relieved.

## Massive pulmonary embolism

(See Chapter 4.)

## Adult respiratory distress syndrome

Although there is usually a latent period of hours or days after hospitalization before this develops the characteristic respiratory disturbance can rapidly become life threatening and it is appropriate to discuss it here. The essential features of this syndrome are:

Severe respiratory distress (dyspnoea, tachypnoea)
Hypoxia despite a high concentration of inspired oxygen
Diffuse shadowing on chest radiograph
Recognized antecedent cause

A wide variety of conditions can cause this syndrome but the unifying pathological event is damage to the endothelium of pulmonary capillaries. This allows leakage of fluid, fibrin, cells and platelets into the alveoli causing 'interstitial oedema' and leading to atelectasis and hyaline membrane formation, which in turn may lead to progressive fibrosis but which may occasionally resolve. The common groups of causes of this syndrome are:

Shock of any cause
Systemic infection, e.g., septicaemia
Respiratory infection, e.g., viral or bacterial pneumonia
Major trauma
Aspiration—gastric acid; drowning
Drug overdosage
Inhalation of fumes

### Management

#### Mechanical ventilation

All patients who have the full adult respiratory distress syndrome will require mechanical ventilation using high inspired oxygen. If hypoxia persists, a trial of increased end-expiratory pressure (PEEP) is justified to try and prevent premature alveolar closure.

#### Fluid management

Over-hydration should be avoided in all patients at risk of developing this syndrome; monitoring of central venous pressure and measurement of pulmonary capillary wedge pressure will assist in maintaining optimum intravascular volume. If the capillary wedge pressure rises despite satisfactory central venous pressure then an intravenous infusion of dopamine is useful.

### Corticosteroids

The value of corticosteroids in ARDS is controversial. Animal experiments suggest they are useful when given before lungs are damaged but there is no evidence of their value in patients with the established syndrome. However in practice they are usually given in high doses.

### Diuretics

These may be useful in patients who are over hydrated or have associated heart failure. The danger of reducing circulating blood volume and worsening the haemodynamic situation must be borne in mind.

### Heparin

Microvascular thromboembolism probably occurs in situ and is always found in patients who die with ARDS. While theoretically attractive there is no clinical evidence of the value of heparin.

## RESPIRATORY DISEASES PRESENTING AS ACUTE MEDICAL ADMISSIONS

### Respiratory failure

Conventionally, respiratory failure is defined as a fall in arterial oxygen tension, breathing air to 60 mmHg (8.0 kPa) or less and/or an arterial carbon dioxide tension of 50 mmHg (6.6 kPa) or above and, in practice, patients fall into one of two categories:

|        | $PO_2$ | $PCO_2$ |
|--------|--------|---------|
| Type I  | ↓ | Normal or ↓ |
| Type II | ↓ | ↑ |

Respiratory failure may be temporary, e.g., in pneumonia or asthma, or permanent, e.g., in chronic bronchitis and emphysema or fibrosing

**Table 5.3 Causes of respiratory failure**

| Neuromuscular | Myasthenia gravis |
|---|---|
| | Guillain–Barré syndrome |
| | Cerebrovascular accidents |
| | Depressed respiratory centre (e.g., drugs) |
| Skeletal | Kyphoscoliosis |
| | Thoracoplasty |
| | Trauma |
| Airways | Chronic bronchitis with emphysema |
| | Asthma |
| | Bronchiectasis |
| | Cystic fibrosis |
| | Upper respiratory obstruction |
| Parenchymal | Pulmonary fibrosis |
| | Pneumothorax (bilateral) |
| | Pulmonary infiltration (malignancy) |
| | Pneumonia |
| Vascular | Pulmonary embolism |
| | Pulmonary oedema |

alveolitis. A practical classification of causes is shown in Table 5.3.

### Physical signs

In severe respiratory failure the following should be observed:
Tachypnoea
Central cyanosis
Overactive accessory muscles
Dilated peripheral veins
Respiratory 'flap'
In addition signs of right ventricular strain/ failure should be found:
Raised jugular venous pressure ('v' wave due to tricuspid regurgitation)
Overactive right ventricle
Accentuated pulmonary second sound
Palpable liver (pulsatile?)
Peripheral oedema

### Electrocardiogram

The ECG shows changes of right ventricular dilatation (strain) relatively late. The earliest sign is tall, peaked P waves seen in leads 2 and 3 and aVF. In lead V1 an rSR pattern and an RS pattern in V5 and 6 are seen late in the course of the disease. T-wave inversion from leads 6 to 8 is common but not specific.

### Chest radiograph

This may show over-inflated lungs with low, flat diaphragms and this may cause underestimation of cardiac diameter. Prominence of the vascular shadows of the hilum suggests established pulmonary hypertension. Changes suggesting an acute precipitating event, e.g., pneumonia, embolism, pleural effusion, should be sought.

### Management

#### Relieve hypoxia

Analysis of arterial blood gas will verify the variety and severity of respiratory failure. This is important because in type I failure, large concentrations of inspired oxygen are necessary to relieve hypoxia with little risk of $CO_2$ retention. In type II failure, with $CO_2$ retention, overzealous administration of oxygen can cause a further rise of $PCO_2$ with increasing drowsiness. The principle of controlled oxygen therapy is to increase the $PO_2$ up to 60 mmHg using the minimum concentration of inspired oxygen without provoking further $CO_2$ retention.

#### Identify the precipitating cause

In a previously healthy person, respiratory failure may be due to pneumonia, asthma, pulmonary embolism, pneumothorax, thoracic trauma or neuromuscular disorder. Much more commonly an acute event is superimposed on a chronic pulmonary condition and the following should be looked for and treated:

Bronchopulmonary infection
Pneumothorax
Pulmonary embolism/infarction
Left ventricular failure
Cardiac arrhythmia

#### Relieve airways obstruction

Measurement of PEFR before and after 5 mg of salbutamol or terbutaline inhaled via a nebulizer will indicate if there is reversible bronchospasm. If improvement occurs this treatment should be given on a regular basis (4-hourly) and an intravenous infusion of salbutamol or terbutaline or aminophylline should be considered. Upper airways obstruction due to mucus impaction,

inhalation or an intrabronchial tumour should also be considered.

#### Treat right ventricular failure

Diuretics in modest doses along with potassium supplements usually remove unsightly peripheral oedema but their effect may take days and the temptation to increase the dose or start with high dosage should be resisted. The right ventricle needs a high filling pressure and if the intravascular volume is reduced by over-vigorous diuresis the patient may feel worse. There is controversy over the use of digoxin because of the risk of arrhythmia due to accompanying hypoxia and diuretic-induced hypokalaemia.

### Management

During early management re-evaluate the patient frequently. Repeated clinical observation and sampling of arterial blood gas allow recognition of a patient who is exhausted and who may need mechanical ventilation. Patients with pneumonia, pulmonary oedema, acute severe asthma or neuromuscular disorder (apart from strokes) should be intubated and ventilated sooner rather than later because of the potential for full recovery. Patients with chronic bronchitis and emphysema, pulmonary fibrosis or chest wall abnormality should be assessed with regard to previous exercise tolerance and lung function, and whether the insult that has produced deterioration is reversible. There is no adequate information to act as a guide to which patients should be ventilated and it is necessary to rely on experienced clinical judgement.

Respiratory drive and elimination of carbon dioxide can be enhanced in patients with type II respiratory failure with doxapram hydrochloride given by intravenous infusion (2 mg/ml). In clinical practice this seems superior to previously used respiratory stimulants such as nikethamide. Management of patients with respiratory disease on a mechanical ventilator is beyond the scope of this chapter.

### Exacerbations of chronic bronchitis and emphysema

Comparisons between clinical and pathological findings suggest that the commonly made division of such patients into 'pink puffers' with predominant emphysema and 'blue bloaters' with predominant obstructive bronchitis is an over-simplification. Most patients have features of both and it seems sensible to use the combined term 'chronic bronchitis with emphysema'. Occasionally emphysema exists in a pure form such as in the condition of hereditary $\alpha_1$-trypsin deficiency.

Most such exacerbations are due to infection, either bacterial or viral, and the majority are easily treated without referral to hospital. Problems arise in patients with severe airways obstruction or who are elderly or debilitated. Such patients may develop severe, wheezy breathlessness and cyanosis. Hypoxia produces constriction of the pulmonary arteries, which in turn produces right ventricular strain and may lead to the peripheral signs of right ventricular failure (cor pulmonale).

## Management

On admission the following investigations should be made.

### Chest radiograph to exclude pneumothorax

Even a small pneumothorax can cause severe respiratory embarrassment in a patient with severe bronchitis and emphysema; an intercostal drain should be inserted more readily in such cases than in the fitter patient.

### Arterial blood gas analysis

If the arterial $PO_2$ is below 60 mmHg (8 kPa) and/or $PCO_2$ is above 50 mmHg (6.5 kPa), the patient is in established respiratory failure and treated accordingly.

### Administer controlled oxygen therapy

The $PO_2$ may be extremely low in severe exacerbations and can rapidly lead to serious disturbance of the heart, brain and kidneys. In such patients, because the respiratory centre has become relatively insensitive to the stimulatory effect of raised $PCO_2$ the hypoxia may be the major drive to ventilation. The principles of controlled oxygen therapy are described in the section on the management of respiratory failure.

### Treat infection

The two most common pathogens identified are *Haemophilus influenzae* and *Streptococcus pneu-*

*moniae* and both are sensitive to ampicillin, 250 to 500 mg, three or four times a day for a week. A satisfactory alternative in people allergic to ampicillin is co-trimoxazole, two 480 mg tablets twice a day for a week. One study has shown that sulfametopyrazine in a single large dose is as effective as ampicillin taken for a week. In severely ill patients, antibiotics may need to be given intramuscularly or intravenously.

### Treat associated bronchospasm

In addition to fixed airways obstruction there may be a small element of reversibility and salbutamol or terbutaline 5 mg (1 ml) in 2 ml of saline should be nebulized and PEFR measured before and after treatment. This therapy may also help humidify the airway and improve the clearance of secretions.

### Long-term oxygen therapy (LTOT)

The WHO have defined corpulmonale as increased thickness of the right ventricle associated with hypoxic pulmonary disease and though not entirely suitable it is currently the best definition available. Clinically patients are in Type II respiratory failure and have peripheral oedema. The prognosis of patients who have suffered an episode of corpulmonale is very poor, only about 30% survive a further five years. It has been shown by two large studies, one conducted by the MRC and the other by the National Institute of Health of the United States, that continuous oxygen given long term considerably improves chances of survival. The mechanism is thought to be due to the relief of hypoxia with reduction in pulmonary arterial vasoconstriction and a fall in pulmonary artery pressure. It was shown that suitable patients needed to take oxygen continuously for at least 15 h per day at a flow rate to be determined by blood gas analysis. The criteria for LTOT in the UK are:

(1) A successfully treated episode of corpulmonale with peripheral oedcma.
(2) Associated left ventricular failure, bronchospasm and bronchial infection should have been adequately treated.
(3) If the above have been satisfied the arterial $PO_2$ at rest breathing room air should be less than 55 mmHg (8 kPa).
(4) The patients should be non-smokers in view of fire risk.

Potentially suitable patients need to be assessed by a respiratory physician and blood gas analysis should be performed with supplemental oxygen at flow rates of 1, 2 and 3 litres to find which flow rate gives optimum improvement in $PO_2$ without exacerbating co-existing hypercapnoea. LTOT is most conveniently and economically delivered by oxygen concentrators but these can only be prescribed by general practitioners on an FP10 form.

There is much evidence that many patients who have concentrators have not been fully assessed and do not comply with the above criteria.

## Sleep apnoea

The pattern of respiration during normal sleep is not uniform. During NREM sleep there is a reduction in tidal volume and frequency. During REM sleep the pattern is more irregular with occasional brief episodes of apnoea with transient and slight episodes of oxygen desaturation. These physiological irregularities are most pronounced in the elderly. An episode of apnoea of 10 s or longer is regarded as abnormal and if more than 30 such episodes occur in one night complications become likely such as increased pulmonary artery pressure, corpulmonale, abnormalities of cardiac rhythm and polycythaemia. The causes of sleep apnoea are classified into:

(a) *Central*. This is absence of movements of the chest wall.
(b) *Obstructive*. This is absence of gas flow due to obstruction usually of the upper airway though chest wall movement continues.
(c) *Mixed*.

The type of sleep apnoea can be diagnosed by laboratory studies during sleep using chest wall electrodes and measurements of nasal air flow. In the majority of cases the apnoea is of obstructive type.

Symptoms which should alert the physician to the presence of obstructive sleep apnoea and which might more easily be obtained from the patients spouse or other friends are daytime sleepiness, personality change or deterioration in intellectual performance, loud snoring and disturbed sleep.

The cause of the upper airway obstruction should always be sought. There are reports of successful surgical procedures to relieve anatomical obstruction. Other patients have abnormal collapsability of the upper airways and may be improved with continuous positive airway pressure ventilation.

## Nocturnal assisted ventilation

It has recently been shown that continuous positive airway pressure ventilation is of great value in patients with a wide variety of diseases leading to respiratory failure. Such patients are particularly prone to hypoxia and hypercapnoea during the REM phases of sleep. After suitable investigation in a centre specializing in this form of ventilatory therapy it has been shown that patients with conditions as various as kyphoscoliosis, previous thoracoplasty, bulbar poliomyelitis and muscular dystrophy, nocturnal assisted ventilation using positive airway pressure via a face mask can correct blood gas abnormalities, reverse pulmonary hypertension and prolong life. Interestingly if blood gas abnormalities are corrected with assisted ventilation during sleep the gases often remain satisfactory during waking hours without the help of a ventilator.

## Pneumonia

This is infective inflammation of lung parenchyma; it may predominantly be alveolar in a segmental or subsegmental distribution (lobar pneumonia) or accompanied by infected intrabronchial secretions in a lobular or multilobular distribution (bronchopneumonia). A useful practical classification is to consider pneumonia either as 'primary' (community acquired; Table 5.4) or 'secondary', occurring either in the presence of pre-existing lung disease or in systemic diseases that impair host resistance (Tables 5.5, 5.6). The division is useful because organisms causing the two sorts of pneumonia tend to be different.

### Diagnosis

The clinical diagnosis of pneumonia is not usually difficult in patients who present with cough, fever and pleuritic chest pain. The severity of the illness should be judged by signs of confusion, respiratory distress and cyanosis. The likelihood of septicaemia should be considered if the patient is cold, clammy and hypotensive. At first, sputum may not be present and the classical physical signs of lobar consolidation may not be apparent. They are:

Reduced percussion note

**Table 5.4 Organisms causing primary pneumonia**

| Organism | Special clinical features | Treatment |
|---|---|---|
| *Strep. pneumoniae* | Classically but uncommonly in lobar/segmental distribution—sputum and blood cultures useful | Benzylpenicillin (i.m./i.v.) Ampicillin (oral) Erythromycin (oral/i.v.) |
| *Mycoplasma pneumoniae* | Radiograph may look worse than patient; sputum unhelpful; diagnosis by rising antibody titre | Tetracycline or erythromycin (oral) |
| *Haemophilus influenzae* | Nil | Ampicillin |
| *Legionella pneumophila* | Severe systemic upset; confusion, gastrointestinal, hepatic, renal abnormalities; diagnosis by rising antibody titres | Erythromycin (i.v. then oral for 3 weeks) |
| *Mycobacterium tuberculosis* | Gradual onset illness; haemoptysis common; sputum Ziehl–Nielsen smear usually positive | Isoniazid, rifampicin, ethambutol, pyrazinamide (triple or quadruple) |
| *Coxiella burnetti* | Occupational (animal contact); 2 weeks incubation period; segmental/lobar on chest X-ray; diagnosis—rising antibody titres | Tetracycline or erythromycin; can be self-limiting |
| *Chlamydia psittaci* | Acquired from birds; severe illness; erythema nodosum and haemolysis occasionally; diagnosis—complement fixation | Tetracycline |
| Viral (influenza, measles chicken pox, respiratory syncytial) | Constitutional symptoms; may be few specific respiratory symptoms; diagnosis—viral studies | Acyclovir; prophylaxis in influenza epidemic |

**Table 5.5 Causes of secondary pneumonia**

*Damaged lungs*
Cystic fibrosis
Bronchiectasis
Fibrosis
Carcinoma
*Epidemic influenza*
*Gastrointestinal aspiration*
Achalasia
Alcoholism
Poor dental hygiene
*Suppressed resistance*
Congenital:
   hypogammaglobulinaemia
Acquired:
   malignancy (e.g., leukaemia)
   iatrogenic (e.g., steroids; chemotherapy;
     immunosuppressives)
   AIDS

Bronchial breathing
Crackles
Whispering pectriloquy
Pleural friction rub
  Widespread crackles may be the only sign of bilateral bronchopneumonia, though patchy bronchial breathing is occasionally heard.

### Chest radiography

This serves to confirm the distribution of consolidation and if lobar in distribution the organism is almost always *Strep. pneumoniae*. In bronchopneumonia, there will be patchy, irregular shadowing, usually of the lower zones; this may be unilateral or bilateral.

### Sputum

This should be sent for Gram and Ziehl–Nielsen staining and culture in all cases of pneumonia. If a patient has received antibiotics before a sample is taken, cultures may not be helpful.

### Blood cultures

These can be positive in a quarter of cases providing they are taken before antibiotics have been prescribed.

### Management

Objective assessment of the degree of systemic hypoxia should be recorded by analysis of arterial blood gas. Most patients with pneumonia admitted to hospital have type I respiratory failure.

**Table 5.6 Organisms causing secondary pneumonia**

| Organism | Special clinical features | Treatment |
|---|---|---|
| *Staphylococcus* | May complicate influenza; thin-walled abscesses; sputum and blood culture useful before antibiotics | Cloxacillin (i.v.) Flucloxacillin (i.v.) Gentamicin (i.v.) |
| *Klebsiella* | Severe illness; high mortality; often upper lobes; abscess formation, haemoptysis common; diagnosis—Gram staining of sputum | Use 2 antibiotics (gentamicin, cephalosporin i.v.) |
| *Pseudomonas aeruginosa* | Predisposition in cystic fibrosis and ventilated patients; chest X-ray—patchy bronchopneumonia | Use 2 antibiotics (gentamicin, carbenicillin, ticarcillin i.v.) |
| *Pneumocystis carinii* | Affects immunosuppressed hosts; induced sputum may be helpful; lung biopsy necessary for certain diagnosis | Co-trimoxazole |
| Anaerobes | Poor dental hygiene, aspiration, predisposing factors; cavitation or slow-resolving disease; sputum often unhelpful; gas liquid chromatography helpful | Penicillin, metronidazole |
| *Escherichia coli, H. influenzae* | Pathogenicity uncertain, frequently commensals or with mixed flora; treat if growth significant | Dependent on sensitivity tests |
| Cytomegalovirus | Asymptomatic infection in healthy patients may be common; immunosuppressed susceptible especially after renal transplants | Gancyclovir |
| Fungi (*Candida, Aspergillus*) | Unresponsive invading and necrotizing pneumonia in the immunosuppressed, e.g., cytotoxic therapy, leukaemia | Amphotericin B, ketoconazole |
| Opportunistic *Mycobacteria* | Often in scarring following *M. tuberculosis*; sputum culture vital | Dependent on sensitivity tests |
| Actinomycosis, *Nocardia* | | Co-trimoxazole |

## Oxygen therapy

This should be prescribed to relieve hypoxia and in practice means inspired oxygen concentrations of at least 35 per cent. It is a mistake to leave administration of oxygen to nurses or physiotherapists because they almost always give 24 per cent inspired oxygen, which could be inadequate, leading to continuous hypoxia of vital organs. Unless the patient is exhausted or has longstanding, irreversible airways obstruction, $CO_2$ narcosis in simple pneumonia is rare.

## Dehydration

In severe pneumonia, patients are often dehydrated and this should be corrected.

## Analgesia

Pleural inflammation is a common accompaniment of pneumonia and unless relieved causes considerable distress.

## Antibiotics

Ideally these should be prescribed according to the results of sensitivity tests made on bacterial cultures. In practice treatment has to be prescribed before this information is available. If a patient has classical lobar pneumonia, benzylpenicillin is the antibiotic of choice. Bronchopneumonia is commoner, however, and the organisms responsible are less predictable. In a previously healthy person the majority of infections respond to erythromycin, which is effective against pneumococcus, mycoplasma and *Legionella*. If the patient is not better in 48 h and sputum and blood cultures have been unhelpful, a change of therapy should be considered in case the infecting agent is 'atypical' due to *Coxiella* or *Chlamydia*.

If the pneumonia is 'secondary' and the patient may be gravely ill it may be necessary to begin broad-spectrum antibiotic treatment. Intravenous cloxacillin or flucloxacillin to cover staphylococcal infection and intravenous gentamicin, carbenicillin, ticarcillin or a cephalosporin to cover Gram-negative organisms such as *Klebsiella* and *Pseudomonas* spp. An outline of treatment for the more unusual organisms is given in the Table 5.6 and in practice should be undertaken with frequent advice from the bacteriology laboratory.

Resolution of fever provides encouragement that the organism is responding to treatment but the antibiotics should be continued for at least a week in all cases and for two or three weeks in special circumstances. The patients usually feel better as the fever resolves, the physical signs may take a little longer and the chest radiograph sometimes takes weeks before completely clearing. Presumably fever and constitutional symptoms resolve as the bacteria are killed but macrophages and other clearance mechanisms take much longer to clear the alveolar exudate.

## Acquired immune deficiency syndrome (AIDS)

Pneumonia is a frequent diagnostic and therapeutic problem in AIDS; it is dealt with in Chapter 3.

## Acute severe asthma

This is an important cause of sudden death in the community. On arrival in hospital, patients should be assessed immediately because cardiorespiratory arrest shortly after admission is a not uncommon tragedy in this condition. Severe asthma may arise from a background of chronic, persistent wheeze or can arise in a patient who has previously been little troubled. It cannot be assumed that an attack is not serious because the patient has never been admitted to hospital before. On the other hand, patients who have had severe attacks requiring mechanical ventilation may require similar management again.

## Assessment

If the patient exhibits some or all of the following features, then immediate treatment is required.

### Cyanosis and/or pallor

This, along with sweating and confusion, is an ominous sign of impending cardiorespiratory arrest.

### Speech

The inability to speak a sentence of moderate length indicates a severe attack.

### Tachycardia

A pulse rate of 120 or more indicates a severe attack and should not be attributed to the previous administration of drugs.

### Pulsus paradoxus

This is due to very high intrathoracic pressure swings and indicates severe airways obstruction. Hypotension is an ominous sign of impending cardiorespiratory arrest.

### Wheeze

Loudness and length of wheeze does not help assess the severity of the attack. Disappearance of wheeze should not be misinterpreted as recovery in the presence of the other signs because it might indicate imminent cardiorespiratory arrest.

A decision about the severity of an attack can therefore be made by simple clinical examination (and a little clinical experience). In most cases, time allows for ancillary investigations to be obtained.

### Investigations

#### Chest radiograph

This is done to exclude a pneumothorax, pneumomediastinum, lobar collapse or pneumonic infection. Although the patient is severely breathless the X-rays are usually of good technical quality because of the accompanying over-inflation.

#### Arterial blood gas analysis

All patients with acute severe asthma are hypoxic and the vast majority have a low $PCO_2$ due to the hyperventilation. A normal or rising $PCO_2$ may be ominous signs of exhaustion. The pH should also be noted.

#### Respiratory function

Such patients are often too breathless to perform a spirogram but a PEFR reading should be made for future reference, even if it is zero.

## Sputum

Examination of sputum in acute, severe asthma is rarely helpful. If infection precipitated the attack it is usually viral and the results of sputum cultures seldom lead to a change of antibiotic.

## Management

### Oxygen

Patients with acute severe asthma usually have type I respiratory failure and oxygen should be administered in sufficient concentrations to raise the $PO_2$ to 60 mmHg (8.0 kPa). Because inequalities in ventilation perfusion usually take weeks to recover, the arterial $PO_2$ remains subnormal for a surprisingly long time after airways obstruction has apparently recovered.

### Rehydration

Acute severe asthma attacks of more than a few hours usually cause some degree of rehydration and an intravenous infusion of saline should be set up to help restore this and to provide access to the circulation.

### Bronchodilator

These may be administered intravenously or by inhalation.

*Intravenous.* Aminophylline, 250 to 500 mg over 10 min, should be given to patients who are critically ill as long as they have not been taking slow-release theophylline preparations orally. If a satisfactory response is not obtained an infusion may be set up delivering 250 to 500 mg 8-hourly in saline. Salbutamol, 200 µg given over 10 min, is an alternative.

*Inhaled.* Most patients will already have taken bronchodilator aerosol before admission. Administration of much larger doses, e.g., salbutamol or terbutaline 5 mg (1 ml in 2 ml of saline) frequently relieves airways obstruction when repeated inhalation from a dose-metered inhaler has not succeeded. Use of $\beta_2$-receptor stimulant, bronchodilator drugs in this dose can be repeated 4-hourly and is surprisingly free of side-effects.

### Corticosteroids

Hydrocortisone, 200 mg intravenously every 6 hours, may be given though it is doubtful if this works any quicker than oral prednisolone as long as this is absorbed. In severe attacks the latter should be started in doses of 30 to 60 mg per day in divided dosage. High doses used over a week or a fortnight cause no significant side-effects and there should be little hesitation in prescribing them.

### Antibiotics

Many asthma attacks are not triggered by infection, and antibiotics are frequently prescribed inappropriately. If sputum becomes infected then a course of ampicillin or co-trimoxazole is indicated.

### Physiotherapy

This has little part to play during the recovery from an attack of acute severe asthma—sputum retention is not due to inability or reluctance to cough but to the sticky nature of the mucus.

### Respiratory stimulants

These should never be used in an acute severe attack of asthma. The respiratory centre is already under maximum drive and if the respiratory effort diminishes, then this is a positive indication for mechanical ventilation.

## Reassessment

The following should be reassessed at frequent intervals during early management.

### Clinical examination

Improvement in colour, tachycardia and pulsus paradoxus are reassuring signs of recovery.

### PEFR measurements

These should be performed 4-hourly before and after inhaled bronchodilator; increasing values reassure that the attack is subsiding.

### Arterial blood gas analysis

If the above measures are not improving in a satisfactory way, then blood gas analysis should be repeated because the patient may become exhausted and require mechanical ventilation.

## Pneumothorax

A practical classification relevant to the management of this problem is as follows.

*Spontaneous*—this occurs in previously fit young people with no underlying lung disease.

*Secondary* to lung disease.

*Airways obstruction*, e.g., asthma, emphysema.

'*Cystic diseases*', e.g., cystic fibrosis, honeycomb lung.

Sub-pleural diseases, e.g., tuberculosis, carcinoma or abscess.

*Trauma*—there may be associated injuries to other vital organs.

Pneumothorax can be divided physiologically into the open and closed type. In the closed type the air leak has sealed but in the open type air continues to leak from intrapulmonary airways into the pleural space. A continuous leak leads to complete collapse of a lung with increasing intrathoracic pressure, reduction of venous return and impending cardiovascular collapse (tension pneumothorax). In most cases there may be a small shift of the mediastinum but the circulation is not embarrassed.

### Symptoms

In a previously fit patient the sudden onset of pleuritic chest pain with or without breathlessness should raise suspicion of a pneumothorax. In a patient with pre-existing lung disease, sudden deterioration of breathlessness along with pleuritic chest pain requires a chest X-ray to exclude pneumothorax—some pneumothoraces occur without symptoms and are discovered as a chance finding on routine radiography.

### Physical signs

In tension pneumothorax a patient is cyanosed, breathless with tachycardia, has displacement of the mediastinum and is hypotensive. In less severe forms the following physical signs are typical:

Unilateral reduction in respiratory movement

Hyper-resonant percussion note compared with the normal side

Diminished or absent breath sounds

### Management

This depends on the degree of lung collapse, the symptoms and the presence of pre-existing lung disease. A pneumothorax occupying only 20 per cent of a hemithorax in a healthy person will cause no distress and usually resolves spontaneously. A pneumothorax of similar size in a patient with lung disease may cause distress and precipitate respiratory failure so intercostal drainage is essential. Even if the patient is asymptomatic, drainage is indicated if it will expedite return to work.

The intercostal drainage tube can be inserted either anteriorly in the second intercostal space or laterally in the fourth or fifth intercostal space. The anterior approach has the advantage that apical pockets of air are more easily drained but its disadvantages are the proximity to the aortic arch on the left side and that the scar on the anterior chest wall may not please some patients. A lateral approach allows easy drainage of accompanying effusion. Opinion is divided about the value of injecting a chemical agent to cause a pleurodesis and prevent recurrence.

If the pneumothorax has resolved radiologically and bubbling through the underwater, sealed drain has ceased, the tube should be clamped and a chest radiograph in expiration obtained; if the lung remains expanded the tube is removed. If the radiograph shows residual air in the pleural space, drainage should continue until it has resolved; if resistant, a continuous, low-pressure suction pump, e.g., a Robertson's pump, will assist complete resolution. If the lung remains resistant to expansion (this usually implies underlying lung disease) referral to thoracic surgeons for pleurectomy should be considered. During transfer to the surgeons the tube should be allowed to drain freely and not be clamped. The bottle should remain below the level of the patient's thorax.

## Lung collapse

Collapse of a lung or part of a lung may produce sudden breathlessness requiring emergency medical admission. The cause is usually bronchial obstruction due to a bronchial carcinoma, a bronchial adenoma or an inhaled foreign body. Classical signs are deviation of the trachea, reduced chest expansion, dullness to percussion and diminished or absent breath sounds. A chest radiograph will confirm deviation of the trachea and mediastinal shift and help differentiate collapse from pneumonia or pleural effusion. If the patient is distressed, then urgent bronchoscopy is indicated. Occasionally, viscid mucus may be responsible postoperatively and can be removed by suction. A foreign body can be identified and removed by a rigid bronchoscope but the usual finding is carcinoma in the trachea or around the carina. At this stage the tumour is inoperable and urgent radiotherapy, which usually shrinks the lesion allowing re-expansion of the collapsed lobe or lung, is indicated.

## Haemorrhage

Intrathoracic haemorrhage causes either haemoptysis or haemopneumothorax. The latter presents in the same way as a pleural effusion and most commonly it is either due to pleural malignancy (primary or secondary) or occurs in the presence of a systemic clotting disorder.

Haemoptysis is a common symptom in acute medical admissions. The causes are briefly reviewed next. They are:

*Cardiovascular disorders*, e.g., left ventricular failure, pulmonary oedema, mitral stenosis, pulmonary embolism

*Lung disease*, e.g. carcinoma, tuberculosis, acute respiratory infection, bronchiectasis or a small mucosal tear (analogous to the Mallory–Weiss tear)

Occasionally patients present with massive haemoptysis (more than 700 ml per day). Here the blood should be grouped and crossmatched in case signs of haemorrhagic shock appear. The most common causes of haemoptysis of this degree are:

Bronchiectasis
Lung abscess
Tuberculosis
Bronchial carcinoma

In bronchial carcinoma bleeding of this degree is usually a terminal event.

The chest radiograph may give a clear indication of the underlying cause but bronchoscopy may also be helpful in identifying the side or lobe of the haemorrhage; urgent radiotherapy to a neoplasm or surgical resection of the bleeding segment may be life saving. If there is doubt about which area of the lung is bleeding, then arteriography via the aorta to outline the bronchial arterial circulation may allow precise identification of the bleeding vessel and it may be possible to introduce therapeutic emboli and thus arrest the haemorrhage.

## RESPIRATORY DISEASES PRESENTING IN OUTPATIENTS

The patient with respiratory disease presents in the outpatients department with a referral letter describing one or a combination of symptoms (see Tables 5.1, 5.2) or because a chest X-ray has shown an unexpected abnormality.

## Breathlessness with or without wheeze

Gradual onset of breathlessness is a common symptom requiring referral for assessment. In determining the cause the most useful points to extract from the history are:
(a) rate of progression of breathlessness;
(b) whether breathlessness is intermittent and unexpected;
(c) has the patient, relative or a doctor heard wheezing?

Clinical history, physical examination, chest X-ray and ECG should exclude cardiac disease, though in some patients cardiac and pulmonary disease may contribute to breathlessness and it may be difficult to decide which is the predominant problem. Simple haematological and biochemical tests will exclude anaemia and metabolic acidosis as a cause of breathlessness. If pulmonary disease is thought to be the cause, then although there is a large number of diseases that may be responsible, in practical terms these can be grouped into two sorts:

Obstructive ventilatory defects
Restrictive ventilatory defects

The flow diagram in Fig. 5.1. is a simple, practical guide to the evaluation of the cause of breathlessness.

### *Obstructive ventilatory defects (air flow limitation)*

The three disease processes that usually cause this are asthma, chronic obstructive bronchitis and emphysema. In some patients, much difficulty may arise in deciding how much of each of these is present in any one case. In practical terms and certainly for the benefit of the patient the following questions need to be answered.

### *Is there objective evidence of airways obstruction?*

Vital capacity is commonly reduced in moderate and severe airways obstruction but the forced expiratory volume in 1s ($FEV_1$; explained in 'Lung function tests' below) will be disproportionately reduced and the simple spirogram using a wedge-bellows spirometer (Vitalograph) is an

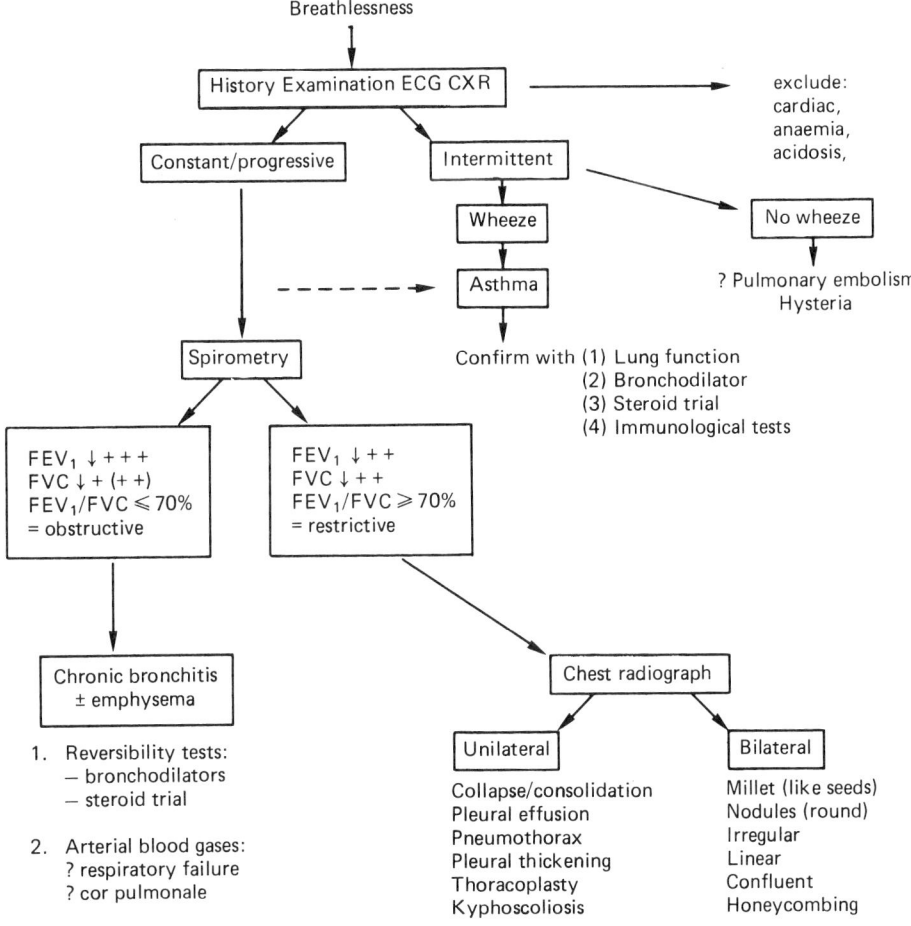

Breathlessness

History Examination ECG CXR → exclude:
cardiac,
anaemia,
acidosis,

Constant/progressive    Intermittent

Wheeze    No wheeze

Asthma    ? Pulmonary embolism
Hysteria

Spirometry

Confirm with (1) Lung function
(2) Bronchodilator
(3) Steroid trial
(4) Immunological tests

$FEV_1 \downarrow + + +$
$FVC \downarrow + (+ +)$
$FEV_1/FVC \leqslant 70\%$
= obstructive

$FEV_1 \downarrow + +$
$FVC \downarrow + +$
$FEV_1/FVC \geqslant 70\%$
= restrictive

Chronic bronchitis
± emphysema

Chest radiograph

Unilateral    Bilateral

1. Reversibility tests:
   − bronchodilators
   − steroid trial

2. Arterial blood gases:
   ? respiratory failure
   ? cor pulmonale

Collapse/consolidation    Millet (like seeds)
Pleural effusion          Nodules (round)
Pneumothorax              Irregular
Pleural thickening        Linear
Thoracoplasty             Confluent
Kyphoscoliosis            Honeycombing

*Figure 5.1*   Flow diagram illustrating the investigation of breathlessness

accurate and reproducible way of measuring this and is more informative than PEFR.

### Is the air flow obstruction reversible?

Repeating the lung function test 10 min after supervised inhalation of a $\beta_2$-agonist bronchodilator may show an increase in both vital capacity and $FEV_1$; if either figure improves by 20 per cent or more, then the air flow obstruction is regarded as partially or wholly reversible, i.e., asthma. If repeat values do not improve significantly with inhaled bronchodilator, then a course of oral corticosteroids should be considered in adequate doses—prednisolone, 30 and 60 mg a day for a week or a fortnight. Lung function testing should then be repeated and if the values have improved by 20 per cent or more the patient should be

regarded as asthmatic. Clearly, oral corticosteroids cannot be continued in this dose and so as it is reduced gradually, inhaled bronchodilator drugs (e.g., salbutamol or terbutaline) and inhaled topically active steroid aerosol (e.g., beclomethasone or budesonide) should be introduced. Particular attention should be paid to the patient's technique of inhaling aerosol; if this is imperfect, alternative methods such as dry powder capsules (rotacaps) or a plastic spacer device might improve the quantity of drug inhaled.

In special circumstances other diagnostic manoeuvres may be helpful. If wheezy breathlessness is particularly troublesome after exertion, a standard exercise test with repeated lung function may produce measurable bronchoconstriction and premedication with either inhaled bronchodilator or disodium cromoglycate may abolish this. If occupational exposure is suspected, then cumulative peak-flow measurements using a portable peak-flow gauge may reveal patterns of bronchoconstriction at work with relief during weekends and holidays. If, despite a trial of bronchodilators and/or oral corticosteroids, the air flow obstruction remains irreversible, further lung function tests (such as volume estimation by gas dilution and gas transfer measurements) may indicate the patient has emphysema in which the lungs will be over-inflated with an increased total capacity, residual volume and functional residual capacity and a low gas transfer. These patients may improve slightly on inhaled bronchodilator drugs but generally inhaled corticosteroid prophylaxis and certainly oral steroids do not produce objective benefit. Oral steroids can produce serious systemic side-effects and should be avoided.

### Restrictive ventilatory defects

These are much less common though more varied than conditions causing airways obstruction; some common causes are:

    Industrial dust disease
    Extrinsic allergic alveolitis
    Cryptogenic fibrosing alveolitis
    Pleural disease
    Skeletal deformity and disease
    Healed fibrotic tuberculosis
    Chronic fibrotic sarcoidosis
    Histiocytosis X of the lung

#### Industrial dust disease

Though likely to become uncommon due to the control of the working environment there are three important conditions—asbestosis, pneumoconiosis and silicosis.

**Asbestosis.** This term should be restricted to interstitial fibrosis developing as a consequence of prolonged inhalation of asbestos fibres. Typically there is irregular nodular and linear shadowing in the lower zones on the chest radiograph. The pleura and pericardium become thickened, clubbing is common and there may be 'asbestos bodies' in the sputum. The diagnosis is usually made on the history of exposure and the presence of a restrictive ventilatory defect on formal lung function testing in the absence of other obvious causes. Lung biopsy may be necessary in some cases, but should not be necessary to assist patients in obtaining compensation.

**Coal worker's pneumoconiosis.** This may occur in coal miners, who may also inhale stone and silica dust, and it used to occur in a more pure form in stokers and trimmers when ships used coal as fuel. A long history of exposure is required to produce the typical X-ray appearances, which consist of irregular, nodular shadowing—this is termed simple pneumoconiosis. Complicated pneumoconiosis is the term used to describe the coalescence of nodules usually in the upper zones leading to progressive massive fibrosis (PMF). In men who have or will develop rheumatoid disease the chest X-ray shows more well-defined, rounded opacities of varying size, which may cavitate or calcify (Caplan's syndrome).

**Silicosis.** This is due to the inhalation of large amounts of silica particles, which overwhelms the normal mechanisms of mucociliary clearance. Nodules enlarge and coalesce, usually in the upper zones. The hilar nodes enlarge and frequently become calcified.

In patients with asbestosis there is an increased incidence of both pleural and pulmonary malignancy. Emphysema is usually present in patients with coal worker's pneumoconiosis (focal) and in silicosis (bullous), and in both conditions cor pulmonale is a common terminal complication.

#### Extrinsic allergic alveolitis

This condition is caused by a type 3 (immune complex) immunological disorder, though cell-mediated immunity is also involved because granuloma formation is a feature. A wide variety of organic dusts causes this type of damage but the common forms in the UK are:

(a) farmer's lung—due to thermophilic organisms which flourish in mouldy hay;

(b) bird breeder's lung—commonly from pigeons or budgerigars;

(c) humidifier fever—due to amoebae and *Micropolyspora faeni* in water and ventilation systems

The disorder can present in one of two ways. Firstly, as an acute illness with malaise, breathlessness (no wheezing) and dry cough after exposure to a large dose of antigen. Typically, crackles are heard in the lungs and the chest X-ray shows fine irregular nodular shadowing. On withdrawal from exposure the disease will remit spontaneously in a week or two though recovery will be hastened by a course of corticosteroids. Re-exposure to a large dose of antigen usually causes a recurrence. Secondly and more sinister is low-dose exposure over a prolonged period so that the patients are not warned by an acute illness. Slowly progressive breathlessness due to fibrosis, most commonly in the upper zones, is the first indication of trouble. When patients present for evaluation the disease may be advanced and the changes are irreversible despite withdrawal from further exposure. Diagnosis depends on specific enquiry about exposure to allergens and a demonstration of precipitating antibodies to the suspected allergens in the patient's blood. Lung biopsy shows interstitial fibrosis with granulomas. If the disease is suspected or proved, a course of corticosteroids should be tried in an attempt to clear inflammatory exudate and halt the progressive fibrosis. This may effect an improvement in symptoms and in the gas transfer measurement but in most cases the radiograph remains abnormal and the patient will always have a degree of dyspnoea on exertion.

## Cryptogenic fibrosing alveolitis

This is a disorder characterized by progressive breathlessness on exertion, high-pitched late inspiratory crackles on auscultation, clubbing and irregular nodular linear shadowing, particularly in the lower zones of the chest X-ray. Lung biopsies show a mixture of fibrosis around and involving alveolar walls and intra-alveolar exudation in which macrophages are prominent. The disease may be rapid, with death occurring between one and two years after presentation (Hamman–Rich syndrome), or it may appear stationary over many years. The blood of some patients may be positive for rhematoid or antinuclear factors; although a lung disorder identical to cryptogenic fibrosing alveolitis has been described in all of the collagen-vascular diseases it is a rare complication of them.

## Pleural disease and skelctal disease and deformity

Exposure to asbestos can cause benign pleural thickening, which is often patchy and may calcify (pleural plaques). Such thickening does not become malignant but occasionally it can become extensive and cause significant restriction to ventilation. Malignant diffuse pleural mesothelioma can cause inexorable restriction of ventilation, often associated with severe pleural pain. The

tumour is not responsive to radiotherapy and chemotherapy but surgery may buy some short-term symptomatic relief.

Significant breathlessness is uncommon in most patients who have ankylosing spondylitis though respiratory failure may occur terminally in a severe case, often associated with recurrent chest infections. Patients with kyphoscoliosis remain relatively free of trouble up to the end of the second and third decades but increasing breathlessness, cyanosis and cor pulmonale become increasingly frequent in middle age and until recently almost inevitably led to early death. At specialist centres, detailed physiological evaluation and the use of the 'iron lung' principle of assisted ventilation with devices that are suitable for home use have undoubtedly changed the course of the disease in selected patients.

## Other chronic fibrosing lung disorders

Pulmonary tuberculosis, even when effectively treated, can lead to extensive pulmonary fibrosis, often in the apices of the lung. Similarly, pulmonary sarcoidosis may lead to bilateral mid-zone fibrosis and patients with either condition would be breathless on exertion. In such cases there may be associated distortion and destruction of the normal bronchial anatomy leading to bronchiectasis and recurrent production of sputum that is often infected—a further complication. If there is significant cavitation these may be colonized by the spores of *Aspergillus* giving rise to aspergilloma.

There are many other rare conditions in which progressive lung fibrosis may become a feature. Virtually all anticancer drugs have been reported as causing pulmonary fibrosis, as has irradiation of bronchial carcinoma. In patients receiving chemotherapy for Hodgkin's disease, non-Hodgkin's lymphoma or leukaemia, breathlessness with increasing pulmonary shadowing may be due to the disease itself, drug-induced fibrosis or an opportunistic infection (usually *Pneumocystic carinii*). Lung biopsy is the only reliable way of deciding the cause of shadowing in this case.

Pulmonary fibrosis associated with a cystic change on X-ray (honeycomb lung) diffusely affecting both lung fields may occur in histiocytosis X (Letterer–Siwe disease, Hand–Schüller–Christian disease and eosinophilic granuloma) and tuberous sclerosis.

## Cough

Irritant receptors lie in profusion throughout the lower and upper respiratory tract so in many respiratory disorders cough as a presenting symptom has little discriminant value. However, close attention to the onset, frequency and productivity of cough may provide important diagnostic clues to the cause. Characteristics of cough most frequently encountered in clinical practice are shown above in Table 5.2.

## Haemoptysis

Coughing of blood from the lungs is often a sign of serious underlying disease and should always be investigated. Firstly, it is important to establish that blood is coming from the lungs. Patients can confuse haemoptysis with haematemesis and bleeding from the larynx or nasopharynx (sometimes self-induced) may provoke cough. In chest clinic practice an identifiable cause for haemoptysis may not be found in many patients. In these it may be due to a small mucosal tear analogous to the Mallory–Weiss tear of the oesophagus.

Haemoptysis may be due to pulmonary or cardiac disease, as follows

PULMONARY
*Acute infection*
Bronchitis
Pneumonia
On chronic bronchitis
*Chronic infection*
Bronchiectasis
Tuberculosis
Lung abscess
Aspergilloma
*Infarction*
*Chest trauma*
*Iatrogenic*
After lung biopsy
*Rare causes*
Goodpasture syndrome
Wegener's granulomatosis
Hereditary haemorrhagic telangectasia
CARDIAC
*Mitral stenosis*
*Acute pulmonary oedema*
*Severe pulmonary hypertension*

If the cause of haemoptysis (such as acute infection) is obvious, then no further investigation may be necessary and the underlying condition is treated. If there has been intrapulmonary shadowing a follow-up chest X-ray should be obtained to ensure complete clearing. If the shadowing persists despite treatment or if there is evidence of chronic disease it may not be possible to exclude the development of further serious disease, such as carcinoma or tuberculosis, and more investigations should be made. Sputum should be examined for tubercle bacilli by smear and culture and a sample sent for cytological analysis for malignant cells. If the chest X-ray shows localized shadowing, then fibre-optic bronchoscopy should be performed and mucosal biopsy and brushings for histological and cytological detection of any abnormality seen should be taken. If the shadowing is beyond the reach of bronchoscopic vision, bronchial lavage or bacteriological analysis and transbronchial biopsy under X-ray control may allow a histological diagnosis to be made. All samples to the bacteriological laboratory should be sent in saline and all tissue for histological processing should be sent in a formalin saline solution.

In most patients who suffer haemoptysis but who have a normal chest X-ray, further investigations fail to reveal any disease process and no explanation emerges on long-term follow up in many of them.

## Chest pain

The history should allow the separation of cardiac pain from other causes of chest pain. The following should be considered in the differential diagnosis of non-cardiac chest pain:
(1) *Tracheitis*—often associated with painful cough and pain on swallowing; common in general practice, not often requiring referral to hospital.
(2) Oesophageal spasm and acid reflux. Pain is retrosternal, often severe and may easily be mistaken for cardiac pain; lack of relationship to exertion and the presence of acid reflux are important clues to the correct diagnosis.
(3) *Pleurisy*. The lancinating pain on deep respiration and coughing is characteristic; it is most commonly caused by pulmonary infection or infarction and is often the presenting symptom of pneumothorax.
(4) *Mesothelioma*. A dull or dragging pain, usually in the lower part of the chest, is a common though undramatic initial symptom of a pleural mesothelioma; the pain may prove

difficult to manage, even with powerful analgesics.

(5) *Chest wall pain:*
  (a) *Ribs*—fractures may be due to trauma or excessive coughing in middle-aged or elderly people. Pain is severe initially and related to deep breathing and movements. Simple analgesia is required but no other specific treatment.
  (b) *Nerves.* Herpes zoster of a thoracic nerve root can cause severe pain and may be difficult to diagnose until the typical rash appears. Rarely, benign neural tumours can cause pain in a segmental distribution; these are extremely difficult to diagnose.

(6) *Cartilage.* Costochondritis is commonly diagnosed to explain vague chest pains though the most florid example, Tietze disease, is rare.

(7) *Nonspecific chest pain.* Pain arising from intercostal muscles, ligaments and costochondral and costovertebral joints is common; it often causes great concern and seldom can an adequate explanation be found. These symptoms are usually self-limiting but patients often require strong reassurance that nothing is seriously wrong. Proven cases of intercostal myalgia due to Coxsackie virus infection, i.e., Bornholm disease, are rare.

## Investigation of chest radiograph abnormality

Every year thousands of chest X-rays are taken on asymptomatic individuals as pre-employment screening for entry to the police force, fire service, council work, hospital work and in recruits to the armed forces. The radiographs are not usually taken for medical reasons but one consequence is the discovery of asymptomatic abnormalities. Some common unexpected abnormalities are shown in Table 5.7 with a brief outline of the likely causes.

## Pulmonary tuberculosis

This remains the commonest form of tuberculosis in the UK, although extrapulmonary tuberculosis is increasingly common in immigrants to this country.

People at highest risk are often to be found in the following groups:

Recent immigrants (especially from the Indian subcontinent)

**Table 5.7 Unexpected changes on chest X-rays and their possible causes**

| Abnormality | Consider |
|---|---|
| Unilateral hilar enlargement | Tuberculosis (especially children), carcinoma, lymphoma, dilated pulmonary artery |
| Bilateral hilar enlargement | Sarcoidosis, lymphoma, Hodgkin's disease |
| Solitary nodules | Carcinoma, adenoma, hamartoma, tuberculoma |
| Reticulonodular shadowing | Dust exposure, sarcoidosis, alveolitis, lymphangitis, miliary tuberculosis |
| Pleural effusion | Transudates—heart failure, hypoalbuminaemia Exudates—infection, infarction, malignancy |
| Pneumothorax | Any underlying lung disease |
| Mediastinal widening | Aortic aneurysm or dissection, carcinoma, lymphoma, Hodgkin's disease |
| Pleural thickening or calcification | Previous history of pneumonia, pleurisy, haemothorax, chest trauma or surgery, asbestos exposure |
| Rib abnormalities | Congenital—bifid ribs, absent first rib Erosions due to metastases; notching due to coarctation |

Close contacts of infectious cases
The elderly (particularly men)
Malnourished
Alcoholics
Diabetics
Previous gastrectomy

### Symptoms

Productive cough often with haemoptysis
Weight loss
Malaise
Fever
Breathlessness
Chest pain (usually pleural disease)

### Physical signs

These are of:
Weight loss

Focal or widespread consolidation
Pleural effusion

## Diagnosis

### Chest radiograph

The X-ray shows confluent or semiconfluent shadowing, commonly at the apices of the lungs and often with cavitation. Bilateral disease is not rare. An effusion is seen in pleural tuberculosis, often with no symptoms of intrapulmonary infection.

### Sputum smear

The diagnosis of pulmonary tuberculosis may be confirmed rapidly by Ziehl–Nielsen staining of sputum when red-staining bacilli will be seen. The stain may be negative despite active disease but the patient can be regarded as non-infectious.

### Sputum culture

Tubercle bacilli will grow in special culture media (Lowenstein) though slowly. A sample must be cultured for six to eight weeks before it can be reported as negative. Further subcultures enable precise identification of the mycobacterium and its sensitivity to antituberculous drugs can be determined. This is important because with appropriate drugs the majority of cases can be cured permanently.

### Pleural aspiration and biopsy

When any pleural effusion is aspirated a sample should be sent for Ziehl–Nielsen staining and culture for tuberculosis. Pleural biopsies usually have the characteristic histological appearances if tuberculosis is the cause of the effusion.

## Management

### Drugs

Rifampicin and isoniazid are the two most effective antituberculous drugs and all the modern treatment schemes contain them. Because a small percentage of bacilli has primary resistance to one of these, a third drug is necessary as a precaution against secondary resistance. The following regimen has been shown in controlled clinical trials to be highly effective at curing infection with virtually no relapse providing the organism is sensitive to two of the drugs.

Rifampicin, 450–600 mg/day for 9 months
Isoniazid, 300 mg/day for 9 months
Ethambutol, 15–25 mg/kg/day for 2 months

### Quadruple chemotherapy

Recent trials have shown the duration of treatment can be reduced to 6 months with the addition of Pyrazinamide to the above regimen with a comparable high rate of cure and low rate of relapse.

If subcultures show that the bacillus is resistant to one of these first-line drugs an alternative must be used. The more commonly used alternate drugs are pyrazinamide and streptomycin. Other antituberculous drugs have more side-effects and are only rarely indicated.

### Admission

Ninety-nine percent of tubercle bacilli are killed in the first two weeks of a treatment that includes rifampicin and isoniazid. Patients become rapidly non-infectious and admission to hospital is not essential, although it may be necessary for the following practical reasons:
(a) to establish diagnosis;
(b) patients are often ill or elderly and require nursing care;
(c) to ensure antituberculous drugs are tolerated;
(d) if there are children under 5 years at home (they are particularly susceptible to the most lethal form of the infection—tuberculous meningitis).

### Prevention

Each patient who is under treatment for tuberculosis must be notified to specialists in community medicine, usually at the area health authority.

Contact tracing will screen the family and other close contacts by chest radiography in adults who have received BCG vaccination and by tuberculin testing (Heaf, Tine, Mantoux tests) and chest radiography in children and adults who have not received BCG. The number of cases of active infection discovered by this scheme is now disappointingly small.

## BCG vaccination

This has been offered to schoolchildren who are tuberculin-negative at the age of 12 to 13 years for over 30 years. Its long-lasting efficacy has been shown (at least in the UK) by several large studies. However, with diminishing numbers of active cases, this mass vaccination campaign is becoming less cost-effective, with an increasing number of vaccinations needed to prevent one case.

## Opportunistic mycobacteria

Also called non-tuberculous mycobacteria these organisms usually infect previously damaged lungs or cause infection in unusual sites. Tuberculosis reference laboratories can usually identify unusual mycobacteria and guide appropriate drug therapy.

## Sarcoidosis

This is a benign and usually self-limiting inflammatory disorder of unknown cause. It is characterized by non-caseating granulomatous infiltration of any organ of the body and, by convention at least, two organs must be involved before the diagnosis is made with certainty. Typically the disease presents between the ages of 20 and 40 years, though cases in younger and older patients have been described. The lungs and intrathoracic lymph nodes are the organs most commonly involved. Though people of any race may be affected it is more common in Blacks and the disease is more likely to progress in them rather than resolve spontaneously.

## Presentation

The disease may either present as an acute illness or more indolently. The commonest presentation is the chance discovery of an abnormal chest radiograph in a relatively asymptomatic person. Some patients report malaise, nonspecific discomfort around the chest or a mild degree of breathlessness. Sarcoidosis is the commonest cause of erythema nodosum in the UK and all such cases should have a chest X-ray. Other modes of presentation are unusual but sarcoidosis should always be considered if patients are being investigated for:

Generalized lymphadenopathy
Hepatosplenomegaly
Non-infectious or 'biochemical' hepatitis
Uveitis
Hypercalcaemia
Fever
Seronegative arthropathy
Cardiac arrhythmias
Bell's palsy

## Radiology

The chest radiograph is used to stage intrathoracic involvement in sarcoidosis as follows:

*Stage I.* Hilar lymphadenopathy with no pulmonary involvement.
*Stage II.* Hilar lymphadenopathy with pulmonary involvement.
*Stage III.* Established fibrosis.

## Diagnosis

The diagnosis may be obvious when a patient presents with erythema nodosum and bilateral hilar lymphadenopathy with or without intrapulmonary shadowing. If a patient has only one of these features, further diagnostic steps are required, as follows.

*Serum angiotensin-converting-enzyme* (SACE) —it is thought that metabolically active granulomas produce this enzyme and its levels are raised in active sarcoidosis and other rare granulomatous diseases. The level falls after the disease becomes quiescent with or without treatment.

*Biopsy* of an involved organ, e.g., liver, lung or conjunctiva, should show the characteristic histological appearances. Granulomas can be found in clinically 'silent' organs but speculative biopsies are not justified.

*Kveim* test—this is positive in about 80 per cent of active cases of sarcoidosis though interpretation of the biopsy requires experience.

## Management

In the majority of cases in the UK the condition resolves spontaneously, although anti-inflammatory agents are useful to control arthralgia and the painful lesions of erythema nodosum. Systemic corticosteroids usually cause rapid resolution of intrapulmonary shadowing but there is no evidence that they pevent pulmonary fibrosis in those patients in whom the pulmonary lesions progress rather than regress. Indications for systemic corticosteroid therapy are:

Breathlessness due to intrapulmonary involvement
Uveitis
Hypercalcaemia
Nervous system involvement
Cardiac disease

## TUMOURS OF THE RESPIRATORY TRACT

### Benign tumours

The following are the most commonly encountered benign tumours:
Bronchial adenomas
Cylindromas
Carcinoid tumours
They present with symptoms and abnormal radiographic appearances that are similar to malignant lesions and are investigated similarly. They are usually treated by surgical resection. Bronchial carcinoid tumours are not truly benign and can metastasise, particularly to liver. If confined to the bronchial tree surgical resection may be curative.

### Bronchogenic carcinoma

This remains the commonest malignant neoplasm in the UK. In parallel with changes in smoking trends the overall incidence in men is falling but rising in women. Although a few hundred cases of lung cancer per year occur in non-smokers, presumably due to atmospheric radiation and other carcinogens, a vast majority of lung cancer sufferers are or have been smokers.

### *Pathology*

The WHO has classified bronchogenic carcinoma into ten different groups. In practice the following four histological types are commonly encountered, i.e. squamous, small cell, large cell and adenocarcinoma. The rare alveolar cell carcinoma does not strictly arise from bronchial epithelium, differs in presentation and radiological appearances and does not respond to any of the three standard forms of therapy.

### *Squamous*

These comprise about 35% of bronchial neoplasms and studies have shown them to have a mean tumour volume doubling time of about 88 days. They are often peripheral, presenting as a solitary nodule, have a tendency to cavitate and to produce parathyroid hormone like protein so that hypercalcaemia may be a feature particularly in its terminal phases. It is the tumour most likely to be amenable to curative surgical resection.

### *Small cell (25% of bronchial neoplasms)*

These tumours have been estimated to have a mean tumour volume doubling time of about 29 days and are the most rapidly progressive of lung tumours. They tend to arise proximally, metastasise early to lymphnodes causing massive mediastinal lymphadenopathy but also metastasise early but silently to other organs. For this reason small cell carcinomas at the time of diagnosis are usually regarded as having spread systemically. The malignant cells are very active metabolically producing a variety of abnormal proteins which are often active endocrinologically, e.g., producing Cushing's syndrome. However, this is usually apparent biochemically rather than morphologically since the classic changes in body habits do not have time to appear in view of the rapid progression of malignancy. It is because the malignant cells are dividing so rapidly that this tumour is most likely to respond to chemotherapy and radiotherapy.

### *Large cell (20% of bronchial neoplasms)*

These tumours have a volume doubling time of about 86 days and may be anaplastic forms of squamous carcinoma, i.e., the cells are of the same size but do not have the characteristic intercellular bridges and cell nest formation. They show little response to chemotherapy or radiotherapy and surgical removal remains the only hope of a cure.

### *Adenocarcinoma (about 20% of bronchial neoplasms)*

These tumours have a mean volume doubling time of about 160 days and therefore are the most slowly progressive of the common lung cancers. It is thought they are probably unrelated to smoking. They too show little response to radiotherapy or chemotherapy.

## Presenting features

### General

Anorexia, weight loss
Anaemia
Clubbing
Hypertrophic osteoarthropathy

### Respiratory

Cough, sputum, haemoptysis
Progressive breathlessness with or without wheeze, due to:
    lobar or lung collapse
    pleural effusion
    bronchial/tracheal stenosis

### Metastases

Brain, spinal cord, Horner's syndrome
Bone pain
Cutaneous
Supraclavicular lymph nodes
Hepatomegaly

### Non metastatic

Neurological
    peripheral neuropathy
    mononeuritis
    dermatomyositis
    cerebellar syndrome
Endocrine
    hypercalcaemia
    inappropriate ADH secretion
    Cushing's syndrome
    gynaecomastia

## Diagnosis

Although most bronchial carcinomas cause characteristic radiographic abnormalities it is wise to seek histological confirmation whenever possible. This has an important influence on the type of therapy chosen and gives information on which to base a prognosis.

### Sputum

Examination of sputum for its cellular content is difficult and time consuming. However, an experienced cytologist may find malignant cells in sputum and confirm the diagnosis without further invasive investigation although precise cellular typing may not be possible. False negative reports are common and alternative investigations should proceed. False positives are rare but occur occasionally. Assessment of bronchial epithelial cells is even more difficult after the bronchial tree has undergone recent instrumentation with bronchoscopy or endotracheal intubation.

### Bronchoscopy

This is the investigation of choice if patients are not producing sputum or cytology has been negative. This procedure and other diagnostic procedures are described earlier.

### Further investigations

These will be necessary in patients being considered for surgical resection or for patients who have symptoms at presentation or during investigation which suggest the presence of metastatic spread. Computerized tomographic examination of the brain, thorax and abdomen may be indicated. If routine biochemical testing shows liver function test abnormalities then an ultrasound examination of the liver should be requested. In patients who have pain suggesting metastases to bone plain radiographs of the skeleton and isotope bone scanning should be requested.

## Management

For the purposes of practical management of lung cancer the different types are divided into two groups:
(a) Small cell lung cancer;
(b) Non-small cell lung cancer.
   The reason for this division is about 70% of small cell tumours show a partial or complete radiological response to chemotherapy. The non-small cell group respond poorly to chemotherapy with any benefits being outweighed by toxicity.

### Chemotherapy

Most chemotherapeutic agents have been shown to be active against small cell cancer. The median survival from the time of diagnosis without treatment is about six weeks. After a complete response to chemotherapy the median survival increases to about nine months. Some patients succumb in the early weeks after diagnosis and treatment but others may have a disease-free survival of up to two years. The agents available have been tried in a variety of combinations and no one scheme has been shown to be convincingly superior to the others.

A typical regimen used is:

| | | |
|---|---|---|
| Vincristine | 1.12 mg/m$^2$ | IV on day one |
| Adriamycin | 40 mg/m$^2$ | IV on day one |
| Cyclophosphamide | 700 mg/m$^2$ | IV on day one |
| Etopozide | 300 mg | Orally on day one, two, three |

The regimen is repeated every three weeks for up to six cycles. Alopecia is invariable. A substantial proportion of patients develop bone marrow suppression and a mid-cycle blood count is mandatory. In patients who get marrow toxicity the blood count is allowed to return to normal then the next cycle is given using 60% of the above doses. All patients should be given prophylactic therapy to prevent nausea during every cycle. Ondansetron though expensive has emerged as the most useful anti-emetic. There is no evidence that more than six cycles of treatment improves the chances of long-term survival. Patients who get a good response have usually done so within the first two cycles of treatment.

Non-small cell lung cancers show disappointingly low response rates to chemotherapy and in view of unacceptable toxicity this form of treatment should be confined to research studies for these kinds of tumours.

### Radiotherapy

This may be administered either in an attempt to obliterate the whole tumour (radical) or be used to relieve symptoms directly attributable to the tumour (palliative) when lower doses are used. There is contention whether radiotherapy cures patients with lung cancer. One has seen five year survivors albeit at the expense of post-radiation pulmonary fibrosis. Patients with non-metastasised peripheral lung cancer may be potentially curable but the tradition has been to refer such cases for surgical resection. This is an area where further research is needed.

Palliative radiotherapy is valuable for the complications of lung cancer and is particularly helpful in controlling haemoptysis, local bone pain due to metastases or infiltration. If given early it may allow re-expansion of a collapsed lobe or a lung thereby relieving dyspnoea. It can relieve stridor due to proximal tracheal or bronchial obstruction and is very effective at relieving superior venacaval obstruction. In patients with cerebral metastases and oedema it can improve a deteriorating conscious level and other neurological deficits albeit relatively briefly.

### Surgery

This represents the best chance of curing a patient with lung cancer but sadly only a small proportion of such patients undergo successful surgical resection. Contraindications to surgery are:

(a) Metastatic spread or infiltration, e.g., recurrent laryngeal nerve or phrenic nerve paralysis as well as evidence of mediastinal involvement and spread to other organs.

(b) Poor lung function; many such patients also have co-existing chronic bronchitis and emphysema and would have inadequate respiratory reserve to sustain life if major pulmonary resection was necessary.

(c) Tumours lying too close to the carina making anastomosis of the bronchial remnant too difficult.

(d) The presence of co-existing disease, e.g., coronary heart disease.

(e) Known small cell cancer.

(f) Age. This in itself is not an absolute contraindication but the very elderly tolerate such major surgery poorly. The ideal patient for surgery is a relatively young, fit man with a squamous carcinoma without metastases but if the physician is in doubt then an opinion of a consultant thoracic surgeon should be obtained.

## INVESTIGATION

### Radiology

An anterior chest radiograph (plate placed against front of patient's chest) 6 ft (approx. 1.8 m) from the X-ray tube in full inspiration is the first investigation required in most respiratory diseases. A technically correct film is essential to exclude over- or under-interpretation of abnormality and the requirements are shown in Fig. 5.2. A lateral radiograph is useful in assessing the anatomical distribution of shadowing, left atrial enlargement, right ventricular enlargement and disease

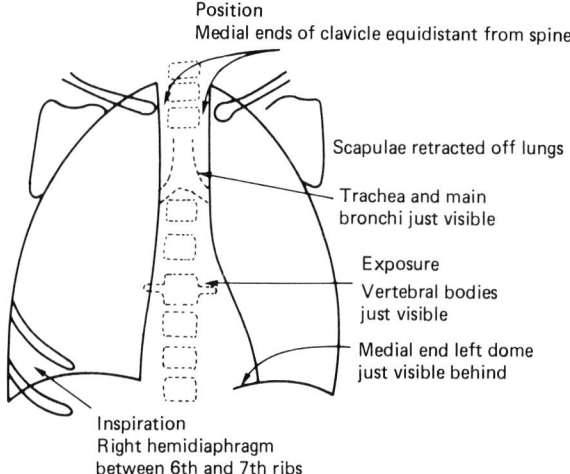

Position
Medial ends of clavicle equidistant from spine

Scapulae retracted off lungs

Trachea and main
bronchi just visible

Exposure
Vertebral bodies
just visible

Medial end left dome
just visible behind

Inspiration
Right hemidiaphragm
between 6th and 7th ribs

*Figure 5.2*  Technical requirements for
anterior chest radiograph

of the thoracic vertebrae. Tomography is useful to
assess:

  Hilar enlargement
  Cavitation
  Calcification
  Precise localization of a lesion before needle
  biopsy
  Other radiographs are indicated in special
circumstances:
(1) *Apical views*—to examine the area behind the
    clavicles.
(2) *Decubitus*—to differentiate pleural fluid from
    thickening or tumour.
(3) *Expiratory*—to exclude a pneumothorax.

### Bronchography

Instillation of radiopaque substances, e.g., Diono-
sil, into the bronchial tree allows accurate assessment of the anatomy of the bronchi and is the
traditional investigation for the diagnosis of bronchiectasis (damaged dilated bronchi, usually with
infection) although computerized thoracic tomography may replace this in the future. The severity
and localization of bronchiectasis are important
because individual diseased lobes can be removed
surgically.

### Computerized thoracic tomography

This is expensive but is now usually available in
many district general hospitals. It is a valuable way

of assessing thoracic diseases. It is of particular
value in the following:
  Presence, degree and nature of pleural thicken-
  ing
  Detection of mediastinal malignancy
  Detection of unsuspected intrapulmonary
  nodules
  Extent and severity of bronchiectasis
  Extent and severity of all fibrosing lung diseases

### Lung function tests

#### Peak expiratory flow rate

This is detected by a small vane in the first 10 ms of
forced expiration into a peak flow gauge following
maximum inspiration. It is a relatively crude test
of lung function, being reduced in many different
lung conditions, but with practice is very reproducible and the gauges or meters are cheap and
mobile. It is particularly valuable when repeated
assessment is needed, such as during recovery
from severe asthma or for detecting variability in
airflow obstruction in nocturnal or occupational
asthma. As with all lung function measurements
the normal value for an individual depends on age,
height, sex and ethnic origin.

#### Spirometry

Vital capacity (VC; maximum volume of air
exhaled after maximum inspiration) is easily measured by an electrically operated, dry-wedge spirometer. In health this volume can be forcibly
exhaled within 3 s (forced vital capacity; FVC) but
takes longer in airflow limitation. The most useful
subdivision is the volume exhaled in the first
second (forced expiratory volume in 1 s; $FEV_1$)
and when expressed as a percentage of VC is a
measure of severity of airways obstruction. Normally the ratio should be 70 per cent or greater.
Ventilatory defects may thus be classified as in
Table 5.8. Typical examples of vital capacities in
disease are shown in Fig. 5.3. In certain conditions
where there is premature small-airway closure

**Table 5.8 Ventilatory defects classified by
$FEV_1$/VC ratio**

|  | VC | $FEV_1$ | $FEV_1$/VC |
|---|---|---|---|
| Obstructive | ↓ | ↓↓↓ | ↓ |
| Restrictive | ↓↓↓ | ↓↓↓ | Normal–↑ |

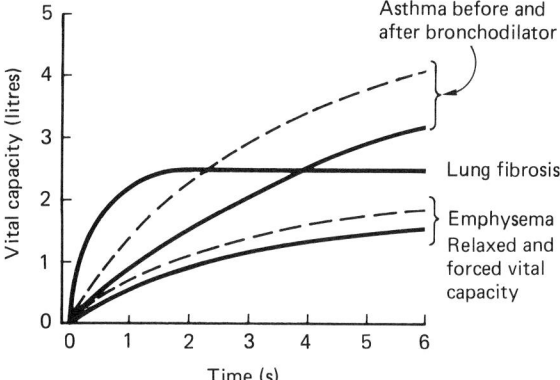

*Figure 5.3* Spirographs of common respiratory conditions

with gas trapping a more relaxed VC measurement may be higher than the FVC and reflect the extent of the trapping. Other derivatives of the spirogram, such as the instantaneous flow rate halfway through exhalation (forced expiratory flow $_{50}$ [$FEF_{50}$] or $\dot{V}_{50}$) or the average flow rate between a quarter and three quarters of the way through expiration ($FEF_{25-75}$), reflect flow through the smallest gas-conducting airways (Fig. 5.4). These measurements as well as plotting flow as a function of exhaled volume (flow volume loop) do not often give additional practical information in managing patients.

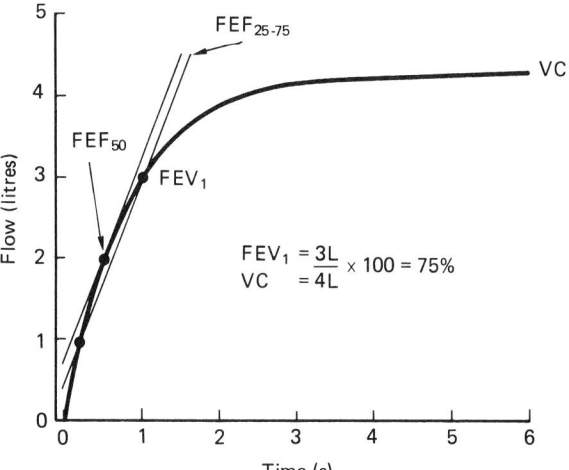

*Figure 5.4* Spirogram illustrating $FEF_{50}$ and $FEF_{25-75}$ as explained in the text

## Lung volumes

Simple spirometry cannot measure total lung capacity because at the end of full expiration about 25 per cent of the total volume remains (residual volume [RV]). Measurement of RV is not necessary in the majority of routine respiratory cases but is useful in difficult diagnostic problems and in following the progression of disease or response to treatment in conditions such as fibrosing alveolitis. There are three ways of measuring RV and, therefore, total lung capacity (TLC). In decreasing order of availability but increasing order of accuracy they are:

Gas dilution technique using helium
Anterior and lateral chest radiographs using planimetry and computer-assisted calculations
Whole-body plethysmography

## Gas transfer

Carbon monoxide is avidly taken up by circulating red cells and when added in tiny concentrations to a closed breathing circuit its disappearance into the circulation is a measure of the efficiency of the gas exchanging surface of the lungs ($D_LCO$). Any condition that upsets the overall balance of ventilation and perfusion of the lungs causes a fall in gas transfer and is valuable in following progression of disease or response to treatment. Typical abnormalities of gas transfer in the common respiratory diseases are shown in Table 5.9.

### Sputum examination

Non-infected sputum is white (mucoid) whereas yellow or green sputum suggests infection (purulent). Asthmatic sputum may be yellow due to eosinophils. The presence of blood (haemoptysis) or rarely other pigments such as coal dust should be noted. A 'fetid' odour might suggest anaerobic infection.

## Staining

A Gram stain may differentiate between pneumococcal or staphylococcal infection (Gram-positive) or *H. influenzae* infection (Gram-negative) before antibiotic therapy. It may allow early diagnosis of the organism causing pneumonia but is of little value in exacerbations of chronic bronchitis. All sputum specimens should have Ziehl–Nielsen stains to exclude tuberculosis.

**Table 5.9  Gas transfer abnormalities in some respiratory diseases**

| Normal | Reduced | Raised |
|---|---|---|
| Asthma | Emphysema | Pulmonary hypertension |
| Non-obstructive bronchitis | Fibrosing alveolitis | Alveolar haemorrhage |
| | Anaemia | Polycythaemia |

### Culture

This is helpful in identifying the organism responsible for pneumonia if taken before antibiotic therapy but is of little practical value in exacerbations of chronic bronchitis or asthma. Lowenstein culture for tuberculosis is not routinely performed unless the Ziehl–Nielsen stain is positive or a specific request is made.

### Cytology

Staining and microscopy of cells in sputum can be a valuable method of diagnosing malignancy in experienced hands. The procedure is time consuming and should only be requested for specific indications (e.g., slow resolving pneumonia, mass on a chest X-ray) rather than be used as a routine or screening test.

### Arterial blood gas analysis

Arterial oxygen ($PO_2$) and carbon dioxide ($PCO_2$) tensions, pH (or $H^+$ concentration) and bicarbonate estimations on breathing room air or a known concentration of inspired oxygen ($FiO_2$) provide a valuable means of assessing severity and response to treatment of many respiratory diseases. Normal values and abnormalities in some common diseases are shown in Table 5.10.

### Immunological tests

These can be divided into two groups relating to reduced or increased immunological activity.

### Reduced immunological activity

Patients who are predisposed to respiratory infection usually have anatomical or physiological defects in bronchial anatomy (e.g., bronchiectasis) or mucociliary clearance mechanisms (smoking or immotile cilia syndrome). Occasionally, recurrent infection may be due to:

Reduced leucocyte count, e.g., leukaemia, aplastic anaemia, cytotoxic chemotherapy

Reduced lymphocyte count, e.g, leukaemia, AIDS, cytotoxic drugs

Reduced IgG, IgA, IgM (myeloma, malnutrition)

Deficiency of components of complement

Cellular immunity may be tested by the injection of antigens that the patient has almost certainly encountered previously, e.g., candidal, mumps, trichophyton, tuberculin (recall antigens); negative responses suggest defective T-lymphocyte function.

### Increased immunological activity

#### Skin prick tests

Skin tests with common environmental allergens, e.g., grass pollen, house dust, animal danders, will identify those people who produce excessive amounts of IgE to these allergens (atopic) and are helpful in diagnosis and management of asthma and rhinitis. Such patients will have elevated total IgE levels and, using the radio-allergosorbent test (RAST), the patient's plasma can be examined for specific IgE to individual allergens.

**Table 5.10  Values for arterial blood gas testing in health and disease**

| | | pH | $PO_2$ | $PCO_2$ |
|---|---|---|---|---|
| Normal | | 7.4 | 90–100 mmHg | 40 mmHg |
| Respiratory failure—type A | Pneumonia; pulmonary oedema; pulmonary embolism; asthma (early) | ↓ or Normal | ↓ | Normal– ↓ |
| Respiratory failure—type B | Chronic bronchitis and emphysema; asthma (late); drugs; neuromuscular diseases | ↓ | ↓ | ↑ |

### Delayed hypersensitivity

Type IV reaction is used to find if patients react to tuberculin. The Mantoux, Heaf and Tine tests inject a tiny amount of tuberculin subcutaneously and a patient who has previously had contact with the tubercle bacillus will have a positive reaction. This does not imply active infection because many people have healed primary lesions (Ghon's focus) or have been given BCG vaccination.

### Specific IgG antibodies (precipitins)

These may be found in the plasma of patients suffering from aspergilloma or bronchopulmonary aspergillosis and from extrinsic allergic alveolitis. The commonest varieties of the latter in the UK are farmer's lung (ask for *Micropolyspora* or thermophilic *Actinomyces* precipitins) or bird fancier's lung (ask for antibodies to pigeons, budgerigars).

### Kveim test

This is a test specific for sarcoidosis (see above). A homogenate of tissue, usually from the spleen of a known case of sarcoidosis, is injected intradermally. The site is biopsied six weeks later and the presence of non-caseating granulomata is good evidence of sarcoidosis. The Kveim test is positive in about 75 per cent of cases of 'acute' sarcoidosis but is frequently negative in chronic cases.

## Bronchoscopy

The bronchial tree may be visualized directly either with a rigid instrument usually under general anaesthesia or a flexible fibre-optic instrument under local anaesthesia. The anatomy, mucosal appearance and presence of bronchial obstruction may thus easily be seen. The flexible technique has the advantage of increased range of vision and biopsy to subsegmental level, particularly in the upper lobes. The disadvantage of this instrument is the narrow suction channel, through which removal of thick secretions and blood clot or control of major haemorrhage is difficult. The biopsies are small and it is not usually possible to remove foreign bodies. For the latter the rigid instrument is the method of choice.

## Biopsy

Multiple but small biopsies can be taken accurately from mucosal lesions under direct vision. Slight haemorrhage (haemoptysis) is common but more serious bleeding is rare.

### Bronchial brushings

Mucosal cells may be removed by rubbing a small brush across lesions and if plated on glass slides (immediately to prevent drying), cytological examination in experienced hands frequently reveals malignant cells from suspicious lesions.

### Bronchial lavage

Bronchial secretions can be collected via the suction channel and submitted to cytological examination; these occasionally give additional information. The instillation of large volumes of isotonic saline into segments or lobes of the lung allows recovery of alveolar cellular content and analysis of this can give useful diagnostic information and can be repeated to follow the progress of diseases such as fibrosing alveolitis, sarcoidosis and asbestosis.

### Transbronchial biopsy

Under radiographic control using an image intensifier, biopsy forceps can be passed beyond direct vision into the periphery of the lung and biopsies containing alveoli can be obtained. This is useful in the diagnosis of fibrosing alveolitis, sarcoidosis and lymphangitis carcinomatosis. This is more hazardous than mucosal biopsy, yet although pneumothorax occurs in about 5 per cent of cases and haemorrhage is also a risk it is the safest of the procedures for biopsy of lung parenchyma.

## Lung biopsy

The following procedures are available for lung biopsy (in increasing order of complexity and risk to the patient).

### Needle aspiration

This is performed percutaneously under radiographic control, the exact location of the lesion having previously been defined; it is best suited for a nodule or a mass. Needle aspiration is best done in collaboration with a cytologist or histologist who can judge whether adequate specimens for diagnosis have been obtained. With training and practice, diagnostic information can usually be obtained from lesions 12 mm in diameter or greater.

## Drill biopsy

This is also a percutaneous technique, usually for larger lesions, using a pneumatic cutting drill. This can be of value in experienced hands but due to increasing experience of needle aspiration techniques is seldom used now.

## Open thoracotomy

One problem with all the techniques outlined above is that samples are small and may be unrepresentative of a diffuse disease, like cryptogenic fibrosing alveolitis, where there may be alveolar desquamation in one part and end-stage fibrosis in another part. It also allows a more representative biopsy of the pleura than can be obtained by percutaneous methods. However, thoracotomy must be regarded as a major operation with all the attendant risk of anaesthesia and postoperative complications and must be undertaken only after full consideration by physicians and surgeons.

## Pleural aspiration and biopsy

Unless the cause of a pleural effusion is obvious (e.g., secondary to pneumonia or heart failure) fluid in the pleural cavity should always be aspirated and samples sent for bacteriological, cytological and biochemical tests. If the effusion might be secondary to pleural or pulmonary disease, then a pleural biopsy should be obtained on each occasion the fluid is tapped.

## Further reading

Baum G. L. (1983). *Textbook of Pulmonary Disease*, 3rd edn. Boston: Little, Brown.

Clark T. J. H. (1981). *Clinical Investigation of Respiratory Disease*. London: Chapman & Hall.

Collins J. V., Dhillon P., Goldstraw P. (1987). *Practical Bronchoscopy*. Oxford: Blackwell Scientific.

Godfrey S., Clark T. J. H. (1983). *Asthma*, 2nd edn. London: Chapman & Hall.

Hodson M. E., Norman A. P., Batten J. C. (1983). *Drill Cystic Fibrosis*. London: Baillière Tindall.

Laszlo G. (1983). *Measurement in Clinical Respiratory Physiology*. New York: Academic Press.

Seaton A., Seaton D., Leitch A. G., eds. (1988). *Crofton and Douglas Respiratory Diseases*, 4th edn. Oxford: Blackwell Scientific.

# 6

# HAEMATOLOGY

Keith Patterson

## GENERAL APPROACH TO THE PATIENT

Certain aspects of the history and physical examination are of particular importance in patients with haematological disease. Anaemia is a feature of many such diseases, and specific questions on exercise tolerance and general tiredness should be asked. The tongue and inner aspect of the lower eyelid should be assessed for pallor.

Examination of the reticuloendothelial system is required in many haematological diseases. Splenomegaly should be investigated using warm hands with the patient relaxed and lying flat, with head on the pillow and hands by the sides. Palpation should start in the right iliac fossa, moving gradually up to the left hypochondrium, in order not to miss the very large spleens that may be found in myelofibrosis and chronic granulocytic leukaemia. Splenomegaly should be quantified by measurement in centimetres from the costal margin vertically above the spleen tip. To localize the spleen and confirm that this is indeed the mass being palpated, check that it moves on respiration and continues beneath the costal margin. The size of the spleen may be an important indicator of clinical response to treatment in the chronic leukaemias, lymphomas and myelofibrosis. Pain in the left hypochondrium in a patient with splenomegaly may indicate an area of splenic infarction. This may be found in sickle cell disease, polycythaemia rubra vera, essential thrombocythaemia, chronic granulocytic leukaemia and myelofibrosis. The pain is often pleuritic in type, and may radiate to the left shoulder due to involvement of the diaphragm in the inflammatory process. A rub may be heard on auscultation over the tender area.

Generalized lymphadenopathy may be a particular feature of chronic lymphocytic leukaemia and lymphomas. Lymph nodes in the axillae and neck provide the best guide to assessing generalized lymphadenopathy. One hand should be placed in the patient's axilla while the patient's arm is supported by the examiner's other hand. The patient's arm is then adducted closer to the trunk, relaxing the axillary skin and allowing exploration of all sides of the axilla. The neck is best examined with the patient sitting up, when the supraclavicular fossae, anterior and posterior triangles and submental areas may be palpated. Measure the size of the enlarged nodes in centimetres and note their consistency and the presence of tenderness. The tonsils should also be assessed. A simple diagram of the physical findings should be made in the patient's notes.

Examination of the mouth may reveal glossitis in iron deficiency or megaloblastic anaemia, ulceration in neutropenia, or gingival enlargement in monocytic leukaemia.

Bone tenderness may be found in leukaemia, myeloma and secondary carcinoma. The palm of the hand should be placed flat on the sternum with the patient lying flat and firm pressure applied. Bone tenderness may also be noted by firm palpation of the spinous processes or iliac crest. When found, enquiry should be made for symptoms of hypercalcaemia, such as thirst, polyuria and constipation.

Neurological examination is indicated when vitamin $B_{12}$ deficiency is suspected.

## BONE MARROW EXAMINATION

The bone marrow may be examined by means of an aspirate or a biopsy. Marrow aspiration may be done from the sternum or anterior or posterior iliac crests. The smears produced allow close

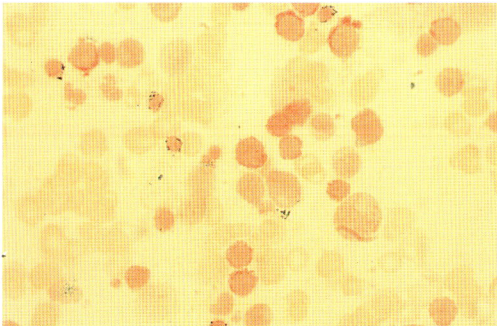

**Plate 6.1.** High power view of bone marrow aspirate stained by Perl's Prussian blue stain for iron, showing normoblasts (counterstained red) some of which have excess iron granules (deep blue) forming a ring around the nucleus – ringed sideroblasts.

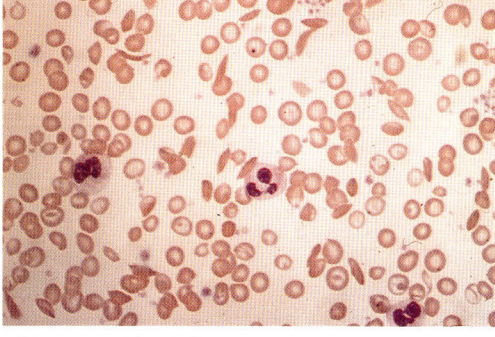

**Plate 6.2.** Blood film in sickle cell anaemia. In addition to the sickled cells, target cells and Howell Jolly bodies are seen. The latter are nuclear remnants resulting from hyposplenism due to splenic infarction.

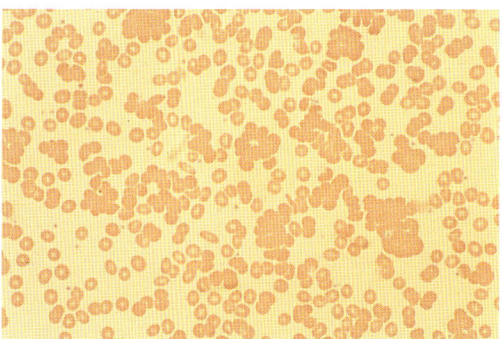

**Plate 6.3.** Blood film showing the appearance of cold agglutinates – haphazard irregular clumps of red cells. These should not be confused with rouleaux, which are branching chains of over-lapping red cells associated with a high ESR.

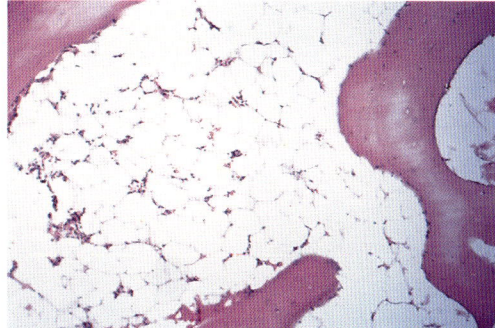

**Plate 6.4.** Bone marrow trephine biopsy in a case of aplastic anaemia, stained by H&E. The marrow spaces between the bony trabeculae are grossly hypocellular, consisting mostly of fat spaces.

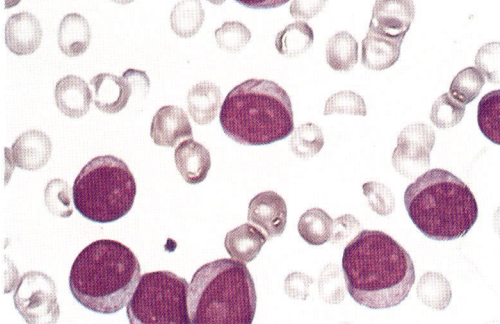

**Plate 6.5.** Blood film in a case of acute myeloid leukaemia showing myeloblasts. The cytoplasm of one of these contains an Auer rod. This pink-staining needle-like structure is diagnostic of acute myeloid leukaemia.

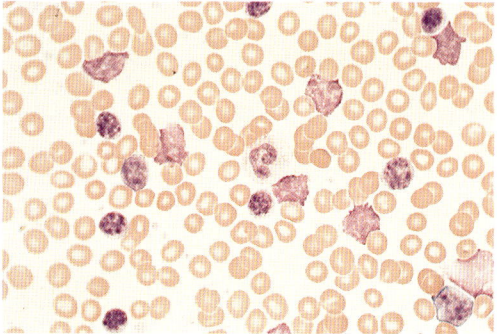

**Plate 6.6.** Blood film in chronic lymphocytic leukaemia. The majority of white cells are small lymphocytes. There are several smear cells – lymphocytes crushed during the making of the film.

examination of individual cells. Trephine biopsy of bone marrow can only be taken from the iliac crest. It is a more uncomfortable procedure than aspiration but produces a cylinder of marrow that is sectioned histologically allowing examination of its structure. Trephine biopsy is indicated in the investigation of secondary carcinoma, lymphoma, Hodgkin's disease and myelofibrosis, and when attempted aspiration has produced a 'dry tap'. The trephine also provides a more reliable estimate of cellularity than marrow aspiration in cases of aplastic anaemia. Marrow biopsy is not generally indicated in the investigation of megaloblastic anaemia unless there is failure to respond to treatment. Previous radiotherapy, for example to the sternum in carcinoma of breast or to the pelvis in Hodgkin's disease, will result in lifelong hypocellularity of that area of marrow.

## ANAEMIA

Anaemia is defined as a haemoglobin less than 11.5 g/100 ml in women, or less than 12.5 in men. Symptoms of anaemia include tiredness, shortness of breath on exertion, palpitations, and ankle swelling, with heart failure in the elderly. There is great variation between individuals in the level of haemoglobin at which symptoms appear. Generally, slow onset of anaemia is tolerated better than rapid onset, and the young tolerate anaemia better than the elderly. Pallor is the major clinical sign, and a compensatory increase in cardiac output may result in a mid-systolic ('haemic') murmur. Clinical examination may reveal clues to the cause of the anaemia, such as koilonychia (brittle, spoon-shaped nails) and angular cheilosis (sore splits at the angles of the mouth) in iron deficiency, and a tinge of jaundice with sore tongue in megaloblastic anaemia. However, the more usual approach to diagnosis of anaemia involves the red cell indices on the blood count. In particular, examination of the mean cell volume (MCV) will allow all anaemias to be classified into microcytic (low MCV), normocytic (normal MCV) and macrocytic (high MCV) types.

### Microcytosis

The common causes of microcytic anaemia are iron deficiency, thalassaemia trait and, in some cases, sideroblastic anaemia and the anaemia of chronic disease.

### Iron deficiency

This is by far the commonest cause of anaemia. Besides a low MCV, the red cells are hypochromic, with a low mean corpuscular haemoglobin (MCH). Most cases of iron deficiency may be diagnosed from the blood count and clinical history. Difficult cases may be confirmed by the finding of a low serum iron and high total iron-binding capacity (TIBC) with a low ferritin. When selecting confirmatory tests it should be borne in mind that the serum iron may be falsely elevated if the patient is taking iron (i.e., stop the iron, then test) and the TIBC is often elevated in pregnancy. The serum ferritin may be falsely elevated in liver disease (released from damaged liver cells) and in the collagen diseases (ferritin behaves as an acute-phase protein). Although the prolonged administration of iron to anaemic patients who are iron deficient should be avoided because of the risk of iron overload, a therapeutic trial of two or three weeks' oral iron is a reasonable course of action in difficult cases.

Enquiry should be made about bleeding (menorrhagia, melaena or blood loss per rectum, nosebleeds, haemoglobinuria). A dietary history should be taken. The drug history should take note of aspirin and non-steroidal anti-inflammatory drugs, which predispose to gastrointestinal bleeding particularly in the elderly. Where an adequate explanation of the iron deficiency is not forthcoming, a barium meal/enema should be given to exclude bleeding peptic ulcer or gastric/colonic carcinoma. A history of weight loss, anorexia, or a high ESR adds urgency to these investigations. A series of three negative tests for occult blood in the stool is reassuring, though positive results may be produced by meat or peroxidase-containing vegetables in the diet. The platelet count may be elevated in iron deficiency, particularly when due to bleeding, and leucopenia may occasionally be found.

Where malabsorption is not present, oral iron therapy produces as quick a haemoglobin response as parenteral therapy without the risk of allergic reactions or skin staining. Start with ferrous sulphate, 200 mg twice or thrice daily. Those patients who suffer gastric upset or constipation may prefer an alternative preparation such as ferrous gluconate or succinate or one of the highly encapsulated, sustained-release preparations of ferrous sulphate. Generally these have less therapeutic effect; a similar alleviation of unwanted side-effects may be produced by reducing the dose of ferrous sulphate.

### Thalassaemia trait

This condition should be suspected when the patient is of Mediterranean or Asian origin, the haemoglobin is not below 9 g/100 ml, and the MCV is unusually low for the level of haemoglobin. When in doubt, the serum iron and TIBC should be measured. In difficult cases, serum ferritin may be measured: this is low in iron depletion, and high in iron overload. In beta-thalassaemia trait an elevated level of haemoglobin $A_2$ is a useful marker of the condition. Alpha-thalassaemia trait is more difficult to prove without studies of haemoglobin chain synthesis. Iron therapy is contraindicated in thalassaemia trait, except where coexistent iron deficiency has been demonstrated.

### Sideroblastic anaemia

The MCV may be high, normal or low in this condition. The diagnostic feature is the presence of ringed sideroblasts (Plate 6.1) in the bone marrow stained by Perls' Prussian blue stain for iron. It may be primary, or secondary to malignancy, collagen disease, alcohol or antituberculous therapy. Marrow iron stores are increased and serum iron is usually high, with a low TIBC. Serum ferritin is elevated.

Management of sideroblastic anaemia involves removal of the cause (if secondary) and administration of pyridoxine, 50 to 150 mg daily, for several months if primary. Symptomatic anaemia may require regular blood transfusions.

### Anaemia of chronic disease

This is usually normocytic and normochromic but may occasionally be mildly microcytic and hypochromic. If the serum iron and TIBC are measured, both will usually be low.

## Normocytic anaemia

The major causes of normocytic anaemia are the anaemia of chronic disease, bleeding, chronic renal failure, marrow disease and sickling.

### Anaemia of chronic disease

This anaemia accompanies chronic medical diseases such as collagen diseases, chronic infection or malignancy. It is often asymptomatic and resistant to all haematinics. When symptomatic, transfusion may be required.

### Bleeding

The response to haemorrhage includes transfer of extracellular fluid into the vascular compartment. This results in haemodilution and anaemia. After a day or so, increased marrow erythropoiesis results in a reticulocyte response. These reticulocytes show polychromasia (grey staining) and anisocytosis on the blood film, and an increased red cell size distribution width (RDW) on the blood count. Chronic bleeding will eventually result in depletion of iron stores and a microcytic anaemia (see above).

Careful history-taking will usually reveal the source of haemorrhage.

### Chronic renal failure

Failure of erythropoietin production by diseased kidneys results in a normocytic, normochromic anaemia. This is generally well tolerated down to levels as low as 7 g/100 ml. When symptomatic, transfusion is required; it should be remembered that this will increase the blood viscosity and may decrease the glomerular filtration rate as there will be less plasma in each millilitre of blood filtered. In the near future more general the use of genetically engineered erythropoietin may obviate the need for transfusion.

### Marrow disease

A reduced platelet and white cell count may often be found when bone marrow disease is causing anaemia. Marrow infiltration may result in a leucoerythroblastic blood picture. This is the presence of nucleated red cells and primitive white cells of any type (e.g., metamyelocytes, myelocytes, promyelocytes) on the peripheral blood film. They can be thought of as being pushed out of their normal habitat in the bone marrow into the blood. There are two major causes, marrow infiltration or early recruitment of cells into the blood in seriously ill patients. Marrow infiltration is commonly due to secondary carcinoma, particularly from carcinoma of breast, prostate, lung, thyroid or kidney. Myeloma, lymphoma and myelofibrosis may also produce a leuco-erythroblastic blood picture.

In acute and chronic leukaemias (see p. 142), leukaemic cells in the blood film will usually make the diagnosis of the anaemia obvious. Rarely, in aleukaemic leukaemia, blast cells are absent from the blood but found in the marrow.

### Sickle cell anaemia

The low oxygen affinity of sickle haemoglobin allows it to give up oxygen to tissues more easily than does haemoglobin A. Consequently the anaemia of sickle cell disease is well tolerated at levels around 8 g/100 ml and anaemia is not usually an indication for transfusion. Patients with sickle cell anaemia suffer repeated splenic infarctions in infancy, resulting in hyposplenism. Patients with sickle cell anaemia should receive prophylactic penicillin, 250 mg twice a day, and be immunized with pneumococcal vaccine. The commonest clinical problem in sickle cell disease is the sickle pain crisis.

### Sickle crisis

Under anoxic conditions, sickle haemoglobin forms long, needle-like tactoids, which deform the red cell into the characteristic sickle shape (Plate 6.2). When large numbers of sickled cells are present in small blood vessels, a 'log-jam' results and impaired blood flow to the tissues causes hypoxia and local acidosis with further sickling of red cells. Sickle pain crisis presents with pain in the trunk or limbs, often poorly localized, and frequently precipitated by infection, dehydration or chilling.

Treatment includes bed rest, rehydration and adequate analgesia. Appropriate antibiotic treatment will usually be required. Exchange transfusion is indicated in sickling of the central nervous system, priapism, lung involvement (chest syndrome), pregnancy and other sickling phenomena unresponsive to conservative treatment.

Rarely, patients with sickle cell disease may present with a much more severe anaemia than usual. This may be due to transient shutdown of marrow erythropoiesis (aplastic crisis) precipitated by intercurrent infection (particularly with the parvovirus) or acute folate deficiency. Another rare cause of severe anaemia in sickle cell

disease is the hyperhaemolytic crisis. when massive sequestration of red cells occurs, usually in the abdominal vasculature. Distinction from aplastic crisis may be made by the higher reticulocyte count and deeper jaundice than is usual for that patient in steady-state.

### Macrocytosis

The megaloblastic anaemias are the commonest cause of macrocytosis, and these are usually due to deficiency of vitamin $B_{12}$ or folic acid. Although megaloblastic maturation of bone marrow cells is characteristic of these anaemias, bone marrow examination is rarely required for their diagnosis. A clotted blood sample for vitamin $B_{12}$ and a folate assay should be taken *before* treatment is commenced.

### Vitamin B₁₂ deficiency

Vitamin $B_{12}$ is found in liver, red meat and fish, so strict vegetarians may develop deficiency. Intrinsic factor, secreted by the stomach, is essential for absorption of vitamin $B_{12}$ in the terminal ileum. Lack of intrinsic factor secretion is the cause of malabsorption in pernicious anaemia. Resection of the terminal ileum or Crohn's disease may prevent absorption of vitamin $B_{12}$, even in the presence of intrinsic factor. Rarely, colonization of small intestinal diverticuli or a blind loop by bacteria that consume the vitamin may prevent adequate amounts being absorbed.

### Pernicious anaemia

This is the commonest cause of vitamin $B_{12}$ deficiency in the UK. Clinical features include pallor, a tinge of jaundice (due to an element of haemolysis), soreness of the tongue and mild diarrhoea. There may be neurological complications of the deficiency, such as subacute combined degeneration of the cord, peripheral neuropathy, dementia and optic atrophy. Commonly there is a family history of pernicious anaemia, and there may be features of other autoimmune diseases, such as myxoedema or vitiligo.

The blood count shows a macrocytic anaemia, with oval macrocytes and hypersegmented neutrophils on the blood film. The leucocyte and platelet count may be moderately depressed, but there is rarely evidence of infection or bleeding. Antibodies to gastric parietal cells are commonly found in the serum but are not specific for pernicious anaemia, being found in normal elderly people. Antibodies to intrinsic factor are found less commonly but are more specific for pernicious anaemia. Serum lactate dehydrogenase is raised; most importantly, the serum vitamin $B_{12}$ is reduced.

The Schilling vitamin $B_{12}$ absorption test should be performed to confirm the need for lifelong therapy; this test may be made when the patient has been established on treatment. The body is first saturated with an injection of 1 mg of cyanocobalamin. A capsule of isotope-labelled vitamin $B_{12}$ is then given by mouth on an empty stomach. If the ability to absorb the vitamin is intact, then it will be taken up, but being superfluous to requirements it will then be excreted in the urine. A 24-h urine collection will contain more than 10 per cent of the ingested dose of radioactivity. Part II of the Schilling test differs only in that intrinsic factor is added in an effort to correct impaired absorption in the part I Schilling.

Initial therapy in vitamin $B_{12}$ deficiency should consist of intramuscular injection of 1 mg of the vitamin on alternate days for a week, then weekly for a month. The recommendation of the World Health Organization for long-term therapy in pernicious anaemia is hydroxycobalamin (better retained in the body than cyanocobalamin) 1 mg intramuscularly every three months. Vitamin $B_{12}$ is relatively cheap and overdosage does no harm. Plasma potassium should be estimated before the therapy and supplements prescribed if hypokalaemia is present, as potassium passes into cells with effective vitamin $B_{12}$ therapy, lowering the plasma level. Carcinoma of the stomach is slightly more frequent in patients with pernicious anaemia, so consideration should be given to yearly endoscopy in young patients with pernicious anaemia. The hypochlorhydria usual in pernicious anaemia results in inadequate splitting of dietary iron from protein, so iron absorption is suboptimal. This may result in iron deficiency supervening shortly after the start of treatment for pernicious anaemia.

### Folic acid deficiency

Folic acid deficiency may occur because of decreased intake, decreased absorption or increased requirements. Decreased intake may be found in alcoholics and in poor or elderly people who have an inadequate dietary intake of fruit and vege-

tables. Malabsorption may be found in coeliac and Crohn's disease. Increased requirements are found in pregnancy and in patients with chronic haemolytic anaemias, such as thalassaemia major, or 'warm' autoimmune haemolytic anaemia. These groups of patients should be on routine folic acid supplements.

Therapy is usually given orally—folic acid tablets, 5 to 15 mg daily.

### Other causes of macrocytosis

#### Liver disease

Interference with the lipid composition of the red cell membrane results in a mild macrocytosis; target cells are seen on the blood film.

#### Alcohol

As well as being a cause of liver disease and dietary folic acid deficiency, alcohol has a direct toxic effect on bone marrow erythroblasts. In the absence of liver disease, the MCV can provide a useful index to cessation of alcohol consumption.

#### Reticulocytosis

Young cells are larger than more mature cells, so that a reticulocytosis may result in an increase in MCV. Polychromasia (grey staining of red cells) may be found on the blood film. The usual cause is haemolysis, or more rarely recovery from a haemorrhage in a young person.

#### Autoimmune haemolytic anaemia (AIHA)

The antibody produced may function best at 37°C ('warm' AIHA) or at room temperature (cold haemagglutinin disease, or 'cold' AIHA). In cold AIHA, agglutinates of red cells may be visible in the blood sample on cooling to room temperature, or on the blood film (Plate 6.3). The direct antiglobulin test, which detects antibody attached to the patient's red cells, is positive. Jaundice may be noted.

Prednisolone is the mainstay of treatment in warm AIHA. When it is ineffective in maintaining a normal haemoglobin, or a maintenance dose over 7.5 mg daily is required, splenectomy is indicated. There is a slight but significant risk of overwhelming septicaemia with organisms such as the pneumococcus, particularly in children, and prophylactic penicillin should be given long-term. Preoperatively, pneumococcal vaccine should be administered. In patients not fit for splenectomy, azathioprine (50–150 mg daily) may help in controlling haemolysis, but will not exert its action for some weeks after starting treatment.

Cold AIHA is relatively unresponsive to steroids, and keeping the patient warm is the mainstay of treatment. Immunosuppression with chlorambucil may be effective in difficult cases. As with all haemolytic conditions, patients with AIHA should be on routine folate supplements.

### Drugs

Cytotoxic agents that interfere with nucleic acid metabolism, such as azathioprine, cytosine arabinoside and hydroxyurea, cause macrocytosis. Methotrexate acts by interfering with the folate metabolism of the cell.

### Myxoedema

This disorder may cause macrocytosis but associated pernicious anaemia should be excluded.

### Haematological diseases

The myeloproliferative disorders (polycythaemia rubra vera, essential thrombocythaemia, chronic granulocytic leukaemia, myelofibrosis) may be associated with macrocytosis, as can myeloma, aplastic anaemia and myelodysplasia.

## LEUCOPENIA

This is usually an absolute reduction in the number of circulating neutrophils, sometimes associated with a reduction in the number of lymphocytes. The major manifestation is increased incidence of infection when the absolute neutrophil count is less than $1 \times 10^9/l$. This is particularly evident at neutrophil levels less than $0.5 \times 10^9/l$.

Leucopenia may be caused by failure of neutrophil production from the marrow, or by increased neutrophil consumption. Bone marrow disease of many types may cause leucopenia, usually with associated anaemia and thrombocytopenia; this is a pancytopenia, considered below.

The commonest cause of leucopenia is drugs. Many of these, for example, the cytotoxics, have a predictable myelosuppressive effect. Others have an idiosyncratic action, such as carbimazole, sulphonamides, thiouracil, isoniazid, phenylbutazone, chloramphenicol and gold. If there is the possibility that a leucopenia is due to drugs, they should be stopped or changed.

Many patients with systemic lupus erythematosus are leucopenic, and antinuclear factor should be looked for when the cause of leucopenia is not clear. Autoimmune neutropenia is also found in association with other collagen diseases. When associated with rheumatoid arthritis and splenomegaly this is Felty's syndrome. Some members of black and Middle Eastern races have a low count of white cells in blood as a racial feature. Their neutrophils are held in the marginating pool in the tissues rather than in the blood. They are able to muster a neutrophilia in response to stress or infection and are therefore not predisposed to infections.

Viral infections such as influenza commonly result in a transient leucopenia. Infection with the human immunodeficiency virus (HIV), the causative agent of AIDS, results in lymphopenia and neutropenia. HIV is lymphocytotoxic to T-helper (T4) lymphocytes and an early manifestation of HIV infection is a decrease in the ratio of helper to suppressor (T4/T8) lymphocytes.

## PANCYTOPENIA

This is a reduction in the numbers of all three cell types in the blood, resulting in anaemia, leucopenia and thrombocytopenia. Bone marrow infiltration by haematological or non-haematological malignancy (see 'leuco-erythroblastic anaemia' above) may result in a pancytopenia. Splenomegaly from any cause may cause a pancytopenia by sequestration of blood cells. Bone marrow biopsy will demonstrate a hypercellular marrow in these circumstances.

### Aplastic anaemia

In aplastic anaemia, the bone marrow is hypocellular (Plate 6.4). This anaemia may result from poisoning of the marrow by drugs (such as cytotoxics, gold, chloramphenicol) or radiation, or after infection by hepatitis viruses. Frequently a cause cannot be found for aplastic anaemia, and it is then termed idiopathic. Some of these patients have serum factors or a subpopulation of lymphocytes that interfere with the growth of bone marrow colonies in culture. This may imply an autoimmune aetiology, particularly as some patients with aplastic anaemia respond to immunosuppressive therapy.

Aplastic anaemia is defined as 'severe' when the haemoglobin is transfusion dependent, the neutrophil count less than $0.5 \times 10^9$/l, and platelet count less than $20 \times 10^9$/l. Supportive treatment in aplastic anaemia will involve blood transfusion, platelet transfusion and antibiotic therapy. Initial treatment may involve attempts to stimulate the bone marrow by anabolic steroids such as oxymethalone. This drug may cause cholestatic jaundice in some recipients. When ineffective, high-dose steroid therapy or antilymphocyte globulin may work. In patients less than 40 years old with a tissue-type compatible sibling, bone marrow transplantation may be a curative option.

## THROMBOCYTOPENIA

A low platelet count predisposes to capillary bleeding, resulting in bruising, nosebleeds, menorrhagia, melaena and haematuria. The usual normal range is 150 to $500 \times 10^9$/l. However, bleeding manifestations are unusual at levels over $70 \times 10^9$/l unless there is a challenge by surgical operation or trauma. Minor bleeding manifestations may occur at levels between 20 and $50 \times 10^9$/l, and these may be severe at levels below $20 \times 10^9$/l. Bleeding episodes at low platelet counts may be precipitated by infection, or therapy with non-steroidal anti-inflammatory drugs or aspirin. Bleeding tendency may be assessed by means of the template bleeding time, which makes a scientifically precise length and depth of cut using a disposable cassette mechanism. This leaves a small scar and so should only be used where it is considered that the investigation will provide valuable clinical information. Normal template bleeding time is up to 9.5 min.

Providing the rest of the blood count is normal, then the common causes of thrombocytopenic are artefactual, idiopathic thrombocytopenic purpura, and drugs. A small clot in the blood specimen is the commonest cause of artefactual thrombocytopenia, and an unexpectedly low platelet count should be repeated before further clinical action is undertaken.

### Idiopathic thrombocytopenic purpura

Many cases of idiopathic thrombocytopenic purpura are discovered at routine blood count made for other reasons. The more advanced blood counters count platelets routinely, and also assess the average size of the platelets (mean platelet volume, MPV). When the MPV is raised in a case of thrombocytopenia it implies that it is due to peripheral consumption of platelets rather than marrow underproduction. Causes of peripheral platelet consumption include idiopathic thrombocytopenic purpura, hypersplenism and disseminated intravascular coagulation (p. 151). Bone marrow in these conditions will show normal or increased megakaryocytes. The majority of cases of idiopathic thrombocytopenic purpura are autoimmune; however, tests for platelet antibodies are technically difficult, particularly when thrombocytopenia is present, and are not usually used except in difficult cases. The antinuclear factor should be sought in the blood in all cases, however, as some patients with systemic lupus erythematosus present with idiopathic thrombocytopenic purpura. An autoimmune thrombocytopenia may also be found in patients with HIV infection.

Treatment of the idiopathic purpura in patients with platelet counts of less than $50 \times 10^9$/l is with prednisolone in a usual dosage of 1 mg/kg/day initially. Cases unresponsive to steroids, or in whom a maintenance dose greater than about 7.5 mg of prednisolone daily is required, may be treated by splenectomy. The spleen is the major site of platelet destruction in this condition. Patients unfit for splenectomy may receive other immunosuppressive agents, such as azathioprine, 50 to 150 mg daily, with the dose adjusted according to the clinical response and white cell count.

When immunosuppression is ineffective and a rapid improvement in platelet count is essential, for example before splenectomy, then high-purity intravenous immunoglobulin may be given. This blocks the sequestration of platelets in the reticuloendothelial system. A suitable regimen is 0.4 g/kg/day by intravenous infusion over two to three hours on three successive days. Side-effects other than mild headache are unusual and the treatment may be given on a day-ward basis. The high cost of this form of treatment has restricted study of its efficacy when administered long-term.

### Drug-induced thrombocytopenia

Drugs may induce thrombocytopenia in several ways, including toxic depression of bone marrow megakaryocytes and antibody-mediated mechanisms. Common examples include sulphonamides (and co-trimoxazole), the thiazide diuretics, rifampicin, paracetamol and quinine. Quinine is usually given for nocturnal cramps, but thrombocytopenia due to intake of quinine as a flavouring in soft drinks has been reported. Prolonged therapy with subcutaneous heparin may also induce thrombocytopenia.

Post-transfusion purpura may result when a rare individual whose platelets are negative for the platelet antigen PlA1 is stimulated to produce anti-PlA1 by transfusion of PlA1-positive blood. Future transfusion of PlA1-positive blood may result in thrombocytopenia 7 to 10 days after transfusion. The patient's own platelets become involved in the immunological reaction and are destroyed, but the mechanism for their involvement is unclear.

Another type of thrombocytopenia occurs after massive blood transfusion, usually during surgery. This is due to dilution and consumption of platelets. Transfusion of platelet concentrate (p. 153) should be used to keep the platelet count over 70 $\times 10^9$/l in the operative period. Blood transfusion for the correction of anaemia in patients who are also thrombocytopenic may worsen the thrombocytopenia as platelets adhere to transfused microaggregates. The use of a microaggregate filter or washed cells helps to prevent this exacerbation of thrombocytopenia.

## LEUCOCYTOSIS

The finding of an elevated leucocyte count should prompt examination of the differential count to determine whether the leucocytosis is due to a neutrophilia or a lymphocytosis.

### Neutrophilia

Pyogenic infection and trauma (such as surgery) are the commonest causes of neutrophilia. In severe cases, slightly immature neutrophils may appear in the blood—described as stab cells, metamyelocytes, or 'neutrophil left shift'. When infection is present, fine violet granules appear in the neutrophils—toxic granulation. A modest neutrophilia, with white cell counts of the order of 10 to 13 $\times 10^9$/l, is usual in pregnancy, perhaps because of the increased production of steroid hormones. The therapeutic use of hydrocortisone or prednisolone may also result in a neutrophilia.

### Lymphocytosis

Viral illnesses commonly result in a lymphocytosis. In childhood, whooping cough is a cause of lymphocyte counts over 50 $\times 10^9$/l (a 'leukaemoid reaction'). In adolescence, glandular fever is a common cause of lymphocytosis, the lymphocytes showing characteristic morphological changes, which have led to their being described as 'reactive mononuclear cells'. Clinically, pyrexia, lymphadenopathy and sore throat are usual. The diagnostic Paul–Bunnell test looks for the presence of heterophil antibodies in the blood. These antibodies have the ability to react with the cells of other animal species, in particular sheep erythrocytes. In middle-aged or elderly persons the commonest cause of a lymphocytosis is chronic lymphocytic leukaemia (see below).

### Leucocytosis of other cell types

An increased count of eosinophils, basophils or monocytes is not usually reflected in an increased *total* leucocyte count.

### *Eosinophilia*

An eosinophilia is frequently found in allergic conditions such as asthma, hay fever, eczema, or drug reactions. It also frequently accompanies parasitic infections, and is recognized to occur in Hodgkin's disease and polyarteritis nodosa.

### *Basophilia*

Basophilia is most frequently seen in association with the myeloproliferative diseases, polycythaemia rubra vera, myelofibrosis, essential thrombocythaemia and chronic granulocytic leukaemia.

### *Monocytosis*

Monocytosis is usually found in association with a neutrophilia. As a single abnormality it may be found in inflammatory bowel disease, myelodysplasia, recovery from cytotoxic chemotherapy, tuberculosis and other chronic infections.

## THE LEUKAEMIAS

The acute leukaemias are characterized by primitive blast cells infiltrating blood (Plate 6.5) and bone marrow. The chronic leukaemias have more mature cells in the blood and bone marrow.

## Acute leukaemias

These are divided into acute myeloblastic and acute lymphoblastic leukaemia. At presentation each may be overtly leukaemic, subleukaemic, or aleukaemic. In overt leukaemia, many blast cells are seen in the blood. In subleukaemic leukaemia, a few blasts are present in the blood, but the total leucocyte count is low. In aleukaemic leukaemia, blast cells are absent from the blood, being found only in the marrow.

The cytotoxic treatment of acute leukaemia is usually divided into three phases: remission induction, consolidation therapy and maintenance.

### Acute lymphoblastic leukaemia (ALL)

Acute lymphoblastic leukaemia is predominantly a disease of children. Besides infiltration of marrow and blood, with consequent anaemia, thrombocytopenia and neutropenia, the lymphoblasts may also infiltrate the central nervous system and the testis. In these anatomical areas, leukaemic cells may escape the effects of antileukaemic chemotherapy. Consequently, craniospinal irradiation and intrathecal methotrexate treatment are used routinely to eradicate disease in the 'sanctuary' of the central nervous system. Three-quarters of children with ALL will go into remission with vincristine and prednisolone treatment. In order to improve long-term results, further cytotoxic drugs have been added, such as daunorubicin and cytosine. Approximately half of all children with ALL can now be cured. Poor prognostic factors are a high white-cell count at presentation, and lymphoblasts with T or B immunological surface markers.

After the successful induction of remission and consolidation, maintenance treatment with vincristine, prednisolone, methotrexate and mercaptopurine is usually continued for two years.

### Acute myeloblastic leukaemia (AML)

Acute myeloblastic leukaemia is a disease predominantly of adults, with less propensity for involvement of the central nervous system than ALL. Effective treatment requires very powerful ablative chemotherapy and the cure rate, defined as five years disease-free survival of treatment, is less than 20 per cent. Induction treatment usually contains various combinations off daunorubicin, cytosine, etoposide and thioguanine. Supportive treatment with broad-spectrum antibiotics and blood and platelet transfusions during the hypoplastic phase after cytotoxic treatment is essential. Maintenance cytotoxic treatment is of no proven value in AML, and in patients under 40 years of age further attempts at curative treatment involve allogeneic bone marrow transplantation from an HLA-matching sibling, or autologous marrow transplantation if such a donor is not available.

## Chronic leukaemias

### Chronic lymphocytic leukaemia (CLL)

Chronic lymphocytic leukaemia is a disease of middle and old age that is commonly discovered as an incidental finding when a blood count is being done for other reasons. There is a lymphocytosis of mature-looking lymphocytes in the blood with smear cells (lymphocytes crushed during the making of the smear) on the blood film (Plate 6.6). In more than 95 per cent of cases the disorder is a proliferation of B lymphocytes. In cases of unexplained lymphocytosis the diagnosis of CLL may be confirmed by the demonstration of an excess of B lymphocytes in the blood (normally two-thirds of lymphocytes are T cells) and showing that these B lymphocytes express only one type of surface immunoglobulin light chain (normally a mixture of kappa and lambda light chain-expressing B cells is found).

The disease progresses through blood lymphocytosis to lymphadenopathy, hepatosplenomegaly and eventually to marrow infiltration resulting in anaemia and thrombocytopenia. The majority of patients have low gamma globulins, even at presentation, and are liable to bacterial and viral infections, including herpes zoster.

Treatment may never be required in asymptomatic cases. Symptomatic lymphadenopathy may be treated by low-dose chlorambucil, 2 to 8 mg daily on a continuing basis, adjusting the dose according to response. Younger patients, or those with more aggressive disease, may benefit from combination chemotherapy with COP (cyclophosphamide, Oncovin [vincristine], prednisolone) or CHOP (cyclophosphamide, hydroxydaunorubicin, Oncovin, prednisolone).

An increased incidence of some autoimmune

phenomena is associated with B-CLL. The most common are warm autoimmune haemolytic anaemia, autoimmune thrombocytopenia, and Sjögren's syndrome.

### Chronic granulocytic (myeloid) leukaemia

Predominantly a disease of middle age, the major manifestation of this is massive splenomegaly, which may present as an incidental finding on routine abdominal examination. The blood shows a massive neutrophilia with left shift; the white cell count is often in the region of 100 to 500 × $10^9$/l. There is commonly a leuco-erythroblastic blood picture and increased numbers of basophils and eosinophils. The platelet count may be low, normal or high. The high white cell count causes an increased blood viscosity and predisposition to thrombosis. This may result in splenic infarction or priapism.

The differential diagnosis in cases without splenomegaly and with white cell counts of less than 50 × $10^9$/l will include a neutrophil leukaemoid reaction. The neutrophil alkaline phosphatase score is low in chronic granulocytic leukaemia and high in reactive neutrophilia. In chronic granulocytic leukaemia, there is a marker chromosome abnormality, the Philadelphia chromosome. Treatment consists of hydroxyurea, 0.5 to 4 g daily, or alkylating agents with allopurinol cover. The majority of cases eventually develop accelerated-phase disease, manifested by increased blast counts in the blood, bone pain, anaemia and thrombocytopenia, anorexia, weight loss and low-grade pyrexia. This may progress to blast transformation, with a blood picture indistinguishable from acute leukaemia and having a poor prognosis.

## MYELOMA AND RELATED DISORDERS

Myeloma is associated with a malignant proliferation of plasma cells in the bone marrow. These produce symptoms by interference with haemopoieisis (anaemia, pancytopenia, leuco-erythroblastic picture) and by the production of a paraprotein and osteoclast-stimulating factors.

A paraprotein is a single type and class of immunoglobulin molecules of identical structure produced by the clone of malignant plasma cells. The immunoglobulin is not usually directed against a known antigen. The clinical manifes-

tations of a paraprotein depend on its physico-chemical properties. It may be a cryoglobulin, or have a tendency to polymerize and cause plasma hyperviscosity. The hyperviscosity syndrome may be found in any type of myeloma, but is commonest in IgM and IgA myeloma. Clinically, these patients have visual disturbances, weakness, anorexia, headache and dizziness, progressing to confusion, fits and coma. They commonly have an associated bleeding diathesis. The plasma viscosity is usually over 4 mPa at 25°C. Plasma exchange may be lifesaving.

The osteoclast-stimulating factor secreted by the plasma cells results in osteoporosis, pathological fractures and hypercalcaemia. The hypercalcaemia may produce nausea, constipation, abdominal pain, weakness, polyuria and polydipsia. Rapid and effective treatment of the hypercalcaemia with rehydration and steroids is important. Mobilization should be encouraged. In resistant cases, diphosphonates, mithramycin or calcitonin may be used.

Renal failure in myeloma is common, due to prerenal problems such as hyperviscosity and dehydration, renal problems such as amyloid, nephrocalcinosis or urate nephropathy, or post-renal problems such as urinary tract infections.

Cytotoxic chemotherapy for myeloma is usually with an alkylating agent such as melphalan, 5 mg/$m^2$ daily for four to seven days. When hypercalcaemia, bone pain, anorexia or thrombocytopenia are present this may usefully be combined with prednisolone, 20 to 40 mg/$m^2$ daily. Cases that become resistant to melphalan treatment may respond to cyclophosphamide, 50 to 100 mg by mouth daily on a continuing basis. Combination chemotherapy may be employed in younger patients or those with resistant disease, e.g., ABCM (Adriamycin, BCNU, cyclophosphamide, melphalan).

### Benign monoclonal gammopathy

The presence of a paraprotein in the serum is not necessarily diagnostic of myeloma. Benign monoclonal bands may be found in the serum of elderly people. They are of low concentration (<20 g/l for IgG paraproteins), their concentration does not increase over time, and they are not associated with a reduction in the levels of the other immunoglobulins (immune paresis) or with clinical manifestations of myeloma, such as bone pain, hypercalcaemia or anaemia. Patients with monoclonal bands of uncertain significance should be reviewed periodically as some cases turn to myeloma.

## Waldenström's macroglobulinaemia

The proliferating cell in this lymphoid malignancy has morphological characteristics of both plasma cells and small lymphocytes. Unlike myeloma, bone pain, hypercalcaemia and renal failure are not features of the disease. Like CLL, these patients have generalized lymphadenopathy and hepatosplenomegaly. Like myeloma, there is a serum paraprotein, almost always of IgM type. Plasma hyperviscosity is common. Treatment is usually with alkylating agents such as chlorambucil.

## POLYCYTHAEMIA

A high haemoglobin or haematocrit results in an increased whole-blood viscosity with predisposition to arterial and venous thrombosis and hypertension. An initial distinction should be made between true polycythaemia and pseudopolycythaemia. True polycythaemia is an increased red cell mass; pseudopolycythaemia is a reduced plasma volume—this may result from dehydration due to diarrhoea, vomiting, pyrexia or diuretics. An increased haemoglobin and PCV is found and these will return to normal on rehydration. Some people maintain a low plasma volume for reasons that are unclear—'stress' polycythaemia. If there is no obvious cause for the polycythaemia, then the red cell mass and plasma volume should be measured, using isotope dilution techniques. If an elevated red cell mass is confirmed, then a cause should be sought.

Chronic hypoxic lung disease will usually be clinically apparent. In doubtful cases, respiratory function tests and blood gases may help in diagnosis. Some patients may benefit from a trial of venesection, particularly when the haemoglobin is over 19 g/100 ml. Smoking will cause a mild degree of polycythaemia in susceptible subjects, particularly if the smoke is inhaled, and the first line of treatment is to stop smoking and review the haemoglobin after a month or two.

Increased pressure within the renal parenchyma stimulates excessive production of erythropoietin, which in turn stimulates marrow erythropoiesis resulting in polycythaemia. Causes include renal cysts, renal tumours, and pyonephrosis. Minimal investigation should include careful palpation of the abdomen for renal masses, urine microscopy and blood urea measurement. Cases without other apparent cause for polycythaemia should have abdominal ultrasonography or intravenous pyelography.

Some tumours produce erythropoietin-like substances, which may cause polycythaemia. These include carcinoma of the kidney, hepatoma, giant uterine fibroids and cerebellar haemangioblastoma.

Rarely, an abnormal haemoglobin with increased oxygen affinity may cause polycythaemia. This may be detected by plotting an oxygen dissociation curve, which is shifted to the left.

Polycythaemia rubra vera is considered below.

## The myeloproliferative diseases

These are grouped together as they frequently share overlapping features, and intermediate varieties of these disorders are found. Polycythaemia rubra vera and essential thrombocythaemia may eventually turn to myelofibrosis. Chronic granulocytic leukaemia is considered above with chronic leukaemias.

### *Polycythaemia rubra vera*

In addition to the erythrocytosis, high haemoglobin and haematocrit, these patients usually have an elevated neutrophil and platelet count. This helps to distinguish polycythaemia rubra vera from secondary polycythaemia. Further aids to differential diagnosis from secondary polycythaemia are the neutrophil alkaline phosphatase score and the ESR. The neutrophil alkaline phosphatase is elevated in primary polycythaemia rubra vera and normal in secondary polycythaemia. An ESR over 2 mm/h is unusual in polycythaemia rubra vera.

The polycythaemia vera study group have established the following criteria for diagnosis:
(a) a raised red cell mass >36 ml/kg (males) or 32 ml/kg (females);
(b) arterial oxygen saturation >92 per cent;
(c) splenomegaly;
(d) platelet count >$400 \times 10^9$/l;
(e) white cell count >$12 \times 10^9$/l;
(f) neutrophil alkaline phosphatase score >100 and serum vitamin $B_{12}$ >900 pg/ml.

The diagnosis is acceptable if (a), (b) and (c) are

present or (a), (b), and any other two criteria from (d) to (f).

Clinically, presentation may be with arterial or venous thrombosis, plethora, or an incidental finding on routine blood count. Associated disorders are gout, peptic ulceration and pruritis. Pruritis may be particularly troublesome after a hot bath and when iron deficiency is present. Iron deficiency is common in patients with polycythaemia rubra vera because a large amount of iron is needed to make a high red cell mass, occult gastrointestinal bleeding is common, and venesection is a common method of treatment.

Venesection is a useful, initial method of treatment, taking a unit of blood daily or on alternate days until the haematocrit is less than 0.48 to 0.50. In patients with a history of cardiovascular disease the venesection should be isovolaemic, with a unit of saline run into one arm whilst a unit of blood is taken out of the other arm. Venesection has the disadvantages that it needs to be repeated, may cause a thrombocytosis, and eventually leads to iron deficiency. Patients with a low MCV and symptoms of iron deficiency, such as tiredness or increased itching, should receive oral iron therapy *and* be venesected. If venesection needs to be repeated more than once a month, or is difficult for some other reason, then other therapy should be considered.

Suppression of bone marrow erythropoiesis by busulphan, hydroxyurea, or $^{32}$P is justified in polycythaemia rubra vera but is generally avoided in secondary polycythaemia because of the slight risk of leukaemogenesis. Intravenous injection of $^{32}$P has the advantage of requiring only one injection for several months' control; the disadvantages are that it is more difficult to obtain, it takes up to four weeks to act, and it is difficult to judge the correct dose.

Busulphan may be administered as single doses of 1 mg/kg/month, or for a few weeks at doses of 2 to 6 mg daily. It should be borne in mind that busulphan continues to exert its myelosuppressive effect for a few weeks after administration is stopped. Recovery of myelopoiesis after treatment with hydroxyurea occurs in a few days, but effective therapy with this drug often requires continuous administration over long periods.

## Myelofibrosis

Massive splenomegaly is the principal clinical feature of this disease. Presentation may be with splenic infarction, manifested by pleuritic pain in the left hypochondrium radiating to the left shoulder and sometimes associated with a rub.

Anaemia is usual, with characteristic tear-drop poikilocytes on the blood film, which is also commonly leuco-erythroblastic (see p. 141). Bone marrow aspirate is a 'dry tap', requiring a biopsy to demonstrate the marrow fibrosis characteristic of this condition. The white cell and platelet count may be high, normal or low. Treatment is generally supportive, with blood transfusions. Symptomatic splenomegaly or unacceptably high or increasing transfusion requirements are an indication for splenectomy. The proliferation of cells in the bone marrow consumes folic acid, so patients should be taking folic acid supplements.

## Essential thrombocythaemia

The major problem in this condition lies in distinguishing it from the causes of a secondary or reactive thrombocytosis. Common causes of secondary thrombocytosis are bleeding, infection, trauma, malignancy and iron deficiency. In essential thrombocythaemia the platelet count is often over $1000 \times 10^9$/l, but platelet counts of this order are unusual in secondary thrombocytosis. The platelets in this disorder may clump spontaneously, causing thrombosis, and fail to clump, causing bleeding.

The spleen may be palpable in some patients, but others have repeated splenic infarction and are hyposplenic. Iron deficiency is frequently present, making the differential diagnosis from secondary thrombocytosis difficult. It is often necessary to perform barium meal and enema in order to exclude a gastrointestinal neoplasm.

The agent of choice for the treatment of essential thrombocythaemia in middle-aged and elderly persons is $^{32}$P. The use of this isotope may increase the risk of leukaemogenesis in the myeloproliferative disorders, and in younger patients, hydroxyurea (0.5–2 g daily) may be less leukaemogenic. This agent also has the advantage that after inadvertent overdosage the resultant thrombocytopenia or leucopenia recovers a few days after stopping treatment. Trials are in progress of α-interferon, 3–8 μg subcutaneously at night, three to seven times weekly, which is an effective antiproliferative agent in the myeloproliferative disorders and may be associated with the least risk of leukaemic transformation.

The aim of treatment is to keep the platelet

count below $500 \times 10^9$/l. Platelet function usually improves once the platelet count is lowered. When the platelet count is very high, thrombocytapheresis on a cell separator may be used to lower the count rapidly. Transient ischaemic attacks may respond to low-dose aspirin, 300 mg twice weekly.

## COAGULATION FAILURE

Clinical history taking in the investigation of coagulation disorders has well-defined objectives. Firstly, careful note should be made of the nature and sites of bleeding. Distinct but overlapping clinical pictures are produced by haemostatic failure due to coagulation factor deficiency and haemostatic failure due to disorders of platelet numbers or function. Coagulation factor deficiency is frequently manifested by deep tissue bleeding (muscle haematoma and haemarthrosis) whereas platelet deficiency is manifested by epithelial surface bleeding (bruising, nosebleeds, and menorrhagia).

The length of bleeding history will indicate whether the disorder is congenital or acquired, and a family history may indicate an inherited deficiency. The drug history should take particular note of aspirin and non-steroidal anti-inflammatory drugs. Initial laboratory screening for a coagulation disorder should include a blood count, including platelet count, prothrombin time, activated partial thromboplastin time (APTT) (or kaolin–cephalin clotting time) and thrombin time.

The prothrombin time detects factor deficiency in the extrinsic system and final common pathway. The APTT detects factor deficiencies in the intrinsic system and final common pathway. The thrombin time tests the final portion of the final common pathway (Fig. 6.1). The thrombin time is the simplest of the coagulation tests. A quantity of bovine thrombin is added to the patient's plasma, converting the fibrinogen to a fibrin clot. This tests only the final part of the coagulation mechanism, and there is a limited number of causes of a prolonged thrombin time. Either the patient has no fibrinogen (defibrination, dysfibrinogenaemia) or there is an inhibitor of the action of thrombin on fibrinogen present. The two common inhibitors are heparin and a high level of fibrin degradation products.

The inherited haemophilias, haemophilia A (factor VIII deficiency), and Christmas disease (factor IX deficiency; haemophilia B) are charac-

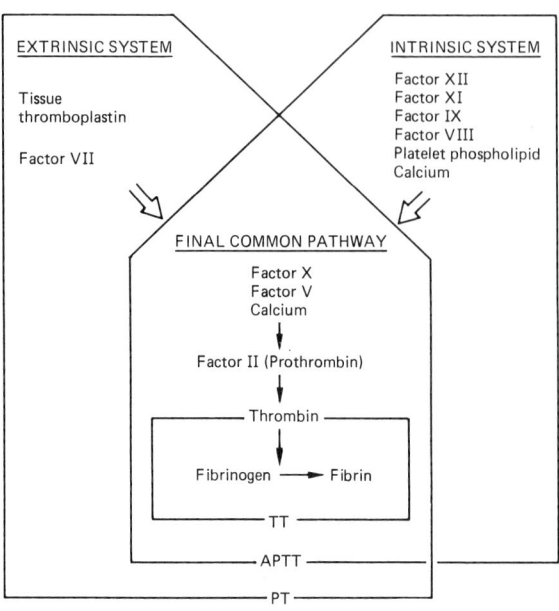

*Figure 6.1* The coagulation mechanism is divided into extrinsic and intrinsic systems, which share a final common pathway. The APTT (see text) tests the intrinsic system and final common pathway. The prothrombin time (PT) tests the extrinsic system and final common pathway. The thrombin time (TT) tests the last part of the final common pathway. The coagulation factors that each test is sensitive to are indicated.

terized by repeated haemarthroses and muscle haematomas, starting in childhood. The inheritance is sex linked, with boys affected and females as carriers. Laboratory investigation shows a prolonged partial thromboplastin time as the only abnormality. Coagulation factor assays are required to demonstrate which coagulation factor is absent.

Liver disease, or treatment with the coumarin (warfarin) anticoagulants, depletes the vitamin K-dependent coagulation factors. These are factors II, VII, IX and X. This causes prolongation of both the partial thromboplastin time and the prothrombin time. In practice, the prothrombin time is used to estimate deficiency of these factors, being technically simpler than the partial thromboplastin time.

### Disseminated intravascular coagulation (DIC)

This is usually manifested by acute haemostatic failure, with severe bleeding manifestations. The cause is release into the circulation of a procoagulant, which promotes blood clotting. After crush injury, and intrauterine fetal death, tissue thromboplastins are released into the circulation. Other obstetric causes of DIC are amniotic fluid embolus and retroplacental haematoma. Some bacterial toxins are procoagulants, so that septicaemia is a potent cause of DIC. Mucus-secreting carcinomas of the gastrointestinal tract produce procoagulant substances, so that handling of these tumours at operation may precipitate DIC.

The laboratory investigation of most cases of DIC shows prolongation of all coagulation times, due to consumption of all coagulation factors. The platelet count is reduced, and fragmented cells and helmet cells are seen on the blood film. These are produced by red cells being chopped up by fibrin strands laid down in the small blood vessels. Young red cells can reseal themselves and continue in circulation as fragmented cells. This is termed a 'microangiopathic blood picture' and is also seen in vasculitis and glomerulonephritis.

When the coagulation system is massively activated, there is usually a corresponding activation of the fibrinolytic system. In the laboratory this may be detected by increased levels of fibrin degradation products in the blood and increased lysis of clots in the test tube. Increased fibrinolysis contributes to the haemostatic defect.

Treatment is directed to removing the cause of the DIC and replacing the coagulation factors. Fresh frozen plasma, which contains all the coagulation factors, should be administered in sufficient quantities to correct the prothrombin time, partial thromboplastin time, and thrombin time to as close to normality as possible. Prolongation of the thrombin time is an indication for fibrinogen estimation. If reduced, cryoprecipitate may be used to supplement the fresh frozen plasma as it contains a relative excess of fibrinogen. Platelet concentrate should be used to keep the platelet count over $50 \times 10^9$/l. Blood transfusion should be used to maintain the haemoglobin, and the coagulation tests repeated every few hours.

The use of heparin in DIC to suppress the consumption of coagulation factors is highly controversial and almost never required. In certain clinical situations where there is a grave risk of DIC, for example during cytotoxic treatment of the promyelocytic variant of acute myeloid leukaemia (M3), low-dose heparin (100 u/h intravenously) may be given prophylactically.

# THROMBOSIS

Predisposition to thrombosis may be caused by factors in the blood or factors in the vessel wall, or frequently by both. The usual abnormality in the vessel wall is atheroma, which will not be considered further here.

Factors in the blood may be divided into those affecting blood flow and abnormal constituents of the blood. Blood viscosity is largely determined by haematocrit, hence polycythaemia predisposes to stagnation and thrombosis. The splenic arterioles contain blood of a higher haematocrit than blood elsewhere in the body, so thrombotic tendencies may manifest by splenic infarction. Stagnation of blood may be found in varicose veins and when an enlarged uterus presses on the pelvic veins. There is increased tendency for the blood to clot after operation and when the platelet count is elevated.

## Anticoagulants

Heparin is an immediate-acting anticoagulant, normally given by the intravenous route. Control is best performed by the partial thromboplastin time, aiming for a ratio of 2 to 2.5 times the control time. When heparin is stopped, the levels decay rapidly over a few hours. In exceptional circumstances the heparin may be reversed by using protamine sulphate.

Once a therapeutic response has been achieved, it is usual to switch to oral warfarin. This requires two days to work, during which heparin should be continued. For an average adult, 10 mg of warfarin is administered on each of three successive nights. When the laboratory uses the British comparative thromboplastin reagents, the prothrombin time will reflect the warfarin effect providing the patient is not over-heparinized. Average daily warfarin dosage is 7 mg, aiming to keep the international normalized ratio between 2 and 4.5 The desired ratio will depend on the indication for anticoagulation.

In the event of accidental over-anticoagulation with warfarin, the action taken should depend on the ratio and the clinical manifestations of bleeding. For ratios of 4.5 to 6, stop the warfarin for one dose and continue with a smaller dosage. For ratios of 7 to 9, stop the warfarin and repeat the prothrombin time daily or on alternate days, only starting wafarin again when the prothrombin time has returned to the therapeutic range. In the event of bleeding manifestations, or ratios over 9, stop warfarin and administer vitamin K and/or fresh frozen plasma. Should it not be required to start warfarin again, then 5 to 10 mg of vitamin K may be given. This will restore the prothrombin time to normal in a few hours. Should it be desired to warfarinize the patient again, then only 1 to 2 mg of vitamin K should be administered, otherwise a profound warfarin resistance will be encountered. For immediate reversal of the warfarin effect, 2 to 4 units of fresh frozen plasma may be used.

## Anticoagulation in pregnancy

Warfarin may cause fetal malformations, particularly of the nasal bones, and should not be given in the first trimester. Because of the risk of haemorrhagic problems at delivery, it is also usual to avoid warfarin in the last trimester. Subcutaneous, low-dose calcium heparin, 5000 to 10 000 u twice daily, is a suitable alternative in most cases, and may be self-administered, using preloaded syringes. The prolonged use of heparin may cause osteoporosis with possible vertebral collapse, so many patients are transferred back on to warfarin during the middle trimester. Patients with some types of artificial heart valves may be at particular risk of emboli, and it is preferred to keep these patients on warfarin throughout pregnancy.

## Thrombophilia

When a predisposing cause for thrombosis or embolus is not evident, particularly in a young person, consideration should be given to screening for a thrombotic tendency. All patients with thrombosis should have a blood count to exclude polycythaemia, with a platelet count to exclude essential thrombocythaemia. The lupus anticoagulant (antiphospholipid antibodies) frequently presents with thrombosis. This may be detected by prolongation of the APTT or by the dilute Russell viper venom test, if available. The fluorescent antinuclear factor test should be done. Congenital deficiency of antithrombin III or of the vitamin K-dependent, anticoagulant proteins protein S and protein C results in a thrombotic tendency that may present in younger patients with a strong family history of thrombotic problems.

## BLOOD TRANSFUSION AND BLOOD PRODUCTS

### Red cell preparations

In chronic haematological diseases associated with anaemia it is usual to attempt to keep the haemoglobin above 10 g/100 ml by transfusion. Blood for the correction of anaemia should be used as packed or plasma-reduced cells. Other action to avoid circulatory overload may include the administration of diuretics (e.g., frusemide, 20 mg by mouth or intravenously before each unit) and a slow rate of transfusion (4–6 h for each unit). Patients with vitamin $B_{12}$ deficiency are at particular risk from circulatory overload, and these patients should receive staged transfusion (e.g., one unit daily) if blood transfusion is unavoidable.

The majority of red cells for transfusion are now issued in optimal additive solutions (e.g., saline adenine glucose mannitol [SAG-M]). These solutions are excellent preservatives of red cells, allowing the unit a 5-week shelf life. They are suitable for replacement of blood volume but contain little protein and few coagulation factors as the plasma has been removed and replaced by SAG-M.

### Blood transfusion reactions

Approximately 15 per cent of patients having a blood transfusion will have some type of unwanted reaction.

The most common is a pyrexia, sometimes with chills or rigors. Often these patients have had transfusions before and the reaction may be due to white cell or platelet antibodies, though in many patients a cause cannot be found. When pyrexia is not over 38°C and is not associated with other symptoms, it is reasonable to take down the offending unit and return to saline until the temperature returns to normal, then go on to the next unit. In some patients with an allergic tendency, urticaria may be noted. Hydrocortisone and chlorpheniramine should be given.

When pyrexia does not settle promptly, or when hypotension or loin pain are present, a full investigation of the reaction should be performed. This will include blood cultures, repeat crossmatch and a direct antiglobulin test. The urine should be examined for haemoglobinuria and the remainder of the blood unit plugged and returned to the laboratory. Serious haemolytic reactions are fortunately rare, and are usually due to clerical errors such as incorrect labelling of the blood sample. Infected blood will produce a similar clinical picture. When a haemolytic reaction is suspected, a coagulation screen and platelet count should be performed to look for DIC. Immediate treatment will include the correction of hypotension by administration of 4.5 per cent albumin or fresh frozen plasma, maintenance of urinary output by mannitol infusion or intravenous diuretics, and correction of electrolyte abnormalities.

Pyrexial blood transfusion reactions due to white cell or platelet antibodies may be alleviated by the use of leucocyte-depleted blood. This has a limited shelf life and is therefore only suitable for elective transfusions. Reduction in the number of leucocytes may also be achieved by spinning the blood in a refrigerated centrifuge to compact the leucocytes into aggregates, then transfusing it through a microaggregate filter.

## Platelet transfusions

Platelet concentrate is prepared from single-donor units or by donor thrombopheresis on a cell separator. Its use is reserved for those patients with thrombocytopenia of less than $20 \times 10^9/l$. Adult patients are usually given six single-donor units or one cell separator pack. Platelet transfusions may improve bleeding manifestations but do not cause a prolonged increase in platelet count. Patients who have received many blood products may become refractory to random platelet transfusions because of the development of anti-HLA antibodies. This may be confirmed by the absence of an increase of more than $20 \times 10^9/l$ in the platelet count one hour after platelet transfusion. An improvement in platelet survival and fewer pyrexial reactions may be obtained by the use of partly or completely HLA-matched platelet donors. Pyrexial reactions to platelet transfusions are common and may be ameliorated by chlorpheniramine, 10 mg intravenously, and hydrocortisone, 100 mg intravenously, before the transfusion and a slow rate of infusion. In severe cases, pethidine, 50 mg by slow intravenous infusion, is effective. The removal of contaminating leucocytes from the platelets by the use of differential centrifugation kits (Leucotrap) or in-line leucocyte filters (Pall) may also decrease the incidence of febrile reactions.

In idiopathic thrombocytopenic purpura the transfused platelets are rapidly destroyed and may also stimulate the production of platelet antibodies. Hence their use in this disease is reserved for haemorrhagic emergencies.

## Human albumin (4.5 per cent)

This isotonic solution (commonly referred to as 'plasma') is the agent of choice for the restoration of circulating blood volume after burns or haemorrhage whilst waiting for crossmatched blood. It contains no clotting factors or antibodies.

## Fresh frozen plasma

This contains all coagulation factors (but not platelets) and normal red cell antibodies and gamma globulins. ABO compatibility must be observed. A frequent use for fresh frozen plasma is the correction of transfusion-induced coagulopathy.

## Further reading

### General

Williams W. J. (1986). Approach to the patient. In *Hamatology* 3rd edn. (Williams W. J., Bentler E., Ersler A. J., Lichtman M. A. eds.) New York: McGraw-Hill, p. 3.

### Anaemia

Cartwright G. E., Deiss A. (1975). Sideroblasts, siderocytes and sideroblastic anaemia. *New Eng. J Med.*, **29**, pp. 185–93.

Cook J. D. (1982). Clinical evaluation of iron deficiency. *Seminars Haematol.* **19**, pp. 6–18.

Erslev A. J. (1970). Anaemia of chronic renal disease. *Arch. Intern. Med.*, **126**, 774–780.

Gordon-Smith E. C., ed. (1989). Aplastic anaemia. *Clinical Haematology*, **2:1**, London: Baillière Tindall, pp. 1–163.

Hoffbrand A. V. (1971). The megaloblastic anaemias. In *Recent Advances in Haematology* (Goldberg A., Brain M. C., eds.) Edinburgh: Churchill Livingstone, p. 1.

Lee G. R. (1983). The anaemia of chronic disease. *Seminars Haematol.*, **20**, pp. 61–80.

Petz L. D., Garratty G. (1980). *Acquired Immune Haemolytic Anaemias*. New York: Churchill Livingstone.

Schubothe H. (1966). The cold hemagglutinin diseases. *Seminars Haematol.*, **3**, 27.

Streiff R. R. (1970). Folic acid deficiency anaemia. *Seminars Haematol.*, **7**, 23–32.

Swisher S. N. (1976). Immune haemolytic anaemia. *Seminars Haematol.*, **8**, 307.

Wu A., Chanarin L., Levi A. J. (1974). Macrocytosis of chronic alcoholism. *Lancet*, **i**, 829–30.

## Haemoglobinopathies

Baughan A. S. J., Hughes A. S. B., Patterson K. G., Stirling L. (1985). Sickle cell diseases. In *Manual of Haematology*. (Patterson K. G. ed). Edinburgh: Churchill Livingstone. ch 7, pp. 40–7.

Fessas P., Loukopoulos D. (1974). The beta thalassaemias. *Clinics Haematol.*, **3**, 411–35.

MacIver J. E. (1961). The aplastic crisis in sickle cell anaemia. *Lancet*, **i**, 1086–9.

Wasi P., Na-Nakorn S., Pootrakul S. (1974). The alpha thalassaemias. *Clinics Haematol.*, **3**, 383–410.

Weatherall D. J., ed. (1974). Abnormal haemoglobins. *Clinics Haematol.*, **3** (No. 2).

Weatherall D. J., Clegg J. B. (1981). *The Thalassaemia Syndromes*, 3rd edn. Oxford: Blackwell Scientific.

## Leukaemias

Galton D. A. G. (1977). The chronic leukaemias. *Clinics Haematol.*, **6**, 1–245.

Goldman J. M., Lu D. P. (1982). New approaches in chronic granulocytic leukaemia: origin prognosis and treatment. *Seminars Haematol.*, **19**, 241–56.

Goldman J. M., Preisler H. D., eds. (1984). Leukaemias. In *International Medical Reviews: Hematology 1* London: Butterworths.

Steinhertz P. G. (1987). Acute lymphoblastic leukaemia of childhood. *Hematol/Oncol Clinics N. Amer.*, **1**, 549–66.

## Blood transfusion

Heaton A., Miripol J., Aster R., Hartmann P., Dehart D., Rzadl B., Grapka A. W., Davisson W., Buchholz D. (1984). Use of Adsol preservative solution for prolonged storage of low viscosity AS-1 red blood cells. *Br. J. Haematol.*, **57**, 467–78.

Mollison P. L., ed. (1987). *Blood Transfusion in Clinical Medicine*, 8th edn. Oxford: Blackwell Scientific.

## Leucocytosis

Carter R. L. (1969). *Infectious Mononucleosis*. Oxford: Blackwell Scientific.

Hardy W. R., Anderson R. E. (1968). The hypereosinophilic syndromes. *Ann. Intern. Med.*, **68**, 1220–9.

Moller G. (1973). T and B lymphocytes. *Transpl. Rev.*, **16**, 3–10.

Wong-Staal F., Gallo R. C. (1985). Human T-lymphotropic retroviruses. *Nature*, **317**, 395–401.

## Haemostasis

Dacie J. V., Lewis S. M. (1984). Investigation of the haemostatic mechanism. In *Practical Haematology*, 6th edn. Edinburgh: Churchill Livingstone, p. 213.

Dacie J. V., Lewis S. M. (1984). Thrombin time of plasma In *Practical Haematology*, 6th edn. Edinburgh: Churchill Livingstone, p. 218.

Hamilton P. J. (1978). Disseminated intravascular coagulation: A review. *J. Clin. Path.*, **31**, 609–19.

Harker L. A., Slichter S. J. (1972). The bleeding time as a screening test for evaluation of platelet function. *New Engl. J. Med.*, **287**, 155–9.

Karpatkin S. (1980). Auto-immune thrombocytopenic purpura. *Blood*, **56**, 329–43.

## Thrombosis

Coon W. W. (1977). Epidemiology of venous thromboembolism. *Ann. Surg.*, **186**, 149–64.

Griffin J. H., Evatt B., Zimmerman T. S., Kleiss A. J., Wideman C. (1981). Deficiency of protein C in congenital thrombotic disease. *J. Clin. Invest.*, **68**, 1370–3.

Schleider M. A., Nachman R. L., Jaffe E. A., Coleman M. (1976). A clinical study of the lupus anticoagulant. *Blood*, **48**, 499–509.

## Myeloproliferative disorders

Lewis S. M. (1976). Polycythaemia vera. *Br. J. Hosp. Med.*, **16**, 125–32.

Tobelem G. (1989). Essential thrombocythaemia. In *Clinical Haematology* London: Baillière Tindall, pp. 719–28.

# 7

# NEUROLOGY

J. G. Llewelyn

## INTRODUCTION

All too often the prospect of having a neurological case for a clinical examination, or even the patient who presents with a neurological problem in the outpatient clinic or as an acute emergency, sends the doctor into despair. This may stem from the too brief attachment that students and postgraduates have with neurology firms. However, with accurate history taking and a good examination technique, especially when focusing on the site of the abnormality, achieving a differential diagnosis will become easier and requesting the appropriate investigations will not only be more fruitful but also more economical.

The scope for treating neurological disorders is increasing, and advances have been made in the important role of rehabilitating affected patients. Caring for the 'neurological' patient depends not only on doctors and nurses but also on the involvement of physiotherapists, occupational therapists, social workers and clinical psychologists, all combining their talents to provide the maximum benefit for the patient.

## TAKING A HISTORY

### General considerations

Two important points to record are as follows:

(1) *Is the patient right- or left-handed?* This is useful to know because when it comes to examining the patient, apparent mild weakness of incoordination of the dominant arm or leg should be considered as significant whereas similar findings in the non-dominant limb may be irrelevant and only lead to confusion.

Up to 98 per cent of right-handed people will have a dominant left cerebral hemisphere (i.e., the hemisphere containing the important centres for language, calculation, speech and writing). The majority of left-handed people (70 per cent) will also have left hemisphere dominance; the remainder having either right hemisphere dominance (20 per cent) or in a small percentage (10 per cent) the distribution is shared.

It used to be common practice to force left-handed children to write with the other hand. To be certain that you don't fall for this, ask the patient which arm they would use to hold a tennis racquet or which leg is used to kick a ball.

(2) *Occupation.* Is the patient working in an environment where the type of work done or exposure to potentially toxic compounds might contribute to symptoms? For example, acrylamide, lead, thallium and solvents such as *n*-hexane can all cause a neuropathy. The nocturnal pain and para esthesias associated with the carpal tunnel syndrome are aggravated by manual work during the day. The office worker who rests on his or her elbows may present with symptoms of ulnar nerve compression. Stressful or tedious jobs may be the cause of tension headaches, as can anxiety about possible unemployment.

The occupation of the patient will influence the examination of the hands and feet; the manual worker would be expected to have strong intrinsic muscles and a suspicion of weakness may carry more significance than similar findings in an office worker. Similarly, because of harder skin from manual work, distal sensation to pin prick and light touch may be impaired so care should be taken before interpreting such signs as evidence of a neuropathy.

## Past medical history

Events from the patient's past can help you expand the differential diagnosis. A detailed account of conditions that can present with neurological features is beyond the scope of this chapter, but the most common are outlined in Table 7.1.

## Drug history

Alcohol is taken to be socially acceptable but in excess its effect on the nervous system can be permanently disabling. Dependence on barbiturates, tranquillizers, hypnotics and narcotic stimulants can, in intoxicating doses, present as 'blackouts' and behavioural disturbance. Convulsions and tremor are seen as part of a withdrawal response when these drugs are omitted suddenly. Many of these problems are the result of poor prescribing.

Table 7.2 lists the more common neurological presentations where drugs can be implicated.

## Family history

The family history can be revealing because many neurological conditions have a genetic basis.

Specific questioning should determine the following facts.

(1) Whether the patients' parents or indeed the patient and spouse are related to each other—this will be of value in identifying recessively inherited conditions.
(2) Which members of the family, if any, are or were affected by any neurological conditions.

(3) If the patient cannot recall a specific diagnosis made on a relative, recording that person's full name and address can be invaluable if further information is required. Living, affected relatives should, if consent is given, be appropriately investigated to confirm the diagnosis.
(4) Where information about the affected relative is sparse, a reasonable description of the disability may provide the necessary clues. Even a statement like 'my grandfather had very odd feet' may, in the context of a suspected inherited neuropathy, be significant.

Knowing that there is a positive family history of a neuropathy or dementia, for example, should not be a reason for taking short cuts with investigations. In fact, it calls for more detailed assessment of the case, because to have the label 'inherited' implies for the majority of adult neurological conditions, with one or two exceptions, that there is no specific treatment with hope of remission or cure. Also, once a patient knows that he or she has an inherited condition, they will want to know the chances of their children developing the same condition. Genetic counselling should, where possible, be provided for the whole family; after extensive discussion about the prognosis, expectancy and quality of life, and the risks to future offspring, the decision whether or not to have more children, or what to tell the children, has to be made. The final decision lies with the patient and spouse, and the genetic counsellor should support their wishes and mobilize the appropriate help required.

**Table 7.1. Common conditions that have a neurological presentation**

| Past medical history | Neurological presentation |
| --- | --- |
| Birth injury | Epilepsy, mental retardation, hemiplegia with impaired development of limb(s) |
| Head injury | Epilepsy, confused or abnormal behaviour, e.g., subdural haematoma |
| Hypertension and ischaemic heart disease | Transient ischaemic attacks, strokes |
| Diabetes | Loss of vision, transient ischaemic attacks, strokes, neuropathy |
| Carcinoma | Headaches, hemiplegia, ataxis, and spinal cord compression due to metastases. Non-metastatic manifestations include cerebellar ataxia, neuropathy, and muscle weakness (Lambert–Eaton syndrome) |
| Organ failure | Tiredness, confusion, and myoclonic jerks are seen with uraemia. Dialysis dementia (? aluminium toxicity). Headaches and drowsiness related to increased $PaCO_2$ in chronic lung disease Encephalopathy and flapping tremor of liver failure |

**Table 7.2. Neurological presentations in which drugs are implicated**

| Symptoms | Drugs implicated |
|---|---|
| Migraine | Food additives/colourings, caffeine, alcohol, oral contraceptives |
| Stroke | Oral contraceptives |
| Tremor | Caffeine, tricyclic antidepressants, bronchodilators, lithium carbonate, aspirin, thyroxine |
| Parkinsonism | Phenothiazines, butyrophenones |
| Involuntary movements | Phenothiazines, dopamine-containing drugs, oral contraceptives, alcohol |
| Neuropathy | Aminoglycosides (deafness), isoniazid, vincristine, metronidazole, alcohol |
| Muscle weakness | Fatigable: streptomycin, penicillin, penicillamine<br>Non-fatigable: $\beta$-blockers, steroids, diuretics, vincristine, alcohol |
| Seizures | Alcohol, phenothiazines, tricyclic antidepressants, oral contraceptives, respiratory stimulants, antibiotics (penicillins, cephalosporins, nalidixic acid), hypoglycaemic agents |
| Visual loss | Alcohol (usually with tobacco), ethambutol, isoniazid, chlorpropamide, streptomycin, digitalis |
| Confusion | Barbiturates, benzodiazepines, phenothiazines, cannabis, narcotics, steroids, diuretics |
| Cerebellar ataxia, nystagmus | Alcohol, phenytoin, carbamazepine |
| Impotence | Alcohol, cannabis, $\beta$-blockers, methyldopa |

Selected neurological conditions with known inheritance patterns are outlined in Table 7.3.

Equally as important as enquiry into possible inherited conditions is information about the age and health of the spouse and children. Looking after a relative who has had an acute stroke, or has been diagnosed as having a progressive disorder (e.g., motor neurone disease) can be difficult both physically and emotionally.

**Social history**

This aspect of the history taking can be the most 'uncomfortable' for the doctor, as it involves asking questions about the personal details of the patient's lifestyle and family. Tension headaches and various other symptoms can be the manifestation of financial worries, or strained relationships between members of the family.

Alcohol is a potent drug, and when taken in excess may be responsible for varied neurological presentations (see Table 7.2). Smoking results in an increased incidence of tumours, in particular lung tumours; their neurological manifestations are outlined in Table 7.4.

In view of the increasing number of cases of acquired immune deficiency disease (AIDS), and considering that 10 to 15 per cent of those will present with neurological problems (Table 7.5), details of homosexual or bisexual behaviour or intravenous drug abuse are important. Although uncommon, there is evidence that infection with human immunodeficiency virus (HIV) in immunocompetent hosts (i.e., those who have not developed AIDS) can present as an encephalitis, meningitis, myelopathy or neuropathy.

**THE NEUROLOGICAL EXAMINATION**

**Speech**

Trying to work out a speech defect can be difficult but the following points should help.

(1) Language disorders arise after damage to the parasylvian region which includes areas of the parietal, temporal and occipital cortex that lie just posterior to the sylvian fissure of the dominant cortex.

(2) Having established that the patient is not deaf, make sure that he or she is able to understand what they are being told, by giving direct instructions like 'lift up your left arm', 'lift up your right arm', 'close your eyes tightly'.

(3) If the patient cannot understand the verbal commands, test the response to written com-

**Table 7.3. Heritable neurological conditions**

| Neurological problem | Inherited disorders |
|---|---|
| Loss of vision | *Leber's optic atrophy*—painless, acute loss of vision; Male:female=8:1; age 15–25 years; majority are auotosomal dominant; optic atrophy, central scotoma, and some may have signs of cerebellar ataxia and neuropathy<br>*Retinitis pigementosa*—progressive night blindness with peripheral field constriction; retinal pigmentation and may be associated with ataxia, deafness, mental retardation, spasticity, myopathy and neuropathy; autosomal dominant |
| Deafness | *Neurofibromatosis*—café au lait skin lesions (>4 spots of 0.5 cm diam. or greater, or one or more with diam. >1.5 cm), cutaneous neurofibromata, bilateral acoustic neuroma; increased incidence of meningioma optic nerve glioma and phaeochromocytoma; autosomal dominant |
| Cerebellar ataxia | *Late onset cerebellar ataxia*–autosomal dominant<br>*Von Hippel–Lindau disease*—cerebellar haemangioblastoma, retinal angiomatosis, polycystic kidneys and pancreas, hypernephroma; increased incidence of phaeochromocytoma; autosomal dominant<br>*Friedreich's ataxia*—onset later than 20 years, with dysarthria, absent knee and ankle jerks, extensor plantars, posterior column sensory loss; kyphoscoliosis and pes cavus; associated with cardiomyopathy and impaired glucose tolerance or diabetes mellitus; autosomal recessive |
| Neuropathy | *Hereditary motor and sensory neuropathy* (HMSN type 1)—(Charcot–Marie–Tooth disease): onset 10–20 years with weakness and wasting distally in the lower limbs initially, but will later involve the hands as well; pes cavus, clawing of feet and hands; all modalities of sensation are impaired distally; associated with ataxia and tremor; autosomal dominant |
| Spastic paraplegia | *Hereditary spastic paraplegia*—autosomal dominant |
| Basal ganglia disorders | *Huntington's chorea*—onset between 20–30 years, with chorea and dementia. Majority of patients die by middle age; gene defect on chromosome 4; autosomal dominant<br>*Chorea with acanthocytosis*—extrapyramidal movement disorder, generalized muscle weakness, ataxia and epilepsy; mild to moderate mental retardation; fresh blood film shows an excess of acanthocytes; autosomal dominant and recessive forms<br>*Wilson's disease*—hepatolenticular degeneration: a treatable condition that should be considered in any young patient with a basal ganglia disorder or ataxia; impaired mentation or behavioural problem may be presenting features; the younger the age of onset, the more likely it is that liver dysfunction will precede the neurological problem; diagnosis is based on the presence of Kayser–Fleischer rings on the cornea (only found with neurological involvement), low serum caeruloplasmin levels (in 95% with neurological involvement—therefore normal levels do not exclude the diagnosis), excretion of >100 $\mu$g of copper in the urine in 24 h or excess liver copper on biopsy; drug treatment: oral penicillamine; abnormal gene on chromosome 13; autosomal recessive |
| Muscle disorders | *Becker muscular dystrophy*—a 'benign' variety with onset around 11 years and most will be able to walk until the age of 30 years; clinically similar to Duchenne dystrophy with proximal myopathy, pseudohypertrophy of calf muscles; 75% have evidence of myocardial dysfunction; mental retardation is also seen; creatine kinase levels are raised in affected males and carrier females; X-linked<br>*Facioscapuloperoneal dystrophy*—onset between 10–30 years; autosomal dominant<br>*Malignant hyperpyrexia*—hyperpyrexia and progressive rigidity during anaesthesia; muscle biopsy and creatine kinase levels unhelpful; autosomal dominant<br>*McArdle's disease* (glycogenosis type V)—onset varies from childhood to adolescence, with muscle cramps on exertion; there is evidence of muscle wasting and weakness; autosomal recessive; M:F=2:1<br>*Myotonic dystrophy*—late onset with wasting and weakness of the face, sternomastoids and distal limb muscles; characteristically associated with frontal baldness, cataracts, gonadal atrophy, cardiomyopathy, diabetes, peripheral neuropathy and mild mental retardation; serum IgG and IgM may be low, and membrane lipids are abnormal; autosomal dominant.<br>*Myotonia congenita* (Thompsen's disease)—muscle hypertrophy with myotonia; autosomal dominant. |
| Epilepsy | *Tuberous sclerosis*—mental retardation, adenoma sebaceum, retinal phakomatoses, hypernephroma and polycystic kidneys, rhabdomyoma; autosomal dominant. |

**Table 7.4. Neurological manifestations of lung tumours**

*Metastatic*
Cerebral metastases
Spinal cord metastases
Meningitis
Drowsiness, confusion or seizures due to hypercalcaemia from bony metastases

*Non-metastatic*
Cerebellar degeneration
Peripheral neuropathy—sensory and sensorimotor
Myopathy, polymyositis, dermatomyositis
Myasthenic syndrome (Lambert–Eaton syndrome)
Drowsiness, confusion, weakness, convulsions and coma due to hypercalcaemia (increased PTH) or hyponatraemia (inappropriate ADH); a myopathy or frank psychosis may be seen with excess ACTH secretion

mands. In a receptive or Wernicke's dysphasia, the lesion lies posteriorly in the parasylvian region. Speech is fluent but the content is abnormal and the patient will use incorrect words in a sentence and in naming objects such as a watch face, strap and buckle (paraphrasia); if severe, everything the patient says is meaningless (jargon aphasia). There is *no* evidence of hemiparesis in those with a purely receptive dysphasia.

(4) Being able to understand written words implies a pure word deafness or auditory aphasia, and the lesion tends to be in the temporal region, with perhaps an associated upper quadrantonopia.

(5) If the aphasia is mainly visual (i.e., a dyslexia), the lesion will mainly occupy the occipital region.

(6) The ability to repeat words or sentences can be impaired in isolation, with normal comprehension and expression. This points to a dominant parietal lobe problem.

(7) If the patient clearly understands verbal instructions but has difficulty with speaking, this is called an expressive or Broca's dysphasia. Naming and writing or impaired but reading is good. In this case as the lesion is in the dominant anterior parasylvian region, close to the motor cortex, there is an associated hemiparesis and dysarthria.

(8) More extensive lesions affecting both dominant frontal and temporal lobes produces a global aphasia (receptive and expressive) with hemiparesis or hemiplegia, hemisensory loss and a visual field defect.

## Cranial nerves

### Smell

Testing the sense of smell is only of value in those who have a history of skull fracture or symptoms of impaired taste. It is important to realise that smell is distorted by all nasal disorders and by cigarette smoke.

### Sight and the visual field

'*Can you read the words on this page?*'
This is adequate to check visual acuity if there is no history of altered vision, in which case accurate recording with a Snellen chart is required.
'*Look at my nose and point to the finger that moves.*'
Stand facing the patient an arms' length away, and with arms extended sideways and lying just above the horizontal plane of vision, move one finger then the other and finally both simultaneously. The movements are then repeated with the arms below the horizontal plane. This will detect any major field defect. If the patient fails to see one of the simultaneous stimuli but clearly sees both when done individually, this is sensory (visual) inattention and usually indicates a lesion of the right parietal or parieto-occipital lobe.

For more detailed assessment, each visual field should be checked separately as follows.

(1) Make sure that the patient is comfortable, and that you are positioned so that your heads are at approximately similar levels.

(2) The patient covers his or her left eye with the left hand and you close your right eye.

(3) With your index finger held out in the lower quadrant of your visual field and equidistant from the patient's eye and your eye, instruct the patient: '*Look into my eye all the time and say "now" when you see my finger moving.*'
Test all quadrants starting at the periphery of your own field.

(4) With the patient's left eye still covered, bring a white pin from the periphery towards the middle in a straight line and locate the patient's normal blind spot or abnormal scotoma.

Check the size of both pupils, and using a bright pen-torch light note the direct and consensual

**Table 7.5. Neurological problems associated with HIV-1 infection**

*Encephalitis*
This is usually due to the direct effect of HIV on brain tissue, and over 30% of AIDS patients will develop a subacute encephalitis; initial clinical features include forgetfulness and difficulty in maintaining concentration, but can progress to a frank dementia; physical examination may reveal a gait ataxia with some weakness in the lower limbs and generalized hyper-reflexia
CT head scan—cortical atrophy with dilated ventricles
EEG—slow-wave activity over both hemispheres
CSF analysis—moderate lympocytosis, raised protein and low glucose
Serum and CSF should be analysed for cytomegalovirus, herpes simplex and zoster titres as these viruses can also cause an encephalitis

*Meningitis*
The fungus *Cryptococcus neoformans* is the commonest cause of meningitis in patients with AIDS; although the usual presentation is an acute or subacute illness, it may manifest itself as chronic headaches with general malaise over months or years; characteristic findings is papilloedema due to direct involvement of the optic nerve head, but with a normal CT head scan. In the more chronic cases, hydrocephalus may be found
CSF usually shows a lymphocytosis with raised protein and low glucose levels, although analysis can be normal
*Cryptococcus* can be stained and cultured from the CSF, and cryptococcal antigen detected in both serum and CSF
Treatment: intravenous amphotericin and oral 5-fluorocytosine.

*Space-occupying lesions*
Abscess—CNS infection with *Toxoplasma* is a diagnostic feature of AIDS, and it may present as an encephalopathy or meningoencephalitis moving the light from one eye to another; it also manifests itself as mild focal deficits due to single or multiple mass lesions that show contrast enhancement on head CT
Toxoplasmosis is treated with pyrimethamine with folinic acid for marrow protection
Tuberculosis and candidal infection are also seen and may have similar CT findings
Tumours—mainly cerebral lymphomas, seen in patients with AIDS

*Myelopathy*
Believed to be as a direct effect of HIV on spinal cord; affected patients have a spastic paraparesis with ataxia

*Neuropathy*
Probably due to HIV infiltration of peripheral nerves, the commonest type is a distal symmetric sensorimotor neuropathy, which is often painful. Other varieties include acute and chronic demyelinating neuropathies and mononeuritis multiplex

*Others*
Retinitis due to cytomegalovirus presenting as visual failure
Progressive multifocal leucoencephalopathy—progressive signs of limb weakness, aphasia or visual field defect
cerebrovascular accident due haemorrhage, infarction or vasculitis

responses. Moving the light from one eye to another, the pupil should stay constricted. If it dilates it implies an afferent pupillary defect on that side (Marcus Gunn pupil).

Pupillary constriction to accommodation depends on the patient being able to focus correctly, and should be tested with their glasses on if they wear them normally.

When examining the fundi, darken the room and first check the red reflex by looking at the eye with the ophthalmoscope from 2 to 3 ft (60–90 cm). Use the right eye to look through the ophthalmoscope at the patient's right eye from the right side of the bed. Likewise, from the left side

of the bed use your left eye. Follow a vessel onto the optic disc. Note the character of the arteries and veins and the pulsation seen in the latter. The disc margins should be distinct, with a pale pink colour. Scan all quadrants of the retinal field.

### Eye movements

'*Look at my finger and follow it with your eyes keeping your head still. Tell me if you see double at any time.*'

Before starting, look for ptosis. Steady the patient's head with your left hand gently placed on the chin, and keeping the guiding finger about 2 ft

(60 cm) away, move it slowly and laterally to the right and left, then up and down.

Look for: impaired movement in any direction; loss of smooth voluntary eye movement; nystagmus.

### Orofacial reflexes, sensation and musculature, including hearing

'*Bite your teeth together.*'

Feel for masseter and temporalis bulk.

'*Push your jaw to the side against my hand.*'

Check for lateral pterygoid strength.

'*Can you feel me touch your face? Does it feel the same on both sides?*'

Use a cotton-wool ball with a light dabbing action, pin prick and temperature in the areas of the three divisions of the Vth nerve. From Fig. 7.1 it can be seen that, in facial sensory loss of trigeminal nerve origin, the angle of the jaw is spared, and that almost the anterior two-thirds of the scalp is involved.

The corneal reflex is tested with a teased wisp of cotton wool placed on the lower lateral aspect of the cornea. To increase the target area, ask the patient to adduct the eye being tested.

As the afferent arc of the reflex is carried in the ophthalmic division and the blink response (orbicularis occuli) by the VIIth nerve, the corneal reflex tests both nerves. The blink response occurs on both sides simultaneously.

'*Lift your eyebrows up.*'

'*Shut your eyes tightly and stop me from opening them.*'

'*Show me your teeth.*'

'*Blow out your cheeks.*'

Look for the symmetry of movement. If you think that one side of the face is weak, ask the patient to blink repetitively and observe the corner of the mouth—in a resolving facial weakness of lower motor neurone origin there may be simultaneous movement of one side of the mouth with each blink. This is the result of aberrant reinnervation and is called synkinesis.

'*Where do you hear the vibration loudest? In front or behind the ear?*'

Use a 512 Hz tuning fork struck on the knee. If Rinne's test is positive (i.e., abnormal) and as bone conduction is greater than through air, look for wax in the auditory canal and check the tympanic membrane before requesting fuller audiometric tests.

'*Open your mouth and say "Ah".*'

Observe palatal movement.

'*Turn your head to the right/left and push against my hand.*'

Palpate the bulk of the sternomastoids.

Observe the tongue as it lies in the floor of the mouth.

'*Show me your tongue and move it from side to side.*'

'*Push your tongue into your right/left cheek and stop me from pushing it in.*'

### Upper and lower limbs

For all parts of the clinical examination, making sure that the patient is as comfortable and as relaxed as possible is important, as a tense patient during a neurological examination makes assessment difficult. It is time worth spending to reassure the patient at the beginning.

Before examining the arms and legs, ask if there is any discomfort or pain in any limb. It will do your confidence no good if during a clinical exam

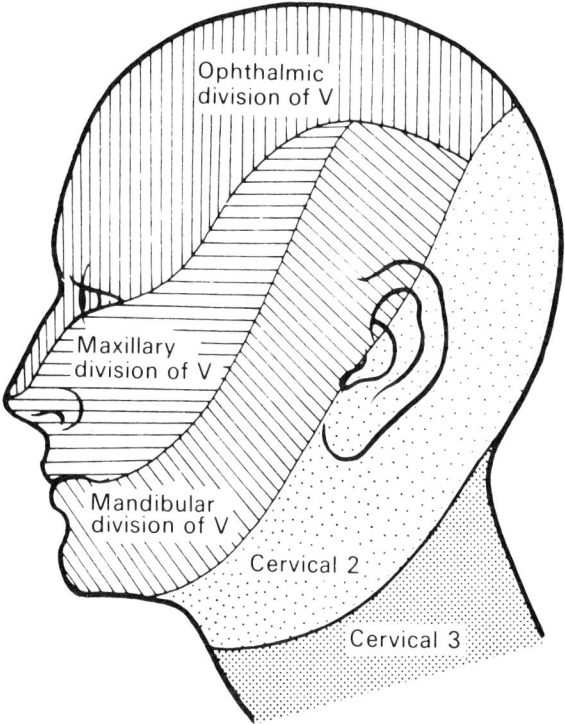

*Figure 7.1. Sensory supply of the head and neck*

you pick up the patient's hand only to hear a wince or scream as the patient tells you that he or she sprained the wrist a few days before! Even worse is that the patient may lose confidence in you, and then the cooperation that is essential between doctor and patient will be lost. If an arm or leg is painful, you can explain (without frightening the patient!) that some of the manoeuvres may make the discomfort worse but that you will be as gentle as possible.

'*Put your hands out straight in front of you (palm upwards), and close your eyes.*'

Look for drifting of one arm: if the arm moves slowly and directly downwards, this is due to an upper motor neurone weakness; if there is slow movement of the fingers (pseudoathetosis), or the hand pronates, this suggests a sensory problem.

With the patient's arms stretched out and palms downwards, say '*Close your eyes. I am going to tap the back of one hand, but try and stop me from pushing it down.*'

With a force strong enough to displace the arm, when the pressure is released suddenly, it normally returns to its original position. In a patient with cerebellar dysfunction there will be rebound and the arm will oscillate upwards and downwards.

### Muscle tone

Grip the patient's hands and pronate and supinate the forearms, and by holding the patient's fingers flex and extend the wrist. If tone is increased, with a 'spastic catch', this may only be felt with the initial movement and may disappear on repetition. The same is true for cogwheel rigidity, but this can be reinforced by asking the patient to move the other arm up and down whilst the tone is being assessed. Cogwheel rigidity is also felt on flexion and extension of the head. In the lower limbs, tone should be assessed by placing your hands on the patient's leg and gently rolling it inwards and outwards when the tone is normal, this is an effortless movement. Then, with your hands on either side under the popliteal fossa, 'flick' the knee briskly upwards. If the patient is tense, lying him or her flat may help. With increased tone (spasticity) the heel will lift off the bed with a kicking sensation.

Clonus at the ankle is tested by putting the leg in a position with the knee flexed to 90°, then briskly dorsiflexing the foot and maintaining the pressure.

### Muscle strength

Examination of muscle strength is done in a systematic manner. The pattern outlined below will cover most of the muscle groups and some of the important individual muscles. There are very few neurological conditions that produce true generalized weakness, the majority being distinctly selective. It is recognizing and focusing attention on this pattern of weakness that enables you to site the lesion.

Again, giving clear, simple instructions is essential; where possible the position of the limb(s) should be demonstrated to the patient. Avoid using 'medical' terminology—most patients will not understand commands like 'abduct your shoulder' or 'flex your elbow'!

Make allowances when testing an elderly patient; or the non-dominant limb; or where pain limits movement. If you are uncertain whether the patient is trying their best or indeed feigning weakness, it is helpful to palpate the muscle being examined and also its antagonist. Look and feel for wasted or hypertrophied muscles, and also for muscle tenderness.

For both recording in clinical notes and in clinical exams, muscle power should be graded according to the MRC scale (Table 7.6). The systemic tests of muscle strength are shown in Table 7.7.

**Table 7.6 Grading of muscle power**

| | |
|---|---|
| 0 | No contraction |
| 1 | Flicker of contraction only |
| 2 | Contraction of muscle, but no movement against gravity |
| 3 | Movement against gravity but not against resistance |
| 4 | Movement against gravity and resistance |
| 5 | Normal power |

Grade 4 can be divided according to degree of weakness against resistance into severe, moderate and mild recorded as 4−, 4 and 4+ respectively.

### Reflexes

Tendon reflexes are useful in localizing the site of focal damage within the nervous system. Because the reflex arc (muscle spindle–peripheral nerve–sensory root–motor root–peripheral nerve) is inhibited by descending pathways like the corti-

**Table 7.7. Systemic testing for muscle strength**

| Instruction to patient | Muscle tested | Nerve supply |
|---|---|---|
| 'Bend your elbows and push your arms sideways. Stop me from pushing down.' | Deltoid | C5 Axillary |
| 'Tuck your elbows into your side, keep your forearm out straight. Stop me pushing your hand in.' | Infraspinatus | C5,6 Suprascapular |
| 'Bend your elbow (to 90°). Pull in against me.' | | |
|    *Arm supinated* | Biceps | C5,6 Musculocutaneous |
|    *Arm pronated* | Brachioradialis | C6 Radial |
| 'Bend you elbow. Straighten out against me.' | Triceps | C7 Radial |
| *Note that it is best to rest the elbow on the bed, supporting it with your hand across the antecubital fossa* | | |
| 'Make a fist and pull your wrist up.' | | |
|    *And in* | Ext. carpi Radialis long. | C6 Radial |
|    *And out* | Ext. carpi Ulnaris | C7 Post. interosseous |
| 'Stop me from pushing against you.' | | |
| 'Bend your fist down. Stop me from pushing it up.' | Flex. carpi Radialis | C6,7 Median |
| 'Fingers straight (palm downwards). Push up against me.' (use the side of your hand) | Ext. digitorum | C7 Radial |
| 'Curl your fingers into your palm. Stop me from prising them open.' | Flex. digitorum superficialis | C8 Median |
| | Flex. digitorum profundus | C8 Ant. interosseous and ulnar |
| 'Spread your fingers out.' (palm down) 'Stop me from pushing them together.' | Interossei | T1 Ulnar |
| 'Lift your thumb up straight.' (palm up) 'Stop me from pushing it down.' | Abductor Pollicis brevis | T1 Median |
| 'Pull your knee up towards your face. Stop me from pushing down.' | Iliopsoas | L1,2 Spinal root and femoral |
| 'Bend your knee.' (to 90°) 'Straighten your leg against me.' | Quadriceps | L3,4 Femoral |
| 'Keep your knee bent and pull your heel against me, towards your bottom.' | Hamstrings | L5; S1 Sciatic |
| 'Keep both legs together. Stop me from pushing them apart.' | Adductors | L3,4 Obturator |
| 'Push your legs out sideways. Stop me from pushing them together.' | Gluteus med. and min. | L4, 5 Superior gluteal |
| 'Keep your legs straight and push your heel into the bed. Stop me from lifting it up.' | Gluteus max. | LS; S1 Inferior gluteal |
| 'Pull your foot up towards your face. Stop me from pulling it down.' (*Dorsiflexion*) | Tibalis anterior | L4,5 Common peroneal |
| 'Push your foot down. Stop me from pushing it up.' (*Plantarflexion*) | Gastrocnemius | S1,2 Tibial |
| 'Keep your heels together and push your feet out sideways against me.' | Peronei | L5; S1 Common peroneal |
| 'Keep your feet together. Stop me from pulling them apart.' | Tibialis posterior | L4,5 Tibial |
| 'Pull your toes up against me.' | Ext. digitorum brevis | LS; S1 Common peroneal |
| 'Pull up your big toe against me.' | Ext. hallucis longus | L5 Common peroneal |
| 'Curl your toes down against my fingers.' | Flex. digitorum longus and Flex. hallucis longus | S1,2 Tibial |

cospinal tracts, any damage to these, either in the cortex, brainstem or spinal cord, will result in brisk reflexes (upper motor neurone lesions). On the other hand, injury to any part of the lower motor neurone system (anterior horn cell, motor and sensory roots and peripheral nerve) will impair or abolish the reflex.

Table 7.8 lists the relevant tendon and superficial reflexes. When eliciting a reflex the limb has to be positioned in a way that the muscle is slightly under tension. The reflex hammer should be freely swung in an arc and once the tendon is struck firmly, the hammer is lifted up as part of one continuous movement.

For the upper limb reflexes the arm should be flexed to 90° at the elbow and rested on the patient's abdomen.

For the *supinator reflex*, strike your index and middle fingers placed on the tendon.

The *biceps* tendon can be placed under slight tension by pressing on it with your thumb, which is then struck with the reflex hammer.

The *triceps* tendon is short and should be struck just above the olecranon process. Otherwise you will hit the muscle directly and produce a contraction that is mistaken for a reflex response.

The *knees* should be supported by the examiner's forearm at an angle of 120°, and the tendon struck firmly.

The *ankle reflex* causes most problems—mainly due to poor positioning of the leg. With the leg abducted and externally rotated, keep the knee and ankle at 90° and apply some pressure to dorsiflex the foot with your non-dominant hand whilst striking the Achille's tendon. If you find that the blow with the reflex hammer is shared between the tendon and the sheet on the bed(!)—it may be helpful if the foot is placed on the lower half of the other shin, giving you unrestricted access to the tendon.

**Table 7.8. Tendon and cutaneous reflexes**

|  | Root | Nerve |
|---|---|---|
| Biceps tendon | C5,6 | Musculocutaneous |
| Triceps | C7 | Radial |
| Supinator (radial) | C5,6 | Radial |
| Finger flexion | C8 | Median, ulnar |
| Knee | L3,4 | Femoral |
| Ankle | S1 | Tibial/sciatic |
| Jaw jerk |  | Trigeminal nerve |

(In a C5,6 lesion, reflexes at this level will be absent or diminished whereas those below [triceps] will be exaggerated; sometimes tapping the biceps tendon will result in triceps contraction [inverted biceps reflex]; finger flexion is seen in states where muscle tone is increased)

*Cutaneous*
| Abdominal |  |
|---|---|
| upper | T7,8,9 |
| lower | T10,11,12 |
| Cremasteric | L1 |
| Anal | S4,5 |
| Plantar | S1 |

(The abdominal reflex should be elicited by stroking each quadrant with a sharp object towards the umbilicus; their loss indicates a corticospinal lesion, and may be the only clinical sign of an upper motor neurone problem; they will not be elicited in the obese, multiparous, or after abdominal surgery)

(A light scratch upwards along the inside of the upper thigh normally produces contraction of the cremaster muscle and elevation of the testicle; its absence indicates a corticospinal tract lesion)

(Contraction of the external anal sphincter following a scratch with a pin of the perianal skin is the anal reflex; it should be performed on all patients with a history of sphincter dysfunction)

(An extensor response in the plantar reflex points to an upper motor neurone lesion, but no response at all may also suggest a similar problem but of a lesser degree)

**Table 7.9. Primitive reflexes**

---

*Pout*: elicited by tapping the lips when lightly closed, with a patella hammer—a positive response consists of protrusion and pouting of the lips; its presence indicates widespread cortical degeneration or a large, frontal lobe, space-occupying lesion

*Grasp*: may be demonstrated by stroking the palm of the patient's hand, and if positive the patient will grip your fingers—sometimes so tightly that you can pull them up from a lying position; if the response is unilateral, it indicates a significant lesion in the opposite frontal lobe

*Palmo-mental*: seen in frontal lobe lesions when there will be a twitching movement of the corner of the mouth on firmly stroking the palm of the hand with a blunt object; as with the grasp reflex, it is of little localizing value when the response is bilateral

---

Remember that you should feel and see the muscle contracting in response to hitting the tendon. If this is not successful, ask the patient to kneel on a chair with his or her legs over the edge and then strike the tendon.

Before you decide that a reflex is absent, a reinforcement manoeuvre is needed—by asking the patient to clench the opposite fist for upper limb reflexes, and by pulling against the flexed fingers (Jendrassik's manoeuvre) for lower limb reflexes.

Eliciting the *plantar response* is an uncomfortable sensation for most patients and you must give an appropriate warning and explanation of what is about to happen. Failure to do this results in a rapid withdrawal that is often misinterpreted as an extensor response. The receptor nerve endings stimulated to produce the plantar response lie in the skin of the S1 dermatome. An 'orange stick' is by far the best implement to use, and it should be drawn along the outer border of the sole and across the ball of the foot towards the base of the great toe. If the patient finds this intolerable, drawing the stick along the outer border of the foot may be better (Chaddock's sign)—but again stimulating within the S1 dermatome. Normally there is flexion of the toes. The extensor response or Babinski's sign has two components—extension of the great toe and fanning of the other toes.

The other *cutaneous reflexes* have been outlined in Table 7.8.

The *jaw jerk* is often forgotten, but is important when you are faced with a patient who has generally brisk reflexes and you have to decide whether the lesion is in the upper cervical cord or the result of bilateral lesions of the cerebral hemispheres. In the latter, the jaw jerk will be brisk, but it will be normal if the problem was in the spinal cord. With the patient's jaw loosely opened, rest your index or middle finger across the jaw and strike it with a downward blow of the reflex hammer.

The *primitive reflexes* (see Table 7.9) are found in patients with lesions of the frontal lobe, when there will be associated behavioural changes and inappropriate emotional responses; also with widespread cortical atrophy when there may be evidence of a dementing process with parkinsonism. Those with cortical atrophy and parkinsonism will also have a positive glabellar response elicited by tapping the middle of the patient's forehead with your finger. This causes a blink reflex in the normal individual, which after the first few taps will stop, whereas it is repetitive in the parkinsonian patient.

## Coordination and fine finger movement

Here we are primarily looking at the functioning of the cerebellum and its connections. These tests will also be impaired by severe loss of sensory ability and joint position sense, but in these cases the performance will be significantly worse when the patient's eyes are closed. Clear instructions, combined with a demonstration, are again essential.

'*With your finger (index), touch my finger and then your nose, and continue backwards and forewards.*' (The patient must be made to stretch his or her arm in order to reach your finger.) This manoeuvre should be performed slowly as rapid movement may disguise an ataxia.

'*Hold out your hands (palm forwards) and turn them quickly from side to side.*'

'*Quickly tap the back of your hand with the fingers of the other hand.*'

'*Put your heel on your knee and slide it down your shin.*'

'*Tap your foot quickly against the palm of my hand.*'

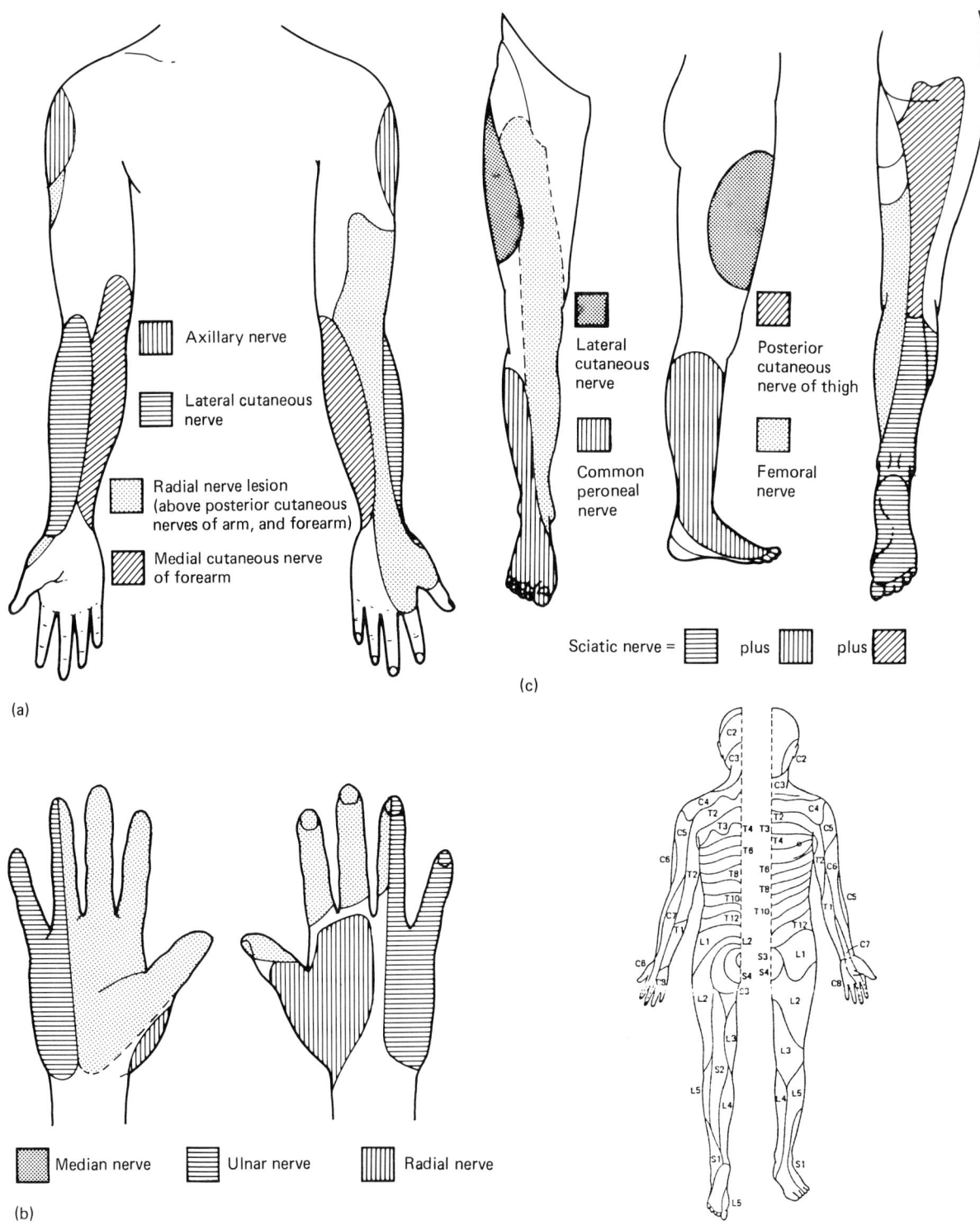

(a)

(b)

*Figure 7.2* Sensory (approximate) in peripheral nerve lesions

(c)

*Figure 7.3* Approximate distribution of segmental dermatomes

Incoordination on one side suggests a lesion of the ipsilateral cerebellar hemisphere. Some patients will have severe truncal ataxia, being unable to sit up from a lying position and having difficulty in walking, with only minimal limb ataxia. In these cases the lesion is in the midline of the cerebellum (vermis) and characteristically there will be an associated dysarthria but no localizing nystagmus as in lesions affecting a cerebellar hemisphere or its connections.

Nystagmus is another sign of cerebellar dysfunction and is discussed later.

## Joint position and vibration sensation

These two test the function of large, myelinated fibres and the posterior columns.

Taking the patient's third or fourth finger, support the distal interphalangeal joint between your finger and thumb and, by similarily holding the tip of the finger, demonstrate clearly to the patient which movement of the joint is up and which is down. The third or fourth digits are chosen for this test because, in the cortical representation of the hand, the thumb, index and fifth digit occupy the largest area reflecting their sensory supply. Abnormality of joint position sense will have to be greatly impaired to be detected in these digits. With smaller cortical representation, the third and fourth digits will give a more sensitive assessment.

*'Close your eyes and tell me which way I move your fingertip, up or down?'* (If the patient appears tired or drowsy, they will fall asleep if their eyes are closed! Therefore allow them to keep their eyes open and shield the movements of the joint with your other hand.)

The joint should be moved through an arc of 2 to 3° only, for accurate testing. The same is done at the third or fourth toes, but here a greater arc of movement (5–10°) is allowed.

If mistakes are made, a more proximal joint can be tried until the responses are correct. Occasionally a patient may give you random replies and as he or she has a 50/50 chance of getting a correct response it is difficult to know whether there is impairment of joint position sense or not. To counteract this, give the patient three choices, 'up', 'down' or 'in the middle'.

Place a 128 Hz tuning fork, struck against your elbow or knee, first on the patient's sternum to confirm that he or she feels the vibrating sensation, then just proximal to the nail of any finger in the hand and the great toe.

*'Do you feel the vibration and does it feel the same on the left and right sides?'*

*'Let me know as soon as the vibration sensation stops.'*

Where there is impaired sensation, the vibrating tuning fork is applied to progressively more proximal sites (styloid process, forearm, olecranon process in the arm and the medial malleolus, mid shin, patella and iliac spine in the leg), until the sensation is normal.

## Light touch, pin prick and temperature sensation

This part of the examination should be reserved for the end of the assessment of the patient on the bed, as it can be both difficult and time consuming. This is especially true for clinical exams where time is important. Having completed the examination as outlined above, you should have a good idea about the diagnosis and the possible areas where sensory loss might be expected. For example, in the patient with a spastic paraparesis you may encounter loss of sensation below a 'level' on the chest or abdomen. Distal weakness, suggesting a lower motor neurone lesion, will probably be associated with sensory loss in a 'glove and stocking' distribution or confined to the territory of a peripheral nerve or nerve root territory (see Figures 7.2 and 7.3). The sensory examination can then be concentrated on these particular regions by starting in the abnormal area and working towards normal.

Use a ball of cotton wool with a soft dabbing action—not stroked across the skin; a disposable pin should be used—hypodermic needles are too sharp and can easily draw blood.

If there are no metal tubes available, the tuning fork can serve as a relatively cold stimulus.

If, for example, sensory loss is confined to the limbs, start by giving a test stimulus on the face to be certain that it is recognized by the patient and then proceed to the limbs. The aim is to compare abnormal area and limb with normal area and limb.

*'Does the cotton wool/pin feel normal?'*

*'Let me know as soon as it becomes normal.'*

*'Does it feel the same on both sides?'*

## Finally

Ask the patient to stand by the bed.

'*Put your feet together. Close your eyes?*' (Romberg's test.)

The aim of this test is to examine the patient's ability to stand upright when deprived of visual clues, so that he or she has to rely solely on proprioception to maintain position. Those who perform worst are those with impaired joint position sense and in these cases Romberg's test should not be done as there is a high risk of these patients falling over and injuring themselves. Those with cerebellar disorder will sway more when their eyes are closed but will not fall.

'*Stand on your tiptoes.*

*Balance yourself on your heels, lifting your toes off the ground.*' (A more accurate test of plantar flexion and dorsiflexion, respectively.)

If there was a suspicion of proximal weakness from the examination on the bed, ask the patient to squat low and then lift himself or herself upright without help. Where there is difficulty with squatting, get the patient to stand up from a seated position in a low chair, without using the upper limbs.

'*Walk normally to the door.*'

Look for:

Walking with a *broad base* (cerebellar).
*Spastic gait*—because of inability to flex the leg at the hip, the patient swings the leg outwards. With an associated hemiplegia, the arm is held flexed at the elbow, wrist and fingers.
*Waddling gait* due to proximal myopathy.
*High steppage* with slapping of the foot onto the ground is due to a sensory ataxia.
*Foot drop*—with characteristic slapping of the foot.
Decreased *arm swing* and flexed posture of parkinsonism.
*Hysterical gait* is completely unpredictable, and the patient often demonstrates great feats of balancing.

'*Walk back towards the bed by putting one heel close in front of the other toe.*'

Heel-toe (tandem) walking enhances a gait ataxia.

### Bedside testing of higher mental function

From the patient's responses to questions when taking a history and during the clinical examination you will have some idea of whether he or she is performing at an adequate or impaired intellectual level, based on what you assess should be normal for that patient. Further information is obtained by checking:

### 1. Orientation

- *Do you know where you are at the moment?*
- *What sort of building is this?*
- *What day of the week is it?*
- *Which month are we in?*
- *Which year is it?*

### 2. Memory

I want you to repeat after me, the following name and address, and I will check later to see if you remember it. *Give the patient a fictitious name and address, and if it can be repeated without mistakes, carry on with other tests, and after two, five and fifteen minutes check the accuracy of recall. Another method is to give the patient five or seven numbers to remember after various time intervals.*

*The Babcock sentence is somewhat more difficult.* 'The one thing a nation must have to be rich and great and that is a large, secure supply of wood.'

*If the patient makes mistakes in repeating the sentence after you, following two or three attempts, there is no point in going on any further to test recall.*

### 3. Intellect

- *Who is the Prime Minister?*
- *Who is leader of the Opposition?*
- *Tell me what has been in the news recently?*
- *Take 7 away from 100, and continue to subtract 7 away from what is left*

The accuracy and speed are recorded – one or two mistakes are allowed if the test is performed in under 60 s.

These are by their nature relatively crude tests, but often provide the first evidence of impaired higher mental function. Formal neuropsychological assessment by a clinical psychologist will detail the nature and site of cortical dysfunction.

## COMMON SYMPTOMS IN NEUROLOGY

### Headache and facial pain

Headache is one of the commonest symptoms in neurology. Despite its predominantly benign nature, headache may be the presenting feature of serious conditions such as cerebral tumour, meningitis, giant cell arteritis and glaucoma. More often than not, the examination will be normal, and therefore a detailed history is critical to enable one to distinguish between a benign and a possibly life-threatening condition.

### History

Are the headaches recent, acute events, or are they a longstanding problem? In a young person with acute onset of episodic headache with no systemic features or loss of consciousness, the most likely diagnosis is a migraine attack. In the elderly with an acute or subacute history, structural causes are more frequently encountered, and cranial arteritis is an important diagnosis to make as it is a treatable condition. Not all patients have tender temporal arteries and the diagnosis is made on the basis of a raised ESR (>80 mm/h) and positive findings in a biopsy of a temporal artery. If there is any delay before the biopsy, treatment with high-dose prednisolone (60–80 mg/day) should be started regardless and the dose titrated according to the ESR.

Headache that has been present for a few weeks only but is getting worse is suspicious of an underlying, space-occupying lesion. It is typically dull and present on awakening. It may be exacerbated by sudden change in position, or by increasing intracranial pressure through coughing, sneezing and straining.

More often than not, the symptoms have been present for a few months or longer. The pain of a migraine headache often begins as a dull ache, intensifying to a throbbing and incapacitating discomfort. A throbbing quality is common to vascular headaches of both migrainous and non-migrainous types, as seen in postfebrile illness and hangover states. Migraine often starts with a unilateral distribution, but may be bilateral or even alternate between sides during an attack. The throbbing is often aggravated by stooping, and may be accompanied by nausea, vomiting and varied visual symptoms. It can occur daily but may be sporadic, lasting from a few hours to one or two days.

The so-called common migraine headache, present in 80 per cent of all migraine sufferers, is not preceded by an aura, though the patient may feel drowsy, tired and irritable for a few days before an attack. Classical migraine does have a well-defined aura, thought to be due to defects in cerebral perfusion. The commonest aura is visual, with fortification spectra and transient sensations of bright, shimmering colours. Zig-zag lines 'marching' across the visual field are characteristic. It should be remembered that any of these abnormalities may be present before, during or after the headache, or indeed in the absence of headache.

To distinguish migraine from tension or muscle spasm headaches and cluster headaches (periodic migrainous neuralgia) the following points should be considered.

(1) Emotional factors are frequently present in those with tension headaches; they tend to be stressed and anxious. Depression is a common feature. Cervical osteoarthritis, dental malocclusion or temporomandibular joint dysfunction can all produce a 'tension' type headache.

(2) The tension headache is described as dull, tight, heavy or squeezing. It is persistent, with periods of severe discomfort and often occurs daily but can persist for weeks, months or even years.

(3) In contrast to migraine, where alcohol aggravates the symptoms, tension headaches may be relieved by alcohol.

(4) Tension headaches tend to occur late in the day and increase in intensity as the day progresses. Migraine does not usually awaken the patient from sleep, and this is in contrast to cluster headaches (a vascular headache), where this phenomenon is more common. With cluster headaches the pain is described as deep or stabbing and is often excruciating, sometimes associated with lacrimation, nasal discharge and facial flushing, usually on the same side as the headache. Patients may notice that one eye appears red, due to dilatation of conjunctival vessels; ptosis and pupillary constriction may also be noted. Cluster headaches are usually episodic, lasting 15 to 90 min and recurring over a period of weeks to months. They are localized mainly behind the eye and nearly always recur on the same side.

(5) A family history of headaches is suggestive of migraine, and if both parents are affected the offspring have a 70 per cent chance of also having migraine. In susceptible people, cluster headaches may be precipitated by vasodil-

ators, including alcohol. Migraine is aggravated by physical and emotional stress as are tension headaches, but also by hormonal changes (contraceptive pill, pregnancy or menopause) and ingestion of foods rich in vasoactive amines (cheese and chocolate containing tyramine and phenylethylamine, respectively).

### Examination

A full general and neurological examination should be performed in all cases. This is a good way to demonstrate to the patient that you take the symptoms seriously. The blood pressure should be recorded. Palpate the back of the neck for evidence of muscle spasm. Auscultate over the site of the headache for a bruit (e.g., arteriovenous malformation). Examine the fundi carefully.

### Investigation of patients with headache

In patients with a typical history of chronic, recurring vascular or tension headaches, extensive investigations are unnecessary. However, if the patient has had only a few episodes, or all the headaches are on one side (which may indicate intracranial arteriovenous malformation), or if the patient has features of transient neurological deficits in the history or any abnormality on examination, then a CT head scan with contrast enhancement are mandatory, together with routine haematological tests, ESR, and serum biochemical investigations.

### Treatment

With vascular or tension headaches, an explanation by a sympathetic doctor of the origin of the symptoms, with firm reassurance, will usually result in a decrease in frequency of the headaches. Precipitating factors should be identified and eliminated when possible. This may involve an elimination diet in order to identify the offending food. As anxiety and stress are often associated with vascular and tension headaches, measures to help the patient relax need important consideration. This may be difficult to implement in certain patients, but if possible, yoga or some form of physical training may be beneficial.

Simple analgesics, such as paracetamol, usually suffice in *tension headaches*. There may be a need for anxiolytics, antidepressants and even formal psychotherapy in individual cases. Treatment may not always be successful and it is therefore worth spending some time discussing the problems with the patient and allowing them to make some modifications to their lifestyle in order to try and treat themselves.

For *migraine*, the frequency of the attacks determines the treatment of choice. If attacks are widely spaced, individual events can be treated with a mild analgesics (aspirin or paracetamol) and an anti-emetic. More severe episodes require an ergotamine preparation at the onset of the prodrome, the dose being repeated after 30 min for maximum benefit. For those with recurrent episodes, despite avoidance of precipitating factors and making dietary changes, prophylactic treatment should be started—feverfew (a herb), taken daily is effective and free of side-effects; pizotifen (a serotonin antagonist) beginning with 0.5 mg daily and increasing the dose in stepwise manner to 0.5 mg, three times a day, or 1.5 mg at night. With some patients it may be necessary to go up to 3 mg/day. Propranolol, tricyclic antidepressants and also nifedipine have also been suggested.

For *cluster headaches*, treatment of individual episodes with ergotamine (1–2 mg), either orally or rectally, should be tried in the first instance. With more difficult cases, propranolol or amitriptyline may be of value, or even prednisolone or lithium if very severe.

### Other causes of headache

Occasionally one is still uncertain at the end of the consultation as to the nature of the headache and it is worth then recalling some other causes of headache and facial pain.

*Trigeminal neuralgia* (tic douloureux) is characterized by brief, excruciating attacks of pain, mainly in the distribution of the second and third divisions of the Vth nerve, occurring in about 10 per cent of cases in the ophthalmic territory. The patient is usually aged 50 years or more and is more likely to be female than male. The condition is only rarely bilateral. The clues to the diagnosis come from asking about 'triggers' such as exposure to cold air, washing, shaving, eating and even talking or swallowing. Examination in the majority reveals no abnormality, although trigeminal neuralgia may be the presenting symptom of multiple sclerosis or acoustic neuroma.

The pain from a *Vth nerve tumour* is more

persistent, with associated facial numbness, impaired corneal reflex and weakness of the masseter and pterygoid muscles. In those with trigeminal neuralgia, it is rare to obtain spontaneous relief that is permanent, and the most effective treatment is with carbamazepine (up to 1.5 g/day). For non-responders, clonazepam may be tried. Where medical therapy fails, alcohol injection into the nerve can be tried. Decompressive microsurgery has been reported to be successful, based on a theory that the neuralgia is caused by vascular compression of the trigeminal nerve root. An alternative that can be of value, especially in the elderly, is transcutaneous nerve stimulation. One should be aware that facial pains may be referred from the eyes, middle ear, sinuses, teeth, temperomandibular joint and from the myocardium.

## Dizziness and episodic loss of consciousness

### Vertigo

Dizziness is a nonspecific term and the doctor's priority is to distinguish, if possible, between a primary central nervous or vestibular problem or indeed a general medical cause like anaemia, dysrhythmia, hypotension and metabolic causes (e.g., hypoglycaemia). Although dizziness is a vague entity, vertigo (defined as 'disordered orientation in space') is a cardinal feature of vestibular disorder. It may be described by the patient in various forms. Firstly, the surrounding world may appear to move, often in a rotatory fashion but sometimes in an oscillatory pattern. Secondly, the patient my feel his or her own body moving—again most commonly in a rotatory manner. Finally, vertigo may be described in terms of unsteadiness, especially of the legs, where they may feel clumsy. If the story is suggestive of vertigo, there are associated symptoms that aid in siting the lesion in the vestibular system. A progressive, unilateral hearing loss with vertigo is suggestive of an underlying acoustic neuroma, which if expanding may produce lesions of the Vth and VIIth cranial nerves. If the symptoms are of sudden onset, with or without unilateral deafness, then a viral or bacterial labyrinthitis should be suspected or a vascular lesion in the inner ear. In between these two presentations, there are the fluctuating symptoms of Menière's syndrome (deafness, tinnitus and vertigo).

The duration of the attacks may also provide a clue to the aetiology, as those of short duration (5–20 s) are secondary to cupulolithiasis; those of Menière's syndrome last up to 24 h and are episodic, whereas a vestibular neuritis (with neither cochlear nor neurological dysfunction) may last for 7 to 10 days or longer. If a diagnosis of vestibular neuritis is made, it must be remembered that no pathological lesion will be demonstrable, and a prolonged follow-up is advisable to exclude the development of other disease features, for example, of multiple sclerosis. Central vestibular lesions produce a gradual onset of continual inbalance. Involvement of the vestibular connecting fibres in either the brainstem or cerebellum will result in a characteristic appearance of symptoms and signs. For example, a tumour in the fourth ventricle (ependymoma or metastases) will commonly produce vertigo precipitated by rapid head movement or change in posture. A plaque of demyelination in the pons will have associated nystagmus and vomiting.

Acute central lesions are usually vascular, and occlusion of the vertebral artery will produce severe, acute vertigo. The lateral medullary syndrome is one such condition, classically due to occlusion of the posterior inferior cerebellar artery, and presents with acute vertigo, hiccup and vomiting. There is an associated ipsilateral Horner's syndrome (ptosis, miosis, enophthalmos), facial pain and numbness to pin prick and temperature. On the contralateral side there will be spinothalamic anaesthesia on the trunk and limbs. Cerebellar signs and paralysis of the soft palate (producing a dysphagia) are found on the same side as the facial numbness. Drugs such as phenytoin and the barbiturates produce giddiness, drowsiness and ataxia by involving both central vestibular and cerebellar connections. The aura of an epileptic attack may be a vertiginous feeling, most frequently in those with temporal lobe epilepsy, and it may be the only manifestation.

### Differential diagnosis

Before embarking on investigations, there are two instances where one can avoid unnecessary studies.

Firstly, *hyperventilation*—a common symptom mainly in young women, who present with a variety of neurological complaints (blackout, giddiness, paraesthesiae, visual disturbance). It can be easily reproduced in the outpatient clinic by voluntary hyperventilation for a minimum of three minutes, and then relieved by slowing the rate of respiration or with brief episodes of breathholding, allowing the arterial $pCO_2$ to rise to normal level.

The second instance is *benign postural vertigo*, which is common after head injury, but more often idiopathic. Giddiness is produced by nonspecific movement of the head, particularly on lying down or looking up. Here again a valuable outpatient test, the Hallpike manoeuvre, may produce the only abnormal physical sign. The patient is asked to lie on the examination couch with shoulders just over the top edge, and the procedure explained. After being raised to a seated position, the patient's head is quickly dropped back to a level 30° below the horizontal and then turned to one side. The procedure is then repeated and the head turned to the other side. In benign vertigo, after a short latent period, the vertiginous feeling and positional nystagmus will appear—though not on every occasion. Even if it is not demonstrated, with a clear history the diagnosis should not be doubted.

Another useful test is Unterberger's test where the patient is asked to 'march on the spot' with eyes closed and arms stretched out in front. If the patient starts to rotate in any one direction, this suggests a vestibular disorder.

### Investigation

Further assessment of the vestibular system involves testing both the vestibulo-ocular and vestibulospinal connections with caloric and gait tests, respectively. Assessment of cochlear function may provide important additional information and should be routinely performed in a neuro-otology or ENT clinic.

### Treatment

The medical treatment of vertigo is not always effective. Those with positional vertigo or vestibular neuronitis can be reassured that the symptoms will eventually regress, although this may take a few years in positional vertigo. A variety of drugs, generally central nervous suppressants, can be used. Betahistine, prochlorperazine and cinnarizine are a few examples. There exists a small group of patients who have severe positional vertigo with nausea ('disabling positional vertigo') and who do not respond to conventional therapy.

### Syncope and seizures

Paroxysmal attacks of faintness and syncope are fairly common. In a syncopal episode, there is a brief loss of muscle tone and strength, so that the patient cannot remain upright, followed by a period of loss of consciousness. The dilemma in such cases is whether or not the patient has had an epileptic seizure. The importance of a witnessed account of the event in question cannot be overstressed. If a witness is not present when the patient attends the clinic, then arrangements should be made for the witness to be interviewed as soon as possible. Occasionally this is not possible and an appropriate questionnaire should then be completed by the witness.

Epilepsy is defined as a 'recurring tendency to epileptic seizures'—the term 'recurring' excluding those with only one seizure.

Some features that help to distinguish a fit from a faint are as follows.

(1) Syncopal episodes are more gradual in onset, with a feeling of faintness, and the patient becomes limp; in an epileptic event, rigidity is usual. If the patient with syncope remains in an upright position, either due to the fact that he or she could not lie flat or to the overenthusiastic help of those in attendance keeping them 'propped up', then rigidity may be seen that progresses to a generalized seizure due to cerebral hypoperfusion. Tongue biting and incontinence are only seen in a fit.
(2) A description of the patient being 'pale and sweaty' tends to favour syncope, whereas during a fit there may be flushing or even cyanosis.
(3) The timing of the attacks can give a clue, in that events occurring during sleep are more often than not epileptic in origin. The patient's spouse may be awoken by abnormal grunting noises or heavy snoring and then find him or her unrousable.
4) If the patient is drowsy after the 'collapse', with some confusion and amnesia for the event, then it is very likely to be a fit. These features are rarely seen with syncope.

The narcolepsy syndrome should always be considered in anyone presenting with an episode of collapse. The patient falls asleep in inappropriate circumstances—for example, during meal times and has episodes of cataplexy, which produces immobilization and collapse, but no loss of consciousness. Cataplexy is characteristically precipitated laughter. Migraine may under certain circumstances simulate and even precipitate an epileptic seizure.

Where the description of an event points to an epileptic origin, the type of seizure should be ascertained. In broad terms, a seizure may either be *generalized* or *partial*.

A. *Generalized*

(1) *Tonic clonic or grand mal seizures.* The patient loses consciousness and falls to the ground. The tonic phase starts with strong contraction of muscle groups with the jaw clenched and there may be incontinence of urine. There may be no respiratory effort apart from grunting noises, and the patient becomes cyanosed with eyes open and rolled upwards. After a few seconds the seizure progresses to the clonic phase with rhythmic shaking of the body and the tongue may be bitten. The breathing is noisy for about 60 s but then returns to normal as the patient sleep. Following this type of seizure, the patient can remain drowsy for a variable period of time.

(2) *Absences or petit mal seizures.* These are very brief, lasting 10 to 60 s and the patient develops a vacant stare, is unresponsive but may continue to use the arms and legs in an apparently purposeful manner. An abnormal EEG recording of generalized spike and wave, occurring at a frequency of 3 Hz, is essential before a diagnosis of petit mal can be made.

(3) *Atonic seizures.* Here consciousness is lost and the patient becomes floppy and falls to the ground. There are no abnormal movements and the rapidity of onset of the collapse and absence of emotion as a trigger distinguishes them from syncope and cataplexy, respectively, although this can be difficult.

B. *Partial*

(1) *Focal or simple partial seizures.* These originate in specific areas of the brain and are highly suggestive of a space occupying lesion. When it involves the motor cortex it is called a *simple motor* or *Jacksonian epilepsy*, and the seizure will most often remain confined to one part of the body. Post-ictally, the affected limb may be weak for several hours – a phenomenon known as *Todd's paresis*. Similarly, if the epileptic focus is in the sensory cortex, the seizure will be manifested as an abnormal sensory sensation of tingling or discomfort in the contralateral part of the body (*simple sensory seizure*). When the patient complains of a sensation of altered smell (usually a burning odour), sometimes so strong that they frantically search for the source, the epileptic focus lies in the temporal lobe (*temporal lobe seizure*). Alternatively or additionally, gustatory hallucinations (usually a bitter taste) or a sensation of epigastric discomfort rising up the body may occur. Vivid recollection of having been in a particular place or carried out a specific task in the past, when these in fact are new experiences, is called *déja vu*, and should be specifically asked about. *Jamais vu* is the opposite sensation, where the patient feels unfamiliar in what should be familiar surroundings. Most people experience déja vu once in a while, but when it occurs more than once every one to two months, then partial seizures of temporal lobe origin are a possible explanation.

In all types of partial seizures, the patient remains fully conscious and is able to give a clear account of events as they occur. It is possible, however, for this type of seizure to become generalized (*secondary generalization*) with the appearance of a tonic-clonic event.

(2) *Complex partial or temporal lobe seizures.* In contrast to simple partial epilepsy, consciousness is impaired in a complex partial seizure. These arise most commonly in the temporal lobe, and the initial event of an abnormal epigastric sensation, or olfactory or gustatory hallucination is known as an *aura*. Following this, behaviour may be very abnormal, with repetitive actions such as chewing or lip smacking being noted. The patient will be amnesic for the period of the seizure, and post-ictally may feel confused or tired. This type of seizure can also develop secondary generalization.

### Investigation

For simple faints a full blood count should be checked to exclude an anaemia. The investigation of a patient with a blackout should include a routine haematological and biochemical screening, including fasting blood glucose and syphilis serology. Cardiac assessment with ECG and 24-h ECG should be done if an arrhythmia is a possibility. The electroencephalogram (EEG) may identify the type of seizure and localize the source, but will not prove or refute the diagnosis of epilepsy. The EEG will in fact be normal in 30 per cent of those with undoubted epilepsy. It has been suggested, however, that the EEG showing interictal epileptiform activity may be diagnostically useful in evaluating patients with suspected epilepsy—the major drawback being that a normal interictal EEG cannot exclude the diagnosis.

Hyperventilation and photic stimulation should be used routinely during the EEG recording to try and stimulate abnormal electrical discharges. Depriving the patient of sleep for one night before an EEG is another method of promoting abnormal electrical activity and is useful in cases where the diagnosis of epilepsy is suspicious but not definite.

For those presenting with epilepsy who are over 30 years of age, or if a focal lesion is suspected clinically or on the EEG of a younger person, a CT head scan should be performed.

Once the patient has been told of the diagnosis of epilepsy, the social consequences should be explained. Currently, the patient has to remain fit free for a period of two years, or only have convulsions when asleep for three years to be eligible to apply for a driving licence. The onus is on the patient to report to the Driver and Vehicle Licencing Centre (DVLC) in Swansea, and his or her insurance company, the fact that he or she has epilepsy. A Heavy Goods Vehicle licence will not under any circumstances be revoked. If a patient has a fit when the medication is altered, either reduced or stopped, after being free of fits for some time, the DVLC will allow 12 months instead of two years as a probationary period. The same conditions apply if, after a 5-year period clear of fits whilst off medication, the patient has a single seizure.

A diagnosis of cataplexy may be supported by clinical evidence of other features of the narcolepsy syndrome (excessive daytime sleepiness, cataplexy, sleep paralysis and pre-sleep dreams). Multiple sleep latency tests confirm the rapid onset of REM sleep in these patients. About 95% will be HLA DR2 positive.

### Treatment

Strong reassurance is all that is usually required for those with simple faints. The choice of medication for epilepsy depends on the pattern and type of seizure, and also on individual preferences. For young women, carbamazepine is preferable as it lessens the risk of teratogenticity and neural tube defects in the fetus. Phenytoin or carbamazepine would be first choice for tonic clonic fits, with sodium valproate as second choice. For complex partial seizures, carbamazepine is effective and should be tried initially, with phenytoin as first reserve. Sodium valproate is probably most beneficial in absence seizures and myoclonic seizures.

The measurement of serum anticonvulsant levels is useful where compliance is in question and also when one needs to increase the dose of a drug to its maximum concentration in order to obtain better control. This can be done for both phenytoin and carbamazepine, but is of limited value for sodium valproate as it is lipid soluble and its serum levels do not reflect CNS levels. If maximal therapy does not produce a good result, a second drug may be added, checking that adequate serum levels are achieved; the first drug is then gradually withdrawn. Monotherapy should be the primary aim and a combination of anticonvulsants only used after good trial with two or three drugs alone has been unsuccessful.

Cataplexy is helped by drugs like clomipramine. CNS stimulants (eg mazindol) are required if narcolepsy is a problem.

### Special circumstances

After one seizure the patient should be reviewed in the clinic in three months time; if there has been no recurrence, anticonvulsant therapy is not indicated—although this point is debatable. Often one encounters a patient who has been fit free for over two years, and a decision is required as to whether or not to stop all medication, providing the patient is in favour of this change. The EEG may be of some value in this instance to see if there has been normalization of previously abnormal recordings before discontinuing treatment. However, the EEG will not predict those who will remain free of fits once the medication has been stopped.

Stopping treatment has to be done slowly in a stepwise manner, and no guarantees can be given to the patient that he or she will remain fit free when off all treatment.

Unfortunately, control is not satisfactory in a proportion of patients, even after adjustment of therapy. In such cases a review of the benefits of previous treatment may be helpful. If the patient is on optimal therapy with no change or an increase in the frequency of seizures, then the original diagnosis of epilepsy must be reviewed. This is often best achieved as an inpatient when the attacks can be documented by the medical and nursing staff. A CT head scan is required to ensure that one is not dealing with a progressive lesion. Hysterical or pseudoseizures, or rage attacks, can be difficult to distinguish from true seizures. Repeated investigations including EEG, sleep-deprived EEG and ambulatory EEG recording for 24-h or longer until an attack is witnessed, with or without simultaneous ECG recording may be necessary. When an attack is witnessed, serum potassium and glucose should be checked immediately; 15 to 20 min after the episode, blood should be taken for prolactin levels—prolactin will be raised after a tonic clonic seizure.

In those patients with epilepsy that is resisted to control with anticonvulsants, but who have a focal abnormality on their EEG, then surgical resection of that focus can be dramatically effective.

## Difficulty walking and muscle weaknesss

For normal muscle contraction, there has to be an uninterrupted pathway from the motor cortex (upper motor neurone) via the corticospinal tract to the lower motor neurone, which starts at the anterior horn cell in the spinal cord and brainstem nuclei to reach the muscle through a peripheral nerve. At the neuromuscular junction, release of acetylcholine alters permeability to sodium and potassium and creates an electrical gradient, which starts a muscle contraction. A lesion in any of these regions will result in a distinct type of muscle weakness.

### Upper motor neurone lesions

Lesions in the corticospinal tract, such as strokes or space-occupying masses, usually result in incomplete weakness affecting certain movement rather than groups of muscles. In the upper limbs, abduction and extension are most affected, whereas flexion is weakest in the lower limbs. Small degrees of deficit may be detectable in these actions, with others relatively well preserved. There will also be an increase in tone, brisk reflexes and extensor plantar response to complete the picture of an upper motor neurone lesion. When both legs are affected, as in lesions of the spinal cord, it is called a spastic paraparesis, or a spastic paraplegia if there is no movement of the legs. If both arms and legs are involved, as in high cervical cord or midline medullary lesions, the terms spastic tetraparesis or tetraplegia are used. A spastic monoparesis of an upper limb is much more likely to be due to a problem in a cerebral hemisphere than in the spinal cord.

A spastic paraparesis in a young adult is most commonly due to multiple sclerosis, and in the elderly due to cervical spondylosis. Other causes are myelitis, spinal cord compression from benign and malignant tumours or epidural abscess, trauma and hereditary spastic paraparesis. Syringomyelia and motor neurone disease will have other characteristic clinical signs. A falx meningioma can produce a spasic paraparesis, as can bilateral cortical lesions—usually cerebrovascular disease; in cerebrovascular disease the patient will show some evidence of dementia, with a brisk pout reflex and grasp response and a brisk jaw jerk.

A hemiparesis as a result of damage to the *cortex* may be associated with ipsilateral, upper motor neurone facial weakness, dysphasia or visual field defect.

If the lesion is in the *brainstem*, there may be contralateral, lower motor neurone facial weakness and sensory changes, ataxia, ophthalmoplegia and nystagmus, and a history of diplopia and vertigo.

In a hemiparesis due to a high *cervical cord* lesion, none of the above symptoms and signs will be present and there will invariably be brisk reflexes or an extensor plantar response on the contralateral side, a sensory level and a history of sphincter disturbance.

### Investigation

Depending on the clinically determined site of the problem, specific investigations should be requested. Urinalysis, routine full blood count and biochemical tests, ESR, syphilis serology, vitamin $B_{12}$, folic acid and antinuclear factor should be checked. Serum proteins should be assayed with an electrophoretic strip. Chest X-ray and ECG are required regardless of the site of the lesion as malignant, inflammatory and ischaemic processes can manifest anywhere. Site-specific investigations include:

(a) *cortex*—CT head scan with contrast enhancement; angiography, if a vascular (meningioma, aneurysm, arteriovenous malformation) or vasculitic lesions need to be excluded;

(b) *brainstem, midbrain, pons*—can be investigated as above, but often MRI (magnetic resonance imaging) is more informative than CT scanning in these regions;

(c) *spinal cord*—plain radiographs of the spine; myelography followed by CT scanning; MRI offers a non-invasive alternative that will in time become the investigation of choice as it has no complications and a prolonged stay in hospital is not needed.

Analysis of cerebrospinal fluid may be required, as the changes in protein, glucose and the number of white cells found can indicate the presence of an infective or inflammatory process. Cytological examination of the fluid may demonstrate malignant cells. The interpretation of cerebrospinal fluid is outlined in Table 7.12 at the end of this chapter.

Electrophoresis of paired samples of cerebrospinal fluid and serum is used to look for oligoclonal IgG synthesis within the central nervous system (and absent in serum) that is characteristically associated with multiple sclerosis. CSF oligoclonal IgG bands can be found in other CNS inflammatory disorders such as neurosarcoidosis.

### Lower motor neurone lesions

Weakness due to lower motor neurone lesions (i.e., anterior horn cell, motor root and peripheral nerve) is, by contrast, limited to specific muscles, with associated hypotonia and depressed or absent reflexes. Sensory abnormalities may also be found, either in root or peripheral nerve distribution, or as a glove and stocking loss in peripheral neuropathy. If the lesion is at the level of the anterior horn cell, fasciculation may be seen. This is an irregular contraction of muscle fibres, which is seen at rest and disappears during voluntary contraction. Although fasciculation is very suggestive of motor neurone disease, it is not pathognomonic of this condition as it can be seen, albeit infrequently, in other types of progressive muscle disorders, and in peripheral nerve or root lesions. Fasciculation should be looked for in the tongue.

### Investigation

Basic investigations are the same as above, together with, when indicated, serum lead and urinary porphyrins for a motor neuropathy. Analysis of cerebrospinal fluid is indicated where an inflammatory or malignant process has to be excluded.

For suspected root compression, myelography followed by CT scanning is required. MRI is the non-invasive alternative.

Confirmation of the diagnosis of neuropathy is achieved by nerve conduction studies, measuring the latency from the stimulus, the amplitude and the condition velocity of both motor and sensory nerves.

Electromyography (EMG) involves sampling muscles with a concentric needle electrode, and will demonstrate the denervation associated with a lower motor neurone lesion and the fasciculation of disease of the anterior horn cells.

Biopsy of a sensory nerve (sural or radial sensory branch) is sometimes required for more detailed information about the pathological process.

### Muscle disorders

The important features of muscle disease (myopathy) include weakness, pain and fatigableness. The weakness occurs in a predominantly proximal and symmetrical distribution affecting the muscles of the shoulder and pelvic girdle, with normal sensation and reflexes. Patients walk in a waddling manner and complain of difficulty in getting out of low chairs or climbing stairs. In any patient with weakness of some duration, one should enquire about muscle pains because the combination of both is characteristic of a myopathic disorder. Pain can arise as a result of muscle cell destruction (polymyositis, alcoholic myopathy) or an arteritis within the muscle (polymyalgia rheumatica). Energy pathway defects (myophosphorylase and phosphofructokinase deficiencies) cause pain that tends to be precipitated by exercise and relieved by rest.

Muscle pain should be distinguished from muscle cramps, as the latter may be a symptom of pyramidal and extrapyramidal disorders as well as of metabolic and endocrine states, such as potassium depletion, uraemia and hypothyroidism. Muscle fatigableness after repetitive contraction suggests a transmitter problem as in myasthenia gravis and myasthenic syndrome (Lambert–Eaton syndrome; see below). Episodic muscle weakness would make one suspect periodic paralysis related to potassium abnormalities.

The hereditary muscular dystrophies include the X-linked Duchenne and Becker varieties: these have similar clinical presentations but the Becker dystrophy is much less severe; the child will be able to walk beyond the age of 13 years and the IQ is normal. Dystrophy of the limb girdle is inherited as an autosomal recessive trait and although it begins in adolescence its progression is very slow and can occasionally be confused with polymyositis. Facial weakness is not found in this dystrophy and the creatine kinase (see below) is only marginally raised. Facioscapulohumeral dystrophy has an autosomal dominant pattern of inheritance and presents initially with symptoms related to facial weakness, marked scapular wasting and weakness and less severe hip weakness.

Myotonia is a painless delay in relaxation of muscle as a result of abnormality in the muscle membrane. This is best demonstrated by asking the patient to 'make a fist' as tightly as possible and then to quickly spread the fingers. Percussion myotonia is elicited by tapping the belly of the muscle following which there will be a temporary dimple in the muscle. Both of these signs will be more marked in the cold, and characteristically seen in myotonia dystrophy.

### Investigation

Specific check should be made of serum electrolytes—$K^+$, $Mg^{2+}$ and $Ca^{2+}$. Creatine kinase is a muscle enzyme and if the levels are raised this indicates muscle cell destruction. The MM band of creatine kinase isoenzyme is specific for skeletal muscle. EMG demonstrates functional activity with characteristic changes in myopathic and neurotransmitter disorders. Muscle biopsy is done on an affected muscle and is helpful in distinguishing a muscle disorder from a neurogenic problem. Inflammatory cells can be seen in a myositis and special histochemical stains may reveal a metabolic or biochemical defect.

The Tensilon test for myasthenia is best done on the ward where atropine should be available, as it involves the intravenous administration of an anti-cholinesterase (edrophonium chloride), starting with a dose of 2 mg and waiting for 30 to 60 s before slowly giving the remainder of the 10 mg. Maximal effect is seen after 20 s in muscles known to be affected clinically, and the improvement will last for 5 min.

Acetylcholine receptor antibodies (AChR) are found in 90 per cent of those with generalized myasthenia gravis.

### Pain, paraesthesiae and numbness

These symptoms may occur in non-neurological conditions like arthritis, claudication, hyperventilation or hysteria, so objective signs, such as absent reflexes, areas of abnormal sensation, muscle wasting, joint abnormalities and atrophic changes, have to be elicited to confirm or exclude a lesion of the sensory pathway. This will be further helped by specific investigations, as discussed later. Lesions at various levels of the sensory pathway have certain characteristics that may help in diagnosis.

At the level of the *sensory cortex*, there may be enormous variability in the patient's response to identical sensory stimuli and this has, on occasions been misleadingly attributed to hysteria. It is the *parietal cortex* that decodes sensory information from the periphery, and a lesion in the parietal lobe leads to the patient being unable to recognize familiar objects (coin or key) placed in the hand with the eyes closed (*astereognosis*), even though pin prick and light touch may be normal. Lesions of the parietal lobe also produce sensory inattention on the opposite side of the body. With the patient lying on the bed, test for this as follows:

'Close your eyes. I want you to tell me which arm/leg I'm touching. Is it the left, right or both together?'

If there is inattention, when touch stimulus is applied to each side individually the responses will be correct, but with simultaneous touch stimulus to the right and left sides, the patient will ignore the stimulus on one side. The commonest finding is left-sided inattention due to a right parietal lobe lesion. Inattention can be demonstrated by asking the patient to copy a picture of a house, or the face of a clock. Figures will be omitted or incorrectly spaced on the one side.

In addition to astereoagnosia, another sign of *right* parietal lobe dysfunction is *agraphagnosia*, an inability to recognize figures drawn on the patient's palm and *apraxia* (see below) of the left arm and leg.

A lesion of the *left* parietal lobe commonly produces *apraxia*, that may affect both sides of the body. Apraxia is an inability to perform intentional movements when there is no evidence of muscle weakness, inco-ordination or sensory loss. Several varieties of apraxia have been described, but the most striking and important one is *dressing apraxia*, where the patient is confused about the sequence of events required to put on items of clothing, and this can easily be demonstrated at the bedside.

An extensive *thalamic* lesion will cause gross impairment of all forms of sensation on the contralateral side of the body, with position sense often more severely affected than cutaneous sensation. This is because the thalamus receives all the posterior column (touch, vibration and joint position sense) and spinothalamic (pain and temperature) fibres, before they are projected to the sensory cortex. The thalamic pain syndrome is usually seen after strokes, where the patient experiences continuous pain on one side of the body, and any form of innocuous stimulus – touch, cold or heat, may induce a prolonged feeling of discomfort (dysaesthesia).

If a lesion is in the region of the *medulla and lower pons*, a characteristic crossed sensory disturbance is found, with contralateral loss of pain and temperature sensation over the body, and ipsilateral sensory loss on the face. This is because the fibres from the three divisions of the trigeminal nerve, enter the nucleus of the trigeminal nerve in the brainstem and then continue up to the medulla and lower pons before they eventually decussate and then project to the thalamus.

Within the *spinal cord*, three presentations of sensory abnormality may be found:

(1) Central grey matter lesions—e.g., syringomyelia, with dissociated sensory loss (loss of spinothalamic but retention of posterior column sensation).

(2) Hemisection or Brown-Séquard syndrome— with hemiparesis on the ipsilateral side and impaired temperature and touch sensation on the contralateral side, usually two spinal segments below the level of the lesion (e.g., meningioma, neurofibroma, cervical spondylosis and may be seen in multiple sclerosis).

(3) Complete transections lesions will result in loss of all sensory modalities below the level that corresponds to the lesion. If this is acute in onset, likely causes are trauma, acute disc prolapse or demyelination, whereas a more gradual onset favours the diagnosis of spinal cord tumour, or tuberculoma, for example.

An expanding lesion may do so either from the outside of the cord towards the centre (extradural or intradural but extramedullary) or in the opposite direction (intramedullary). The direction of expansion will produce a different pattern of sensory loss, as the pain and temperature fibres are placed on the periphery of the cord. Also remember that the sacral fibres are situated in the outer perimeter of the cord and progressively more medially will be lumbar, thoracic and cervical fibres, so that an extradural expanding mass may produce an ascending sensory level, first seen at the sacral level, then the lumbar and then the thoracic; if the lesion is high in the cord a cervical sensory level will be evident.

When there is an acute onset of motor paralysis with spinothalamic loss below a level (usually T8–10) but with preserved function in the posterior column, this is likely to be due to infarction of the anterior spinal artery.

When patients describe feelings of 'tightness' or 'like having my legs wrapped in bandages', this suggests a lesion affecting the posterior columns— for example, multiple sclerosis or cord compression.

*Dorsal nerve root* pain and paraesthesiae are referred along the appropriate segmental dermatome and the pains are of a lancing or shooting nature. They are often aggravated or precipitated by movements that increase intraspinal pressure, such as coughing and sneezing or straining, and more often than not are caused by root compression from disc protrusion. The symptoms improve with bed rest, with or without some sort of traction therapy. Root pain that is not relieved or is aggravated by bed rest is more sinister and a malignant infiltration around the roots has to be excluded. Involvement of the dorsal root alone will produce appropriate segmental sensory loss with reflex changes (see Table 7.8). If the ventral root is also involved, then weakness and muscular wasting may be seen. Radicular pain may also be found with herpes zoster infection and diabetes.

At the level of the *peripheral nerve*, two types of neuropathy are encountered. Firstly, a polyneuropathy that is symmetrical and usually associated with metabolic (diabetes mellitus) or systemic disorders (amyloidosis), deficiency (vitamin $B_{12}$) and toxic states (alcohol, drugs). As it is the longest fibres that are affected, initial sensory symptoms may consist of burning pains, paraesthesiae, shooting pains and numbness that begin in the feet and ascend up the leg. Clinical signs are found in the feet, with a variable degree of wasting and weakness. There will be loss of ankle before knee jerks and sensory loss in a 'stocking' distribution. Similar changes are later found in the upper limbs starting at the fingertips. These neuropathies are of a subacute onset over a period of weeks or months. Many of the hereditary neuropathies are more chronic, slowly progressing over many years. The second type of neuropathy encountered is that of a mononeuropathy, as seen in entrapment syndromes, vasculitic or granulomatous processes and peripheral nerve tumours. Those with an ischaemic origin—for example, rheumatoid arthritis, diabetes and polyarteritis nodosa—are often painful in the acute stage, as in diabetic femoral neuropathy. In the diabetic patient, both polyneuropathy and mononeuropathy may coexist.

The relative involvement of predominantly motor or sensory fibres or the presence of a mixed neuropathy will provide some clue as to the possible aetiology. Most, in fact, of the mixed sensorimotor type. Predominant sensory loss should make one think of diabetes mellitus, amyloidosis, or leprosy as possible causes. Vitamin $B_{12}$ deficiency will produce an almost pure sensory neuropathy, as will some of the hereditary sensory neuropathies. A sensory neuropathy may also be the initial manifestation of an occult malignancy. When motor involvement is predominant, then Guillain–Barré syndrome or porphyria are the most likely cause.

The condition of 'restless legs' and 'painful legs and moving toes' bears the eponym Eckbom's syndrome; it may be confused with a sensory neuropathy, but on examination and investigation no significant nerve or muscle abnormalities are found. This condition is said to be associated with iron deficiency anemia and uraemia. The patient experiences an unpleasant deep aching pain or tingling in the feet, often associated with cramp, and has an uncontrolled desire to move the legs. These symptoms are often worse when the patient is relaxed, either when sitting in a chair or typically in bed at night. Such patients may respond to clonazepam or chlorpromazine at night.

In those with a predominantly sensory neuropathy there will be sensory impairment and loss of tendon reflexes, but in some cases allodynia (pain in response to a non-noxious stimulus) or hyperpathia (unpleasant feeling after a noxious stimulus) may be encountered.

Tremor is also a rare accompaniment of neuropathy, mainly those associated with paraproteinaemia and hereditary motor and sensory neuropathy. Where a neuropathy is longstanding, limb deformities such as pes cavus and toe and finger clawing may occur. Pes cavus may be distinguished from a high arch by pressing the palm of your hand against the sole of the patient's foot; if daylight is seen when looking from the side this suggests a true pes cavus. A simple examination, which should routinely be performed on anyone with a neuropathy, is nerve palpation. Although difficult to assess, it may suggest nerve thickening, alerting one to the possibility that the neuropathy may be due to amyloidosis or leprosy. Neurofibromatosis or a neurilemmoma can result in localized nerve thickening. The easiest nerves to palpate are the greater auricular nerve in the neck, the ulnar nerve just above the elbow, the common peroneal nerve as it crosses the neck of the fibula and the superficial peroneal nerve over the anterior aspect of the ankle.

In all patients with a somatic peripheral neuropathy, an assessment of *autonomic function*, both in the history and examination, is mandatory as both somatic and autonomic neuropathy may coexist, for example in diabetes, and amyloidosis and Guillain-Barré syndrome. There are three heart-rate tests (response to Valsalva manoeuvre, to standing up and to deep breathing) and two blood-pressure tests (responses to standing and to sustained handgrip) that are commonly used to assess autonomic neuropathy. Values for the three tests that can be carried out in the clinic or on the ward are given in Table 7.10, and outlined below.

*Heart rate response to standing*: the patient is attached to an ECG recorder and, after baseline recordings while lying flat, is asked to stand up and the heart rate further recorded for 45 s. From the time of standing up you find the 15th beat and measure the shortest R–R interval around that time. Next locate the 30th beat and measure the longest R–R interval around that time. The ratio of the longest to the shortest times is recorded (30:15 ratio).

*Heart rate response to deep breathing*: the patient is asked to breathe in and out over 5 s each. This is repeated six times. The maximum and minimum heart rates are recorded for each 10-s cycle and the difference recorded.

*Blood pressure response to standing*: record the blood pressure with the patient lying down and again approximately one minute after standing.

**Table 7.10. Cardiovascular tests of autonomic function**

|  | Normal | Borderline | Abnormal |
| --- | --- | --- | --- |
| Heart rate variation (R–R interval) during deep breathing (max–min HR) | >15 beats/min | 11–14 | <10 |
| Heart rate response to standing (30:15 ratio) | >1.04 | 1.01–1.03 | <1.00 |
| BP response to standing (fall in systolic BP) | <10 mmHg | 11–29 | >30 |

## Involuntary movements

The commonest movement disorders likely to be encountered are those of benign essential tremor and parkinsonism, but others to be recognized include chorea, dystonia and tardive dyskinesia. In order to assess the possible aetiology of involuntary movements, questions should be asked to ascertain:

(1) Age of onset and rate of deterioration—the commonest are those that arise in late middle age and are likely to be degenerative (Parkinson's disease), vascular or neoplastic in origin. Those of vascular origin will have an acute onset whereas the degenerative conditions result in a slower rate of development.
(2) Medication and toxic exposure—phenothiazines (Parkinsonism tardive dyskinesia), oral contraceptives (chorea), alcohol and exposure to manganese (tremor) are a few factors to consider.
(3) Past medical and family history—ask about birth hypoxia, rheumatic fever, liver disease and systemic lupus erythematosus. A positive family history may be found in cases with essential tremor and Huntington's chorea.

During the examination, the movements should be observed and specific instructions given to amplify them. In the first instance, ask the patient to hold the hands out in front with the palms turned upwards, and to keep this position with the eyes closed. Finger–nose testing and performing tasks of increasing difficulty, like playing an imaginary piano and doing and undoing buttons, will add to the picture. By this stage one will know whether the involuntary movements are present at rest or exacerbated by movement; whether they are rhythmic, non-purposeful, semipurposeful, complex or simple, and whether they are slow or rapid, brief or prolonged.

*Essential tremor* is dominantly inherited and characterized by being of variable amplitude (7–11 Hz), aggravated by stress and relieved by alcohol. Propranolol and other non-cardioselective β-blockers may reduce or even abolish the tremor in many cases. If the tremor is not causing much distress to the patient, the possible side-effects of the drug should be considered relative to their potential benefit. The tremor of idiopathic Parkinson's disease is slower (6 Hz) and coarser in amplitude. It initially involves the thumb, index and middle fingers—so-called pill-rolling tremor. There may be confirmatory signs of basal ganglia disturbance, such as lack of facial expression, increased tone and bradykinesia.

*Myoclonus* is a brief muscle jerk being irregular or rhythmic, often occurring repetitively in the same muscle. Myoclonus does occur in normal individuals as they enter a sleeping state and in this situation strong reassurance is all that is required. More seriously, it is found with all types of epilepsy, encephalopathy due to organ failure and alcohol withdrawal. Sodium valporate or clonazepam maybe effective.

A *tic* is again due to a brief muscle contraction, but is repetitive and can usually be supressed voluntarily or during sleep. Tics are aggravated by anxiety; they stand to involve blinking, facial grimacing or shoulder shrugging and do not interfere with normal movement.

*Dystonia* is a sustained muscle spasm that distorts the body into characteristic postures including torticollis (wry neck), writer's cramp, equinovarus deformity and blepharospasm. Again, dystonias are exacerbated by anxiety and disappear during sleep.

*Choreiform movements* are purposeless, continuous and irregularly timed muscle jerks, occurring in the resting state and disappearing during sleep. Chorea may be associated with drugs (neuroleptics, levodopa, contraceptive pill), ageing, pregnancy, rheumatic fever, stroke and systemic lupus erythematosus, Huntington's disease and Wilson's disease. Athetosis may be difficult to distinguish from chorea, and both may coexist.

When indicated, treatment with dopamine receptor blockers (e.g., phenothiazines, haloperidol) and drugs that deplete presynaptic dopamine levels (e.g., tetrabenazine) may control the chorea.

*Athetoid movements* are slow, sinuous and purposeless, resulting in an inability to maintain parts of the body in one position. They often result from perinatal brain injury.

*Tardive dyskinesia* is caused by exposure to drugs that bind with, and block dopamine receptors; such as, antipsychotics (phenothiazines and butyrophenones) and antiemitics (metoclopramide). The symptoms of persistent, repetitive rapid movements, may affect the face (chewing, grimacing), the trunk and the distal parts of the arms and legs. Tardive dyskinesia is thought to be due to dopamine receptor hypersensitivity, and is usually resistant to treatment.

### Investigation

Investigation of those with posture tremor should include thyroid function tests. For intention tremor, liver function tests and a CT head scan looking specifically for cerebellar abnormalities are appropriate. Serum copper levels should be checked in any young person that presents with parkinsonian features to exclude Wilson's disease. Diagnosis of rapid involuntary movement can be difficult—the differential being between myoclonus, tic, epileptic or voluntary contractions. There are clinical distinguishing factors, as discussed above, but EEG and EMG will be of value in making the diagnosis.

## SPECIFIC CONDITIONS

### Transient ischaemic attack and stroke

Transient ischaemic attacks (TIAs) and strokes are acute episodes of focal cerebral dysfunction of acute onset, that differ in the duration of the attack, in that a TIA lasts less than 24 h. Together, they make up the most common disorder of the nervous system that presents to an acute medical team.

*Clinical presentation of TIA*
This depends on whether the TIA occurs in the carotid (80%) or vertebrobasilar (20%) territory, except that hemiparesis and hemianopia can occur in either.
*Carotid TIAs* are additionally associated with transient monocular blindness (amaurosis fugax) and dysphasia if the event is in the dominant hemisphere.
*Vertebrobasilar TIAs* may present with diplopia, vertigo, nausea and vomiting, dysarthria, ataxia and cortical blindness.

Most TIAs are embolic, due to platelet aggregates. Occasionally, they are caused by hypotension, in which case symptoms will be precipitated by change in posture. The significance of a TIA is that it is associated with a 5% annual risk of stroke for that patient.

*Clinical presentation of stroke*
Whether the cause is infarction or haemorrhage, the onset is acute and the signs depend on the blood vessel territory affected. A haemorrhagic cause is more likely to be associated with a severe headache and altered level of consciousness. The most common presentation involves the middle cerebral artery resulting in a hemiplegia, homonymous hemianopia and if it is the dominant hemisphere, aphasia. Marked weakness of the leg with relative sparing of the arm suggests a lesion in the territory of the anterior cerebral artery, with additional frontal lobe signs of change in affect, incontinence, grasp and pout reflexes and apraxia.

In certain situations a stroke does not produce a hemiplegia – a lesion of the posterior cerebral artery may result in an isolated hemianopia; a lesion of the dominant parietal lobe may cause a receptive aphasia with no weakness. Occlusion of a small penetrating arteriole produces a *lacunar stroke*, and although many of these occur in clinically silent areas of the brain, discrete lacunar syndromes have been described, including a pure hemisensory stroke. Lacunar strokes are invariably associated with hypertension.

A gradually progressing hemiparesis may result from an evolving infarct, but is more likely to be caused by a tumour, and therefore warrants urgent investigation.

In the clinical history, *risk factors* have to be

identified, and these are similar for both TIA and stroke – previous cerebral infarction/TIA, neck trauma, cardiac disease, vascular claudication, hypertension, diabetes, lipid disorders, arteritis, coagulation disorders, smoking, alcohol, oral contraceptive and a positive family history.

### Investigation and management

The investigations include full blood count and ESR; electrolytes, liver function tests, fasting lipids, cholesterol and glucose; syphilis serology; autoantibodies (in young patients) including anti-cardiolipin antibodies and a detailed clotting screen, chest X-ray and ECG. Younger patients (less than 45 years of age) should have an echo-cardiogram. After consultation with a neurologist, a CT brain scan may be indicated if it helps in the management – for example, in patients under the age of 40 years, or if there is doubt regarding the clinical diagnosis, or if treatment with aspirin or anticoagulation are contemplated (to exclude haemorrhage).

Additional investigations in selected cases would be carotid ultrasound to detect occlusive disease, and in cases with a greater than 70 per cent stenosis, intra-arterial digital subtraction angiography would be justified.

*Treatment*
(1) Of TIA – Aspirin (150–300 mg per day), and if this fails to stop attacks, anticoagulation with warfarin should be tried over a period of 3 to 6 months. Ticlopidine may be more effective than aspirin. Provisional data from large European and North American studies, suggest that carotid endarterectomy is beneficial in reducing the incidence of stroke in those cases with carotid stenosis of greater than 70%. This is dependent on the operation being performed only in centres with expertise in carotid artery surgery.
(2) Of stroke – This is determined by the size and cause of the stroke. In those who have made a good recovery from a small ischaemic stroke, aspirin is likely to be of benefit in reducing the risk of recurrence. For strokes due to cardiogenic emboli, including atrial fibrillation, anticoagulation should be started 10 days after the event.

Hypertension should only require treatment in the acute stage if it is very high, and then it should be cautiously reduced to levels of 170 mmHg systolic and 110 mmHg diastolic. In the convalescent stage, persistent hypertension can be treated more aggressively.

Neurosurgical intervention may be required for evacuation of moderately large intracerebral haematomas with associated deterioration in level of consciousness, which is usually due to raised intracranial pressure. Therefore fluid restriction, intravenous mannitol infusion (0.25 to 1.0 g per kg every 2 to 6 h), and artificial over-ventilation ($pCO_2$ at 25 mmHg) may help to stabilize the patient prior to surgery.

In the UK the incidence of stroke is about 200 per 100 000 of the population, and of these a third will not recover sufficiently to reach a stage of functional independence. The role of the physiotherapist, speech therapist, occupational therapist and social worker cannot be overstressed as it is they who guide such patients through their stay in hospital and prepare them to face the outside world. This team should be introduced to the patient as soon as possible, even though the patient may require bed rest for the first five to seven days after a haemorrhage. It will boost the patient's morale when he or she realizes that expert help is available to deal with not only a newly acquired physical disability but also to sort out financial and social difficulties that may arise whilst in hospital. Before discharge a home visit may be required to assess whether the patient's home is suitable. Are there steps to climb to the front door? Are the doors wide enough to cope with a walking frame or wheelchair? Is the bathroom upstairs? Is there adequate heating?, and so on.

The general practitioner's health care team will be notified before discharge and district nursing help organized as required. If there is no close family or friend to help with convalescence, or if the home is unsuitable, alternative residential accommodation will have to be arranged and this may take several weeks or months, depending on availability.

The patient should be given an outpatient clinic appointment for about four to six weeks time following discharge. After the initial rapid improvement, things may seem to be fairly static and the patient may become depressed. Further reassurance and advice for the patient and family is initially all that may be necessary, but if the symptoms and signs of depression persist it should be treated with initially small doses of amitriptyline (25–50 mg daily).

## Parkinson's disease

The diagnosis of Parkinson's disease is made when the following triad of clinical features are present:

- *Bradykinesia*: slowness of movement and difficulty in initiating movement; e.g., expressionless face, poor arm swing on walking. Look for bradykinesia by getting the patient to perform *rapid* finger and hand movements such as playing an imaginary piano, repetitively tapping the index finger on the thumb or pronating and supinating the forearm. In Parkinson's disease, both the speed and amplitude of the movement will be impaired.
- *Rigidity*: an increase in muscle tone that can affect all muscle groups, but is usually more obvious in the arms than in the legs. Examine tone by flexing and extending the wrist and supinating and pronating the forearm.
- *Response to levodopa*: all patients with idiopathic Parkinson's disease show some improvement after starting levodopa treatment. If there is no clinical response, another form of parkinsonism should be suspected.

Other features that may be present include:

*Tremor* – this is the commonest presenting symptom of Parkinson's disease and is present at rest, mainly affecting the hand and arm. In the early stage of the disease, the tremor is often asymmetric. The pill-rolling tremor is composed of alternating flexion and extension of the thumb and fingers with a rotatory movement at the wrist. As the Parkinson's disease progresses, the tremor becomes bilateral and will involve the lower limbs and the head. It is the combination of tremor and rigidity that gives the cogwheel sensation when examining muscle tone.

*Flexed posture and abnormal postural reflexes* – patients have a stooped posture, the neck is flexed and the arms held in a flexed position. Turning becomes difficult and they lose the ability to correct momentary losses of balance (righting reflex) when changing the direction of walking or if they are pushed, resulting in many falls.

*Symptoms* – of muscle aches and pains, lethargy and depression.

## Differential diagnosis

(1) Multisystem atrophy, Shy-Drager syndrome. This is parkinsonism with autonomic dysfunction (postural hypotension, urinary incontinence and decreased sweating).

(2) Steele-richardson-olszewski syndrome. Here there is parkinsonism with dementia, and striking abnormality of eye movement, with an inability to down gaze due to a supranuclear palsy.

(3) Drug-induced. For example, phenothiazines.

## Treatment

As a general rule, drug treatment need only be started when the symptoms interfere with the patient's normal life.

*Anticholinergics* have little to offer in the treatment of Parkinson's disease because of complications which include blurring of vision, constipation and confusion. They may also precipitate urinary retention and glaucoma.

*Levodopa/carbidopa* (Sinemet) or *levodopa/benserazide* (Madopar) combinations are the most beneficial drugs. It is a good policy to use the minimal effective dose, and starting, for example, with Sinemet Plus or Madopar 62.5 one tablet three times a day and increasing slowly according to the clinical response. If more levodopa is required, these preparations can be replaced by stronger ones (Sinemet 275 or Madopar 250). Slow release preparations are also now available. Nausea, vomiting, postural hypotension, confusion, hallucinations and involuntary movements are the commonest side effects.

If the patient does not respond to levadopa, then the likelihood is that the patient has some other disorder affecting the basal ganglia (see above).

*Selegiline* (Eldepryl) is a monoamine oxidase-B (MAO-B) inhibitor, and causes accumulation of dopamine in the striatum. Unlike MAO-A inhibitors, it can be safely given with a levodopa preparation, although the side effects of levodopa may be enhanced. Selegiline can be used as first line therapy, starting with a dose of 5 mg twice daily. There is evidence to suggest that selegiline may slow down the degeneration of the nigrostriatal pathway and therefore the progression of Parkinson's disease. This finding has yet to be confirmed, but if it is the case, then treatment should be started early.

*Amantadine* was initially introduced as an antiviral agent, but was found to have anti-parkinsonian properties. Amantadine can be used as the initial treatment in early Parkinson's disease, or in combination with other drugs. Confusion, hallucinations and skin pigmentation are recognized side effects.

*Bromocriptine* and, more recently introduced pergolide, are dopamine receptor agonists. Postural hypotension is more readily induced than with levodopa – containing drugs, otherwise side effects are similar. They are used as adjunctive treatment to levodopa and should be introduced gradually.

*Apomorphine* is a dopamine agonist. Because the large oral dose required produced unacceptable nausea, vomiting and renal impairment, its use in the treatment of Parkinson's disease was abandoned. With the development of non-centrally acting antiemetics (domperidone), and the discovery that apomorhine could be administered subcutaneously, it can now be successfully used in selected patients who fluctuate from being akinetic to having severe drug induced dyskinesias on levodopa. The patient, or relative, have to be able to manipulate a continuous infusion pump. The amount of apomorphine and the duration of the infusion has to be adjusted according to the clinical requirement. Apomorphine can also be given by multiple single subcutaneous injections via a penject, at times of bradykinesia. This is similar to the administration of insulin by a diabetic.

### Other treatment

(1) Regular exercise and physiotherapy.
(2) Social support for those with more advanced disease (home help, district nurse visits, arrangements for respite care etc).
(3) Although implantation of fetal dopaminergic tissue has been performed in a limited number of cases, this form of treatment for Parkinson's disease is still in the experimental stage and has no role in the current management of patients with Parkinson's disease.

### Multiple sclerosis

The characteristic of multiple sclerosis (MS) is the occurrence of disseminated demyelination in the central nervous system with resulting clinical abnormalities. The majority of young patients have a relapsing and remitting course of their disease, whereas in those with onset over the age of 40 years, almost 50% will have a progressive form.

Its aetiology is uncertain, but there is evidence of an immunological component with involvement of circulating suppressor T lymphocytes, activated T lymphocytes infiltrating the central nervous system, and deposition of IgG and complement components in central nervous tissue, levels of which are reflected in the cerebrospinal fluid. Genetic factors may also be important as a high proportion of patients with multiple sclerosis (in the Northern hemisphere ) have HLA tissue types DR2, DW2 and B7.

The condition can be aggravated by the patient's moods, severe physical exercise and hot baths. Although it is believed that the risk of a relapse is raised within the first 6 months after delivery, pregnancy is not contraindicated.

Diagnosis of multiple sclerosis is made from:

(a) a history of relapsing and remitting neurological deficits in a patient aged between 10 to 40 years old;
(b) documented abnormal neurological signs attributable to more than one site in the central nervous system;
(c) confirmatory investigations (see below).

MS can affect any part of the nervous system, but the common sites of initial involvement are the optic nerve, brainstem/cerebellum and cervical cord.

Acute optic neuritis is almost always unilateral, and presents as a painful eye with some degree of visual (especially colour) failure. It may be associated with a central scotoma. The optic disc is usually normal (retrobulbar neuritis), but a lesion at the head of the optic nerve may cause blurring of the disc margin (papillitis). Even with normal visual acuity, pupillary response to direct light may be impaired (afferent pupillary defect). The majority of cases with advanced disease will have nystagmus, but an earlier sign is failure of smooth pursuit eye movement. Diplopia is usually associated with a lesion in the medial longitudinal fasciculus – internuclear ophthalmoplegia. This is manifested clinically as eye movements that are out of synchrony; on lateral gaze there is failure of adduction of one eye and nystagmus in the fully abducted eye (ataxic nystagmus). Acute onset of vertigo and vomiting are common in multiple sclerosis. L'hermitte's sign of an electric discomfort down the back of the legs on flexing the neck is in context, very suggestive of cervical cord demyelination, although the phenomenon can be elicited in patients with other forms of cervical cord damage.

Progressive weakness of the lower limbs is a common symptom. With an acute relapse the onset of weakness may be more rapid. A spastic paraparesis with brisk tendon reflexes and bilateral extensor plantar responses is the common clinical picture in those with moderately advanced disease. This can progress to produce severe spasticity with painful extensor spasms. Transient sensory symptoms or paraesthesiae affecting any part of the body are common at all stages of the condition. On clinical examination however, sensory loss is rarely a prominent feature early on, and even in advanced cases it is joint position sense and vibration impairment distally in the legs that is usually found with only minimal change in cutaneous sensation.

With severe multiple sclerosis of long duration, dementia is common and in these cases euphoria may be an additional feature.

### Investigation

The diagnosis of multiple sclerosis is predominantly a clinical one but the following investigations can help to confirm the diagnosis.

(1) Evoked potentials—visual, somatosensory and brainstem auditory.
(2) Analysis of cerebrospinal fluid for an oligoclonal IgG banding pattern. A serum sample must also be analysed to confirm local, central nervous production of IgG.
(3) MRI of the brain and/or spinal cord. The characteristic distribution of periventricular and discrete abnormalities of the white matter can be seen in 99 per cent of patients with a clinical diagnosis of multiple sclerosis. MRI is useful in those patients who have a history of several neurological episodes but in whom clinical examination is either normal or abnormalities are confined to one site but other investigations are normal. If the MRI is abnormal and the clinical history and examination is strongly suggestive of MS, there is no need to examine the CSF or obtain evoked potentials.

Conditions such as SLE, sarcoidosis, Behçet's disease, polyarteritis nodosa and neurosyphilis can produce multiple CNS lesions, and have to be excluded.

When signs are confined to the spinal cord, for example a spastic paraparesis with a sensory level and with no recovery, the spinal cord must be imaged either with MRI or myelography.

### Management

Only when there is no doubt regarding the diagnosis should patients be told that they have multiple sclerosis. Although one episode of neurological deficit may not be enough to be called multiple sclerosis, patients may ask whether they have the condition or not. In this circumstance the possibility has to be raised. It is however difficult to give individual patients information on prognosis, but signs favouring a more benign course include young age at onset of the disease and complete remission after the first episode which consisted of purely sensory symptoms. Conversely, motor deficit and cerebellar ataxia in the first attack, early onset of progression and late age of onset with a progressive course indicate a less favourable prognosis.

Acute attacks of demyelination are probably shortened by the use of steroids prescribed as:

prednisolone E.C., 60 mg/day for three days, then reducing by 20 mg every three days;
ACTH or its synthetic analogue, 1 mg/day intramuscularly for three days and reducing by 0.25 mg every three days;
methylprednisolone, 3 g given as 1 g intravenously on alternate days.

Steroids, however, do not influence the long-term course of multiple sclerosis. No other forms of treatment have been shown to be of any benefit. A diet high in polyunsaturated fatty acids taken as sunflower seed oil or evening primrose oil may be recommended.

Whilst physiotherapy is the most important aspect of treatment in the recovery phase, drugs may be required for:

(a) spasticity of the limbs—baclofen, dantrolene sodium and diazepam;
(b) sphincter disturbance—urodynamic studies may be needed initially to confirm a spastic bladder that can be treated with bladder training and detrusor muscle relaxants (anticholinergic agents: propantheline, oxybutynin and terodiline). Cholinergic drugs (carbachol,

bethanecol) are used to stimulate detrusor contraction when there is hesitancy or retention of urine.

(c) constipation—lactulose (20 ml) given daily; intermittent enemas or even manual evacuation may also be needed;

(d) dysarthria—speech therapy;

(e) sensory symptoms—present as paraesthesiae or burning pain in the limbs or as trigeminal neuralgia. These are difficult to treat but carbamazepine is sometimes helpful; transcutaneous nerve stimulation is another option.

(f) depression.

All the help that social services can provide for the patient at home should be investigated by the social worker and occupational therapist.

## Motor neurone disease

Motor neurone disease is characterized by degeneration of motor neurones in the corticospinal tract and brainstem and of anterior horn cells. It is a disease of middle and late life that manifests clinically as either lower or upper motor neurone weakness, or a mixture of both.

Motor neurone disease occurs throughout the world with a constant incidence of 1–2 per 100,000, and is slightly commoner in males than females (1.5:1). No cause has been identified, but studies on familial cases, which make up about 10% of all cases (autosomal dominant inheritance) have suggested an abnormality on chromosome 21.

The three main clinical types are: *amyotrophic lateral sclerosis* (mixture of upper and lower motor neurone features) – presenting usually with localized wasting and weakness of the anterior tibial compartment of one leg or of the small muscles of one hand. Dysphagia or dysarthria are signs of bulbar involvement and this may be the presenting feature in about 30% of cases. The weakness gradually becomes more widespread. Muscle fasciculation is common and often noted by the patient. There are no sensory signs, but symptoms of muscle pain and cramp may be an early feature. Bladder and bowel control remain normal even in advanced disease. *Progressive muscular atrophy* (lower motor neurone manifestation) – initially there is global wasting and weakness of the small muscles of both hands, but the weakness spreads to involve the respiratory muscles. The frequent involvement of bulbar weakness will help to distin-

guish this type of motor neurone disease from spinal muscular atrophy which usually an inherited disorder and begins at a younger age. *Progressive bulbar palsy* (brain stem motor nuclei affected) – dysarthria and dysphagia are the main symptoms and are usually due to both upper and lower motor neurone involvement giving rise for example, to a spastic and wasted, weak tongue. There is often associated upper and lower motor neurone signs in the limbs.

### Investigation

Diagnosis is based on clinical findings supported by EMG studies showing denervation and fasciculation of the muscle. If upper motor neurone signs are confined to the limbs, a spinal cord lesion has to be excluded by myelography or MRI.

### Management

The prognosis is poor, with death occurring in the majority within five years of diagnosis. Those with predominantly lower motor neurone involvement, and those with early onset of disease survive longest have a slightly better prognosis. The outlook is worst for those with bulbar symptoms and because of problems with aspiration and nutrition, feeding through a gastrostomy may be necessary.

There is no effective treatment. Open discussion with the patient and family about the diagnosis and long-term problems is important. Physiotherapy is rewarding and social services will need to be mobilized with visits from the district nurse when the time is appropriate.

### Investigation

At the stage where there is meningism a lumbar puncture is all that is required. The virus may be isolated or antibody titres against the virus raised in the cerebrospinal fluid. Serum from the patient should also be checked for herpes simplex and other viral antibody titres because, if they are raised in both serum and cerebrospinal fluid, the diagnosis of herpes simplex encephalitis is less convincing.

There is always an increase in the lymphocyte count ($50–200/mm^3$) in the cerebrospinal fluid, with normal glucose and protein levels.

EEG may show focal abnormalities, and CT head scan may reveal temporal lobe changes, but it is not unusual for these latter investigations to be normal. MRI may show changes at an earlier stage.

The definitive diagnostic procedure is a brain biopsy, but this is often not undertaken, the patient being treated on the strength of the clinical diagnosis.

## Management

A patient suspected of having encephalitis needs regular neurological observation (4 hourly or more often) by nursing and medical staff. If the level of consciousness deteriorates the patient should be transfered to an intensive care unit.

Acyclovir inhibits viral replication and therefore has to be administered early on in the illness in order to be effective. Once lesions have been demonstrated in the cortex on CT scanning, the chances of treatment being successful are small. Acyclovir is administered intravenously at a dose of 10 mg/kg body weight 8 hourly for 10 days. Its only significant side-effect is thrombophlebitis at the site of infusion in some patients. Although cerebral oedema may be seen on the CT scan, there is no evidence that steroids improves the clinical situation. Untreated, herpes simplex encephalitis has a mortality of 80 per cent.

## Inflammatory polyneuropathy

The Guillain–Barré syndrome or acute inflammatory demyeliating polyneuropathy is an immune-mediated condition. Antimyelin antibodies are present in serum and CSF of patients. There is also evidence that cytotoxic T cells contribute to the immune response. In about two thirds of cases there is a history of a prodromal illness of sore throat, cough and ''flu-like' symptoms within 6 weeks of onset. This is followed by a progressive weakness beginning in the feet and then the hands. Facial weakness (unilateral or bilateral) is found in half of the cases, and muscle weakness may progress to involve the chest wall and affect swallowing and speech. Paraesthesiae affecting the feet and hands and back pain may be prominent symptoms but sensory deficit on examination is usually mild, with a glove and stocking distribution. Tendon reflexes are absent. Patients can have severe swings in blood pressure and pulse, with cardiac arrhythmias as a result of an autonomic neuropathy.

## Investigation

The protein level of cerebrospinal fluid is raised in 80% of cases and although the CSF is usually acellular, there may be 10 to 20 white blood cells/mm$^3$ (mainly lymphocytes).

Nerve conduction studies show slowing of motor and sensory conduction velocity, although these can be normal in a small percentage (10%) of patients.

## Management

Regular recording of the vital capacity is essential in these patients as ventilatory function can deteriorate over a period of a few hours. If the vital capacity falls below one litre, ventilatory support is required. Most patients with this syndrome will recover spontaneously, but because of the suggested immune aetiology, plasma exchange should be offered (if available) to those in whom neurological deterioration is rapid and who are unable to stand without support. There is no fixed regimen for plasma exchange in Guillain-Barré syndrome—but three or four exchanges each of 2 to 3 litres on alternate days seems appropriate. Current evidence suggests that steroids are not useful, but intravenous gammaglobulin (0.3 mg/kg body weight daily for 5 days) may be as effective as plasma exchange. Subcutaneous heparin (5000 units twice daily) should be given to all patients confined to bed. ECG monitoring may detect cardiac arrhythmias, secondary to an auto immune neuropathy.

For less severely affected patients, general medical and nursing care with gradually increasing amounts of physiotherapy is the treatment required.

The Miller-Fisher syndrome is a variant of the Guillain-Barré syndrome and has the clinical features of ophthalmoplegia, ataxia and areflexia. It has a benign course with usually complete recovery. Protein concentration in the CSF is raised in most cases.

## Myasthenia gravis

Circulating antibodies to the acetylcholine receptor (AChR) on the postsynaptic membrane cause a depletion of receptors and the clinical manifestation of abnormal fatigableness. The fluctuation of symptoms and signs often results in the diagnosis being missed. Ptosis is the commonest presenting symptom, often associated with diplopia. Because of the asymmetrical involvement of the extraocular muscles the patient may appear to have an internuclear ophthalmoplegia. The face and neck are weak in nearly all cases. Chewing and swallowing may become difficult. Limb weakness is predominantly proximal but, as with other muscles, it is the fatigableness that is characteristic.

Reflexes are present and sensory testing normal.

Myasthenia gravis must be distinguished from the myasthenic or Lambert–Eaton-syndrome, again an autoimmune disorder where the release of acetylcholine at nerve endings is reduced. In this syndrome, ocular involvement is unusual and tendon reflexes are absent. A careful search for an underlying tumour (mainly small cell carcinoma of the lung) should be made. The clinical suspicion of myasthenia gravis can be confirmed by assessing improvement in muscle strength and diplopia following an injection of an anticholinesterase drug (Tensilon test, see page 176).

### Investigation

Antibodies against the AChR are found in about 90 per cent of those with myasthenia gravis, but may be normal in 25 per cent of those with the disease confined to the eyes. Antibody titres bear no relationship to the severity of the disease. Other investigations required included a chest X-ray, with a CT scan of the chest looking for thymic enlargement as myasthenic patients have a 15 per cent incidence of thymoma, an incidence that is further increased in the older patient. Other autoimmune diseases and certain tissue types (HLA–B8 and DRW–3) are also associated with myasthenia gravis, and the patient should be screened for these.

The myasthenic conditions can be clearly distinguished on EMG because repetitive nerve stimulation produces a reduction in the size of the muscle action potential in myasthenia gravis, whereas in the Lambert–Easton-syndrome the action potential will be greater than normal.

### Management

Treatment with an anticholinesterase (pyridostigmine, 60 mg in 3 to 6 doses daily) is only symptomatic, and therefore immunosuppressive treatment, which may alter the disease process, is required. This is achieved through thymectomy and administration of azathioprine or prednisolone in low, maintenance doses. Thymectomy should be considered in most cases if they are fit for surgery, regardless of age or sex, although the young tend to have a better response clinically. A good response after thymectomy means that the dose of anticholinesterase can be reduced. If the response is not good, then treatment with prednisolone and azathioprine is started and the dose tapered to appropriate maintenance levels, remembering that steroids may cause initial deterioration in symptoms.

Drug treatment may not completely alleviate diplopia or ptosis, and wearing an eye patch or an eyelid crutch on the inside of glasses can help. If dysphagia remains a problem, the patient should be advised to take small portions of liquidized food more frequently. The patient's home and furniture may have to be modified, and the occupational therapist's assessment is invaluable.

A *myasthenic crisis* is a medical emergency. The onset of a crisis should be suspected if the patient is experiencing recurrent brief episodes of dyspnoea with inspiratory stridor. Once respiratory distress is present, the patient has to be ventilated immediately and all medication stopped, as it can be difficult to distinguish clinically between a myasthenic crisis and overdosage of anticholinesterase by the patient because of increasing weakness (cholinergic crisis). Atropine can be given for distressing cholinergic symptoms. The cause (for example, infection, drugs such as diazepam or steroids, hyperthyroidism and emotional stress) can then be determined. Treatment, other than ventilation, is by plasma exchange; in the absence of infective or metabolic abnormalities, high dose steroids (2 mg/kg/day) can also be added.

If signs remain confined to the eyes for three years, the patient has a variant called ocular myasthenia, and after this time spread of myasthenia to bulbar muscles and the limbs is very unusual. In those with generalized myasthenia, the severity of the disease gradually decreases after the first 7 years, and 20% of patients will go into spontaneous remission at some stage over the following 13 years. When remission is achieved, anticholinesterase drugs should be very gradually withdrawn.

### Herpes simplex encephalitis

This is the commonest sporadic form of encephalitis, in which the herpes simplex virus replicates in the brain. It occurs in all age groups but predominantly in those between 20 and 40 years. It is a treatable condition and clinical awareness has to be heightened to its protean manifestations. The onset is usually mild with symptoms of malaise, headache and a low-grade pyrexia. There may also be some change in personality. This clinical picture can persist for up to 14 days before meningism, nausea and vomiting develop. After this stage the deterioration can be rapid, with acute neurological disturbance such as seizures, hemiparesis and behavioural disorder, leading to coma.

## Coma and brain-stem death

From the Glasgow Coma Scale (Table 7.11) the comatose patient is one who shows no eye opening, cannot express words and fails to localize painful stimuli. For the relatives and medical staff it is important to try and establish at a reasonably early stage what the prognosis will be for the patient.

**Table 7.11. Glasgow Coma Scale**

*Eye opening*
1. Nil
2. Pain
3. Verbal
4. Spontaneous

*Motor response*
1. Nil
2. Abnormal extension
3. Abnormal flexion
4. Weak flexion
5. Localizing
6. Obeys commands

*Verbal*
1. Nil
2. Incomprehensible
3. Innappropriate
4. Confused
5. Orientated

The history of events before coma is vital and should be obtained from witnesses. Having established adequate circulation and ventilation, a careful routine examination, recording the basic signs (temperature, pulse, blood pressure and respiratory pattern) will yield important information as to the probable cause of coma, and direct the next

stage of management. The smell of the breath may provide clues – alcohol, ketones and hepatic fetor. Skin texture may show evidence of dehydration and skin colour may indicate anaemia, jaundice, cyanosis or the cherry-red discolouration of carbon monoxide poisoning. Bruising may point to a bleeding disorder. Meningococcal septicaemia may produce a rash. Blisters over pressure areas suggests a deep coma, often seen in barbiturate overdose.

Valvular heart disease and endocarditis have to be excluded. Abdominal examination for enlargement of the liver, spleen and kidneys and the presence of other masses.

The neurological assessment will necessarily be limited in the comatose patient, but important observations to be made are as follows:

(i) The position of the patient and whether there are any spontaneous movements such as myoclonus.
(ii) The presence or absence of neck stiffness.
(iii) The presence or absence of papilloedema.
(iv) Examine the ears for tympanic membrane perforation.
(v) Examine the mouth and fauces for signs of infection and bleeding.
(vi) Assess the level of consciousness (Glasgow Coma Scale).
(vii) Examine tendon reflexes and plantar responses.
(viii) Assess brain-stem reflexes:
   - *Pupillary size and reactions.* Pontine lesions cause miosis with normal light reflexes. Mid-brain lesion cause unresponsive pupils, fixed in mid-position.
   - *Corneal responses.*
   - *Spontaneous eye movements.* In light coma, there is involuntary roving of the eyes and this is a normal phenomenon. Involuntary deviation of both eyes away from a paralysed limb suggests a cortical lesion, whereas if the eyes deviate towards the paralysed side a brain-stem lesion would be suspected.
   - *Reflex eye movements*, oculocephalic and oculovestibular (see below).
   - *Gag reflex.*
   - *Respiratory pattern.* Hiccough indicates a brainstem disturbance, as does Cheyne-Stokes respiration. If the medulla is also compromised, ataxic breathing may be seen.

In summary, coma associated with focal brainstem or focal cerebral signs indicates cerebral haemorrhage, infarction, tumour or abscess. Coma without focal signs can be due to diffuse cerebral anoxia, epilepsy, metabolic disturbance, drug overdose or septicaemia. The presence of meningism would suggest meningitis, encephalitis or subarachnoid haemorrhage.

Investigation should include FBC, ESR, urea and electrolytes, liver function tests, glucose, cardiac enzymes, amylase, and a drug screen. Arterial gases should be checked. ECG and chest X-ray. If the blood tests exclude a metabolic cause, a CT head scan is required and if this is normal the CSF should be examined (see Table 7.12). An EEG may help to exclude subclinical status epilepticus.

Discussions with the patient's family should take place in a quiet room, and always in the presence of the staff nurse or sister who is caring for the patient at that time. Providing the relatives with information about prognosis is difficult in the early stage of coma, and they should be given regular updates of the results of investigations and on the clinical situation. Patients who remain comatose after 10 days will either enter a persistent vegetative state or die. If the prognosis is poor, the patient should be managed on a general ward, and after full discussion with the next of kin, a decision to withhold active medical intervention (for example antibiotics for infection, or cardiac resuscitation) has to be made.

Making a diagnosis of brain death is usually done by the consultant or senior registrar, but the guidelines should be familiar to all. First, the patient must be in a state of apnoeic coma due to irreversible brain damage. Secondly, drug intoxication and a metabolic or endocrine cause must be excluded, and the rectal temperature must be higher than 35°C to rule out hypothermia. Thirdly, five brainstem tests are required to confirm brainstem death—these are as follows.

(1) No pupillary response to strong light. Pontine and brainstem lesions result in pinpoint pupils with little response to light. With the exception of opiates and glutethimide, drugs and most metabolic disorders do not affect the pupils.
(2) Absence of a corneal response following firm corneal pressure with a sterile swab.
(3) If there is no evidence of injury to the cervical spine, dolls-eye movement can be looked for by holding the eyelids open with your thumbs and rapidly turning the head from side to side. In the unconscious patient with an intact brain-stem, the eyes will lag behind the initial head movement but will catch up and adopt a fully adducted/abducted position, in the opposite direction to head movement (oculocephalic reflex). Absence of dolls-eye movement indicates severe brain-stem dysfunction.

For caloric responses (oculovestibular reflex), having first checked that the auditory canals are free of wax, 50 ml of ice-cold water is injected into each ear. In brain-stem damage, there is no eye-movement response. If the patient is comatose and there is deviation of the eyes towards the stimulated side, this would indicate a cortical lesion.

**Table 7.12. Interpretation of cerebrospinal fluid**

| CSF findings | Cells | Diagnosis |
|---|---|---|
| Thousands of WBCs, low glucose, high protein | Polymorphs | Bacterial meningitis, ruptured CNS abscess |
| >200 WBCs/mm$^3$, normal glucose, high protein | Polymorphs | Partially treated meningitis, bacterial meningitis, chemical meningitis |
| 10–200 WBCs/mm$^3$, low glucose, protein normal or raised | Polymorphs | Bacterial meningitis |
| | Lymphocytes | Tuberculosis, sarcoid, meningovascular syphilis cysticercosis |
| 10–200 WBC/mm$^3$, normal glucose and protein | Polymorphs | Neoplastic, *Cryptococcus*, early bacterial meningitis |
| | Lymphocytes | Early TB meningitis, viral encephalitis, neoplasia |

CSF glucose should normally be 40–60 per cent of serum level taken at the same time.

(4) Firm pressure over the supraorbital area or firm nailbed pressure should produce no motor response in the brain dead patient. Flexion and external rotation of the arms with extension and internal rotation of the legs in response to a painful stimulus indicates decorticate rigidity. Strong extension of both arms and legs suggests decerebrate rigidity.

(5) There should be no gag reflex to bronchial stimulation from a suction catheter passed down the trachea.

These five basic tests of brainstem reflexes must be repeated before a diagnosis of brainstem death can be made. Finally, it must be established that no respiratory movements occur during disconnection from the ventilator by ensuring that pre-oxygenation with 100 per cent oxygen is done 10 min before, and that following this, the patient breathes 5 per cent carbon dioxide in 95 per cent oxygen for 5 min before dissconnection to raise the $PaCO_2$ to 5.3 kPa. This should rise to 6.65 kPa before the patient is deemed to be brain dead according to the UK code.

The EEG has no role in the UK code of diagnosis of brain-stem death and on the whole has no prognostic value. All of the tests mentioned above have to be repeated by an independent consultant or senior registrar, and this can be done within four hours of the initial examination. With possible drug overdoses, it is best to allow a few days between examinations as the half-life of certain drugs can be extremely variable.

The next of kin should be informed of the results of the brain-stem tests, and if ventilatory support is to be discontinued, the possibility of organ donation should be sensitively raised at the earliest opportunity, to allow the relatives adequate time for discussion amongst themselves and with medical staff.

## Further reading

### General neurology textbooks

Rowland L. P., ed. (1989). *Merritt's Textbook of Neurology*, 8th edn. London: Lea & Fabiger.

Spillane J. D., Spillane J. A. (1982). *An Atlas of Clinical Neurology*, 3rd edn. Oxford: Oxford University Press.

Swash M., Oxbury J., eds. (1991). *Clinical Neurology*, Vols I and II, London: Churchill Livingstone.

### Neurological examination

*Aids to the Examination of the Peripheral Nervous System* (1986). London: Baillière Tindall.

Harrison M. J. G. (1987). *Neurological Skills. A guide to examination and management in neurology.* Oxford: Butterworth–Heinemann.

De Jong R. N. (1979). *The Neurological Examination*, 4th edn. Hagerstown: Harper & Row.

# 8

# RHEUMATOLOGY

Paul Davies

On the general ward, despite the presence of musculoskeletal problems, the locomotor system is frequently neglected. This neglect arises from blinkered attention to the 'current' problem without regard to the 'whole patient' and may, particularly in elderly patients, lead to musculoskeletal problems not being recognized until near to the time of discharge, hence delaying their return home.

The diversity of rheumatic disorders and the systemic nature of the connective tissue disorders is such that there is frequent overlap with 'general medicine', e.g., ruptured Baker's cyst mimicking a deep vein thrombosis and systemic lupus erythematosus presenting with pleuritic chest pain. As a result of this and the plethora of physical signs in rheumatic diseases, the examination candidate is likely to be confronted by a rheumatological case in the clinical part of medical examinations. Accordingly, the ability to examine the musculoskeletal system competently is important.

This chapter first goes through the history taking and examination of patients with rheumatic diseases with emphasis on the important clinical clues that can be gained. Those two sections are followed by a brief account of some of the more common rheumatic conditions and their management. The management of acute monoarthritis is then discussed and the chapter finishes with an outline of commonly used rheumatological investigations.

## HISTORY

### Age and sex

Rheumatic disorders can affect people of all ages and either sex. Rheumatoid arthritis, for instance, may start at any age, though seropositive disease is unusual before the age of 5 years. The peak incidence is between 25 and 55 years of age and the female to male ratio is 3:1.

Consideration of the age and sex of the patient may occasionally be of diagnostic value as is the case with gout and gonococcal arthritis. The aphorisms of Hippocrates (460–357 BC) on gout still hold true: 'Eunuchs do not take the gout. A woman does not take the gout, unless her menses be stopped. A youth does not get gout before sexual intercourse.'

Accordingly, a diagnosis of gout may effectively be ruled out in prepubertal boys and menstruating females. Gonococcal arthritis is usually confined to females because their asymptomatic genital infection may go untreated. In contrast the urethritis in males usually leads to early treatment but gonococcal arthritis may be seen in homosexuals where occult rectal or pharyngeal infection is the septic source.

## Race

Osteomalacia and tuberculosis are still frequently seen in the UK immigrant population, especially in the Asian community. Sickle cell disease also occurs in immigrant populations, particularly blacks from Africa and the New World. It often causes painful crises involving bone and joint, and leading to aseptic necrosis and transient synovitis.

## Symptoms

In musculoskeletal disorders, symptoms may arise from joints, bone or muscle. Pain, stiffness, swelling and the resulting disability are the hallmarks of joint disease. The joints involved, and the duration, frequency and intensity of symptoms, may give rise to a pattern that allows a differentiation to be made between the various forms of arthritis.

## Pain

This is the symptom that troubles patients most. Some patients, in addition to experiencing pain on movement, may describe rest pain. Such pain is particularly troublesome at night and is characteristic of periarticular disorders of the shoulder (e.g., frozen shoulder), advanced osteoarthritis of the hip and knee, and osteoid osteoma.

In the case of backache, night pain raises the possibility of malignant secondary deposits.

## Stiffness

Stiffness is a sense of resistance to free movement and subjectively is closely linked with pain. Early morning stiffness of one or more hours' duration is a characteristic feature of inflammatory rheumatic disorders, such as polymyalgia rheumatica and inflammatory arthritis. In contrast, morning stiffness in osteoarthritis is short-lived, being seldom longer than 30 min. The duration of morning stiffness is shortened by exercise, heat and drug therapy, particularly non-steroidal anti-inflammatory agents and steroids. Its precise cause is unclear but is thought to be due to congestion of the synovium and para-articular tissues (joint capsule, ligaments and muscle). Clinically, a tight joint effusion is frequently the explanation for a particularly 'stiff joint'. During the day, patients often find that their affected joints feel stiff after resting (e.g., sitting). This phenomenon is known as 'gelling' and occurs not only in osteoarthritis but also in inflammatory arthritis.

## Locking

Joint locking characteristically occurs in meniscal lesions of the knee when the loose fragment causes a block in extension. Locking can also be caused by loose bodies and may therefore be seen in osteochondritis dissecans, osteochondromatosis and osteoarthritis. Spinal flexion sometimes induces 'locking', whereby the victim is temporarily immobilized with severe back pain and associated muscle spasm.

## Pattern of joint involvement

A clear outline of the temporal and anatomical pattern of joint involvement is important in history taking.

The temporal aspect is best exemplified by acute gout in which the sufferer is typically woken in the night by severe pain in the metatarsophalangeal joint of the big toe (podagra). The joint becomes hot, red and swollen and the patient is often unable to tolerate even the weight of bedclothes on the affected foot. After 2 to 14 days the joint returns to normal. Episodic arthritis may also be seen in pseudogout, palindromic rheumatism, intermittent hydrarthrosis and familial Mediterranean fever.

Some patients describe a migratory arthritis in which the symptoms move from one joint to another. The flitting arthritis of rheumatic fever is well recognized but it may also be seen in gonococcal and Lyme arthritis.

Which joints are involved, their number and the symmetry of involvement are also important. An acute monoarthritis is typical of crystal arthritis, infective arthritis and haemophilia (see later). Some diseases run an oligo- or pauciarticular pattern (four or fewer joints involved) such as pauciarticular juvenile arthritis, Reiter's disease, psoriatic arthritis and the peripheral arthritis of ankylosing spondylitis. Typically the arthritis is asymmetrical in these conditions.

Sometimes, however, the peripheral joint involvement in Reiter's disease, psoriatic arthritis and ankylosing spondylitis is symmetrical and polyarticular (more than four joints). Symmetrical polyarthritis of this kind though is more typical of rheumatoid arthritis and systemic lupus erythematosus.

## Constitutional symptoms

Fever, malaise, lethargy and weight loss are common systemic effects of inflammatory disease, be it infective or autoimmune in origin. Accordingly, they are a not infrequent accompaniment of inflammatory rheumatic disease, particularly rheumatoid arthritis and the connective tissue diseases. Less commonly they may occur in the crystal-induced arthritides and the seronegative spondarthritides. High fevers are usually associated with septic arthritis and rheumatic fever. A swinging pyrexia (remittent fever) is typical of systemic juvenile chronic arthritis (Still's disease) but may also occasionally be found in the connective tissue diseases.

It should be remembered that patients with inflammatory arthritis and connective tissue disease are more susceptible to infection. Therefore the presence of high fever and rigors should still suggest articular or extra-articular infection; blood cultures and other appropriate investigations should therefore be undertaken. In the connective tissue diseases it is sometimes extremely difficult to differentiate between an infection and a true flare of the disease.

## Extra-articular features

Extra-articular manifestations are clinical features that span both history and examination but as some of these manifestations may no longer be extant when the patient is seen they are here discussed under history. Clinically, by adopting a 'wide-angle lens' approach, the astute physician will often be able to clinch the diagnosis by finding, for example, a tophus or patch of psoriasis.

As patients are unlikely to associate, for example, an attack of uveitis with their current back pain, it is important to enquire into their previous medical history and to complete a systems review by direct questioning, as follows.

## Eyes

The ocular tissue involved may vary from disease to disease (see Table 8.1). The dry, gritty eyes of keratoconjunctivitis sicca occur as part of Sjögren's syndrome and are seen in various autoimmune conditions, particularly rheumatoid arthritis. Rheumatoid arthritis is also the most common rheumatic condition in which episcleritis and scleritis may be seen. Such patients usually have longstanding seropositive disease and may have other extra-articular features, e.g., vasculitis. Various different kinds of scleritis may affect the eye in rheumatoid arthritis, of which scleromalacia perforans is the best known. This is a necrotizing scleritis without apparent adjacent inflammation in which a greyish-yellow, necrotic scleral nodule develops and later separates, leaving bare choroid with consequent risk of rupture.

Uveitis is a relatively common disorder. An association between acute anterior uveitis and the seronegative spondarthritides has long been recognized; in recent years, studies have shown that approximately 50 per cent of patients presenting with acute anterior uveitis carry the HLA B27 antigen. Not surprisingly, many of these patients have ankylosing spondylitis or go on to develop features of the disease at a later date.

Uveitis is not found any more often in rheumatoid arthritis than in the non-rheumatoid population. However, occasional patients with severe

**Table 8.1 Rheumatic disorders and the eye**

|  | Conjunctivitis | Kerato-conjunctivitis sicca | Episcleritis | Scleritis | Uveitis | Retinal vasculitis |
|---|---|---|---|---|---|---|
| Juvenile chronic arthritis |  |  |  |  | + |  |
| Rheumatoid arthritis |  | + | + | + |  |  |
| Systemic lupus erythematosus | + | + | + | + | + (rare) | + |
| Progressive systemic sclerosis |  | + | + | + |  |  |
| Polymyositis/dermatomyositis |  | + | + | + |  | + |
| Mixed connective tissue disease |  | + |  |  |  |  |
| Polyarteritis nodosa | + | + | + | + | + (rare) | + |
| Wegener's granulomatosis | + |  | + | + | + (rare) | + |
| Relapsing polychondritis | + |  | + |  | + | + |
| Ankylosing spondylitis |  |  |  |  | + |  |
| Reiter's disease | + |  |  |  | + |  |
| Psoriatic arthritis | + |  |  |  | + |  |
| Colitic arthritis |  |  |  |  | + |  |
| *Yersinia* arthritis | + | + |  |  | + |  |
| Sarcoidosis |  |  |  |  | + | + |
| Behçet's syndrome | + |  | + |  | + | + |

episcleritis or scleritis may have secondary inflammatory changes in the uveal tract.

In contrast to the pain, redness and blurring of vision in acute anterior uveitis, the chronic iridocyclitis of juvenile chronic arthritis is an insidious disorder in which visual acuity is gradually lost. It is mainly seen in pauciarticular, antinuclear antibody-positive cases and such patients must have regular slit-lamp examinations so that any early signs of iridocyclitis may be detected and treated.

Retinal vasculitis causes vascular occlusion and retinal oedema. In systemic lupus erythematosus, retinal microinfarcts give rise to cotton-wool spots (cytoid bodies) but visual impairment is uncommon. There is though, a high risk of visual loss in temporal arteritis due to involvement of the branches of the ophthalmic artery.

When patients with established rheumatic disease develop eye symptoms the possibility of iatrogenic disease needs to be considered. Steroids are known to cause posterior subcapsular cataracts and antimalarials are associated with reversible keratopathy and irreversible retinopathy.

### Skin and mucous membranes

#### Subcutaneous lumps and nodules

Rheumatoid nodules occur in 20 to 30 per cent of patients with rheumatoid arthritis; they are virtually confined to seropositive disease (Fig. 8.1). They are most frequently found over pressure points—ulnar border of the forearm, olecranon, occiput, sacrum and Achilles tendon. Similar nodules have rarely been described in systemic lupus erythematosus. Like rheumatoid nodules, the subcutaneous nodules seen in rheumatic fever are located over bony prominences and tendons. They differ from rheumatoid nodules in tending to be smaller and less persistent.

Nodular swellings are also a feature of multicentric reticulohistiocytosis and hyperlipidaemia (Type II and III), and may be confused with rheumatoid nodules when over the hands and elbows. Occasionally tophi may look like rheumatoid nodules, though usually the chalky-white, crystalline monosodium urate monohydrate can be seen through the thinned, shiny skin, allowing differentiation (Fig. 8.2). The diagnosis can easily be confirmed by aspirating the tophus and looking for urate crystals by polarizing microscopy. Tophi are commonly found in periarticular tissues, bursae, tendon sheaths and the pinna of the ear.

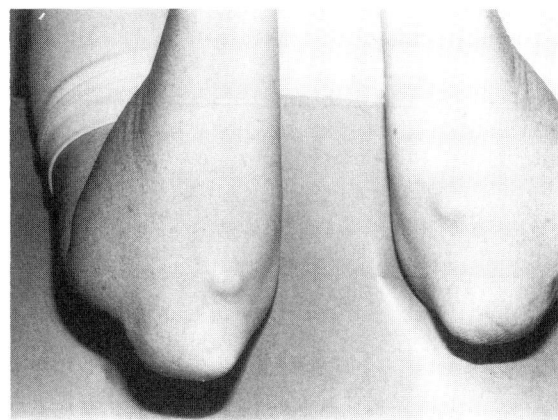

Figure 8.1 Subcutaneous rheumatoid nodules on the extensor aspect of the forearms of a patient with seropositive rheumatoid arthritis.

Heberden's nodes (osteoarthritis) and fluctuant swellings of the tendon sheath seldom give rise to diagnostic difficulties.

### Nails

Nail abnormalities occur in 80 per cent of patients with psoriatic arthritis compared with 20 per cent of patients with psoriasis alone. The commonest changes are nail pitting and onycholysis. The subungual hyperkeratosis leading to onycholysis is also occasionally seen in patients with Reiter's disease. Vasculitis, particularly rheumatoid vasculitis, may cause small cutaneous infarcts in the nail fold: 'nail-fold lesions'; (Fig. 8.3); in dermatomyositis, characteristic nail-fold telangiectasis

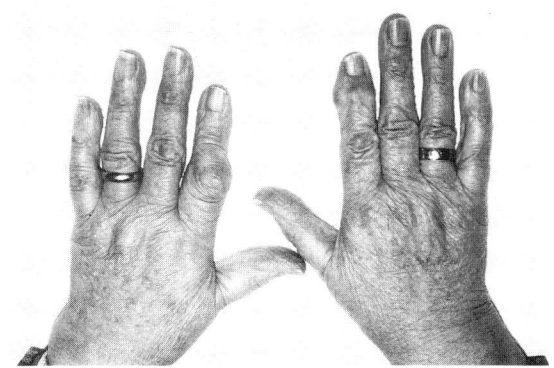

Figure 8.2 Chronic tophaceous gout in the hand.

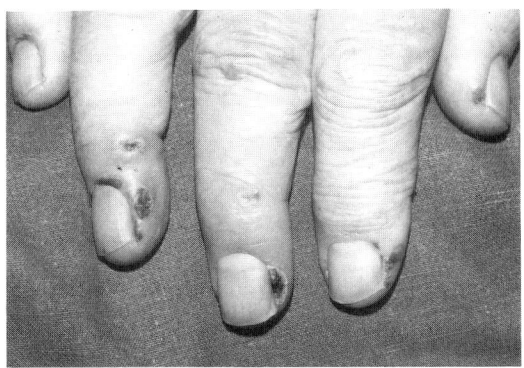

*Figure 8.3* Vasculitic nail-fold lesions in a patient with rheumatoid arthritis.

may be present. Whilst the physician may expect to see the occasional case of finger clubbing associated with hypertrophic pulmonary osteoarthropathy, the nail-fold coral beading of multicentric reticulohistiocytosis and the hypoplastic nails of the nail–patella syndrome would be rare events.

### Hair

Alopecia is a frequent accompaniment of systemic lupus erythematosus and often mirrors the activity of the disease. Diffuse rather than patchy alopecia is the commoner pattern. Diffuse alopecia is also seen in mixed connective tissue disease, dermatomyositis and after drug therapy, e.g., cyclophosphamide.

### Skin

A variety of rashes may be associated with rheumatic diseases. Psoriasis is distinctive when it occurs in plaques over the extensor surfaces. However, the lesions may be scanty and then examination of the scalp, behind the ears, the navel and the natal cleft can be rewarding. There is an interesting overlap both clinically and histologically between keratoderma blenorrhagica (Reiter's disease) and pustular psoriasis. Typically in Reiter's disease the vesiculopustular rash is seen on the soles and palms (Fig. 8.4) but in severe cases there may be hyperkeratotic plaques over the scalp and trunk.

The bacteraemia in gonococcal and meningococcal infection may be associated with skin lesions and arthritis. In gonococcal bacteraemia the lesions are initially vesiculopustular and later become haemorrhagic, whilst the meningococcal rash is more purpuric. An extensive maculopapular purpura is also the hallmark of Henoch–Schönlein purpura, typically involving the buttocks and extensor surfaces. In these diseases the purpura is vasculitic in origin and a similar pattern may occasionally be seen in polyarteritis nodosa (Fig. 8.5). More commonly, though, other changes of cutaneous vasculitis, namely livedo reticularis, digital infarcts and vasculitic ulcers, are seen in polyarteritis nodosa. Similar vasculitic changes may be found in rheumatoid vasculitis and systemic lupus erythematosus but photosensitivity and the 'butterfly' facial rash are more classical skin manifestions in the latter. Dermatomyositis and scleroderma are easily recognized by characteristic skin changes. The typical rash in dermatomyositis is a purplish, sometimes scaly erythema on the face, particularly the upper eyelids ('heliotrope rash') with violaceous plaques on the backs of the knuckles ('collodion patches' or 'Gottron's papules').

Scleroderma is characterized by skin thickening, tethering and tightness, involving particularly the hands, face and anterior chest wall (Fig. 8.6). Later in the disease, facial telangiectasia is common. Interestingly, subcutaneous calcinosis is seen in both diseases.

Various important skin eruptions are associated

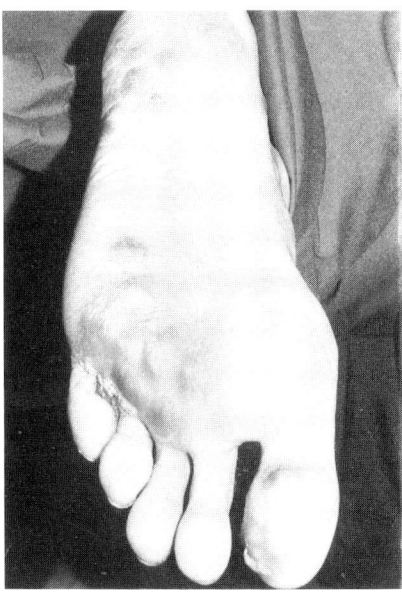

*Figure 8.4* Keratoderma blenorrhagica.

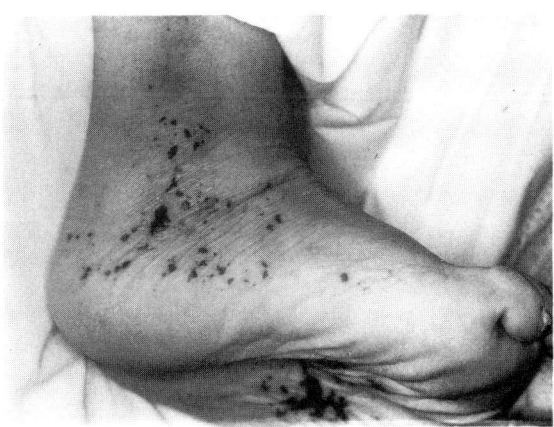

Figure 8.5 Vasculitic purpura in polyarteritis nodosa.

with rheumatic diseases. Erythema nodosum appears over the shins and is often associated with arthritis. The most common cause is sarcoidosis. Erythema marginatum is now rarely seen but is of diagnostic importance in rheumatic fever. The erythematous rash of systemic-onset, juvenile chronic arthritis (Still's disease) is an evanescent maculopapular rash over the trunk and limbs, best seen at the time of the evening fever.

When faced with a new skin eruption the possi-

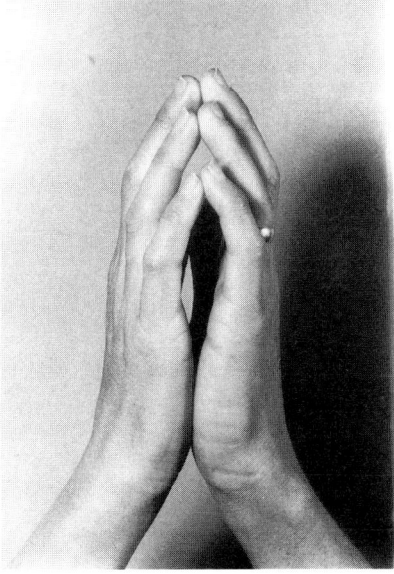

Figure 8.6 Flexion contracture of the fingers in progressive systemic sclerosis. This is a result of skin tightening and tendon involvement.

bility of a drug reaction should always be considered (e.g., fenbufen, allopurinol, gold, penicillamine and antimalarials).

### Orogenital lesions

The oral ulceration that occurs in systemic lupus erythematosus and Reiter's disease tends to be asymptomatic, whilst in Behçet's syndrome the ulceration is often painful. Similarly, the genital lesions in Reiter's disease ('circinate balanitis') are usually painless whilst the vulval and scrotal ulcers of Behçet's syndrome are painful. The urethritis of Reiter's disease is usually, but not always, symptomatic.

### Cardiovascular manifestions

These may be divided into peripheral and cardiac manifestations. The peripheral manifestations are Raynaud's phenomenon and arteritic changes such as cutaneous vasculitis (small vessels; see the foregoing section on 'Skin'), gangrene and claudication (large and medium-sized arteries as in Takayasu's and giant cell arteritis). Raynaud's phenomenon is particularly common in progressive systemic sclerosis, occurring in up to 90 per cent of cases. Both in this disease and in mixed connective tissue disease, Raynaud's phenomenon is often severe, resulting in repeated, small infarcts with loss of fingertip pulp and tuft resorption (see Fig. 8.6). Raynaud's phenomenon is also seen in systemic lupus erythematosus, rheumatoid arthritis, Sjögren's syndrome, dermatomyositis and polymyositis.

The main cardiac manifestations associated with the different rheumatic diseases are detailed in Table 8.2. Most of these cardiac lesions are uncommon with the exception of rheumatoid and lupus pericarditis, which have been found on echocardiography in half or more of cases. An important cardiovascular complication not listed in the table is hypertension, which is a frequent accompaniment of renal involvement in the connective tissue diseases and is also common in Hurler's syndrome.

Occasionally, rheumatic problems are secondary to cardiac diseases, e.g., atrial myxoma and subacute bacterial endocarditis.

### Respiratory manifestations

The pulmonary features that may be seen in various rheumatic diseases are shown in Table 8.3.

Such patients may have typical respiratory symptoms, such as dyspnoea, pleuritic chest pain, cough and sometimes haemoptysis. It should be remembered, however, that through reduced mobility arthritic patients may not experience shortness of breath until the respiratory disease is fairly advanced. Many patients with connective tissue diseases develop lung infiltrates associated with fever (see Table 8.3) and in such cases infective causes must be excluded by appropriate microbiological investigation. Differentiation cannot reliably be made by X-ray appearance alone. Similarly, confusion may occur when the nodular lesions of rheumatoid arthritis and Wegener's granulomatosis cavitate, mimicking tuberulous lesions. However, in erythema nodosum and hypertrophic pulmonary osteoarthropathy the chest X-ray may be diagnostic.

Patients with connective tissue diseases are more prone to infections, particularly respiratory infections. This is certainly the case in Sjögren's syndrome, where reduction of bronchial secretions may play some part in the increased vulnerability these patients have to respiratory infections. In progressive systemic sclerosis and polymyositis, aspiration pneumonia is a potential complication of the dysphagia that these patients may have.

Pulmonary changes may also occur as a complication of drug therapy in rheumatic diseases.

Aspirin is known occasionally to precipitate asthma in sensitive individuals; cytotoxic drugs and gold may rarely cause pulmonary fibrosis. A few cases of Goodpasture's syndrome have been reported in patients taking penicillamine.

Changes in the upper respiratory tract may be seen in rheumatoid arthritis and relapsing polychondritis. In rheumatoid arthritis, involvement of the crico-arytenoid joint may cause hoarseness and more rarely dyspnoea and stridor. Epiglottic and laryngeal involvement in polychondritis will produce similar symptoms, and collapse of the tracheal and bronchial rings causes breathlessness and wheezing.

### Nervous system

Paraesthesiae are a common complaint in rheumatological practice and are frequently due to root involvement from disease of cervical or lumbar discs. Carpal tunnel syndrome is also a common cause of paraesthesiae, through compression of the median nerve at the wrist by inflammatory synovitis, e.g., rheumatoid arthritis and psoriatic arthritis.

Less commonly, paraesthesiae may be due to a peripheral neuropathy secondary to a vasculitic illness such as polyarteritis nodosa, Wegener's granulomatosis, systemic lupus erythematosus

**Table 8.2 Cardiac manifestations associated with various rheumatic diseases**

| | Juvenile chronic arthritis | Rheumatoid arthritis | Systemic lupus erythematosus | Progressive systemic sclerosis | Dermatomyositis/polymyositis | Polyarteritis nodosa | Temporal arteritis | Relapsing polychondritis | Ankylosing spondylitis | Reiter's disease | Psoriatic arthritis | Rheumatic fever | Marfan's syndrome | Hurler's syndrome |
|---|---|---|---|---|---|---|---|---|---|---|---|---|---|---|
| Conduction defects | | + | + | + | + | + | | + | + | + | | + | | |
| Pericarditis | + | + | + | + | + | + | | + | + | + | | + | | |
| Heart muscle disease | + | + | + | + | + | + | | | | | | + | | |
| Myocardial infarction | | + | + | | | + | + | + | | | | | | |
| Aortic incompetence | | + | + (rare) | | | | | + | + | + | + | + | + | + |
| Other valvular lesions | | + | | | | | | + (rare) | + (rare) | + | | + | + | + |

**Table 8.3 Respiratory manifestations of various rheumatic diseases**

| | Juvenile chronic arthritis | Rheumatoid arthritis | Sjögren's syndrome | Systemic lupus erythematosus | Progressive systemic sclerosis | Polymyositis/dermatomyositis | Polyarteritis nodosa | Wegener's granulomatosis | Ankylosing spondylitis | Reiter's disease | Rheumatic fever |
|---|---|---|---|---|---|---|---|---|---|---|---|
| Pleurisy | + | + | + | + | +<br>(rare) | | | + | | + | |
| Pleural effusion | + | + | + | + | +<br>(rare) | + | | + | | | |
| Pulmonary fibrosis | + | + | + | + | + | | + | + | + | | |
| Lung infiltrates/pneumonitis | +<br>(rare) | +<br>(rare) | +<br>(rare) | + | | | | + | | + | + |
| Nodules | | + | | | | | | + | | | |
| Asthma | | | | | | | + | | | | |

and rheumatoid vasculitis. The picture is usually that of a mononeuritis multiplex but, through multiple nerve involvement, a symmetrical sensorimotor pattern may result. In rheumatoid patients, sensory symptoms may be the first indication of cord compression secondary to cervical subluxation. However, it is frequently not until there is motor involvement with spastic tetraparesis or paraparesis that the diagnosis is made.

### Renal manifestations

Renal impairment is a not uncommon accompaniment of rheumatic disease; it may be due to the disease itself or drug-induced. Fortunately, severe renal disease is infrequent, but when present is of adverse prognostic significance. The development of glomerulonephritis in systemic lupus erythematosus, polyarteritis nodosa, Wegener's granulomatosis and Henoch–Schönlein purpura is well recognized and may present as proteinuria, haematuria, nephrosis, acute nephritis or just as deteriorating renal function. In rheumatoid patients, glomerular disease due to rheumatoid arthritis per se is surprisingly rare, whilst glomerular involvement from gold, penicillamine (membranous nephropathy) and secondary amyloid is more frequently recognized. Renal amyloid may also be a late development in patients with anky-

losing spondylitis and juvenile chronic arthritis. It usually presents with heavy proteinuria and may be diagnosed either indirectly through rectal biopsy or directly through renal biopsy.

Renal tubular defects are seen in Sjögren's syndrome (renal tubular acidosis). The tubules also bear the brunt of the damage in urate nephropathy, interstitial nephritis and analgesic nephropathy. Interstitial nephritis following the use of non-steroidal anti-inflammatory drugs is rare but has been the subject of several case reports in recent years.

### Causative factors

The cause of a particular rheumatic problem is often apparent from the history, e.g., a meniscal lesion after a football injury or the development of a polyarthritis in a young woman who has just recovered from rubella. However, a history of trauma, infection or exposure to infection is not always forthcoming and then direct questioning may be needed. Enquiry into the possibility of sexual contacts may be necessary and must be handled tactfully.

### Drug history

Certain rheumatic conditions may be precipitated or sometimes exacerbated by drugs (Table 8.4).

The precipitation of acute gout by diuretics is a frequent occurrence, whilst drug-induced lupus is relatively rare.

Clearly, as well as documenting all current medication, previous antirheumatic therapy and any adverse reactions should be recorded as this will influence further therapeutic strategies. With gold, penicillamine, steroids and cytotoxic drugs it is important to ascertain when the drug was used, in what dosage and the reason it was stopped (lack of effect or toxicity).

Finally, any history of drug allergy should be noted in the usual way.

## Previous medical history

Any previous or concomitant disease such as peptic ulceration or ischaemic heart disease should be documented as it may influence future drug and surgical treatment, respectively. All orthopaedic operations and their dates should be noted.

**Table 8.4 Drugs precipitating rheumatic disorders**

*Drugs and toxins that may precipitate acute gout*
Diuretics (especially thiazides)
Pyrazinamide
Ethambutol
Aspirin (low dose—<2 g/day)
Allopurinol
Uricosuric drugs
Cytotoxic therapy
Alcohol
Chronic lead poisoning
*Drugs that may cause a disease flare in SLE*
Oral contraceptives
Penicillin
Sulphonamides
*Drugs that may induce a lupus-like syndrome*
Hydralazine
Procainamide
Isoniazid
Phenytoin
Ethosuximide
Propylthiouracil
Penicillamine
*Serum sickness type of drug reaction*
(causes arthritis rash and fever)
Penicillin
Aspirin
Streptomycin
Sulphonamides
Thiouracils
Carbamazepine

## Family history

A positive family history may be present in several rheumatic disorders (e.g., gout and nodal osteoarthritis) and this may be helpful diagnostically. Patients with seronegative spondarthritis often have a family history of uveitis, colitis, psoriasis, Reiter's disease or ankylosing spondylitis.

That occasional clustering of rheumatoid cases occurs within families has been appreciated for some time and in recent years tissue-typing studies have shown a strong correlation with HLA DW4 and HLA DR4, confirming a genetic component.

Certain inherited diseases are associated with rheumatic problems: haemophilia A and B (X-linked recessive), sickle cell disease (recessive), haemochromatosis (recessive), ochronosis (recessive), osteogenesis imperfecta (the commonly seen variety is Type 1—dominant) and pachydermoperiostitis (dominant). Where these inherited diseases arise from spontaneous mutations (up to 25 per cent of cases in haemophilia A) there will not be a positive family history.

The family history is not only important in looking at genetic factors but also at the possibility of exposure to pathogens through other family members, as in the case of tuberculosis.

## Social history

Illness affects not only the 'whole person' but also the whole family. An awareness of this and the subsequent handling of it is just as important as making a diagnosis and prescribing medication. The degree of disability and its interaction with the family, home and work environment needs to be assessed.

The patient's ability to carry out various activities of daily living (ADL) should be inquired into. By getting an assessment of the patient's ability to dress, wash, bathe, manage in the toilet, manage housework, cook, eat and walk, a picture of the level of disability can be built up. When mobility is compromised, the position of the toilet, bathroom and bedroom will need consideration and if significant problems are revealed, the help of the occupational therapist should be sought. Additionally, the level of social support should be noted—home help, meals on wheels, etc.

A patient's occupation may occasionally play some causative role, e.g., de Quervain's tenosynovitis in operators of visual display units, Caplan's syndrome in miners and acro-osteolysis in workmen who clean reactor vessels containing the polymerizing agent vinyl chloride.

## EXAMINATION

### General points

All patients with rheumatic problems should have a full medical examination so that important extra-articular manifestations such as splenomegaly and gouty tophi are not missed and any concomitant medical problem such as ischaemic heart disease or chronic bronchitis may be assessed. Consideration of such medical problems becomes particularly important when orthopaedic operations are being considered.

An orderly system of examination of the locomotor system is mandatory, so as not to miss any important physical clues that may be present. The time-honoured sequence of inspection, palpation and movement (look, feel, move) should be followed.

### Inspection

Before looking at individual joints, much may be gained from general observation of the patient's movements, gait and posture; a process that begins on the entry of the patient into the consultation room.

When examining a joint, the overlying skin should be inspected for erythema, as may be seen with an acutely inflamed joint (e.g., septic arthritis, acute gout and palindromic rheumatism). Also tell-tale scars from previous joint surgery or old osteomyelitic sinuses may be present.

Muscle wasting and joint swelling are usually self-evident or can be identified by comparison with the other side. The presence of deformity in either the axial skeleton (e.g., kyphoscoliosis) or peripheral skeleton (flexion deformities, subluxations and valgus/varus deformities) should be noted. The position of the deformity will suggest whether it is in the bone (e.g., fracture and Paget's disease) or whether it is a joint deformity.

### Palpation

Plunging straight into palpating what may be an extremely tender joint is unlikely to endear the doctor to the patient or to an examiner. Accord-ingly, it is wise to enquire of the patient whether or not the joint is tender beforehand and during the examination to watch the patient's expression to see if he or she is in discomfort or not.

The joint should first be felt for any increased warmth using the back of the fingers and comparing with the other side. It is important not to be misled by the increased warmth that is present over a joint when it has just had a splint or elasticated support removed.

Next the joint itself may be palpated along the joint line and around the periarticular structures. Tenderness may be diffuse as with an inflamed arthritic joint or localized over a ligamentous or muscular insertion or origin, e.g., the medial collateral ligament of the knee and the lateral epicondyle of the elbow (in tennis elbow). When palpating a joint the type of swelling may be determined. The hardness of bony swelling is easily recognized but the 'boggy' feel of inflamed synovium ranges from the obvious to the subtle. The presence of a joint effusion may be similarly easy or difficult to detect (cross-fluctuation being the usual characteristic). Around the joint other swellings may be found, such as nodules, bursae and effusions of the tendon sheath. Palpation of muscles may be relevant and any tenderness or swelling should be noted.

### Movement

Proper assessment may inevitably involve some painful movements of the joint but it is still possible for the doctor to be both thorough and considerate. Active movement may be limited by pain or weakness and in peripheral joints passive movement should be studied as well, in order to determine the range of articular movement. Movement can be measured using a goniometer (Fig. 8.7) (peripheral joints) or tape measure (axial skeleton). The normal anatomical position is taken as the zero position, with the exception that the palms of the hands are against the thigh in the sagittal plane. The elbow, knee and interphalangeal joints have no natural extension beyond the zero position and any presence of hyperextension is suggestive of hypermobility (see below). At the opposite end of the spectrum is joint ankylosis (complete loss of motion of a joint).

During joint movement a fine or coarse grating sensation (crepitus) may be felt or even heard. (Crepitus may also be felt over tendon sheaths and

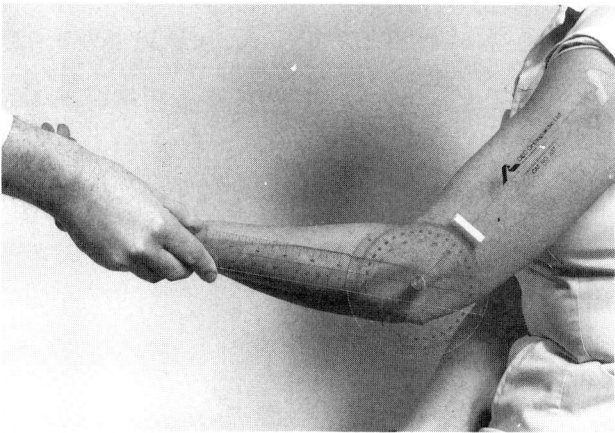

*Figure 8.7* A goniometer, which is used for measuring the range of movement in large joints.

is a particular feature of progressive systemic sclerosis.)

### Hypermobility

The range of movement of an individual joint varies from person to person and diminishes with age. It shows a Gaussian distribution in the normal population. In general, women have more lax joints than men; and joint laxity is more marked in Asians than Africans or Europeans. Joint hypermobility may be due to a familial tendency or be caused by certain inherited diseases, e.g., Marfan's syndrome, homocystinuria, osteogenesis imperfecta and Ehlers–Danlos syndrome.

The presence of hypermobility is assessed using a standard set of manoeuvres (passive), as follows.

| | | |
|---|---|---|
| (1) | Bending the little finger back to 90° or more | 2 points (one for each hand) |
| (2) | Flexing the wrist and placing the thumb against the ulnar aspect of the wrist | 2 points (one for each thumb) |
| (3) | Hyperextending the elbow by more than 10° | 2 points (one for each elbow) |
| (4) | Hyperextending the knee by more than 10° | 2 points (one for each knee) |
| (5) | Placing the hands flat on the floor while standing with the knees straight | 1 point |

This gives a total potential score of 9 points; a patient is regarded as being hypermobile if the score is 5 or more. The clinical importance of hypermobility lies in its association with nonspecific aches and pains and affected subjects seem to be more prone to early osteoarthritis and pyrophosphate arthropathy. Possible extra-articular associations include hernia, varicose veins, pneumothorax and prolapse of the mitral valve.

### EXAMINATION OF THE AXIAL SKELETON AND PERIPHERAL JOINTS

A method for examination of the axial skeleton and the various peripheral joints follows. Detailed noting of precise joint movements may be restricted to those that are obviously deformed or limited.

### The axial skeleton

Before individual parts of the spine are examined, the posture of the whole spine should be noted whilst the patient is standing. Any obvious lordosis, kyphosis, gibbus or scoliosis and the level at which it occurs should be observed.

### Cervical spine

For musculoskeletal purposes the neck is best viewed from behind and any tilt (torticollis), swelling or muscle wasting noted. The neck should be palpated for lymph nodes as their presence may be directly relevant, e.g., acute lymphadenitis may cause torticollis in children. The supraclavicular fossae should be examined for possible cervical ribs and sometimes the hard craggy mass of an advancing Pancoast's tumour may be felt.

Lastly, any tenderness over the spinous processes, paracervical or trapezius muscles should be noted.

Both active and passive movements of the neck should be tested in: flexion (45°), extension (50°), lateral flexion (60°) and rotation (70°).

In cervical disc disease, side bending and lateral extension may precipitate root symptoms and is a valuable confirmatory sign (foraminal compression test).

Evidence of compression at the thoracic outlet can be conveniently sought at this stage by feeling the radial pulse for any diminution or obliteration while carrying out one or both of the following manoeuvres:

(1) Shoulder bracing—the patient's arms are raised to 90° in abduction and then externally rotated with the elbows flexed to 90°.

(2) Pulling down on each of the patient's arms in turn whilst he or she is standing.

These manoeuvres sometimes reproduce the patient's symptoms.

### Thoracic spine

Any deformity should be noted. Fixed scoliosis is associated with twisting of the thoracic cage so that the ribs on the convex side of the curve are more prominent posteriorly. Palpation of the spine may reveal local tenderness. Such a finding may relate to spinal disease (e.g., spinal tuberculosis and vertebral collapse due to secondary deposits or osteoporosis), but more frequently is nonspecific.

The main movement of the thoracic spine is rotation (70°; Fig. 8.8). The patient is examined seated, in order to anchor the pelvis, and then asked to twist round first one way and then the other (with the arms folded). Any pain on movement should be documented, particularly if it reproduces the patient's pain as may be the case in thoracic disc disease. Symmetrical diminution in rotation would favour a diagnosis of ankylosing spondylitis.

In assessing a patient with ankylosing spondylitis, chest expansion should be measured as this frequently becomes limited due to costovertebral involvement. The arms should be elevated to 90° to raise the scapulae out of the way and then, with a tape measure around the chest at nipple level, the difference between full inspiration and expiration should be measured. Accurate measurements are more difficult in the female but should read 5 cm or more in either sex.

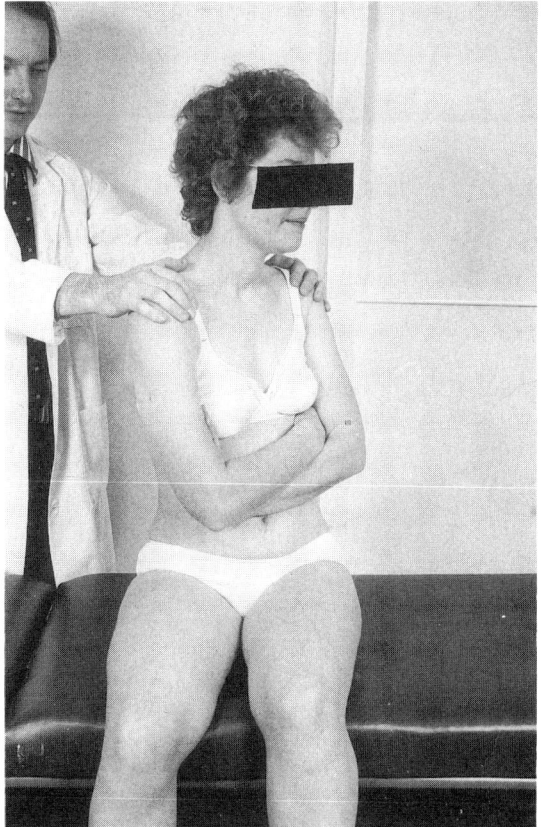

*Figure 8.8* Thoracic rotation. With the patient seated to fix the pelvis, the shoulders are then rotated.

### Lumbar spine

Inspection and palpation of the lumbar spine is usually done concurrently with that of the thoracic spine and the same points apply. The spinous processes of the lumbar spine should be palpated not only to locate any tenderness but also to ascertain if there is any 'step-up' suggestive of spondylolisthesis (usually at L4/5 or L5/S1). Either side of the spinous processes should also be palpated and may provoke radicular pain in cases of prolapsed intervertebral disc. Sometimes tenderness is localized to the area between L5 and the iliac crest over the iliolumbar ligament.

Flexion is examined by standing behind the patient whilst he or she bends forward to 'touch the toes'. With a postural scoliosis the abnormal curvature disappears on full flexion whilst in the case of a fixed structural scoliosis the deformity becomes more obvious. The persistence of a scoliosis on flexion may also be seen in compensatory scoliosis (due to unequal limb length) and sciatic scoliosis. Some patients have a transitory scoliosis on straightening up from flexion (a 'mechanical wiggle'), which may be seen in association with instability, particularly spondylolisthesis. A patient's ability to touch the toes is a measure not only of spinal mobility but also of hip mobility and hamstring tightness. More objective measurements of spinal flexion may be made using the modified Schober's test (Fig. 8.9). In this test, a line is drawn 10 cm above and 5 cm below the level of the dimples of Venus (lumbosacral junction), with the patient standing. Then, on flexion, the distance between the top and bottom mark is remeasured with a tape measure—an increase by at least 5 cm is usual.

Having assessed flexion, the examiner should then go on to test extension and lateral flexion (side bending).

All patients with back pain, particularly those with a history of sciatica, should have their straight leg raising and lower limb neurology assessed. In Lasègue's test (straight leg raising) the subject lies flat on their back and the leg to be tested is raised passively with the knee straight (normal 90°; Fig. 8.10a). This manoeuvre pulls on the dura and sciatic nerve roots and in the presence of a disc prolapse will induce pain and contraction of the hamstring muscles, thereby limiting the degree of straight leg raising. If the leg is then lowered slightly and the patient's foot dorsiflexed (sciatic stretch test; Fig. 8.10b), root irritation may again be provoked, with pain radiating down the leg and up into the lumbar region.

The specificity of Lasègue's test in the diagnosis of root compression (L5, S1) is much greater when the straight leg raising is limited to 45° or less. The precipitation of back pain alone during these tests is of dubious diagnostic value as it may be due to movement of the lumbar spine as the pelvis rotates and the lumbar spine flattens.

Straight leg raising may also be limited by tight hamstrings and is usually a bilateral finding, with the patient complaining of a tight discomfort behind the knee.

Sometimes patients with a prolapsed lower

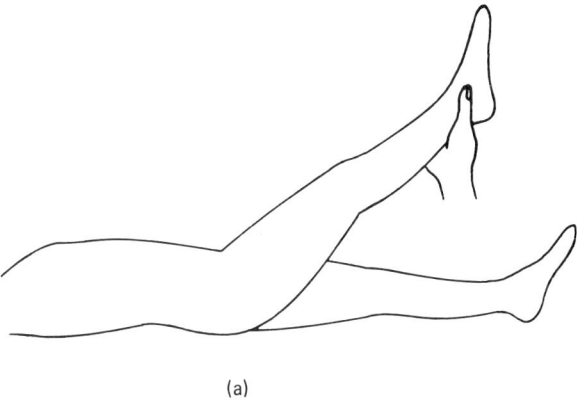

(a)

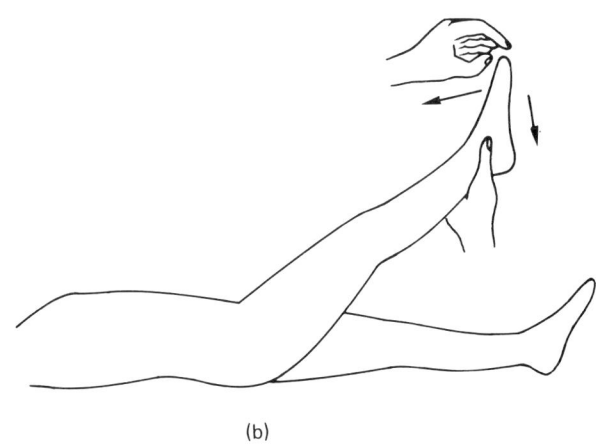

(b)

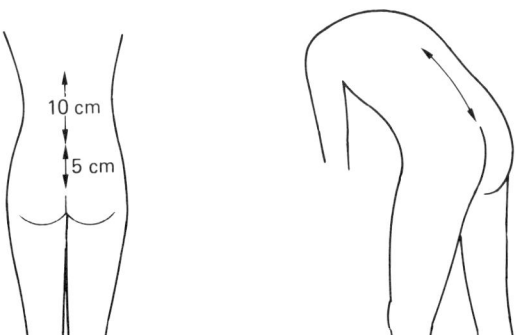

Figure 8.9  The modified Schober test. A line is drawn from 10 cm above the dimples of Venus to 5 cm below. The distance between these two points is then remeasured on full flexion.

Figure 8.10  (a) Lasègue's test (straight leg raising). (b) Sciatic stretch test. The leg is lowered slightly from the limit of straight leg raising and the foot dorsiflexed precipitating pain down the leg and in the back.

lumbar disc have pain down the symptomatic leg, precipitated by raising the good, contralateral leg. This 'cross-sciatic reflex' is highly specific for disc lesions. If whilst performing straight leg raising the patient appears to overreact, the validity of the test may be checked later in the examination by observing if the patient is able to sit at 90°, with the legs outstretched, or not.

Root tension in the upper lumbar roots (L2, 3, 4) is tested with the patient lying prone and then flexing the knee and if no pain is provoked, extending the hips as well (femoral nerve stretch test; Fig. 8.11). Pain down the anterior thigh denotes a positive test.

### Sacroiliac joints

Mechanical pain from sacroiliac joints is a rare event as they are capable of little movement.

However, pain resulting from inflammatory involvement of the synovial joint is not unusual, e.g., ankylosing spondylitis and tuberculosis.

There are two sacroiliac stress tests that are of discriminatory value in sacroiliitis. In both these tests it is important that the patient localizes the pain to the sacroiliac joints just below the dimples of Venus for it to score as a positive test. In the first test, with the patient lying prone, firm pressure is applied over the centre of the sacrum using the ulnar border of the hand (Fig. 8.12a). In the second test the patient is supine and downward pressure is applied over the anterior superior iliac spines (Fig. 8.12b). Sacroiliac tenderness is not as discriminatory as these two stress tests.

### Sacrococcygeal joint

Pain arising from this joint is not uncommon (coccydynia). The joint is best examined between

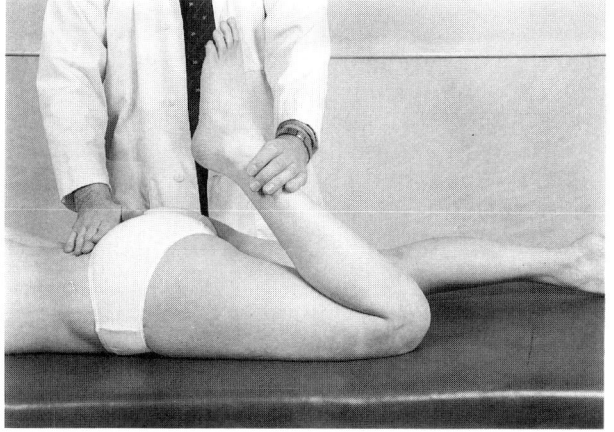

(a)

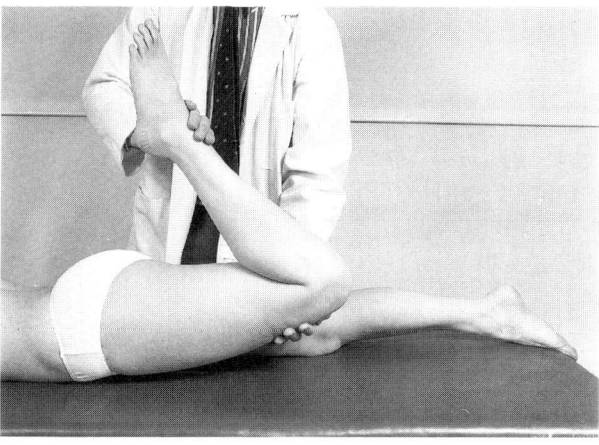

(b)

*Figure 8.11* Femoral nerve stretch test. If knee flexion (a) fails to provoke a positive test then further femoral root tension (b) may be applied by gently extending the hip as well.

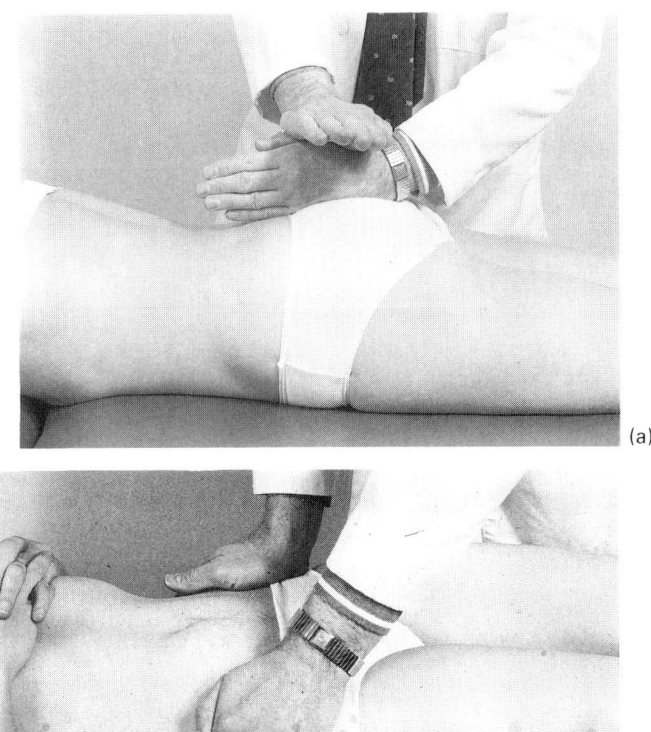

(a)

(b)

*Figure 8.12* Sacroiliac stress tests. In two separate tests downward pressure is applied over the centre of the sacrum (a) and over the anterior superior iliac spines (b).

the index finger and thumb whilst performing a rectal examination.

### Peripheral joints

#### Temporomandibular joint

This joint lies just anterior to the tragus and any tenderness or crepitus may be apparent whilst palpating the moving joint. Joint movement may be limited and this can be recorded by measuring the gap between the upper and lower incisors.

#### Shoulder

This is a complex 'joint' comprising the sternoclavicular, acromioclavicular, scapulothoracic and glenohumeral joints. The glenohumeral joint is a multiaxial joint; the other joints of the shoulder girdle allow elevation, depression, protraction and retraction.

Sometimes the sternoclavicular joint is unduly prominent due to subluxation and occasionally it is the site of infection and inflammatory arthritis.

The acromioclavicular joint may become subluxed or dislocated as a result of trauma and is often the site of osteoarthritis in elderly patients. The examination of this joint is best considered in conjunction with the rest of the shoulder.

On inspection, the two shoulders should be compared. Muscle wasting is best seen from the back and joint swelling from the front. Small effusions are usually not apparent because of the overlying musculature and for similar reasons synovial thickening is usually not discernible in inflammatory disease. On palpating the shoulder any tenderness around the long head of biceps, the acromioclavicular joint or over the supraspinatus tendon should be sought.

As active movements may be limited by pain, weakness or ruptured tendons, passive movements should also be studied. Abduction of the shoulder involves both scapulothoracic and glenohumeral movement from the start. As the glenohumeral joint is the one most frequently involved in disorders of the shoulder it is important to be able to assess its movement separately. This can be done by fixing the inferior angle of the scapula between the thumb and index finger of one hand whilst abducting the arm with the other (Fig. 8.13). The maximum abduction that may occur at the shoulder joint is 180° of which 80 to 90° takes place at the glenohumeral joint. During active abduction pain may occur in a 'painful arc' between 60° and 120° and is typical of supraspinatus tendinitis. Pain during the latter part of abduction (90–180°) is a feature of acromioclavicular disease: it is in this range that most movement of the acromioclavicular joint takes place. Adduction (50°) is tested by bringing the arm across in front of the chest. Extreme adduction stresses the acromioclavicular joint and may provoke pain in an abnormal joint. Full forward flexion (180°) involves both glenohumeral (80–90°) and scapulothoracic movement. Backward extension (60°) is mainly glenohumeral movement.

External and internal rotation are most easily assessed by asking the patient to touch the back of the neck and the small of the back respectively and seeing how far down or up he or she can reach. Alternatively, rotation may be examined with the arm by the side or abducted to 90° and the elbow held at a right angle, indicating the degree of movement (Fig. 8.14).

### Elbow

Inspection and palpation of the elbow may reveal nodules (see Fig. 8.1), tophi or a bursa. In addition, local tenderness should be sought over the medial (golfer's elbow) and lateral epicondyles (tennis elbow). The ulnar nerve can readily be palpated in the groove between the medial epicondyle and olecranon. Synovial swelling may make palpation of the nerve difficult but usually such swelling is more apparent on the radial side between the lateral epicondyle, olecranon and radiohumeral joint.

A fixed flexion deformity of the elbow is associated with an increase of the carrying angle (compare the two sides). The usual range of flexion is 0

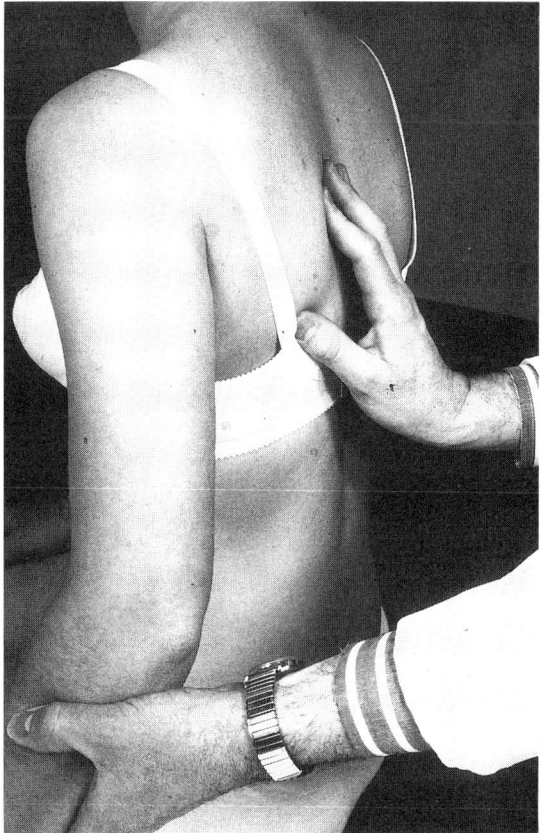

*Figure 8.13* 'Fixing' the scapula before assessing glenohumeral abduction.

to 150°. Any extension beyond 0° is labelled as hyperextension.

Pronation (80°) and supination (90°) involve the radiohumeral and superior and inferior radioulnar joints. These movements should be examined with the elbow flexed to 90° and the thumb uppermost.

### Wrist

The wrist joint is frequently the site of inflammatory arthritis and the diffuse synovial swelling is usually easily detected by inspection and palpation. More discrete swellings, such as ganglia (usually over the dorsum) and nodules, may also be apparent.

Tenderness should be sought in the anatomical 'snuff box' (fractured scaphoid), over the base of the thumb (osteoarthritis of the first carpometacarpal joint) and over the tendons of the abductor pollicis longus and extensor pollicis brevis beside

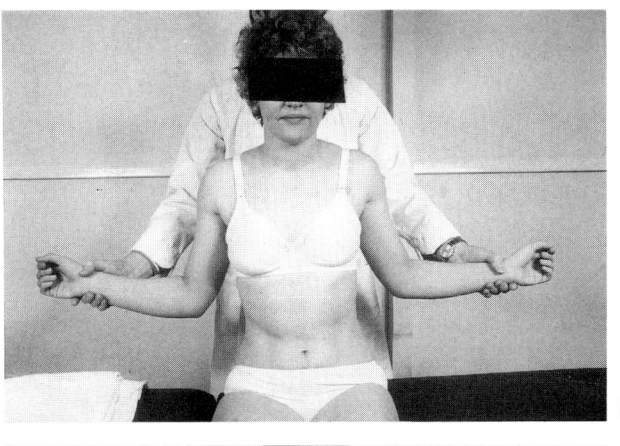

(a)

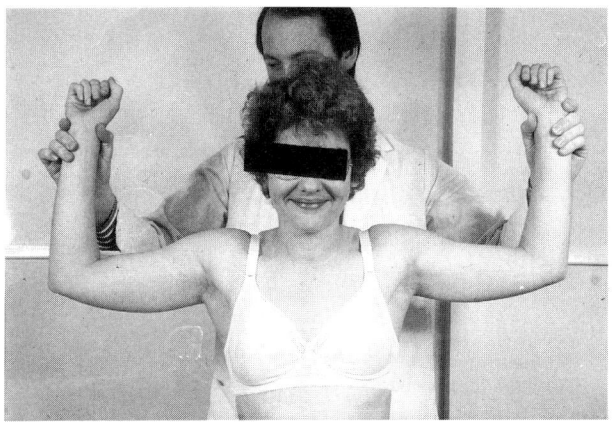

(b)

*Figure 8.14* External rotation of the shoulders with the upper arms held in (a) neutral and (b) abducted positions.

the radial styloid (de Quervain's tenosynovitis). The pain of de Quervain's tenosynovitis can usually be reproduced by resisted abduction of the thumb and/or by passive adduction of the wrist and thumb (Finkelstein's test).

Extension (70°) of the wrist is best compared and studied by asking the patient to adopt a prayer position with the hands and to raise the elbows (Fig. 8.15a). Similarly, flexion (70°) may be examined with the hands back to back (Fig. 8.15b). Radial deviation (20°) and ulnar deviation (30°) should also be examined.

### Hand

The hand is first inspected for any subcutaneous lumps (e.g., nodules and tophi) and any skin changes such as psoriasis or vasculitic nail-fold lesions should be noted. The nails should be examined for clubbing, pitting and onycholysis, and the two hands compared for muscle wasting. The presence and pattern of joint swelling is usually highly informative. In osteoarthritis the combination of Heberden's nodes, Bouchard's nodes and squaring of the hand due to involvement of the first carpometacarpal joint is classical (Fig. 8.16). The typical pattern in rheumatoid arthritis is symmetrical involvement of the metacarpophalangeal (MCP) and proximal interphalangeal (PIP) joints of both hands; involvement of the terminal interphalangeal (TIP) joint is uncommon. In contrast, joint involvement in psoriasis is usually asymmetrical and includes the TIP as well as the MCP and PIP joints.

Flexion deformities of the fingers may be seen in scleroderma (see Fig. 8.6), diabetic cheiroarthropathy, Dupuytren's contracture and inflammatory arthritis. The 'Z-shaped' thumb, 'swan-neck' and 'boutonnière' deformities, along with subluxation

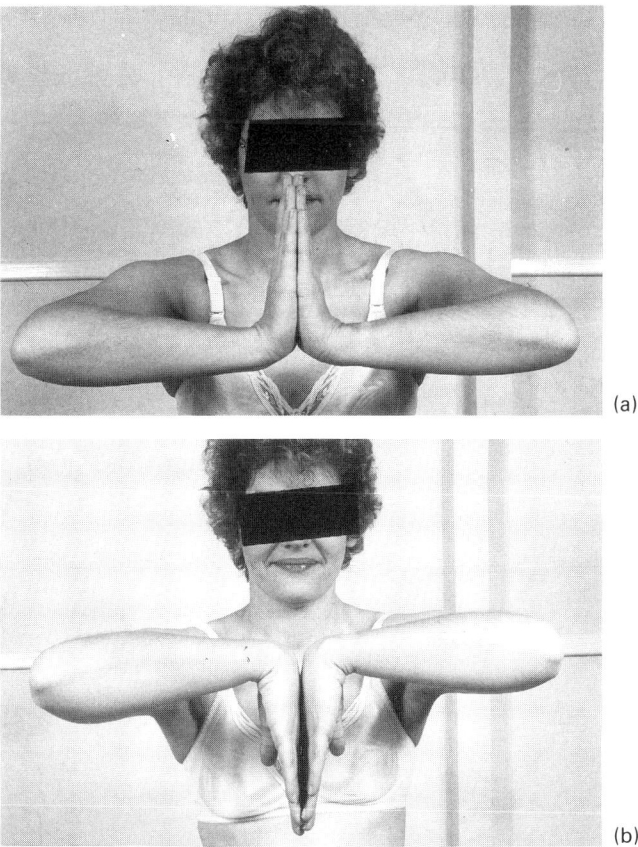

(a)

(b)

*Figure 8.15* An easy method for the comparison of wrist extension (a) and flexion (b) on the two sides.

of the MCP and ulnar deviation, are typical of rheumatoid arthritis.

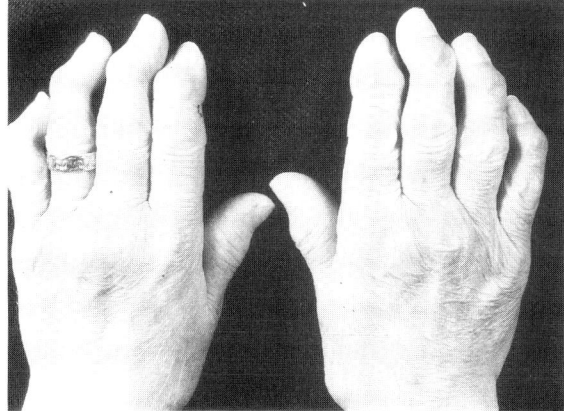

*Figure 8.16* Osteoarthritic changes in the hands with Heberden's nodes, Bouchard's nodes and squaring of the hand.

After examining each joint in turn for tenderness or swelling (bony or synovial), both active and passive flexion and extension of the fingers and thumb should be examined. Active movements may be tested by asking the patient to make a fist and then opening the hand flat again. On opening the hand a trigger finger may be revealed (flexor tenosynovitis) and in the case of ruptured extensor tendons the patient's inability to extend the affected fingers may be noted. Thumb opposition, abduction and adduction should also be tested, remembering that thumb abduction and adduction occur in the plane at right angles to the palm. Examination of passive movement allows any limitation of movement due to articular disease to be differentiated from a neurological or tendon lesion. Having examined the hand in this way an assessment of the global function of the hand may be gained from testing grip strength. This may either be done subjectively by asking the patient to grip the examiner's middle and index finger or objectively by using a rolled-up sphygmomanometer cuff inflated to 30 mmHg.

Finally, as lesions of the ulnar and median nerve (carpal tunnel syndrome) may also affect the function of the hand, neurological examination should be included.

### Hip

Hip pain may be due not only to hip disease but also to sacroiliitis and disorders of the lumbar spine. Accordingly, the lumbar spine and sacroiliac joints should always be carefully examined in cases of hip pain. Trochanteric bursitis, ischial bursitis and adductor tendinitis also enter the differential diagnosis.

With the patient supine both hips should be inspected and any scars, muscle wasting or swellings noted. Psoas abscess and swelling of an iliopsoas bursa are rare; swelling of the hip joint itself is not seen because of its deep-seated position. Any deformity should be sought by first making sure the anterior superior iliac spines are level and then observing the leg for any deformity of shortening, rotation or adduction. The front of the hip should be palpated but tenderness here is often nonspecific. Local tenderness may be found over the insertion of the adductor muscles (adductor tendinitis), greater trochanter (trochanteric bursitis) and ischial tuberosity (ischial bursitis).

Next, with the patient still supine, passive hip movements are tested. Loss of extension may result in the development of a fixed flexion deformity, which may be hidden by a compensatory exaggeration of lumbar lordosis. To detect it the contralateral hip is flexed until, with one hand beneath the patient's lumbar spine, the lordosis is felt and seen to have been abolished. If there is a flexion deformity, the thigh on the affected side will become flexed and the amount may be measured (Thomas' test) (Fig. 8.17). Hip flexion (115°) is carried out with the knee flexed while holding the contralateral thigh down to anchor the pelvis. Then, with the anterior superior iliac spines level and a hand holding the pelvis, abduction (50°) and adduction (45°) are assessed. Internal rotation (45°) and external rotation (45°) are tested either with the leg (and patient) flat or with the hip flexed to 90° (and also the knee flexed to 90°; Fig. 8.18). In the former position the patella indicates the degree of rotation and in the latter position the tibia acts as the marker.

The remaining movement, extension (30°) is tested with the patient lying prone. Each thigh is lifted in turn to the limit of its range at which point pelvic rotation may be seen or felt. Shortening of the lower limb should be sought and may be true or apparent (Fig. 8.19). Before measuring true shortening it is important to get the anterior superior iliac spines level and the legs straight. In a fixed adduction deformity, for example, this may not be possible unless the good limb is similarly adducted. Measurement is made from the base of the anterior superior iliac spine to the lower border of the medial malleolus and the two sides compared. Apparent shortening is measured, with the two legs parallel, from the xiphisternum to the bottom edge of the medial malleoli. Shortening here in the absence of true shortening of the leg is

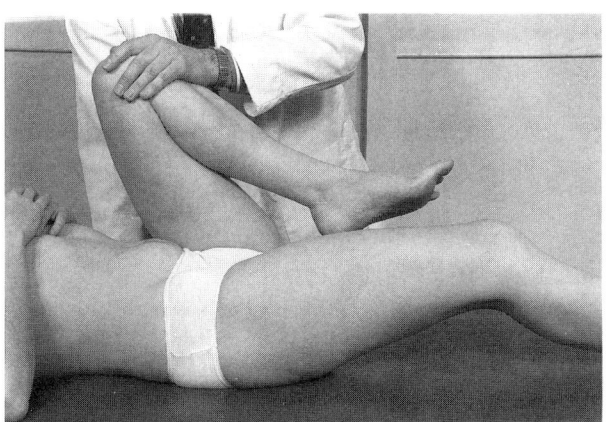

*Figure 8.17* Thomas' test for detecting flexion deformity of the hip. As the contralateral hip is flexed, abolishing the lumbar lordosis, any flexion deformity of the hip is revealed.

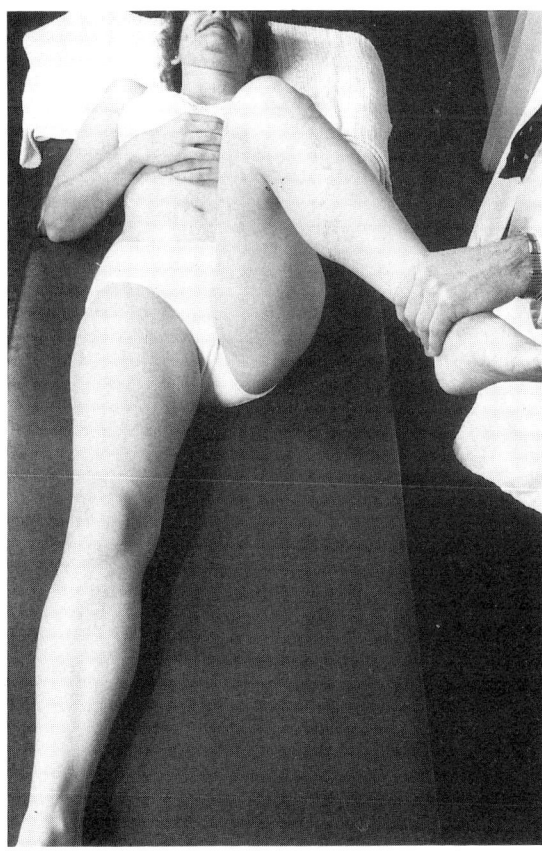

Figure 8.18   Internal rotation of the hip. The tibia indicates the degree of rotation.

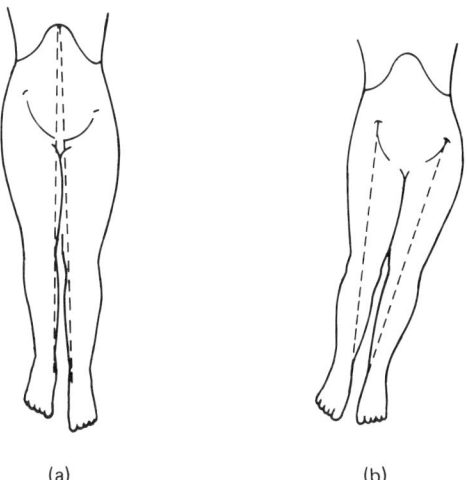

(a)                                    (b)

Figure 8.19   Apparent and real limb length inequality. In (a) there is apparent limb length inequality due to scoliosis. This is assessed by comparing the distance between the xiphisternum and medial malleoli on the two sides. In (b) the lack of true leg shortening is shown by first getting the limbs square with the pelvis and then measuring the distance between the anterior superior iliac spine and the medial malleoli on both sides.

the result of pelvic tilt secondary to scoliosis or a hip adduction deformity.

The Trendelenburg test completes the examination of the hip (Fig. 8.20). The patient stands on one leg and when this is the affected side it may result in the unsupported hip sagging, which is the reverse of normal. A positive test may be due not only to hip disease but also muscle weakness (e.g., myopathies and polio).

### Knee

On inspection of the knee any erythema, deformity or swelling should be noted. When varus or valgus deformity is present, it is important to examine the knee with the patient both lying and standing, as the degree of deformity will be greater when weight bearing. Occasionally, in severe rheumatoid and osteoarthritic cases, a varus deformity of one knee and a valgus deformity of

the other knee is seen, giving a 'windswept' appearance. Discrete swellings of the knee, such as lateral meniscal cysts and pre- and infrapatellar bursae, can usually be differentiated from the more diffuse swelling of synovial thickening and fluid by virtue of their positions.

On palpation, the warmth of the two joints should first be compared. Then each joint should be systematically palpated around the patella, tibial tubercle and joint line. The presence and site of tenderness may be important diagnostically—for instance, the tenderness of the tibial tuberosity in Osgood–Schlatter disease and of the joint line in meniscal tears.

On feeling the joint, it should be possible to distinguish between bony swelling, synovial swelling and that due to an effusion. A moderate or large effusion can usually be detected by cross-fluctuation or by the patella tap sign. This sign is elicited by pushing the patella directly down and obtaining a palpable 'clunk' as it taps the underlying femoral condyles. When only a moderate effusion is present these signs may only be found if the fluid in the suprapatellar pouch is first 'milked' into the main compartment. Small effusions are

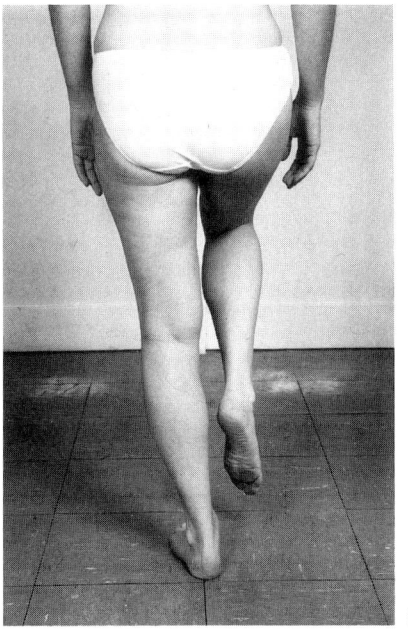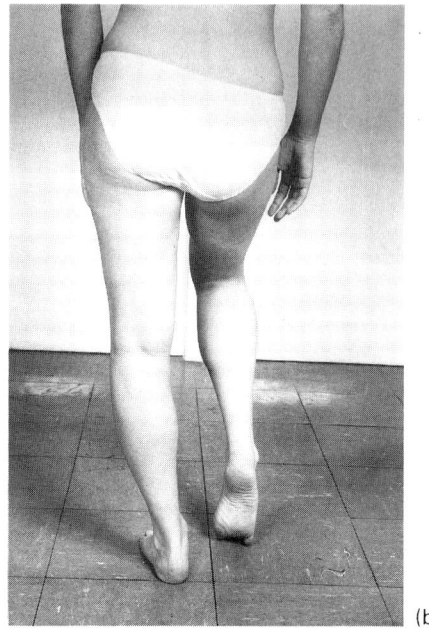

(a)　　　　　　　　　　　　　　　　　　　(b)

*Figure 8.20* Trendelenburg test. The patient is asked to stand on first one leg and then the other. (a) Normally the pelvis tilts up slightly on the non-weight bearing side (negative Trendelenburg test). (b) In the presence of hip disease or weak hip abductors the unsupported side of the pelvis drops (positive Trendelenburg test).

best detected by stroking the fluid away from the medial side of the knee and occluding the suprapatellar pouch with one hand (Fig. 8.21). Then, whilst watching the medial side of the joint to see if a bulge appears, the other hand strokes the fluid back from the lateral side to the medial side (bulge sign).

The popliteal fossa should also be palpated and any swellings such as a Baker's cyst or popliteal aneurysm noted. Lastly, the knee should be felt during flexion/extension for crepitus.

Before examining movement the stability of the joint should be assessed. The collateral ligaments are tested with the knee flexed 10° and then alternately applying a valgus (medial ligaments) and varus (lateral ligaments) force (Fig. 8.22). To test the cruciate ligaments it is essential that the quadriceps and hamstring muscles are relaxed otherwise instability may be missed. With the knee in 10° of flexion the leg is grasped either side of the knee and anterior/posterior distraction of the joint attempted (Lachman's test). The integrity of the cruciate ligaments may also be tested with the knee at 90°. In this position, the alignment between the patella and the tibial tuberosity should first be studied as the tibia may be subluxed

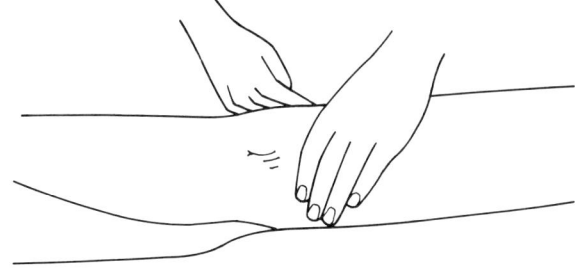

*Figure 8.21* Bulge sign. Having emptied the medial side of the joint and occluded the suprapatellar pouch, fluid is milked from the lateral to the medial side to produce a visible bulge.

posteriorly in association with a ruptured posterior cruciate ligament. The examiner then sits on the patient's foot and with the examiner's hands just below the knee draws the tibia anteriorly and posteriorly (Fig. 8.23). This tests the anterior and posterior cruciate ligaments, respectively. If the tibia is already subluxed posteriorly a spuriously positive anterior draw sign may be obtained as it moves forward to a neutral position: hence the importance of checking the tibial position beforehand.

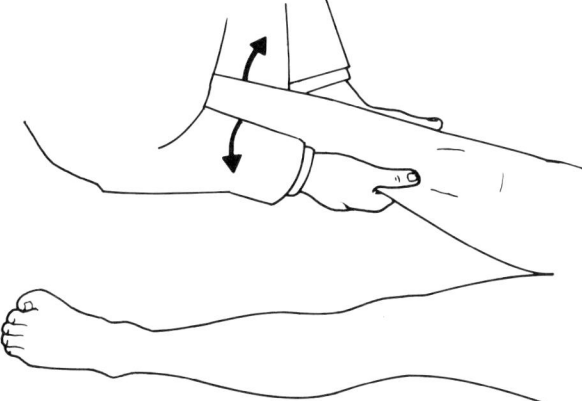

Figure 8.22 Testing collateral ligament stability.

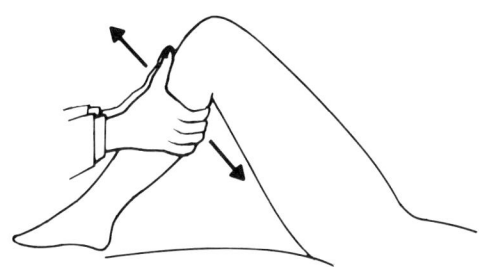

Figure 8.23 Testing the cruciate ligaments of the knee.

In recent years the lateral pivot shift test has become accepted as a useful test of anterolateral stability (anterior cruciate ligament and posterolateral capsule). The patient's foot is held under the examiner's arm with the tibia internally rotated and knee extended. In this position, the lateral tibial condyle is subluxed forwards when anterolateral instability is present. A valgus force is then applied and the knee slowly flexed until, at 20° to 30° of flexion, the lateral tibial condyle suddenly flicks back to its correct position.

Meniscal integrity is traditionally tested by McMurray's test in which the knee is rotated in varying degrees of flexion and then straightened. A positive test is marked by an audible or palpable

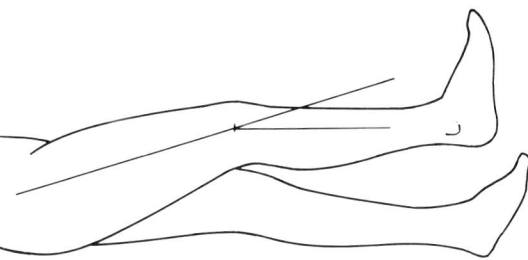

Figure 8.24 Quadriceps lag.

click associated with pain. The test is probably best avoided when the diagnosis of a torn meniscus is not seriously in doubt, as it may be extremely painful and occasionally the patient's knee may become locked.

Flexion (135°) is the main knee movement, any extension beyond 0° being hyperextension. Examination of the knee should include assessment of muscle power, particularly the quadriceps muscle. Normally the leg can be elevated with the knee straight. However, in the presence of severe arthritis of the knee and particularly after surgery, quadriceps weakness may be such that a small amount of flexion occurs at the knee (often <10°) before the whole leg is raised ('quadriceps lag'; Fig. 8.24).

Lastly, patello-femoral irritability should be looked for by pushing the patella from side to side and in addition getting the patient to contract the quadriceps muscle whilst holding the patella down against the femur.

### Ankle and subtalar joint

Swelling of the joint is usually obvious but differentiating between a mild synovitis and a naturally podgy ankle may be difficult. Ankle deformity may be either congenital (e.g., talipes equinovarus) or acquired (e.g., valgus deformity of the hind foot in rheumatoid arthritis). It is best appreciated by observing the ankle from behind, with the patient standing.

On palpation, skin temperature is assessed and any tenderness of the joint is noted. In addition, tenderness should be sought at the insertion of the Achilles tendon into the calcaneum. Tendinitis here is sometimes found in Reiter's disease and ankylosing spondylitis.

Ankle movements take place at the mortise and subtalar joints. Dorsiflexion (20°) and plantar flexion (50°) occur at the mortise joint and the two sides may be compared simultaneously. Inversion (5°) and eversion (5°) take place at the subtalar joint and are examined by abducting and adducting the heel.

## Foot

The medial and longitudinal arches of the foot should be inspected with the patient standing and any accentuation (pes cavus) or flattening (pes planus) noted. The toes should also be observed for any deformity (hallux valgus, claw toes and hammer toes).

Bony thickening of the first metatarsophalangeal (MTP) joint due to osteoarthritis is common, but inflammatory changes in the toes may also occur, such as the 'sausage' digit that may be seen in psoriatic arthritis.

The plantar aspect of the foot should be palpated in search of tenderness under the medial aspect of the calcaneum (plantar fasciitis). Tenderness of the MTP joint may be present in various polyarthritides and may be elicited by gently squeezing the forefoot. More specific localization of this tenderness is detected by palpating each MTP joint in turn, between the thumb and index finger. At the same time any thickening or subluxation of the joint may be appreciated.

Movements occur at the midtarsal, MTP and individual toe joints. To examine the midtarsal joints one hand fixes the patient's heel whilst the other inverts (30°) and everts (20°) the forefoot. Flexion/extension of the MTP and interphalangeal joints should also be tested.

## OSTEOARTHRITIS

Osteoarthritis is a degenerative disease of hyaline articular cartilage and is the commonest form of arthropathy worldwide. Classically it is divided into primary and secondary forms. Primary osteoarthritis is of unknown aetiology but secondary osteoarthritis may be a consequence of previous trauma, inflammatory joint disease or metabolic disease such as haemochromatosis and ochronosis.

Osteoarthritis is mainly a disease of later life, being unusual under the age of 50 years. Overall it is seen slightly more commonly in women than in men.

## Clinical features

Joint pain is the predominant symptom. There may be morning stiffness but this seldom lasts for more than half an hour. Patients often describe 'gelling' in which the joints become stiff after a period of rest, e.g., after sitting.

Generalized nodal osteoarthritis is the commonest subset of primary osteoarthritis. It is typically seen in middle-aged women about the time of the menopause and is characterized by firm swellings over the distal interphalangeal joints (Heberden's nodes) and proximal interphalangeal joints (Bouchard's nodes) of the hands. Involvement of the base of the thumb (the first carpometacarpal joint) is frequently seen in association with the nodal form of disease, giving rise to squaring of the hand. Other joints that may be involved in this disease subset include the uncovertebral joints in the neck, the apophyseal joints of the spine, the knees and first metatarsophalangeal joints.

An effusion may appear during the acute exacerbations of the disease in the knee but, in contrast to inflammatory disease, the joint is usually cool.

Pain in the knee may be the only symptom in patients with osteoarthritis of the hip but more frequently the pain is felt in the groin and lateral buttock. It is an important cause of the pain and disability in the elderly and is more commonly seen in males than females, suggesting that it may represent a separate subset.

## Investigations

Blood tests (including the ESR and tests for rheumatoid factor) are usually normal. Synovial fluid is typically clear and viscous (non-inflammatory).

## X-rays

The radiological changes in osteoarthritis are characterized by loss of joint space, osteophytes, subchondral bone sclerosis and juxta-articular bone cysts.

## Management

Patients should be advised to maintain a level of activity that they find comfortable, though individual joints may need to be rested during acute exacerbations. Overweight patients will need to be encouraged to slim, especially if they have weight-bearing joints involved.

The drug treatment of osteoarthritis is limited to analgesics and non-steroidal anti-inflammatory drugs (NSAIDs). In most cases simple analgesics plus explanation and reassurance suffice. Paracetamol alone or in combination with dextropropoxyphene (co-proxamol) is a good deal safer with regard to gastrointestinal complications than NSAIDs, especially in the elderly, who, of course, make up the majority of sufferers. Physiotherapy is helpful in improving mobility and controlling the pain of acute exacerbations. Walking aids should be provided and a home assessment made if necessary.

Surgery (e.g., hip and knee replacements) is indicated when conservative treatment has failed.

## RHEUMATOID ARTHRITIS

Rheumatoid arthritis is a polyarticular inflammatory joint disease of unknown aetiology. It has a prevalence of about 3 per cent with a female preponderance (F:M 3:1). There is little geographical or racial difference in prevalence, though countries with warmer climates do appear to see less severe disease.

The aetiopathogenesis of rheumatoid arthritis remains unsolved, but genetic factors have been shown to be important. The HLA antigen DR4 is present in 60 per cent of patients with rheumatoid arthritis compared with a rate of only 30 per cent in the normal population. The trigger for the onset of the disease in such genetically susceptible individuals is unknown despite intensive research. An infective agent is regarded as being the most likely candidate. Whatever the trigger the main pathological change is the development of chronic inflammatory changes in the synovial membrane, which results in proliferating granulation tissue (pannus) eroding both bone and cartilage as it spreads across the joint.

Rheumatoid factors (antiglobulins) of different immunoglobulin classes are produced by plasma cells in lymphoid tissue and the synovial membrane itself. They play an important part in the humoral immunopathology and are found in the circulating immune complexes of patients with rheumatoid arthritis (see later under 'Investigations').

### Clinical features

Disease of the joints is the main clinical manifestation; it usually presents as an acute symmetrical polyarthritis though sometimes has a more insidious onset. Some cases start with just mono- or oligoarticular disease but with the passage of time most of these cases will become polyarticular. A rare form of presentation is palindromic rheumatism in which there are intermittent, recurring attacks of acute arthritis in one or two joints. The episodes are usually short-lived, lasting from only a few hours to a few days before subsiding.

As well as pain and swelling of joints, patients complain of morning stiffness which if untreated lasts for at least an hour. Systemic symptoms such as tiredness and anorexia are common. There may be accompanying weight loss and a few patients run a low-grade fever. The wrists, hands (MCP and PIP joints), knees, ankles and feet are the usual joints to be involved. The shoulder and elbow joints are also frequently affected whilst involvement of the hips, neck and temporomandibular joints occurs less often. Tenosynovitis is common, e.g., swelling of the dorsal tendon sheath at the wrist and 'triggering' of the flexor tendons in the hands.

As the disease progresses, characteristic deformities develop in the hands (MCP subluxation, ulnar deviation, 'Z' thumbs, boutonnière and swan-neck deformities). In the feet, subluxation of the MTP joints with subsequent claw toe deformity and hallux valgus is the typical picture.

Rheumatoid involvement of the neck is often mild, giving rise to little more than intermittent pain and stiffness. However, the possibility of more significant disease due to atlanto-axial or subaxial subluxation should always be borne in mind in patients with longstanding disease.

As well as joint involvement many patients have extra-articular manifestations. Indeed some systemic features, such as rheumatoid nodules, pulmonary fibrosis and Felty's syndrome, can predate the onset of articular symptoms. However extra-articular features are more usually seen in patients with established seropositive disease (Table 8.5).

### Investigations

#### Full blood count

A normochromic, normocytic anaemia (anaemia of chronic disease) is commonplace in rheumatoid arthritis. Not infrequently an associated iron

**Table 8.5 Extra-articular manifestations of rheumatoid arthritis**

| | |
|---|---|
| *Eyes* | Keratoconjunctivitis sicca (as part of Sjögren's syndrome) |
| | Episcleritis |
| | Scleritis |
| *Skin* | Palmar erythema |
| | Vasculitis (nail-fold infarcts and arteritic skin ulcers) |
| | Subcutaneous nodules |
| *Tendons* | Nodules |
| | Attrition rupture |
| *Muscle* | Polymyositis (uncommon) |
| *Cardiovascular system* | |
|   Peripheral: | Raynaud's phenomenon |
| | Small vessel vasculitis (skin, vasa nervorum) |
| | Arteritis (rare)—coronary, cerebral, renal |
|   Cardiac: | Pericarditis |
| | Myocarditis |
| | Valvulitis |
| | Conduction defects |
| *Respiratory system* | Hoarseness (crico-arytenoid joint involvement) |
| | Pleurisy |
| | Pleural effusions |
| | Pulmonary nodules |
| | Fibrosing alveolitis |
| | Caplan's syndrome |
| | Obliterative bronchiolitis |
| | Increased risk of bronchial infections (as part of Sjögren's syndrome) |
| *Nervous system* | Cervical cord compression (atlanto-axial and sub-axial subluxation) |
| | Mild sensory peripheral neuropathy |
| | Mononeuritis multiplex |
| | Entrapment neuropathies, e.g. carpal tunnel syndrome |
| *Renal* | Amyloid |
| | Glomerulonephritis (rare) |
| *Blood and reticuloendothelial system* | Anaemia—anaemia of chronic disease ± mild iron deficiency anaemia |
| | Thrombocytosis |
| | Felty's syndrome |
| | Hyperviscosity syndrome |
| | Lymphadenopathy |
| *Sjögren's syndrome* | |

deficiency anaemia may complicate the picture because of gastrointestinal blood loss (secondary

to use of NSAIDs). In this situation, checking the serum iron and total iron binding capacity or alternatively the ferritin is helpful. The white cell count is usually normal but, if low, Felty's syndrome or drug-induced leucopenia should be considered. The platelet count is often elevated, its height mirroring the disease activity.

The ESR and plasma viscosity are commonly raised, especially in active disease.

### Biochemistry

Routine biochemical tests show raised globulin levels and, in active disease, the alkaline phosphatase is frequently elevated (mainly liver in origin and mirrors disease activity).

### Autoantibodies

The latex and Rose–Waaler tests are positive in 70 per cent of cases. The antinuclear antibody is positive in 40 per cent of cases. DNA antibodies are, however, absent.

### Synovial fluid

Typically the synovial fluid is 'inflammatory' and is of low viscosity with a cloudy-yellow appearance. It has a high white cell count, the majority of which are polymorphonuclear leucocytes.

### X-rays

X-rays of the hands (including wrists) and feet should be taken in order to assess progress of the disease. Other films may be necessary (e.g., flexion/extension views of the cervical spine) when clinically indicated.

The characteristic radiological changes in rheumatoid arthritis are (a) narrowing of the joint space; (b) juxta-articular osteoporosis; (c) marginal joint erosions.

### Management

Having made the diagnosis and informed the patient it is important that some immediate counselling is undertaken as the diagnosis of rheumatoid arthritis often conjures up considerable dread in the minds of patients. Whilst it can be a crippling disease, the majority (65 per cent) of patients get on reasonably well with proper treatment.

## Rest and splints

In active cases, bed rest is of immense value in allowing inflammatory joints to settle. Splinting of wrists and knees allows the joints to be rested in a functional position.

## Physiotherapy

The aim of physiotherapy is to help control pain by physical means and to maintain function of the joints. Advice on the use of heat (hot baths and hot-water bottles) and of cold (packs of frozen peas) is helpful to patients on their return home. Hospitalized patients will need their joints put through a passive range of movement when resting and help in mobilization once the synovitis has settled—hydrotherapy is very useful in this regard. Once better, patients should be advised to maintain a level of activity with which they feel comfortable.

## Occupational therapy

Patients should be referred to the occupational therapy department for functional assessment of their ability to manage not only in the home but in the place of work, so that appropriate advice and/or aids can be provided.

## Drug treatment

(See the *British National Formulary* for prescribing details.)

### Analgesics

Whilst simple analgesics can be a useful adjunct to antirheumatic therapy they are seldom adequate as the sole form of drug treatment. Paracetamol and paracetamol-containing compounds such as co-proxamol and co-dydramol are the most widely used. The more powerful opiates are restricted to short-term usage only.

### NSAIDs

This group of drugs is the mainstay of treatment for patients with inflammatory arthritis. Their effectiveness in relieving pain and stiffness varies from individual to individual and according to how active the disease is. Concern continues to centre on their safety, particularly with regard to gastrointestinal side-effects. Nevertheless, the vast majority of patients tolerate NSAIDs well and are helped by them.

Contraindications to NSAID therapy are active peptic ulceration, history of previous peptic ulceration, renal failure and concurrent anticoagulant therapy. Asthmatic patients should be advised to stop therapy if their asthma worsens.

Aspirin is no longer widely used because it is less well tolerated and less easy to handle (too many tablets) than newer NSAIDs though some formulations, e.g., Benoral (10 ml, twice a day) have overcome this latter problem.

Of the other NSAIDs, ibuprofen, naproxen, diclofenac and indomethacin are widely used. There is little to be gained by combining NSAIDs of different types, though the addition of slow-release medications or suppositories (e.g., diclofenac and indomethacin) are often helpful in the relief of morning stiffness.

### Disease-modifying drugs or second-line agents

These drugs can suppress disease activity in the majority of patients but do not totally halt progression as judged radiologically by changes in the extent of erosion. They are given in conjunction with NSAIDs and analgesics but their onset of action is slow, varying between two and six months before clinical benefit is seen. The precise mode of action of these agents is ill-understood but they are thought to modulate the immunopathological process, resulting not only in fewer active joints but also a reduction in ESR, C-reactive protein and rheumatoid factor. These drugs are usually given to patients with persistent or progressive articular disease and are now being used earlier, with the aim of 'controlling' the disorder before erosive changes are seen on X-ray.

Sulphasalazine, gold and penicillamine are the most commonly used second-line drugs. Close monitoring of full blood counts is necessary throughout treatment and, in the case of the latter two drugs, urine testing for protein is needed as well. Antimalarials (chloroquine and hydroxychloroquine), although well tolerated, have not gained widespread acceptance because of the risk of ocular toxicity and the resultant need for regular ophthalmological screening (every three to six months). Cytotoxic agents (azathioprine, cyclophosphamide, chlorambucil and methotrexate) are less frequently used, being mainly reserved for cases where other second-line agents have failed to control articular progression and for the treatment of aggressive extra-articular disease such as severe vasculitis and necrotizing scleritis. These drugs too require regular monitoring of full blood counts. Their use should be avoided in women of child-bearing age because of their adverse effect on gametogenesis and the potential for teratogenicity.

### Steroids

The use of steroids in rheumatoid arthritis is controversial. They are extremely potent in the short term and are particularly valuable in association with cytotoxics in the management of vasculitis and other rheumatoid complications. The difficulty revolves around their use in articular disease. Rheumatoid arthritis is a chronic disorder and though the acute exacerbation may have settled with steroids, patients find it difficult to reduce or stop such treatment because of the breakthrough of more pain and stiffness in their joints as the dose comes down. This leaves the patient at risk to all the attendant problems of long-term steroid therapy.

For articular disease the dose of prednisolone should be restricted to a maximum of 10 mg daily with a view to decreasing the dose to 7.5 mg or less. This regimen can be of undoubted value in elderly patients whose independence is being threatened by pain and stiffness whilst waiting for second-line agents to take effect.

High-dose, pulse therapy with steroids using intravenous methylprednisolone (1 g) has a place in dampening aggressive disease (articular or extra-articular) whilst at the same time starting disease-modifying drugs such as penicillamine or azathioprine.

Intra-articular steroids are of immense benefit in treating individual active joints. (For details on injecting and aspirating joints see 'Further Reading'.)

### Medical synovectomy

Various agents have been given by intra-articular injection in an attempt to achieve a lasting suppression of local synovitis. Yttrium-90 for the knee joint and Erbium-169 for the small joints are the most widely used.

### Plasmapheresis

This is of no proven value.

### Total lymphoid irradiation

This form of therapy may have a limited role in the treatment of refractory cases of severe rheumatoid arthritis. The regimen is similar to that used in Hodgkin's disease but the dosage of radiation is lower.

### Surgery

Orthopaedic surgery has an important part to play in the overall management of rheumatoid arthritis. The aims are to relieve pain and improve function and the development of hip and knee replacements has been a great breakthrough in this regard. A combined approach is needed between physician and surgeon on timing and selection of patients for orthopaedic surgery.

## SYSTEMIC LUPUS ERYTHEMATOSUS (SLE)

SLE is a chronic inflammatory multisystem disease. The prevalence of this disorder seems to be increasing, possibly because of the detection of milder cases through serological testing. Reported prevalence rates vary between 1:250 to 1:10 000. There is a racial variability in prevalence rates, it being nearly three times more common in West Indian and American black females than in their white counterparts. SLE is most frequently seen in females during the third and fourth decades; the female to male ratio is about 9:1.

### Clinical features

SLE commonly presents in an acute fashion with malaise, fever, arthralgia, rash and pleuritic chest pain.

*Joints*: commonly there is more arthralgia than arthritis. However, a symmetrical polyarthritis mainly involving the hands, wrists and knees may occur. It is rarely erosive but joint deformities may develop (Jaccoud-like arthropathy).

*Skin*: the classical malar 'butterfly' rash, non-specific erythema, photosensitivity, vasculitic rashes and alopecia are the commoner cutaneous manifestations. Livedo reticularis is a mild manifestation of skin vasculitis but palpable purpura, ulcers, nail-fold lesions and even digital gangrene may be seen. Raynaud's phenomenon is seen in about 20 per cent of cases and is rarely severe.

*Muscles*: myalgias are common and occasionally polymyositis may develop.

*Kidneys*: renal disease is found in approximately half of patients and is associated with a poor prognosis. Asymptomatic proteinuria is the commonest manifestion but kidney disease may present as nephrotic syndrome, acute nephritis or renal failure.

*Lungs*: pleurisy with or without a small effusion is seen in half of patients with SLE. Diffuse pulmonary infiltrates and pulmonary fibrosis with areas of basal collapse (the disappearing lung syndrome) are less common.

*The heart*: acute pericarditis may be a presenting feature. Myocarditis is rarely seen and Libman–Sachs endocarditis is seldom detected clinically. Lupus patients seem to be at an increased risk of developing atheromatous disease of the coronary arteries.

*Nervous system*: nonspecific features, such as headaches and mood disturbance, are commonplace in lupus patients. More florid psychiatric and neurological disorders are occasionally seen, such as fits, strokes, cranial nerve lesions and peripheral neuropathy (mononeuritis multiplex). Not surprisingly, severe cerebral lupus carries a poor prognosis.

*Miscellaneous*: other systemic features include Sjögren's syndrome, lymphadenopathy, hepatomegaly and splenomegaly.

Patients with SLE have an increased tendency to spontaneous abortion and thrombosis. This is thought to be mediated through anticardiolipin antibodies (lupus anticoagulant). Pregnancy may be complicated by increased disease activity in the postpartum period.

## Investigations

### Full blood count

A mild normochromic normocytic anaemia is commonplace. More rarely a Coombs'-positive haemolytic anaemia is seen. Leucopenia is a recognized feature: in particular lymphopenia is common in active disease (due to antilymphocyte antibodies). The platelet count is often low but severe thrombocytopenia is rarely encountered.

The ESR is usually elevated in active disease. The C-reactive protein, however, is often normal and, if elevated, would suggest an intercurrent infection (see 'Investigations').

### Biochemistry

Routine biochemical tests should be undertaken to screen renal function. As with rheumatoid arthritis a slightly elevated alkaline phosphatase may be found and there may occasionally be some elevation of the transaminases, in which case the possibility of drug-induced liver damage should be considered (e.g., aspirin).

### Urine testing

Routine 'stix' testing of urine should be performed and a mid-stream and 24-h urine collection sent for analysis if necessary.

### Autoantibodies

Antinuclear antibody is present in 95 per cent of affected patients. Tests for rheumatoid factor are positive in about 40 per cent of cases.

### DNA antibodies

Antibodies to double-stranded DNA are highly specific for SLE and in general their levels correlate with disease activity.

### ECG and chest X-ray

These should be done as part of the general assessment of acute cases.

## Management

The majority of patients with lupus have an excellent prognosis and they should be reassured accordingly. In the majority, the predominant symptom is articular and can be treated with NSAIDs alone. Aspirin should be avoided as in high doses it is hepatotoxic. Caution needs to be exercised when prescribing NSAIDs for patients with impaired renal function as these drugs may lead to further deterioration in renal status.

In cases where NSAIDs alone are insufficient to control the arthritis then antimalarials (chloroquine and hydroxychloroquine) are indicated. This group of drugs is also particularly valuable in patients with skin disease.

Patients with more systemic features, such as fever, pericarditis and pleurisy, will need corticosteroids. Having controlled the disease with 30 to 40 mg of prednisolone daily the dosage should be reduced to the lowest needed to maintain control. Higher doses of prednisolone (40–60 mg/day) are needed when treating severe vasculitis, nephritis or neurological disease. Pulse treatment with intravenous methylprednisolone is an alternative in aggressive disease of this kind and cytotoxics (e.g., azathioprine or cyclophosphamide) are indicated in such seriously affected patients.

## ACUTE MONOARTHRITIS

This represents an important rheumatological emergency (Fig. 8.25). Whilst the diagnosis often lies between septic and crystal-induced arthritis other possibilities enter into the differential diagnosis, such as trauma, haemophilia and various inflammatory disorders (palindromic rheumatism, Reiter's disease, psoriatic arthritis and acute sarcoidosis). In children, pauciarticular juvenile chronic arthritis and juvenile ankylosing spondylitis (especially in males) have to be added to this list and crystal arthritis removed. Gout is extremely rare in childhood and when present tends to be due to an inborn error of purine metabolism or due to secondary causes, e.g., chemotherapy in acute leukaemia.

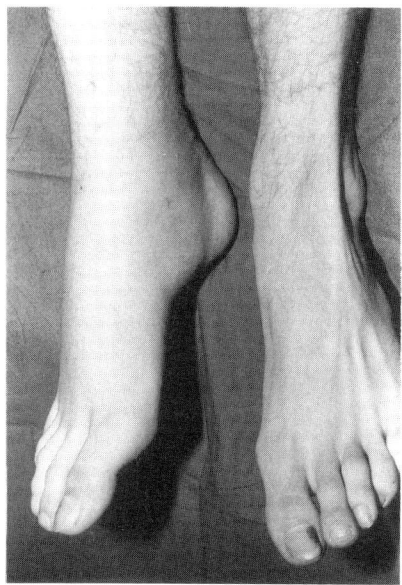

*Figure 8.25* An acute arthritis of the ankle (following enteric infection with *Campylobacter jejuni*—reactive arthritis).

### History

The site, duration and intensity of symptoms should be ascertained and inquiry made into whether the patient has had any similar attacks in the past. Any past or current history of rash, urethritis, uveitis or diarrhoea should be sought. The history may uncover possible precipitants, such as recent use of diuretics, trauma and surgery in the case of crystal-induced arthritis, and gastroenteritis in the case of postdysenteric Reiter's disease. Other possible precipitants may only be unearthed after more specific inquiry— low-dose aspirin (gout), extramarital sexual exposure (Reiter's disease) and intravenous drug abuse (septic arthritis).

### Examination

This should be full and not confined to looking at the joint and asking the nurse to check the patient's temperature. Many important clues may be picked up, such as tophi, nodules and skin lesions (e.g., psoriasis, erythema nodosum or the vesiculopustular lesions of gonococcaemia).

### Investigation

Blood should be taken for full blood count, ESR, biochemical profile (including calcium, phosphate and alkaline phosphatase), uric acid, latex or Rose–Waaler test and antinuclear antibodies. Blood and urine should be sent for culture. If there is a history of diarrhoea, stool cultures should be done; when gonococcal infection is suspected, cultures from the urethra, cervix, anorectal region and pharynx are indicated.

The single most important investigation is aspiration of the joint and analysis of the synovial fluid so obtained. For a detailed account of joint aspiration see 'Further Reading'. Arthrocentesis should be done without delay and the fluid sent for a total and differential cell count, crystals and culture. Much may be gained from the appearance of the synovial fluid. In osteoarthritis and traumatic disorders of the joint the fluid retains its normal straw colour and clarity. Conversely, inflammatory fluid is cloudy (turbid) and may even be frankly purulent. The aspiration of frank blood (traumatic haemarthrosis, haemophilia, anticoagulants and pigmented villonodular synovitis) is usually easy to differentiate from the patchy blood-staining of a traumatic tap.

Fluid for cell counts should be placed in an

EDTA bottle, whilst plain sterile containers should be used for crystal examination and microbiological investigation. On emptying the syringe full of synovial fluid into the various bottles, some assessment of viscosity may be made. Non-inflammatory fluid has a high viscosity in contrast to the more watery viscosity of inflammatory fluid. The high viscosity of non-inflammatory fluids relates to the large amount of hyaluronic acid present.

The cell count tends to be in the range of 200 to 2000 cells/mm³ for non-inflammatory fluids; 2000 to 50 000 cells/mm³ for inflammatory conditions and greater than 50 000 cells/mm³ in cases of sepsis. However, the overlap is such (Table 8.6) that this cannot be relied upon to decide whether or not sepsis is present.

If possible, the fluid should be promptly studied for crystals as the finding of crystals of urate or calcium pyrophosphate will often obviate the need for admission to hospital.

The results from culture of the joint fluid will take one or two days, but a quick indication as to the possibility of joint sepsis may be gained from the lactate level in synovial fluid (if available locally) and Gram staining. Both false-positive and false-negative results may occur with these two tests but if organisms are identified by Gram staining, it allows the physician to make a more enlightened choice of antibiotic.

If gonococcal or anaerobic infection is suspected the microbiologist's attention should be drawn to it on the request form so that the culture may be set up on the appropriate media and incubated under appropriate conditions. As well as looking for pyogenic organisms, joint fluid should routinely be sent for mycobacterial culture. As they are of no diagnostic value, tests for rheumatoid factor, antinuclear antibody and/or complement levels in synovial fluid have no clinical relevance. For a more detailed account of the examination of synovial fluid see 'Further Reading'.

Radiographs should be taken of both the affected and contralateral joint. They are often non-contributory at this early stage but sometimes chondrocalcinosis may be seen (Fig. 8.26). Mild osteoarthritic changes are too ubiquitous in late middle-aged and elderly patients to be of much diagnostic significance in the context of an acute monoarthritis. A chest X-ray should also be routinely ordered as the presence of pulmonary disease may be relevant, e.g., bilateral hilar lymphadenopathy and pulmonary infection (tuberculous or pyogenic).

**Table 8.6 Total white cell counts in synovial fluid**

| White cells/mm³ | Diagnosis |
|---|---|
| <2000 (non-inflammatory) | Normal |
| | Osteoarthritis |
| | Traumatic joint disorders |
| 2000–50 000 (inflammatory) | Connective tissue diseases |
| | Rheumatoid arthritis |
| | Seronegative spondarthritides |
| | Gout |
| | Pseudogout |
| | Septic arthritis |
| >50 000 (septic) | Rheumatoid arthritis |
| | Reiter's disease |
| | Gout |
| | Pseudogout |
| | Septic arthritis |

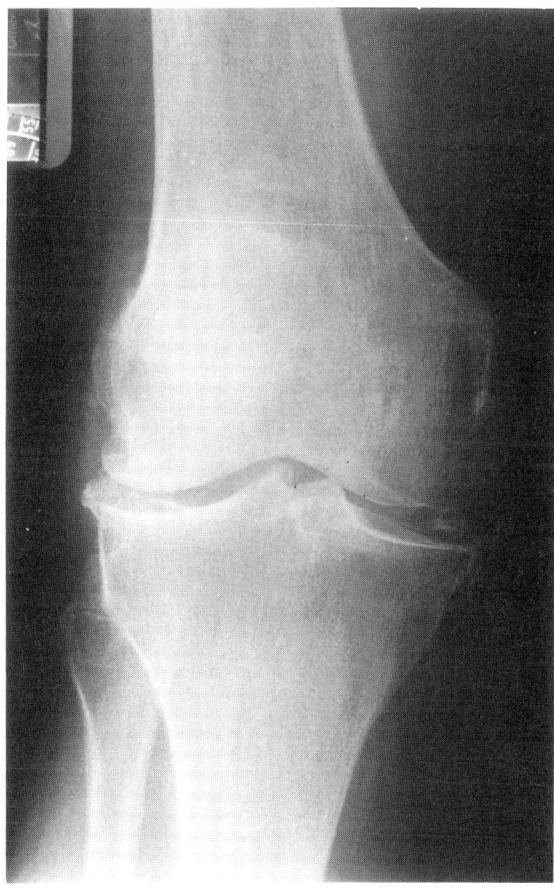

*Figure 8.26* Chondrocalcinosis in an osteoarthritic knee.

## Management

If infection is suspected the patient should be admitted and started on parenteral antibiotics (Table 8.7). The antibiotics may need changing when the organism and sensitivities are known. If polarizing microscopy reveals crystals, then the patient may be treated as an outpatient with an NSAID and rest. In the case of gout, NSAIDs should be given in high dosage at first, e.g., indomethacin, 50 mg four times a day. Patients with acute, crystal-induced arthritis should be reviewed in clinic not more than one week later with the results of the various investigations. It is important that the culture report is secured as there have been occasional cases in which crystals and micro-organisms have coexisted.

**Table 8.7 Chemotherapy in septic arthritis when the organism is unknown**

| Age | Commonly involved organisms | Antibiotic |
|---|---|---|
| 0–6 months | Gram-negative bacilli | Gentamicin and |
|  | Staphylococcus aureus | flucloxacillin |
| 6 months–2 years | Haemophilus influenzae | Amoxycillin |
| 2–15 years | Staphylococcus aureus | Flucloxacillin and |
|  | Streptococcus pneumoniae | amoxycillin |
|  | Streptococcus pyogenes |  |
| 16–50 years | Neisseria gonorrhoeae | Amoxycillin and |
|  | Staphylococcus aureus | flucloxacillin |
| >50 years | Staphylococcus aureus | Flucloxacillin and |
|  | Streptococcus pneumoniae | amoxycillin |
|  | Streptococcus pyogenes |  |

*NB* In patients aged 6 months or more gentamicin should be added if Gram-negative infection is suspected or if Gram-negative bacilli are seen on Gram stain.

Despite the above investigations the diagnosis may remain unclear and if the arthritis remains active a synovial biopsy should be performed. The tissue should be sent for culture (including for mycobacteria) and histology. In the case of the knee this may be conveniently done arthroscopically.

## INVESTIGATIONS USED IN RHEUMATOLOGICAL PRACTICE

### Erythrocyte sedimentation rate (ESR)

Most patients attending with a rheumatological problem merit having an ESR (or plasma viscosity) performed. An elevation in the ESR is largely determined by the increase in the level of immunoglobulins and fibrinogen found in inflammatory disorders. Accordingly, its value lies in distinguishing between inflammatory and non-inflammatory disease. However, occasional patients are seen with a normal ESR but who yet have an active inflammatory disease. Polymyositis is notorious in this regard, about half of cases having a normal ESR.

### C-reactive protein (CRP)

CRP is an acute-phase protein and its level broadly mirrors the ESR but is more sensitive to changes in disease activity. It is less good than the ESR as a screening test, being normal in myeloma and macroglobulinaemia. The reason for this disparity is that an acute-phase reaction is not found in these two conditions but the changes in plasma proteins that occur give rise to a high ESR. Some of the connective tissue diseases, such as SLE, produce only a small rise in CRP but during intercurrent infections the CRP level becomes considerably elevated.

### Rheumatoid factor

Rheumatoid factor is also referred to as antiglobulin because it is an antibody against determinants on the Fc fragment of human or animal IgG. Rheumatoid factors may be of all five immunoglobulin classes but it is IgM rheumatoid factor that is measured in the widely used latex and Rose–Waaler tests. In the latex test, human IgG-coated latex particles are used, which on the addition of the patient's serum will become agglutinated if rheumatoid factor is present. The Rose–Waaler test is similarly an agglutination test in which rabbit IgG-coated sheep red blood cells are used rather than human IgG-coated latex particles.

The latex test is more sensitive but less specific than the Rose–Waaler test. Seventy per cent or more of patients with rheumatoid arthritis have IgM rheumatoid factor in their serum. It confers a less good prognosis and a greater chance of developing erosions, nodules and other extra-articular features. IgM rheumatoid factor may also be found in other autoimmune disorders (Table 8.8), many infectious disorders (e.g., infectious mononucleosis, viral hepatitis, subacute bacterial endocarditis, malaria, kala-azar and schistosomiasis) and various other disorders—fibrosing alveolitis,

**Table 8.8 The frequency (%) of positive rheumatoid factor and antinuclear antibody tests in various autoimmune diseases**

|  | Antinuclear antibody | Rheumatoid factor |
|---|---|---|
| Systemic lupus erythematosus | 95 | 40 |
| Rheumatoid arthritis | 40 | 70 |
| Progressive systemic sclerosis | 80 | 35 |
| Sjögren's syndrome | 60–70 | 75–100 |
| Chronic active hepatitis | 50 | 20 |
| Cryptogenic fibrosing alveolitis | 30 | 30 |

chronic liver disease, sarcoidosis and Waldenström's macroglobulinaemia. A positive latex or Rose–Waaler test may also occur in around 5 per cent of normal individuals and this frequency increases with age. It is usually of low titre.

IgG rheumatoid factor is quantitatively the most important rheumatoid factor but its measurement is not in common clinical usage.

## Antinuclear antibody test

This test has superseded the LE cell test. It is less time consuming and because of its greater sensitivity acts as a valuable screening test for SLE.

The test is done by taking a cryostat section of unfixed tissue (e.g., rat liver) and incubating it with dilutions of the patient's serum. After washing, a fluorescein-labelled antihuman IgG antibody is applied, which will react with any IgG from the test serum that has become attached to the section. Having washed the section once more it is viewed by ultraviolet-light microscopy and any staining observed.

Various antinuclear staining patterns are recognized. Homogeneous staining is the commonest pattern and represents antibody to deoxyribonucleoprotein (DNA-histone). It is mainly seen in SLE and to a lesser extent in rheumatoid arthritis, Sjögren's syndrome and drug-induced lupus.

Peripheral staining correlates with native, double-stranded DNA and is highly specific for SLE. Speckled staining is due to antibody against soluble, non-histone proteins (extractable nuclear antigens) and is seen in mixed connective tissue disease, scleroderma and SLE. Lastly, a nucleolar

staining pattern (anti-RNA) is occasionally seen and is mainly associated with scleroderma.

As with tests for rheumatoid factor, the test for antinuclear antibody is nonspecific and a positive test (25 iu/ml or more) may be seen in various conditions in addition to those in Table 8.8, such as polymyositis, dermatomyositis, juvenile chronic arthritis, myasthenia gravis, infectious mononucleosis and mixed connective tissue disease.

## Anti-DNA antibodies

The nuclear antigens giving these staining patterns and other nuclear antigens have in recent years been more closely characterized (see Hughes [1984] and Bernstein [1987]—'Further Reading'). Antibodies to double-stranded DNA are highly specific for SLE. There are two methods in common usage for detecting these antibodies. The Farr ammonium sulphate precipitation of antibody to radiolabelled double-stranded DNA (DNA binding) is the more commonly used technique. The other method is an immunofluorescent test against the double-stranded DNA containing kinetoplast of *Crithidia luciliae*. Antibodies to double-stranded DNA are found in 70 per cent of cases of SLE and high levels of antibody in general correlate well with increased disease activity. However, there are some patients with SLE who remain clinically well despite high levels of antibody.

## HLA typing

Study of the histocompatibility antigens has greatly increased our understanding of the spondarthritides (HLA B27) (Table 8.9) and also of rheumatoid arthritis (HLA DR4). Whilst, at the present time HLA typing has no part to play in the investigation or management of rheumatoid arthritis, it does, however, under two circumstances have some diagnostic value in patients with possible B27-associated disorders. Firstly, in young patients with a seronegative oligoarthritis; secondly, in young patients with back pain, in whom the history and examination is suggestive of spondylitis but there are no supporting radiological changes and the diagnosis remains unclear. In both of these circumstances, though, it must be remembered that 7 per cent of the normal Caucasian population carry the B27 antigen and thus

**Table 8.9 HLA B27 antigen frequency in seronegative arthritis and normal controls (Caucasian population)**

|  | Antigen frequency (%) |
|---|---|
| Normal controls | 7 |
| Ankylosing spondylitis | 95 |
| Reiter's disease: |  |
| sexually acquired | 75 |
| post-dysenteric | 85 |
| Inflammatory bowel disease with spondylitis | 65 |
| Psoriatic arthritis: |  |
| peripheral arthritis | 25 |
| spondylitic | 80 |
| Anterior uveitis | 55 |

there is always the possibility of a false-positive result.

Asking for HLA B27 typing in clearcut cases of ankylosing spondylitis, Reiter's disease or psoriatic arthropathy is a waste of resources and money.

## Radiology

Radiographs are of great value in rheumatology not only in diagnosis but also in following the progress of disease. Plain X-rays are the most commonly requested and when a peripheral joint is involved the contralateral joint should also be filmed to allow comparison. Patients with polyarthritis should have radiographs of both hands (including the wrists) and feet taken at the outset. Those patients who continue to have active disease, especially rheumatoids, should have follow-up films taken to monitor the development or progression of any erosive change.

More specialized radiological investigations are also used. Arthrography in demonstrating synovial leaks (e.g., ruptured Baker's cyst) and double-contrast arthrography in delineating meniscal lesions in the knee joint. Lumbar radiculograms and CT scanning are widely used to define disc lesions and spinal stenosis. In addition, computed tomography is valuable in examining other areas, such as the sacroiliac and sternoclavicular joints.

Bone scans allow the early detection of metastases and avascular necrosis. Autologous Indium-111 labelled leucocyte scans and Gallium-67 scans have proved of value in localizing infection and thereby allowing infection of joint prostheses to be distinguished from loosening.

Magnetic resonance imaging is an exciting new non-invasive technique and is proving to be the method of choice for imaging menisci, tendons, ligaments and intervertebral discs.

## Further reading

Bernstein R. M. (1987). Antibodies to cells and connective tissue diseases. *Reports on Rheumatic Diseases* (Series 2). London: The Arthritis and Rheumatism Council.

Currey H. L. F., ed. (1986). *Mason and Currey's Clinical Rheumatology*. Edinburgh: Churchill Livingstone.

Dieppe P. A., Doherty M., Macfarlane D. G., Maddison P. J. (1985). *Rheumatological Medicine*. Edinburgh: Churchill Livingstone

Hughes G. R. V. (1984). Autoantibodies in lupus and its variants: experience in 1000 patients. *Br. Med. J.*, **289**, 339–42.

Jayson M. I. V., ed. (1976). Diagnosis and assessment. *Clinics Rheum. Dis.*, **2**, 1–297.

Jeffery M. S., Dick W. C., eds. (1983). The role of the laboratory in rheumatology. *Clinics Rheum. Dis.*, **9**, 1–285.

Kelley W. M., Harris E. D., Ruddy S., Sledge C. B., eds. (1989). *Textbook of Rheumatology*, 3rd edn. Eastbourne: Holt-Saunders

Waddell G. (1982). An approach to backache. *Br. J. Hosp. Med.*, **28**, 187–219.

Williams P., Gumpel M. (1980). Aspiration and injection of joints (1). *Br. Med. J.*, **281**, 990–2.

Williams P., Gumpel M. (1980). Aspiration and injection of joints (2). *Br. Med. J.*, **281**, 1048–9.

# 9

# ENDOCRINOLOGY

Anthony P. Weetman

Endocrine disorders can produce a wide variety of non-localizing signs and symptoms because the effects of abnormal levels of circulating hormone are reflected in the response of the target organs. Therefore, examination and investigation of a patient with these diseases depend upon awareness of this diversity in presentation. Endocrine disorders may be common (thyroid dysfunction, diabetes mellitus) or rare (acromegaly, Addison's disease) but, irrespective of prevalence, cases turn up in examination after examination. This is the result of rather static physical signs (even successfully treated acromegaly does not regress rapidly) and the importance of recognizing the major endocrine problems, which are so amenable to treatment.

Another distinctive feature of endocrinology is the heavy reliance placed on laboratory testing in this speciality. The broad principles of testing endocrine function are (a) screen for abnormal hormone secretion and then do more detailed testing to define the exact aetiology; (b) if hyperfunction is suspected, see if the relevant hormone can be suppressed normally, and if hypofunction is suspected, see if the hormone can be stimulated normally. Too often inappropriate or superfluous testing is undertaken for suspected endocrine disorders, when a more logical approach would save time, money and effort.

In this chapter I will concentrate only on the practical aspects of diagnosis and management of the major endocrine disorders of adulthood encountered in general medical practice; in particular, disorders of growth and sex differentiation and detailed investigation of infertility and virilism will not be discussed. Where values are given for hormone levels, these are only as a guide; each laboratory will provide its own reference range.

## SPECIFIC ASPECTS OF THE GENERAL EXAMINATION IN ENDOCRINOLOGY

There is no straightforward way to examine the 'endocrine system' in the way that there is for the heart. Clues to an endocrine disease may be obtained from the patient's general appearance. The facies of acromegaly, Cushing's syndrome, hypothyroidism and thyrotoxicosis are characteristic. The patient's skin may be pigmented as in Addison's disease or Nelson's syndrome, pale due to hypopituitarism or yellowish due to carotene accumulation in myxoedema. Loss of body hair and testicular atrophy are characteristic of hypopituitarism.

Examination of the hands can reveal acromegalic changes, the tremor, moistness and occasional palmar erythema of thyrotoxicosis, and the short fourth metacarpal of pseudohypoparathyroidism. Carpopedal spasm, spontaneous or induced, occurs with hypoparathyroidism. Thyroid acropachy is a form of clubbing usually seen in association with Graves' ophthalmopathy. While examining the hands, you should check the skin thickness on the back of the hand; this is increased in acromegaly and decreased in Cushing's syndrome and hypopituitarism. The lower limb may show pretibial myxoedema in Graves' disease or the skin lesions of diabetes—'hockey-stick' shins, foot ulcers and necrobiosis lipoidica.

A goitre demands full assessment—diffuse or nodular, mobile or fixed, hard or soft—and associated lymphadenopathy should be sought.

Examination of the eyes can reveal the changes of Graves' ophthalmopathy, the calcification of hyperparathyroidism, and the cataracts and retinopathy of diabetes. Pituitary tumours have important effects on the optic chiasm and less commonly the IIIrd, IVth and VIth cranial nerves, and in all such patients careful examination of the visual fields and eye movements is essential.

Prolactinomas may produce galactorrhoea that is not apparent without manual expression; this can be demonstrated by gently massaging the milk towards the nipple. Other signs suggestive of endocrinopathy may only come laterally from examining other systems. In particular, peripheral vascular disease and a variety of neuropathies may be due to diabetes mellitus, and atrial fibrillation may be due to thyrotoxicosis.

## DIABETES MELLITUS

This has a prevalence of about 2 per cent in the UK. The major primary forms are type I (usually juvenile- or adolescent-onset patients who require insulin; probably due to autoimmunity) and type II (late-onset patients who often do not require insulin, due to relative insulin resistance as well as reduced secretion; there is a stronger family history than in type I but the exact nature of the defects is unknown). Type III diabetes (phasic insulin-dependence or tropical diabetes) is a major type of diabetes mellitus worldwide, usually occurring in adolescents with preceding severe malnutrition. Secondary diabetes arises from pancreatic disorders or excessive production of diabetogenic hormones, e.g., growth hormone, cortisol and glucagon. This section will deal only with the main presenting features and management problems of diabetes, although much of the current interest in the field lies in attempts to uncover the pathogenesis, which should allow prevention or cure.

### Presentation

There is a spectrum of presentation. In the older patient the diagnosis is often made by routine urine testing when investigating a related disorder, e.g., peripheral vascular disease. Symptoms in this group may include blurred vision, skin infections and thrush (vaginitis or balanitis). The classic presentation in type I diabetes is with polyuria, polydipsia and polyphagia progressing to ketoacidosis but in many the course is subacute and there may be a history of weight loss and lack of energy over the preceding one or two months. Rarer presenting symptoms may be related to neuropathy (especially impotence) or nephropathy.

### Diagnosis

Glycaemia, like blood pressure, is a continuous variable and the cut-off point between normal and abnormal is to some extent arbitrary. However, a single clearly elevated blood glucose (>8 mmol/l fasting or >11 mmol/l random) with symptoms is sufficient to establish the diagnosis of diabetes mellitus. The diagnosis can be made without any need for an oral glucose tolerance test (OGTT) in over 80 per cent of patients merely by checking blood glucose.

An OGTT is required when the fasting glucose is equivocal, is less than 8 mmol/l but diabetes is strongly suspected because of complications, or when screening for gestational diabetes (e.g., in women with a strong family history, previous large babies, multiple stillbirths or polyhydramnios). In the OGTT, the patient is given 75 g of glucose solution (most tolerably as 'Lucozade', 350 ml) in the morning after a 12-h fast. There should be no carbohydrate restriction at least three days before the test. It is customary to take a glucose sample before the glucose loading and thereafter at 30 min intervals for two hours. In diabetes mellitus, the 2-h glucose is >11 mmol/l and in subjects with impaired glucose tolerance, 8 to 11 mmol/l; in either group intermediate values may rise above 11 mmol/l. Asymptomatic subjects with impaired glucose tolerance normally fare better than those with frank diabetes (and some may subsequently have a normal OGTT), but this is not the case in patients with impaired glucose tolerance and symptoms. Moreover, impaired tolerance in pregnancy also demands close attention because it worsens obstetric risk and is associated with an increased incidence of subsequent diabetes.

### Management
#### Diabetic emergencies

There are two common diabetic emergencies: diabetic ketoacidosis, in which there is hyperglycaemia and a metabolic acidosis with raised ketone levels and non-ketotic hyperosmolar coma, in which uncontrolled hyperglycaemia is not associated with significant ketosis. However, these should be regarded as extremes of a continuous spectrum. Ketoacidosis occurs with previously undiagnosed diabetes or in established diabetics who have an added illness (infection, myocardial infarction) or who omit insulin, often because of an associated health problem such as vomiting. Clinical features are variable but include confusion progressing to coma, Kussmaul respiration, dehydration, nausea, vomiting and abdominal pain. Diagnosis may be apparent from the smell of ketones in the breath and should be confirmed rapidly by testing the blood for glucose and ketones by appropriate indicator strips. Blood gases, urea and electrolytes, chest X-ray, ECG and cultures from the blood and urine should be obtained and treatment instituted promptly as in Table 9.1. Added complications such as hypotension, aspiration, hypothermia and deep vein thrombosis should be anticipated and ideally prevented, as should iatrogenically-induced hypoglycaemia, hypokalaemia and heart failure.

**Table 9.1 Management of diabetic ketoacidosis**

*Aims*:
    Rehydration
    Replace potassium
    Restore normoglycaemia gradually
    Correct acid-base balance (bicarbonate rarely
        needed)
    Treat underlying illness

*Initial treatment*:

| | |
|---|---|
| Insulin | 6 units i.v. followed by |
| | 6 units/hour by i.v. infusion |
| Fluids | 0.9% saline 1 litre in 30–60 min then |
| | 1 litre/hour for 2 hours then |
| | 1 litre/4 hours |
| | (If Na >150 mmol/l, give 1 litre of 0.45% saline initially) |
| Potassium | 20 mmol KCl to each litre of saline (provided $K^+$ <6 mmol/l) |
| | Keep $K^+$ between 4–5 mmol/l |

Monitor blood glucose hourly and electrolytes at 2 and 5 hours

*Consider*:
    Bicarbonate (if pH <7.0) : give 100 mmol Na $HCO_3$
                            with 20 mmol KCl over
                            1 hour
    Blood or plasma (if systolic BP <80 mm Hg)
    Oxygen (if hypoxic)
    Heparin (if elderly or unconscious)
    Antibiotics (if infection suspected)
    Nasogastric tube, CVP line, urine catheter

*Later treatment*:
    Replace saline with 10% glucose plus 10 mmol KCl (1 litre/4–8 hours) when blood glucose <14 mmol/l. Reduce insulin to 3 units/hour by infusion and convert thereafter to subcutaneous insulin.

Non-ketotic hyperosmolar coma characteristically occurs in older patients with previously undiagnosed type II diabetes. In such patients dehydration is more severe due to impaired recognition of thirst but ketosis is prevented by the presence of sufficient insulin to prevent ketogenesis (although it is insufficient to avert hyperglycaemia). Patients present with a range of symptoms but commonly are very dehydrated and have an altered level of consciousness. Kussmaul breathing is absent. Their management is generally the same as for those with ketoacidosis but the elderly withstand fluid overload less well and caution is required in correcting dehydration. Measuring the plasma osmolality is important and in extreme cases 0.45% saline may need to be used as initial fluid replacement.

Lactic acidosis is a rare complication in diabetes and is almost always seen in patients taking the biguanide metformin. This is much less likely to cause the problem than phenformin, now withdrawn. Renal and hepatic failure demand reduction of the dosage of metformin. Failure to appreciate this, or accidental overdosage account for most cases of lactic acidosis. The patient usually presents in coma with acidotic breathing but without hyperglycaemia or ketosis. Treatment is rehydration and infusion of sodium bicarbonate but the mortality is high.

### Primary treatment

Type I diabetics need insulin, which should be given twice daily. The best regimen for most patients is a short- plus intermediate-acting insulin, e.g., Actrapid plus Monotard, Humulin S plus Humulin Zn, although fixed combination preparations, e.g., Mixtard, may work in some. Insulins can be either human or porcine. There is little to choose between them except cost, although human soluble insulin is absorbed faster than porcine and may be less immunogenic. In the future, recombinant human insulin is likely to become the standard. Small doses of insulin (up to 20 u total daily) should be given initially, split to give equal amounts of short- and intermediate-acting components, with two thirds of the daily total in the morning and one third in the evening. Doses are adjusted thereafter by regular premeal monitoring of blood glucose. Careful instruction in injection technique, including the need to rotate sites, is mandatory; injection into the abdomen is easy to master and absorption from there is not affected by exercise as it is after injection into the leg or arm.

Glycaemic control can be improved by several methods. The simplest is to increase the number of injections, although patients are often reluctant to do this. A convenient method is to give a 'blanket cover' of long-acting Ultratard in the evening supplemented by Actrapid before each meal. This is now best done with a portable multidispensing device like the NovoPen and Penject, which can be easily carried, are simple to use and, besides giving good control, allow greater flexibility in meals, e.g., eating out. If nocturnal hypoglycaemia or matinal hyperglycaemia is a problem, the evening dose of intermediate insulin should be given before going to bed rather than before dinner. Continuous, subcutaneous infusion of insulin by a portable pump appears to offer the best possible opportunity for normalizing blood glucose but precise indications for its use are not yet established. The patient must be highly motivated and there must be adequate clinical back-up. Trials suggest that this delivery system can reduce complications but the same is probably true for intensified conventional treatment.

Diet is important in type I diabetes. Total intake should avoid weight gain, and calorie intake should be distributed between regular meals to avoid large swings in blood glucose. The emphasis is now on a low-fat, high-fibre intake, which has rendered obsolete ideas of carbohydrate restriction; complex carbohydrates should make up the energy balance produced by a reduction in fat intake.

In type II diabetes, diet is usually the first line of treatment; this should aim to produce weight loss and reduce the elevation of glucose after meals. While total energy intake is a key factor, the postprandial glucose peaks can be reduced by a high-fibre intake supplemented by guar gum sprinkled on the food, if the patient will tolerate this. A low-fat intake should also be recommended and again guar may provide extra control of hyperlipidaemia. If diet, alone or with guar, is inadequate, hyperglycaemia may be controlled by oral hypoglycaemic agents, but the effect of these is often less than expected, particularly over a long period of time. Glibenclamide is usually used, starting at a dose of 2.5 mg/day (up to a maximum of 15 mg); in the elderly tolbutamide (up to 500 mg, three times daily) is preferable because its shorter action runs less risk of producing hypoglycaemia. Metformin may be added to sulphony-

lureas, particularly in obese patients, but may produce lactic acidosis and is contraindicated in patients with impaired hepatic, renal or cardiac function. Its use is limited and should always be carefully monitored. Although type II diabetes is frequently termed 'non-insulin-dependent', this is misleading and insulin should always be given if hyperglycaemia remains a problem. In the elderly, less rigorous control than in type I diabetics is often adequate and so a single daily injection of a long-acting insulin, e.g., Monotard, should be tried.

### General follow-up

Patients need education about their disorder and the need to achieve good glucose control. They also need sympathy and time, which are often short in a busy diabetic clinic. New diabetics on insulin or tablets must inform both the DVLC at Swansea and their car insurance company of their disorder. Safe driving demands education, good glucose control and preparation before driving any distance. A Medic-Alert bracelet or similar device is a sensible precaution and patients should be made aware of the benefits of joining the British Diabetic Association. Advice is also needed about smoking (i.e., stop at all costs), alcohol (only in moderation), foot care and contraception (the low-dose combined oral contraceptive is suitable; patients should let their clinic know as soon as possible after becoming pregnant). All patients attending a clinic should have at least an annual assessment for possible complications (see below) including screening for creatinine, hyperlipidaemia, and abnormalities on ECG. A baseline chest X-ray should be done on new diabetics.

Glycaemic control is best monitored in two ways:
(1) *Home blood glucose monitoring.* This should be done before each meal one or two days a week in most cases, although in very well-controlled patients or those with mild diabetes (on diet or oral agents) this need not be so frequent. It is a mistake to believe that non-insulin dependent diabetics need only use urine testing as a measure of control. This is an inaccurate method that will not provide the necessary information, i.e., whether the patient requires additional measures to control glucose; modern blood sampling devices (e.g., 'Autolet') are not painful to use and the

method is less of a problem for many patients than urine testing. Unless life expectancy is short, patients should be persuaded to perform home blood glucose monitoring if possible. Although visual assessment of the monitoring strips (e.g., BM-Test glycemie) is usually adequate, some patients prefer to buy a meter that accurately reads the glucose value. A meter should also be used to manage pregnant diabetics.

(2) The *integrated glycaemic control* over the preceding four to six weeks can be checked in the clinic using glycosylated haemoglobin (HbA$_{1c}$) or serum fructosamine.

## Chronic complications of diabetes

### *The eye*

Regular (annual) examination of the eyes is essential in all patients. The visual acuity in each eye should be recorded, if necessary with a pinhole or lenses (or glasses) to correct refractive errors. Cataracts should be sought (10+ dioptre lens on ophthalmoscope) and any new vessels on the iris (rubeosis) identified. Then with the pupils dilated a systematic examination of the fundus is made (Fig. 9.1). Changes can be grouped as follows.

(1) Background retinopathy with microaneur-ysms, small haemorrhages and scattered hard and cotton-wool exudates. Veins and arteries may be irregular.

(2) Diabetic maculopathy: the same lesions are situated near the macula and threaten vision. It is subdivided into three types according to the predominant lesion: exudative, oedematous and ischaemic.

(3) Preproliferative retinopathy; severe changes with intraretinal microvascular abnormalities, that is, tortuous dilated vessels in the retina.

(4) Proliferative retinopathy, with new vessel formation. These vessels can bleed, producing a vitreous or subhyaloid haemorrhage, or they may be associated with fibrous tissue, which can cause retinal detachment.

Minimal background retinopathy requires careful follow-up in the diabetic clinic but more active retinopathy should be referred to a specialist eye centre, urgently if there is new vessel formation or macular involvement. Full assessment will then consist of indirect ophthalmoscopy, retinal photography and fluorescein angiography to determine the need for and extent of treatment. Photocoagulation should be given before severe deterioration because by then it may be too late to achieve good results; hence the emphasis on regular screening in asymptomatic patients.

Photocoagulation is usually performed with an

(a)
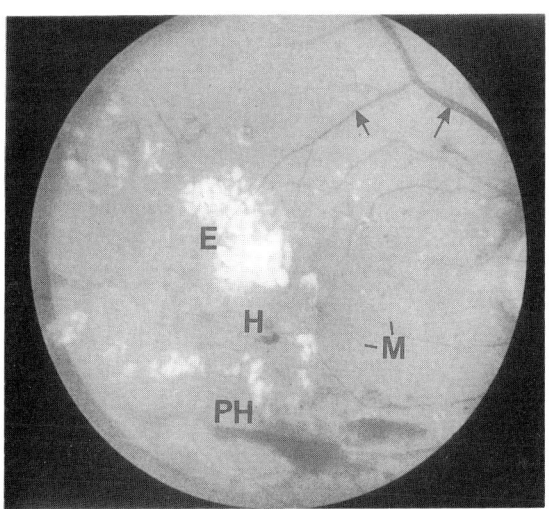

(b)
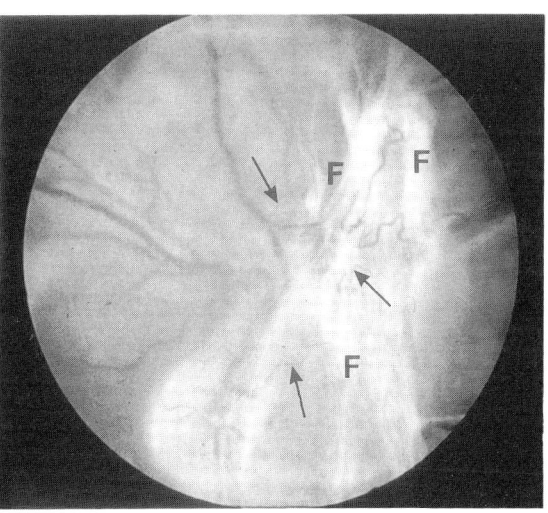

*Figure 9.1* Diabetic retinopathy. (a) Hard exudates (E) near the macula with microaneurysms (M), deep blot haemorrhages (H), pre-retinal haemorrhages (PH) with fluid levels, and venous dilatation (arrowed). (b) Extensive fibrous tissue (F) with new vessel formation (arrowed) (photo courtesy of Dr G. Williams).

argon laser, which requires only local anaesthesia. This treatment in exudative maculopathy aims to seal leaky vessels near the macula by making burns of small diameter over the vessel or exudate. Oedematous maculopathy is usually treated with a 'grid' of burns around the macula because the lesion is more generalized. Ischaemic maculopathy responds relatively poorly to treatment. For proliferative retinopathy, new vessels may be coagulated directly but a more effective approach for new vessels arising from the periphery or the disc is panretinal photocoagulation. At least 2000 burns are placed over the retina, avoiding the macula, and this destruction of ischaemic areas prevents new vessel formation by removing the source of factors inducing angiogenesis. More treatment can be given if vessels fail to regress.

Surgery is required in diabetic eye disease for cataract, and vitrectomy can be performed for retinal detachment and vitreous haemorrhage. However, the vitreous haemorrhage is usually first treated expectantly with bed rest if the patient has both eyes functioning. Surgery is done only if the haemorrhage fails to resolve after several months.

## Nephropathy

Microalbuminuria assessed by radioimmunoassay is a good predictor of subsequent nephropathy and precedes the appearance of proteinuria as detectable on routine screening. Diabetics should at the least have dipstick testing for proteinuria every three to six months. Demonstrable proteinuria should be followed by careful microscopy of the urine, culture and estimation of the creatinine clearance. Absence of retinopathy suggests a non-diabetic cause for proteinuria and a coincidental renal lesion should be sought. Overt proteinuria goes on to chronic renal failure in 5 to 15 years. These patients require careful control of blood glucose and blood pressure to minimize the rate of deterioration, and if urinary protein losses are not excessive (e.g., with the nephrotic syndrome) protein restriction may also help.

Haemodialysis is not well tolerated by diabetics and chronic ambulatory peritoneal dialysis is preferable. Insulin can be given by this route and glycaemic control may improve. Renal transplantation, especially from a living donor, offers the best prospects in diabetics with chronic renal failure.

## Neuropathy

A variety of neuropathies may occur in diabetes (Table 9.2). Apart from the clinical features, autonomic neuropathy can be diagnosed by simple bedside tests, the easiest of which is to perform an ECG while the patient performs deep breathing or stands up from lying. In both cases the R–R interval (i.e., beat to beat heart rate) fails to vary in autonomic neuropathy. It is important to document autonomic neuropathy because this is associated with increased mortality from cardiovascular arrest and caution is required giving general anaesthesia to these patients. Unfortunately, there is little treatment that benefits diabetic neuropathy, although mononeuropathy and radiculopathy usually recover spontaneously.

**Table 9.2 Diabetic neuropathy**

| Type | Signs and symptoms |
| --- | --- |
| Radiculopathy | Pain and sensory loss in a dermatome |
| Mononeuropathy (may be multiple) | Pain, weakness and sensory loss; reflex change—may affect cranial nerves, especially the oculomotor nerve |
| Polyneuropathy | Glove and stocking sensory loss, later loss of pain and muscle weakness; absent reflexes and impaired vibration sense |
| Autonomic neuropathy | Impotence, postural hypotension, peripheral oedema, reduced sweating, gastric atony, incontinence, diarrhoea, Argyll Robertson pupil, sudden death |
| Amyotrophy | Pain over the anterior thigh and weakness of proximal leg muscles—responds well to improved glucose control |

## Peripheral vascular disease

This is a clinically detectable manifestation of the increased incidence and earlier presentation of atherosclerosis in diabetics. All diabetics should have their feet checked regularly for ischaemia, neuropathy and infection. In the ischaemic foot, pulses are absent and it feels cold and painful (contrasting with the warm and numb foot in neuropathy). Night pain, relieved by dangling the legs over the side of the bed, is a common symptom.

The ischaemia predisposes to infection, which can easily become chronic and deep-seated. This is aided by dulling of pain sensation if the patient has an associated neuropathy that allows trauma to pass unnoticed. Trophic ulcers must be avoided by advising on chiropody, shoes (loose fitting and made-to-measure) and general precautions (do not walk barefoot). Patients should stop smoking, maintain a normal weight and try to achieve near-normal glycaemia. Beta-blockers should be avoided and oedema treated. Once established, ulcers should be treated early with rest, including elevation of the foot to improve venous drainage, systemic antibiotics, analgesia and regular dressing.

Patients presenting with intermittent claudication should be treated expectantly and encouraged to exercise to tolerance limits, so that the collateral circulation may be optimized. Angioplasty, vessel reconstruction or grafting are required in patients with (a) severe, established claudication; (b) ulcers that don't respond to medical treatment; and (c) gangrene, which requires not only amputation but also increased blood flow to ensure its successful abolition. Gangrene confined to the toes may be treated with local or ray excision (Fig. 9.2). However, in many patients, major amputation is required to deal with spreading gangrene or deep-seated infection, when arterial reconstruction is not possible.

### Surgery in diabetes

Diabetics need an adequate period of preoperative glucose assessment for optimum management. Patients on a diet with reasonable control before surgery require only frequent glucose assessment after the operation; conversion to insulin should be prompt if control deteriorates. In all but minor surgery, patients on oral hypoglycaemics should be started preoperatively on twice daily insulin and this is continued until full recovery. An all-round regimen for managing insulin and glucose control during surgery is given in Table 9.3, assuming an operation first on the morning list (which should be aimed for wherever possible). A refinement of this regimen is to give the insulin by a separate infusion pump. While providing greater flexibility, it also demands much closer attention.

### Pregnancy in diabetes

Meticulous glucose control is essential to avoid increased fetal mortality, congenital malformations and high birth weight. Referral should be made to a combined medical/obstetric ante-natal

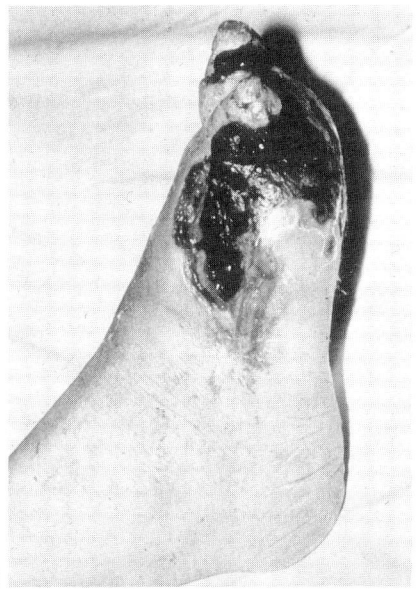

(a)

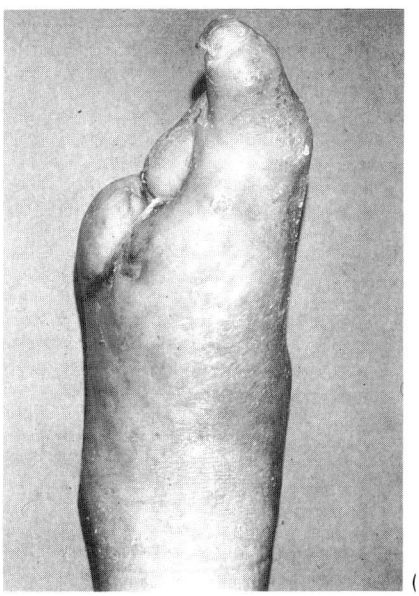

(b)

*Figure 9.2*   (a) Severe peripheral vascular disease in a diabetic with gangrene. (b) A good result was obtained in this patient by ray excision (photo courtesy of Dr G. Williams).

**Table 9.3 Insulin regimen for surgery in diabetes**

No subcutaneous insulin on the day of surgery
*08.00* Set up intravenous infusion of 500 ml 10 per
    cent glucose containing 15 u Actrapid and 10 mmol
    KCl: give over 5 h
*10.00* Check blood glucose:
if 5–10 mmol/l—continue
if <5 mmol/l—change to 5 u Actrapid*
if >10 mmol/l—change to 20 u Actrapid*
if >20 mmol/l—change to 25 u Actrapid*
Repeat blood glucose every 3–4 h
Check K$^+$ twice during day:
if >5 mmol/l—stop KCl*
if <4 mmol/l—increase KCl to 20 mmol*
Continue infusion until feeding—then back to insulin
    twice daily

\* Other constituents of infusion and its rate remain the
same.

clinic. Patients with mild impaired glucose tolerance, discovered during pregnancy, may be tried
on a diet and regular home blood glucose monitoring. However, in any patient who fails to respond
to this, or in whom the HbA$_{1c}$ reveals poor
control, insulin should be started early. In such
patients three preprandial boluses of Actrapid
(e.g., using a NovoPen) are usually satisfactory.
Patients on regular, twice daily insulin also benefit
from a more intensive regimen; remember that
insulin requirements may double during the third
trimester.

Delivery should be planned according to
obstetric evidence of fetal well-being; the optimum time appears to be 38 weeks. Admission
before induction is helpful to stabilize control and,
during labour, this can be achieved by subcutaneous insulin and infusion of glucose, although the
protocol in Table 9.3 is probably preferable in all
cases where it can be adequately monitored. The
same regimen is also used for cover of caesarean
section, which should be done promptly in diabetics with any obstetric complications or whose
labour fails to progress.

## HYPOGLYCAEMIA AND INSULINOMA

### Presentation

The acute symptoms of hypoglycaemia are sweating, palpitations, tremor and tachycardia, often
accompanied by hunger, headache and weakness.
These symptoms may disappear spontaneously if
sufficient glucose is mobilized by the release of
adrenaline. Prolonged hypoglycaemia may result
in a variety of psychiatric symptoms and progress
to other forms of central nervous system involvement: increased reflexes, hemiplegia, coma and
finally death.

### Investigation and management

Iatrogenic and factitious causes of hypoglycaemia
are the most common. To make the diagnosis of
hypoglycaemia in insulinoma, the patient should
be tested by fasting. An overnight fast will often
be sufficient to confirm hypoglycaemia (<2
mmol/l) but if this fails, fasting should continue at
least for 48 h in hospital. The diagnosis depends on
proving Whipple's triad: (a) symptoms produced
by fasting with (b) biochemical evidence of hypoglycaemia and (c) reversal of symptoms by glucose. Insulin should also be checked at the time of
hypoglycaemia; an inappropriately high level confirms an insulinoma. The tumour may be localized
by arteriography or CT screening. Treatment is
primarily surgical but if this proves impossible
diazoxide or streptozotocin can be used.

## HYPERTHYROIDISM

### Presentation

This is a common disorder. In the classic epidemiological survey of Whickham in the North-
East of England, the prevalence was 2 per cent in
women, a ten-fold excess over men, with a mean
age at presentation of 48 years. Most cases (>80
per cent) are due to Graves' disease. Less commonly the cause is toxic multinodular goitre or
toxic adenoma; other causes (Table 9.4) are rare.
The typical patient complains of heat intolerance,
sweating, weight loss despite a good appetite,
tremor, fatigue and dyspnoea. Palpitations, pruritus, amenorrhoea and thirst may also be prominent. The patient or family may also be aware of
sleeplessness, irritability and other mood changes.

Early thyrotoxicosis may be much less obvious
and in the elderly the diagnosis can be notoriously
obscure; apathy, isolated atrial fibrillation or heart
failure may be the only clues.

### Examination

The patient's appearance may be characteristic
(Fig. 9.3). Systemic signs of any form of thyrotoxi-

**Table 9.4  Main causes of hyperthyroidism**

*Common*
Graves' disease
Toxic multinodular goitre
Toxic adenoma
Thyrotoxicosis factitia (ingestion of T3 or T4)
*Infrequent*
Transient thyrotoxicosis in subacute or postpartum
  thyroiditis
*Rare*
Struma ovarii: ectopic thyroid tissue in ovary
Hydatidiform mole or choriocarcinoma (very high
  levels of chorionic gonadotrophin behave like
  excess TSH)
Malignancy: ectopic TSH
Pituitary adenoma producing excess TSH
Rare follicular cell carcinomas
Jod–Basedow phenomenon: iodine ingestion in
  previously iodine-deficient patient

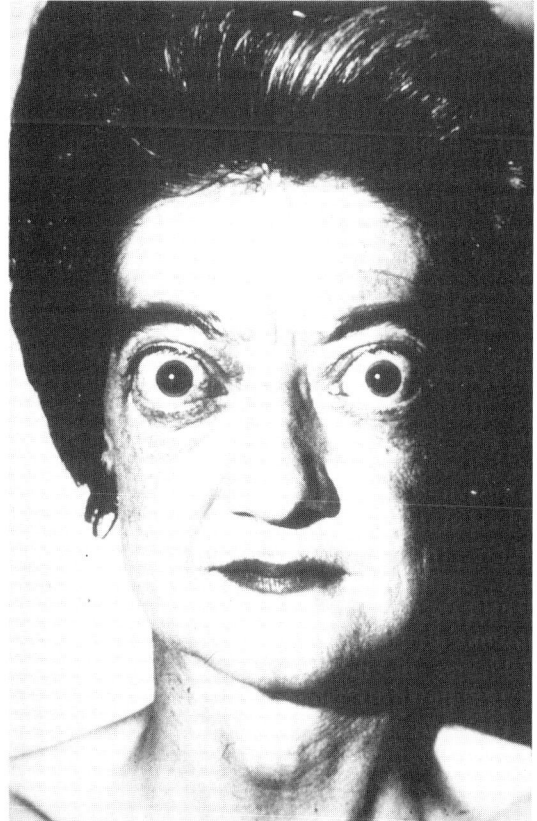

*Figure 9.3*  Typical facial appearance in thyrotoxicosis.

cosis include tremor, best assessed by palpation of the outstretched and spread fingers, warm and moist palms (a good distinguishing feature from anxiety states in which this is not found) and tachycardia (or atrial fibrillation). The patient may be obviously wasted and tendon jerks are brisk. Ankle oedema, not necessarily due to heart failure, and onycholysis are also features in some cases.

Thyroid palpation usually reveals a smooth diffuse goitre in Graves' disease, which contrasts with the nodular or multinodular swellings in the thyroid with toxic adenoma or toxic multinodular goitre. The goitre may be difficult to feel in men with Graves' disease. Having the patient slowly drink a glass of water may be useful; keep your fingers still beside the trachea to feel the gland as it moves up and down. The normal right lobe is usually the bigger of the two and it enlarges more in Graves' disease.

Graves' disease may be associated with a variety of eye signs (Fig. 9.4). Patients who have the eye signs of Graves' disease but are biochemically euthyroid are said to have ophthalmic Graves' disease: this dichotomy is a good indication that these two conditions are in fact separate although usually closely linked. The signs include lid lag (the inexperienced examiner often tests for this too fast: get the patient to follow your horizontal index finger slowly) and lid retraction, exophthalmos (the same as proptosis), periorbital oedema, chemosis (oedema of the conjunctiva, mild cases of which can be demonstrated by pushing the

lower lid gently over the lateral sclera, which causes a bulging of swollen conjunctiva at the lid margin), ophthalmoplegia, and rarely congestive ophthalmopathy. Lid retraction makes the sclera visible between the cornea and upper eyelid; exophthalmos makes it visible below. Proptosis can be measured easily using a Hertel exophthalmometer to provide a numerical record of eye changes. Because exophthalmos may prevent complete lid closure, exposure keratitis can develop. Always check that the patient can close the eyes properly. Proptosis, in particular, may be a sign confined to one eye only in Graves' ophthalmopathy and can be confused therefore with a retro-ocular tumour. Ophthalmoplegia causes double vision and this is most frequent when testing upward and outward gaze (superior rectus involvement); changes may then occur sequentially in upwards inward, lateral, medial and inferior directions. On extreme lateral and medial

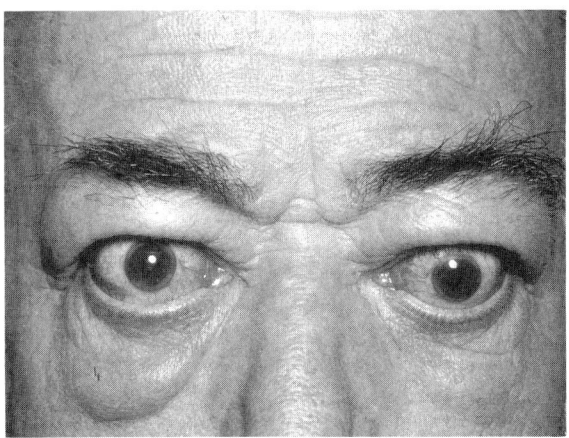

*Figure 9.4* Graves' ophthalmopathy. Note the proptosis (sclera visible below pupils), conjunctival injection and chemosis and periorbital oedema. Ophthalmoplegia is also present: there is asymmetry of the reflection of light from the pupils, indicating inability to elevate the left eye properly.

gaze, the inflamed insertions of the medial and lateral recti may be seen.

In congestive ophthalmopathy most of these features are present to an alarming degree; chemosis can be so severe that there is prolapse of inflamed conjunctivae between the lids. Although corneal ulceration may result, the most worrying complication of congestive ophthalmopathy is compression of the optic nerve, resulting in defective colour vision, scotomas, constriction of the visual fields or finally blindness.

Rarely (5 per cent) patients with Graves' disease develop pretibial myxoedema. Typically the skin is thickened and purple but with no pitting; other forms include an appearance like erythema nodosum (but not tender) and definite nodules. The main site is the shin but it can occur elsewhere, related to points of trauma or pressure. Thyroid acropachy is like clubbing, but without nail-fold oedema, and often occurs in patients with pretibial myxoedema. Other features sometimes found in Graves' disease are splenomegaly, lymphadenopathy, and evidence of other autoimmune diseases, e.g., vitiligo.

## Investigation

Newer hormone assays are supplanting standard investigations but, in some hospitals, the diagnosis of thyrotoxicosis still depends largely upon a raised serum total T4. Rarely only T3 (tri-iodothyronine) is increased (T3 toxicosis) so in a clinically thyrotoxic patient with normal T4, a T3 assay is indicated. Serum total T4 depends mainly upon the concentration of T4 bound to carrier proteins rather than the free effective fraction (<0.02 per cent of total) and is therefore of little value if the patient has a protein-binding anomaly. The commonest of these (1 in 2000) is excess T4-binding globulin (TBG) and these patients are euthyroid (normal free T4) but have a high total T4. This can be diagnosed by using the free T4 index or the more recently developed assays that measure only the free T4. Free T4 assays are simple to perform so these may soon replace total T4 assays but there are still pitfalls in their interpretation (Table 9.5). Another useful recently introduced test measures the serum thyroid-stimulating hormone (TSH) with assays sensitive enough to detect the low values that occur in thyrotoxicosis as the result of feedback suppression by the high levels of T3 and T4. Thus estimation of free T4 and sensitive TSH appear to be the future tests of choice for the diagnosis of most thyroid disorders. In the absence of a sensitive TSH assay, difficult cases can be diagnosed by the TRH test. The subject is given 200 µg TRH intravenously and the TSH is checked before and 20 min after the injection. Subjects with thyrotoxicosis fail to show any rise in TSH but so do some patients with acromegaly, Cushing's disease, ophthalmic Graves' disease or non-toxic, diffuse goitre.

Patients with Graves' disease usually have detectable autoantibodies to thyroglobulin and/or microsomes and these can be measured easily. However, the autoantibody that actually produces the thyrotoxicosis is a TSH-receptor antibody that stimulates thyroid hormone synthesis. Although these antibodies can be measured for research purposes, they have no routine clinical value. The best test to distinguish Graves' disease from other forms of thyrotoxicosis is thyroid scanning, usually with $^{99m}$Tc. Solitary or multiple toxic areas can be distinguished from the diffuse scan given by a Graves' thyroid. This test may also be valuable in patients with postpartum or subacute thyroiditis, in which destruction of the gland gives rise to temporary thyrotoxicosis but a reduced uptake of isotope (more accurately quantified by measuring uptake of $^{131}$I).

Graves' ophthalmopathy can usually be diagnosed on clinical grounds, but ophthalmic Graves'

**Table 9.5 Biochemical tests in thyrotoxicosis and disorders that can cause confusion with this**

| Condition | Total T4 | Total T3 | Free T4[a] | TSH |
|---|---|---|---|---|
| Thyrotoxicosis | ↑ | ↑ | ↑ | ↓ |
| T3 toxicosis | N | ↑ | N | ↓ |
| Increased thyroxine-binding globulin (genetic, pregnancy, oestrogens, hepatitis) | ↑ | ↑ | N | N |
| Abnormal albumin or pre-albumin[b] | ↑ | N | ↑ | N |
| T4-antibodies[b,c] | ↑ | N | ↑ | N |
| Amiodarone[b,d] | ↑ | N or ↓ | ↑ | N |
| Severe illness[b] | ↑, N or ↓ | ↓ | ↑, N or ↓ | ↑, N or ↓ |
| Peripheral or pituitary thyroid hormone resistance[b] | ↑ | ↑ | ↑ | N or ↑ |
| Iodine-containing contrast media[b] | ↑ | ↓ | ↑ | N or ↑ |

↑ = increased, ↓ = decreased, N = normal.
[a] Measured by single-step analogue method, e.g., Amerlex.
[b] These patients are euthyroid clinically and do not require treatment.
[c] T4 antibodies may occur in autoimmune thyroiditis.
[d] Permanent hyper- or hypothyroidism can also occur.

disease, particularly if unilateral, may present a problem. The differential diagnosis is from a retro-ocular tumour, including lymphoma or pseudotumour, an arteriovenous malformation behind the eye, and a frontal sinus mucocele. Positive thyroid autoantibodies may favour the diagnosis of ophthalmic Graves' disease but these are common in the population; a suppressed TSH by sensitive assay or a flat TSH response to TRH may also be found in some patients. However if there is any doubt, a CT scan of the orbits must be made to rule out any of the previously mentioned diagnoses. In Graves' ophthalmopathy the main finding is enlargement of the muscle bellies (Fig. 9.5) with sparing of the tendinous insertions; the whole muscle and its insertion are enlarged in orbital pseudotumour.

## Treatment

It is worth distinguishing cases of Graves' disease from the other causes of thyrotoxicosis because about 40 per cent of these patients will have a remission of their disease with antithyroid drugs (carbimazole, or less frequently propylthiouracil). There are two methods of treatment. The first is to start with high doses of carbimazole, 40 to 60 mg/day, and follow the patient regularly, reducing the dose progressively towards 5 to 10 mg daily as the patient becomes hypothyroid. The second is the blocking replacement regimen, which is much more convenient and probably more effective. The patient is given 40 mg carbimazole daily (divided in two doses for convenience but this is

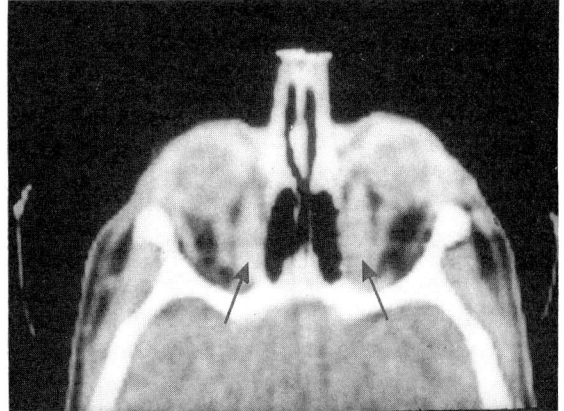

Figure 9.5 CT scan of the orbits in Graves' ophthalmopathy. There is symmetrical enlargement of the bellies, but not tendons, of the medial recti (arrowed). In some patients changes may be confined to one eye and the resulting unilateral proptosis must be differentiated from a retro-ocular tumour.

not essential pharmacologically) and after a month started on 100–150 μg T4 daily to maintain euthyroidism. This strategy requires less frequent follow-up and does not have to be tailored to each patient. Treatment in both cases is usually given for a period of one to two years, but there is no compelling evidence that this is more successful than a 6-month course of high-dose treatment, as in the blocking replacement regimen. All patients should be warned to report fever or sore throat immediately because this may herald agranulocytosis (less than 1 in 500 patients); this usually occurs in the first three months of treatment. With such symptoms the antithyroid drug should be stopped and a white cell count checked. Other side-effects include rashes, fever and arthralgias. Propylthiouracil is usually given to patients intolerant of carbimazole—for example, if it causes a skin rash.

In over half of patients with Graves' disease, antithyroid drug therapy fails to produce a long-term remission but, as there is no way to predict outcome, it is current practice to treat all new Graves' patients with a course of antithyroid drugs and then follow up at regular intervals to check for relapse (most occur in the first year after stopping treatment). There is no reliable prospect of remission after a second course of antithyroid drugs in these patients and destructive therapy, either surgery or radioiodine ($^{131}$I), should be recommended. This also applies to patients with toxic adenoma or multinodular goitre at initial presentation who will never be cured by antithyroid drugs. However, in all three groups, euthyroidism should be restored with carbimazole while definitive therapy is being arranged; this will normalize thyroid function as long as it is taken. Carbimazole should be stopped at least three days before giving $^{131}$I to allow uptake of the isotope.

Partial thyroidectomy is probably still indicated in women of child-bearing age and in those who wish a rapid cure of their disease; patient preference is also important. Radioiodine is becoming much more popular in all groups of patients as its long-term safety becomes established, and it is used for almost all patients in some clinics. There is little doubt that it is the treatment of choice for patients over 40 years of age and for those in whom surgery has failed. There is a certain failure rate (i.e., recurrent thyrotoxicosis) with both forms of treatment but this depends largely on the surgical or radiotherapeutic techniques used. Hypothyroidism is also a problem and is almost inevitable after radioiodine, even if the dose used is selected on the basis of gland size or tracer uptake to maintain euthyroidism. Such a regimen results in hypothyroidism in 10 per cent of patients at one year and 3 per cent per year thereafter; this should obviously be discussed with the patient before treatment. A rational extension of this observation is to render the patient hypothyroid by deliberately ablating the thyroid with a large dose (>550 MBq) of $^{131}$I and then restoring euthyroidism with T4, usually 100–150 µg/day. The advantages of this approach are that the patient requires little follow-up except to check that replacement is being maintained, recurrent hyperthyroidism does not occur and the gland can be at no risk from thyroid carcinoma. However, such an approach demands very careful discussion with the patient and communication with the general practitioner. In the elderly in particular, any form of radioiodine treatment may release so much stored hormone that severe thyrotoxicosis ensues. This can be avoided by giving carbimazole in the month before treatment. Propranolol may also be used to relieve milder symptoms.

Thyrotoxic storm is a rare and serious medical emergency, with sudden worsening of thyrotoxicosis, usually in already known cases. It may be brought on by any form of physical stress, such as surgery in patients who are not rendered euthyroid preoperatively, childbirth and severe infection. Most of the symptoms of thyrotoxicosis are prominent, with fever (up to 41°C) a major feature; thyroid storm may also produce abdominal pain, vomiting and diarrhoea. Propylthiouracil not only blocks synthesis of thyroid hormone but also blocks peripheral conversion of T4 to T3 and is therefore preferred to carbimazole in this condition. It should be given in doses of 200 mg 4-hourly. To inhibit release of already synthesized hormone, this should be supplemented with Lugol's iodine (saturated potassium iodide) 8 drops 6-hourly, but this should only be started an hour after propylthiouracil, to prevent new hormone being synthesized in response to the iodine. Many symptoms can be relieved with propranolol, 40 to 80 mg 6-hourly, and it is usual to give hydrocortisone, 300 mg intravenously followed by 100 mg intramuscularly 8-hourly; both agents inhibit conversion of T4 to T3. Parenteral fluids, antibiotics and treatment for heart failure may also be needed.

Mild degrees of Graves' ophthalmopathy usually cause only discomfort and cosmetic problems and in more severe cases, where exophthalmos and ophthalmoplegia are prominent, the disease is usually self-limiting. Methyl cellulose eye drops relieve the feeling of grittiness and guanethidine eye drops may be given to help lid retraction but these are uncomfortable to use and offer little benefit to most patients. Suturing the lateral portions of the eyelids (tarsorrhaphy) may prevent exposure keratitis from severe exophthalmos and improve the appearance. Protection of the eyes from dusty environments and wind is also sensible. Mild diplopia may be tolerated by some patients or improved in others by Fresnel prisms; however, corrective surgery of the eye muscles in the stable phase of the disease is now very successful and should be considered in all patients whose diplopia is a problem.

As mentioned above, congestive ophthalmopathy is a serious emergency that can progress with alarming speed. Expert joint medical and ophthalmological management is essential. Optic nerve involvement is an indication for steroids in high doses, e.g., dexamethasone 5 mg 6-hourly. Such a regimen runs the risks of infection and peptic ulceration; very close observation is necessary. If there is a good response, steroids are tailed off after a week and withdrawn after three months. If there is no improvement in 48 h, orbital decompression is needed, and in some centres this is performed in all patients because of the risks from high-dose steroids. Other forms of treatment, such as radiotherapy or immunosuppressants, have been tried but no clearly superior therapy has yet emerged.

## HYPOTHYROIDISM

### Presentation

The prevalence of hypothyroidism is over 1 per cent of the general population, with women affected 10 times more often than men. In about 80 per cent of cases this is the result of autoimmune hypothyroidism; it follows destructive therapy for thyrotoxicosis in most of the remainder. Other causes are rare in the UK but include congenital absence of the thyroid, dyshormonogenesis, Reidel's thyroiditis and the usually temporary hypothyroidism of subacute thyroiditis. It is worth remembering that iodine deficiency is still the major cause of goitre worldwide and can lead to hypothyroidism as well as endemic cretinism in severe cases. This is surely the most easily treated of all disorders, whose eradication has largely been prevented by an international lack of social and political will.

Hypothyroidism has been classified into three categories:
(1) *Subclinical*: no symptoms. There is marginal thyroid destruction and failure but increased pituitary secretion of TSH compensates and maintains a normal serum total T4.
(2) *Mild*: nonspecific symptoms only such as

tiredness. Again TSH is elevated and the T4 is around the lower limit of normal.
(3) *Overt* (myxoedema): there are clear symptoms, raised TSH and low T4. Patients complain of energy loss, constipation, anorexia, cold intolerance, loss of hair, flaking dry skin, weight gain, hoarseness of the voice, menorrhagia and, occasionally, carpal tunnel syndrome. Rarely, effusions occur into a wide variety of cavities: pleural, pericardial, peritoneal, middle ear and joints. Psychiatric changes range from common (nonspecific depression) to rare (organic psychoses, so-called myxoedema madness). Myxoedema coma is an extreme presentation, with hypothermia and hypoventilation. It is usually precipitated by cold exposure, infection or phenothiazines.

### Examination

Facial puffiness is often an obvious feature, accompanied by thinning of the scalp hair, periorbital swelling, dry flaky skin (often yellowish from carotene accumulation) and a hoarse voice (Fig. 9.6). The thyroid may be enlarged (usually in Hashimoto's thyroiditis, but large goitres occur in dyshormonogenesis), or impalpable (in primary atrophic thyroiditis), but always check for a thyroidectomy scar. In overt cases there is bradycardia and delayed relaxation of tendon reflexes. This latter sign is often best appreciated using the biceps rather than the Achilles tendon reflex. Rarer features include vitiligo, ascites, pleural effusions and deafness (due to serous otitis media but remember Pendred's syndrome: an autosomal recessive, iodine organification defect with deafness—this is the commonest form of dyshormonogenesis).

### Investigation and treatment

From the above classification it is clear that exclusion of hypothyroidism depends on the serum basal TSH. A sensitive type of assay is not necessary, and although intravenous TRH will give an exaggerated TSH response, it is totally superfluous to perform a TRH test. The basal T4 will define how low the thyroid hormone secretion has fallen and if below normal is a clear indication for treatment. Difficulty arises in those patients with nonspecific symptoms in whom increased TSH secretion is maintaining a T4 within low

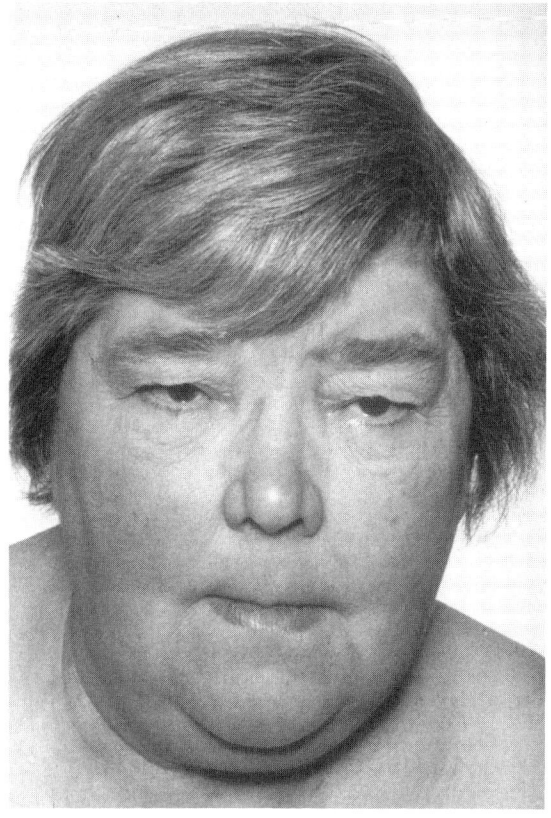

Figure 9.6 Typical facial appearance in clinical hypothyroidism.

normal limits. These patients clearly run the risk of going on to develop overt thyroid failure as autoimmune destruction of the gland continues. The risk of this happening is much higher in patients with circulating thyroglobulin and/or microsomal autoantibodies. It is therefore sensible to treat these patients, and those whose symptoms may be due to mild hypothyroidism, with thyroxine. In patients whose TSH is mildly elevated but who have a normal T4 and no thyroid autoantibodies, follow-up is probably all that is required.

Confusion may arise if the T4 is low but the TSH is normal. The commonest cause for this is a reduction in thyroxine-binding globulin, either inherited (X-linked) or due to protein loss (e.g., nephrotic syndrome), but it can also occur in patients taking phenytoin, salicylates or phenobarbitone. The normal TSH indicates euthyroidism and there is no need for treatment. Any severe systemic illness can produce lowering of T4 by a

combination of mechanisms, although it is not yet clear whether this is beneficial, irrelevant or detrimental. Replacement therapy is not normally given unless the TSH is elevated, but in this setting hypopituitarism must also be excluded.

The usual replacement dose of T4 is 100 to 150 µg daily. Elevation of the serum TSH provides a good index of underreplacement or lack of compliance. The serum T4 is often checked in patients on replacement to assess its adequacy but there may be large fluctuations in serum T4 depending on the time of sampling after ingestion of T4 and the result provides little information about compliance. At best a persistently elevated T4 is a sign that too much T4 is being given, but with sensitive TSH assays now also capable of assessing this (by detecting suppressed TSH levels), this test alone should provide the means to follow up T4 replacement in primary hypothyroidism.

A final caveat is the management of hypothyroidism in the postpartum period. It is now well recognized that many women (5–10 per cent) may experience a transient form of autoimmune thyroiditis after delivery and this can produce a hypothyroidism that is usually temporary (as discussed above, other women with the syndrome may have transient thyrotoxicosis). This is often neglected because symptoms are mild but if symptoms are prominent the condition warrants T4 replacement, particularly because the patient needs all the energy she can muster at this time. Attempts should be made after a sensible period (e.g., six months) to stop replacement gradually. This condition recurs in subsequent pregnancies and some women go on to develop permanent thyroid failure.

Myxoedema coma still has a fairly dismal outcome and should be prevented at all costs. At presentation, large doses of T4 are required (500 µg intravenous bolus on one occasion; further doses of T4 are not required in the next week). A more refined approach is to give 250 µg T4 intravenously immediately, plus 100 µg 24 h later, together with 25 µg T3 intravenously 12-hourly until the patient is able to take oral replacement. Meticulous general medical attention is also needed: ventilation is often required for respiratory acidosis, gradual rewarming is necessary, fluid and electrolyte balance must be maintained and infections require prompt treatment. Intravenous hydrocortisone is also given, 100 mg 8-hourly, to treat any unsuspected adrenal insufficiency.

## THYROID TUMOURS

Thyroid nodules are common and may be an incidental finding in the general medical clinic, so warrant a brief consideration here. Up to 10 per cent of nodules found by chance are malignant; all nodules need investigation. Symptoms such as pain or voice hoarseness, and signs such as lymphadenopathy, hardness of the nodule with fixation, and stridor all suggest malignancy.

The serum T4 is usually normal but if elevated suggests a toxic adenoma, virtually excluding thereby a malignancy. All nodules should be scanned, preferably with $^{123}$I, and in many centres they are subjected to fine-needle aspiration biopsy. If a functioning nodule (i.e., one which takes up isotope) is revealed, there is no need for surgery. A non-functioning ('cold') nodule requires further investigation; in experienced hands diagnosis by the fine-needle biopsy may prove over 90 per cent accurate, and certainly if a cyst is revealed, simple aspiration (with cytological examination of fluid) and close follow-up are probably all that is required. However, many centres still rely on open biopsy of the nodule for final diagnosis. If this reveals a carcinoma, management consists of selecting the appropriate regimen for the tumour type, in conjunction with surgeon and radiotherapist.

Thyroidectomy is usually indicated in almost all cases, together with external radiation for anaplastic carcinoma and lymphoma. If papillary or follicular cell carcinoma cannot be dealt with by surgery alone, radioiodine can be used to ablate residual thyroid tissue and, on the basis of repeated body scans, any metastases. Recurrence can also be monitored by measuring serum thyroglobulin, which should be undetectable if the thyroid has been ablated and there are no metastases. Patients will require replacement of T4 but this should be in large enough doses (up to 300 µg daily) to completely suppress TSH, which can be a trophic factor for some tumours.

## ACROMEGALY

### Presentation

This is an uncommon disorder (4 per 100 000) with no sex or racial predisposition; rarely it may be part of a multiple endocrine neoplasia syndrome (type 1), along with parathyroid and pancreatic adenomata. Very rarely ectopic production of growth hormone-releasing hormone by tumours can result in acromegaly; this hormone was recently sequenced from such material. Onset before epiphyseal fusion produces gigantism (less than 1 per cent of all cases), but in most patients the disease has an onset between the ages of 30 and 50 years, usually detectable by a retrospective review of family photographs. Attention is drawn to the condition in a roughly equal manner by (a) the patient noticing altered facial features or the size of hands or feet—excessive sweating and carpal tunnel syndrome are other common complaints; (b) symptoms produced locally by the pituitary adenoma, in particular headache, defects of the visual field and hypogonadism as the result of pressure on adjacent normal pituitary (cells producing thyrotrophin (TSH) and adrenocorticotrophic hormone (ACTH) are relatively more resistant to pressure effects than the gonadotrophs producing luteinizing hormone (LH) and follicle-stimulating hormone (FSH)—nonetheless, TSH and ACTH deficiency can occur in severe or longstanding cases); and (c) recognition by medical staff in the course of investigation for another complaint, for example acromegaly-associated hypertension.

### Examination

Typical acromegalic features are shown in Fig. 9.7. There is coarsening of the features, with a protruding jaw, prominent brow, and enlarged nose, ears, tongue and lips. Prognathism may prevent the patient being able to bite the fingernails. Skin tags are common on the neck and trunk and the skin may darken. Hands and feet also enlarge; check rings and shoes. Skin thickness is increased: this can easily be assessed by taking a fold of skin from the back of the patient's hand between your right thumb and index finger while simultaneously comparing with your own skin thickness by performing the same manoeuvre on the back of your right hand with your left thumb and index finger. This is surprisingly sensitive and can be refined further by using a suitable normal age- and sex-matched control, if available (really only worthwhile in the elderly).

Other organs may be detectably enlarged—including the heart, the liver and the thyroid (diffuse or nodular goitre). The ribs enlarge because of growth at the cartilage–bone junction, producing a chest that is sometimes too large for

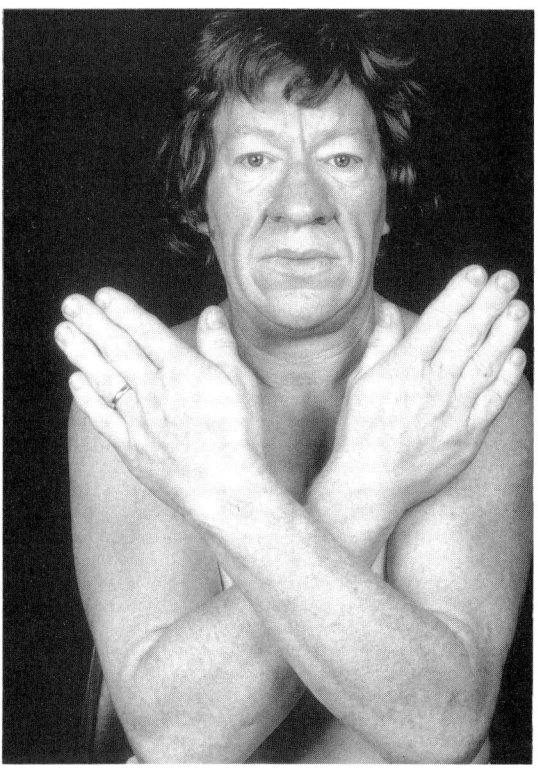

*Figure 9.7* Physical appearance in long-standing acromegaly (photo courtesy of Prof. G. F. Joplin).

a conventional X-ray film. Kyphosis may accompany the chest abnormalities. Carpal tunnel syndrome has been mentioned as a presenting feature and appropriate changes should be sought. In all patients, testing the visual fields is essential. This can be performed by confrontation in an examination setting but plotting with a Goldman perimeter or Bjerrum screen is required for routine management, so that an accurate record is maintained.

## Investigations

Due to fluctuations in basal levels, a random measurement of growth hormone is inadequate to exclude the diagnosis. In all patients in whom the diagnosis is suspected a glucose tolerance test is required. Growth hormone is measured on samples taken before and at 30-min intervals after the patient is given 50 g of glucose in solution (best given as 235 ml 'Lucozade'); the level should suppress to below 4 mU/l at some time during the 2-h period after the drink. Simultaneous measurement of glucose levels may reveal the impaired glucose tolerance found in 30 to 50 per cent of patients. A plain lateral radiograph of the skull may show expansion and destruction of the pituitary fossa but this is now rarely performed with the advent of CT scanning and magnetic resonance imaging.

Acromegaly can be a fatal disease; patients have double the expected death rate, usually from cardiovascular problems (although there are hints that neoplasia may also be more frequent). Moreover, major complications can arise from the local effects of the pituitary tumour. Thus treatment is indicated for active disease in almost all cases. Further investigations are required for management, which should be performed in a specialized centre. Before any therapeutic intervention, the remainder of pituitary function should be assessed, most readily done using the protocol in Table 9.6. The size of the tumour is best assessed by CT scanning or magnetic resonance imaging, which will localize microadenomata and document the extent of any suprasellar extension.

## Treatment

The mainstay of current treatment is ablation of the pituitary tumour with surgery or radiotherapy. Surgical removal is by the transsphenoidal route in all but the largest tumours but there is disagreement regarding the extent of surgery. Partial or total hypophysectomy rather than selective adenomectomy offers the better chance of complete tumour removal but at the expense of residual hypopituitarism in many patients (however, even 'total' hypophysectomy does not always lead to hypopituitarism because sufficient tissue may remain to resume normal function).

Radiotherapy may be considered if there is evidence of persisting tumour after surgery or in those cases in which surgery would be dangerous. It may also be used in some centres as principal therapy. There is no mortality and little morbidity (provided the dose and fractions are suitable; up to 45 Gy as daily fractions of 2 Gy maximum), but the disadvantage is the slow (effects may continue up to five years) and often only partial response. Accelerated particle or proton radiation and local implantation of $^{90}$Y seeds are used in some specialized centres but offer little advantage over conventional (photon) radiotherapy and may have their own problems.

## Table 9.6 Combined pituitary test

*Preparation*
ECG and history to exclude myocardial ischaemia and epilepsy
Fast patient from midnight
Give a reasonable account to the patient of expected symptoms
Insert butterfly cannula: keep patent with heparin–saline solution
Have intravenous glucose ready

*Test*
Take basal samples 30 min after inserting cannula
Give insulin:
   if probably hypopituitary—0.1 u/kg
   if probably normal—0.15 u/kg
   if probably acromegalic or Cushing's syndrome—0.3 u/kg
*plus* thyrotrophin-releasing hormone (TRH) 200 μg
*plus* gonadotrophin-releasing hormone (GnRH) 50 μg
   (all intravenously)

*Samples*

| Time (min): | 0 | 30 | 60 | 90 | 120 | Normal response |
|---|---|---|---|---|---|---|
| Glucose | √ | √ | √ | √ | √ | <2 mmol/l |
| GH | √ | √ | √ | √ | √ | >15 mU/l |
| Cortisol | √ | √ | √ | √ | √ | rise by 170 nmol/l; max >550 nmol/l |
| TSH | √ | √ | √ | | | should rise; adequate |
| LH/FSH | √ | √ | √ | | | levels depend on laboratory reference range |

*Notes*
The patient must achieve adequate hypoglycaemia marked by sweating and a blood glucose of less than 2 mmol/l. Give more insulin after 45 minutes if this is not the case. The patient must be supervised throughout and given breakfast at the end.

Medical treatment of acromegaly has to date been disappointing but now that long-acting analogues of somatostatin (the hypothalamic peptide that normally inhibits the secretion of growth hormone) are available, there may be scope for such therapy in the near future.

## PROLACTINOMA

### Presentation

Although galactorrhoea is usually considered a key feature of prolactinomas, it is actually found in less than half of cases and even then can often only be disclosed by the patient or physician on manual expression of the breast. More commonly, the periods are absent, irregular or scanty; in some women the periods are regular but fertility is a problem (due to an inadequate luteal phase or anovulation). Rarely, weight gain, acne and hirsutism may occur, related to polycystic changes in the ovaries. Dyspareunia may occur as a result of the vaginal dryness produced by hypogonadism; this is due either to decreased secretion of gonadotrophin from the local effects of tumour or a direct interference with the action of gonadotrophin by prolactin at the ovarian level.

In men, galactorrhoea is less common still and it is important to note that prolactinomas *per se* do not cause gynaecomastia, which is only the result of excess oestrogens or reduced androgens. The common presentation is decreased libido or impotence. In men and women, local progression of the tumour and hypopituitarism may also be presenting features.

### Investigation

Elevation of prolactin (>400 mU/l) on two occasions in an unstressed patient will usually confirm the diagnosis of hyperprolactinaemia. A careful history is required to eliminate drugs (e.g., phenothiazines, metoclopramide, methyldopa) as a cause; hypothyroidism and renal failure should also be excluded. A prolactinoma is likely with high levels of prolactin (>2000 mU/l) and may be diagnosed by CT scanning or magnetic resonance imaging. Lower but nonetheless elevated levels of prolactin, in the absence of radiographic evidence, may be due to very small prolactinomas or may be functional. Specialist referral is indicated for further assessment. All patients with macroadenomas should have a combined pituitary function test to assess other hormonal reserves (see Table 9.6).

### Treatment

Tumours of less than 1 cm in diameter are microprolactinomas. These are best treated with the dopamine agonist bromocriptine given in a gradually increasing dose, usually up to 7.5 mg daily; it should be given with food to avoid nausea and dizziness. Fertility is rapidly restored in most cases. Management of prolactinomas in pregnancy is best handled by a specialist team of endocrinologist and obstetrician because rarely (in less than 5 per cent of cases) macroadenomas may enlarge due to oestrogen stimulation. Some centres advocate transsphenoidal surgery for microadenomas but this should probably be reserved only for those patients intolerant of bromocriptine.

With the larger macroadenomas (>1 cm diameter) complications in pregnancy are more likely and the tumour may already be causing local symptoms. However, bromocriptine usually produces rapid shrinkage of the tumour, and it is best to assess the patient's response to bromocriptine before considering ablative therapy. Surgery is unlikely to produce a permanent remission and so for more aggressive tumours external radiotherapy is used with bromocriptine treatment until the radiotherapy takes effect.

## HYPOPITUITARISM

### Presentation

Pituitary failure may result from several processes (Table 9.7), the commonest of which is a functional or functionless pituitary tumour. These may in turn produce their own symptoms, including headache and disturbances of the visual field, which occur by superior extension of the tumour and compression of the optic chiasm. Commonly the defect is a bitemporal hemianopia but earlier, more subtle defects can be demonstrated by accurate charting and testing for defective colour vision. Inferior extension of the tumour may produce cerebrospinal fluid rhinorrhoea and lateral extension (usually unilateral) may produce IIIrd and more rarely IVth and VIth cranial nerve palsies.

The endocrine manifestations of hypopituitarism depend on the age and sex of the patient and the extent of hormone loss. Dwarfism is clearly a major paediatric problem. In the adult, partial

**Table 9.7 Aetiology of hypopituitarism**

Pituitary tumours:
   functional or functionless
   metastases or local invasion (e.g., meningioma)
   craniopharyngiomas
Iatrogenic: pituitary surgery or irradiation
Traumatic: following head injury
Infiltration: sarcoidosis, histiocytosis,
   haemochromatosis
Ischaemia: postpartum (Sheehan's syndrome)
Autoimmune pituitary disease
Infection: tuberculosis, syphilis

hormone loss is common and tumour progression usually impairs secretion of gonadotrophin and growth hormone first. Loss of gonadotrophins produce amenorrhoea or impotence and azoospermia. Full-blown hypopituitarism may result in coma, the combined result of hypoglycaemia (increased insulin sensitivity due to loss of growth hormone and cortisol), hypothyroidism, sodium depletion and water retention (cortisol is required for effective vasopressin activity).

### Examination

The patient is characteristically pale and this is not simply the result of accompanying anaemia, as witnessed by depigmentation of the nipples and inability to tan (as a result of ACTH deficiency). Body hair is scanty or absent and the skin is thin and finely wrinkled. The white lunula of the fingernail bed may be lost. The testes may be small and soft; in women the breasts may atrophy. Other features that may be apparent are hypotension and signs of hypothyroidism (see above).

### Investigation

The mainstay of investigation is the combined pituitary test which will test reserves of all relevant hormones (see Table 9.6). However, if hypopituitarism is suspected, a basal estimation (9 a.m.) of cortisol before testing is indicated. If this is already low, insulin could be dangerous and in this case an estimation of ACTH should be made to distinguish between secondary (pituitary) and primary (adrenal) causes; the ACTH is low in the former and high in the latter.

A cause for hypopituitarism may be obvious from the history. Imaging may help to diagnose a pituitary tumour, craniopharyngioma or tuberculoma and a chest X-ray may reveal a primary tumour that has produced metastases. The possibility of sarcoidosis is also worth appropriate investigation.

### Treatment

This should obviously be directed to the primary aetiology if possible. Emergency presentation in coma requires prompt resuscitation with intravenous fluids (isotonic saline and/or dextrose), a single dose of hydrocortisone, 200 mg intravenously, and 50 to 100 mg hydrocortisone intramuscularly, 8-hourly. Hypothermia should be treated with appropriate blankets and signs of infection sought; antibiotics should be started promptly.

Long-term management depends upon exact definition of the various potential hormone deficiencies. Gonadotrophin failure is best treated in women by cyclical oestrogen and progesterone and in men by testosterone injections (e.g. Sustanon 250 intramuscularly every three to four weeks). Fertility can be restored by gonadotrophin therapy; this requires specialist referral. Thyroxine (T4: usually 100–150 µg daily) is given for failure of TSH but, if cortisol is also deficient, should be withheld until hypocortisolaemia is first corrected. Dosages of cortisol vary and may require individual tailoring; 20 mg very first thing in the morning and 10 mg around 4 to 5 p.m. are often suitable. Sometimes the second dose is taken too late and checking this can relieve evening symptoms of lethargy and later insomnia. With pituitary (but not adrenal) causes of hypoadrenalism, mineralocorticoids are not needed because these are not under ACTH control. Finally, the patient must be fully conversant with the steroid regimen and the need to continue it at all times, increasing the dose with stress (e.g., infections) and seeking immediate medical help if infections are more than trivial. A properly carried steroid card or Medic-Alert bracelet is mandatory.

## DIABETES INSIPIDUS

### Presentation

Shortage of vasopressin leads to polyuria (up to 20 l daily) and polydipsia. The condition may be caused by (a) a primary or secondary tumour—pituitary tumours only rarely produce diabetes insipidus and even after trauma or surgical removal of the pituitary it is usually temporary because the hypothalamus can secrete vasopressin directly into the circulation; (b) infiltration of the neurohypophysis, e.g., sarcoidosis, histiocytosis; and (c) idiopathic (some may be autoimmune).

### Investigation

The cause of diabetes insipidus may be obvious, e.g., after pituitary surgery, but in many cases the diagnosis requires exclusion of other causes of polyuria. Dilute urine (<200 mosmol/kg) provides a good clue in favour of diabetes insipidus but does not exclude compulsive water drinking. Firm diag-

nosis depends on a fluid deprivation test. The patient is given a light breakfast (no tea or coffee) and then is fluid deprived for eight hours. No smoking is allowed and careful supervision is required to prevent occult consumption of fluid or dangerous dehydration. The patient is weighed before testing and at four, six, seven and eight hours (stop test if weight falls by more than 3 per cent) while urine is collected hourly for the first hour and between four and eight hours. Plasma is taken at the mid point of each urine collection. In diabetes insipidus the urine osmolality remains below 270 mosmol/kg throughout and the urine: plasma osmolality ratio on paired samples never exceeds 1.9. The test can be repeated after vasopressin (DDAVP; see below) administration to distinguish cranial diabetes insipidus from the nephrogenic form; patients with the latter do not respond to DDAVP by concentrating their urine.

### Treatment

The synthetic long-acting analogue of vasopressin, desmopressin or DDAVP, is given intranasally, 10 to 20 µg daily, in one or two doses. Remember that diabetes insipidus is usually temporary after trauma (including surgery) so the need for continued therapy must be reassessed in these patients.

## CUSHING'S SYNDROME AND DISEASE

About 80 per cent of cases of Cushing's *syndrome* are caused by a pituitary lesion—these patients have Cushing's *disease*. Only call the condition Cushing's disease if the cause has been established and distinguished from the other aetiologies of Cushing's syndrome, namely ectopic production of ACTH and primary adrenal disease.

### Presentation

Cushing's syndrome presents more commonly in women (sex ratio 4:1) usually aged 30 to 50 years. The change in appearance is the main reason for seeking attention and this is discussed below. Less frequent complaints include back and bone pain, polydipsia and nocturia, headache, psychiatric changes and menstrual disturbances.

### Examination

The face is red and rounded, accompanied by hirsutism, acne, increased pigmentation and thinning of the scalp hair (Fig. 9.8). There is truncal obesity with wasting of the limb muscles and purple-coloured abdominal striae are found in 60 per cent of cases. The skin is thin, and bruising, leg ulceration and ankle oedema can occur. Spinal osteoporosis can produce kyphosis, pathological fractures and loss of height. A proximal myopathy is usually best demonstrated by asking the patient to get up from a squatting position. Hypertension occurs in 85 per cent of patients and there is an increased incidence of venous thrombosis.

When Cushing's syndrome is the result of ectopic production of ACTH, the condition usually progresses rapidly so that these features may not have a chance to evolve. High levels of ACTH can produce deep pigmentation and the patient may be generally thin and wasted as a result of the underlying tumour. Ankle oedema is common.

## Investigation

With the full-blown syndrome the clinical diagnosis is easy and simple testing will confirm increased cortisol production. However, in some cases the diagnosis is much more difficult because cyclicity is an occasional but well-documented phenomenon in this disease. Such periodic fluctuations in the overproduction of the hormone may or may not be accompanied by temporary remission of symptoms, usually with a cycle length between two weeks and three months; over time this interval becomes shorter. Very early cases may provide another potential source of missed diagnosis, so an open mind should be kept if clinical suspicion is high and tests should be repeated. Investigation should be in two stages: first document the presence of the syndrome and then determine the cause.

Daytime plasma cortisol varies considerably and may well be normal in Cushing's syndrome; a random cortisol is therefore of no real value. The best outpatient screen is of the free cortisol, in 24-h urine, which is elevated in nearly all cases of Cushing's syndrome; two samples are usually tested. Make sure the patient is not pregnant or on oral contraceptives and has normal renal function. Stress can also affect the result. Inpatient screening should include estimation of the plasma cortisol at midnight, which is much less subject to fluctuation than the daytime value. Cortisol normally drops to below 250 nmol/l by midnight but this circadian fall is lost in Cushing's syndrome. Pregnancy, oral contraceptives and stress interfere with the interpretation.

If the diagnosis is in doubt an overnight dexamethasone test should be performed. The patient is given 2 mg dexamethasone by mouth at midnight and the plasma cortisol is measured at 9 a.m. Normally this high dose of exogenous steroid, which does not interfere with the cortisol assay, will suppress ACTH and hence cortisol. In most cases of Cushing's syndrome, cortisol is not suppressed but there is a problem in determining the cut-off point, i.e., the level of plasma cortisol selected for normal suppression. Setting this level too low will increase the chance of diagnosing Cushing's syndrome but will also increase the number of false positives, particularly in obese or chronically ill subjects. The more complicated,

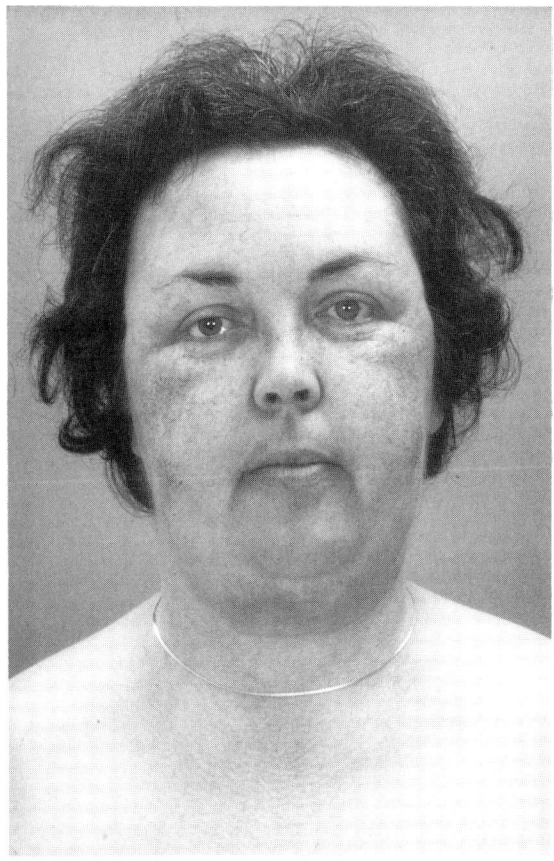

*Figure 9.8* Typical facial appearance in Cushing's syndrome, in this patient due to Cushing's disease (photo courtesy of Prof. G. F. Joplin).

multiple-dose dexamethasone suppression test is reserved for patients in whom the diagnosis remains equivocal. The patient is given 0.5 mg dexamethasone 6-hourly for eight doses starting at 9 a.m., and the response can be assessed in two ways. The first is to measure the plasma cortisol at 9 a.m. on day 3 (six hours after the last dose of dexamethasone); a value below 170 nmol/l excludes Cushing's syndrome. Alternatively, free cortisol in the 24-h urine can be measured on day 2 and this should be suppressed to less than 60 nmol/24h.

Alcoholism can produce the typical appearance and biochemical changes of Cushing's syndrome, so-called pseudo-Cushing's syndrome. Distinction can be made from the true syndrome by performing the insulin part of the combined pituitary test (see Table 9.5) and assessing the cortisol response, which will be a rise in pseudo- but not true Cushing's syndrome. This test may also be useful in depressed patients who can also display some of the biochemical features of Cushing's syndrome.

Having confirmed the diagnosis the aetiology must be discovered. Although this can be clear using the tests described below, there are still cases in which the diagnosis is incorrectly made despite compelling laboratory evidence. Full expert assessment is needed in Cushing's syndrome. The best test is the 9 a.m. plasma ACTH, which is suppressed and thus undetectable with an adrenal cause of Cushing's syndrome (adenoma or carcinoma) but is normal or elevated in Cushing's disease or the ectopic ACTH syndrome. Special precautions are required because ACTH binds to glass: samples are usually transferred immediately to ice and plasma then separated quickly. Very high levels of ACTH favour an ectopic ACTH syndrome rather than Cushing's disease.

Two other biochemical tests are very helpful:
(1) *The metyrapone test.* Metyrapone (750 mg, 4-hourly for 24 h) inhibits 11 β-hydroxylase, which reduces cortisol output and hence stimulates the pituitary production of ACTH. This rise in ACTH can be measured directly in the plasma or indirectly by measuring the subsequent increase in the steroid precursors up to the 11 β-hydroxylase block, usually assessed as the 24-h excretion of urinary 17-oxogenic steroid. Urine samples are collected daily before, during and after the 24-h metyrapone test because the rise may be maximal in the day after metyrapone. In the ectopic ACTH syndrome, metyrapone has little or no effect as the ACTH source is extrapituitary. In adrenal adenomas or carcinomas, pituitary ACTH is usually suppressed by the autonomous cortisol production and again there is no rise in ACTH or 17-oxogenic steroids in response to metyrapone. However, in Cushing's disease there is a normal or exaggerated response due to increased pituitary production of ACTH. Unfortunately some patients with ectopic ACTH syndrome and less commonly some with an adrenal adenoma may show a normal response to metyrapone.

(2) *High-dose dexamethasone test.* In a sense this is the opposite of the metyrapone test because it tests the ability to suppress pituitary production of ACTH by the feedback mechanism; clearly in the pathological state high doses of exogenous steroid are required to do this as the set-point for feedback is much higher in Cushing's disease. The patient is given 2 mg dexamethasone 6-hourly for two days and the plasma or urinary cortisol checked. These are reduced by more than half in typical Cushing's disease but in the ectopic ACTH syndrome or in adrenal causes of Cushing's syndrome there should be no suppression of cortisol. This is the most fallible of the three tests described.

Imaging plays a major part in diagnosis. An abdominal CT scan will rapidly exclude an adenoma or carcinoma. CT scanning can also reveal the presence of a small percentage of pituitary tumours in Cushing's disease. Search for an ectopic source of ACTH should be made. Half of these are small cell bronchogenic carcinomas and another 15 per cent are thymic carcinomas or bronchial carcinoid tumours, so a careful review of the chest X-ray is essential. CT scanning may supplement the search for a thoracic tumour.

### Treatment

Untreated patients have a 50 per cent mortality in five years. Cushing's syndrome can be a major management problem: in severe cases the patient is frail and weak, susceptible to infection and unable to heal wounds. In these patients, initial management should be with metyrapone (or ketoconazole) to allow sufficient recovery from hypercortisolaemia for definitive treatment. This is directed to the source of the problem. The best treatment for Cushing's disease is still a matter of debate but bilateral adrenalectomy is no longer indicated unless treatment of the pituitary fails. This is because, left untreated, the pituitary adenoma may enlarge causing local space-occupying problems and Nelson's syndrome, in which skin pigmentation is increased due to very high ACTH levels. As in acromegaly, the pituitary therapy selected will be dictated by local experience and by the individual patient. Selective removal of the adenoma, partial or total hypophysectomy or irradiation all produce reasonable results in over 70 per cent of patients, although external beam irradiation is probably less effective than other modes. Medical treatment is usually required in patients given irradiation because its effects may not be apparent for several years. Adrenal tumours should be treated surgically, and treatment supplemented with *o,p'*-DDD (a specific adrenolytic agent) for metastases if the lesion is an adrenal carcinoma. The source of ACTH should be removed if possible in the ectopic ACTH syndrome; depending on the lesion, surgery, radiation or chemotherapy may be indicated. If the tumour cannot be removed and yet has a good prognosis, bilateral adrenalectomy may be indicated.

## ADDISON'S DISEASE

### Presentation

This is a rare (prevalence 1 in 25 000) but serious disease, more commonly affecting women, due to the preponderance of an autoimmune aetiology in the UK. Presentation depends upon the natural history. In slowly progressing adrenal failure, pigmentation, tiredness, dizziness and depression may be prominent features, as are gastrointestinal complaints of anorexia, nausea, vomiting and diarrhoea. Weight loss is common and amenorrhoea occurs if there is associated autoimmune oophoritis. Acute adrenal failure can present with extreme weakness, nausea and vomiting and the patient may rapidly progress to coma.

### Examination

Pigmentation distinguishes primary from secondary (i.e., pituitary-dependent) adrenal failure. Although generalized, there is especially enhanced pigmentation in the skin creases on the palm of the hand, on the insides of the cheeks, on the elbows and in recent scar tissue. Hypotension,

especially postural, is another cardinal feature. In women the adrenal is the main source of androgen so body hair may be lost. Vitiligo, alopecia, thyroiditis and pernicious anaemia may be associated with autoimmune Addison's disease.

### Investigation

A random plasma cortisol is only useful in excluding Addison's disease if the patient presents with acute illness. Under these conditions the stress of illness should normally elevate cortisol to more than 600 nmol/l but this fails to happen in Addison's disease. A sample should be stored before any emergency treatment in suspected cases so the diagnosis can be confirmed retrospectively. Addison's disease can be diagnosed by two tests:

(1) Elevation of plasma ACTH in the face of a normal or low plasma cortisol; this also distinguishes primary from secondary hypoadrenalism.

(2) *Synacthen test.* The patient is given 250 µg synthetic ACTH (tetracosactrin [Synacthen]) intramuscularly and the cortisol measured 45 min later; a normal response is a level of greater than 600 nmol/l, which is not achieved in any form of hypoadrenalism. This test can be used if the patient has already begun steroid replacement, provided this is for a period of less than three weeks and consists of dexamethasone for the 48 h preceding the test. Primary hypoadrenalism can be distinguished from the secondary form by a prolonged test in which 2 mg of a depot preparation of long-acting tetracosactrin is given and cortisol is checked after 4 and 24 h. The normal response is for a peak in cortisol to occur at 4 h; in secondary hypoadrenalism this is delayed until 24 h whereas no rise at all is seen in the primary form.

Adrenal antibodies may be tested to confirm an autoimmune aetiology and active tuberculosis should be excluded. Adrenal calcification (on plain X-ray or the more sensitive CT scan) is usually due to tuberculosis and excludes an autoimmune aetiology but lack of adrenal calcification does not exclude tuberculosis. In up to 24 per cent of cases of Addison's disease due to tuberculosis the disease is confined to the adrenal and if the aetiology is in doubt a CT scan of the abdomen should be performed; in addition to calcification the adrenals are often enlarged with tuberculosis of short duration but shrunken with autoimmune disease. Sometimes overzealous screening in a recently diagnosed patient will turn up a low T4 but this does not necessarily indicate associated hypothyroidism; in some patients the T4 returns to normal after a few weeks of steroid replacement. Replacement of T4 should only be started after careful assessment.

## Treatment

Acutely ill patients need prompt resuscitation and this should not wait for the results of cortisol estimations; as indicated the diagnosis can readily be confirmed retrospectively. Treatment of these patients is the same as for acute hypopituitarism, namely intravenous fluids and parenteral hydrocortisone.

Replacement therapy requires cortisol, usually 20 mg in the morning and 10 mg in the early evening, but this dose may need adjustment and a 4-hourly profile of plasma cortisol will sometimes help. Aldosterone also needs replacement with fludrocortisone, 0.05 mg daily. If hypotension persists the dose can be increased but watch for overtreatment, showing itself as hypertension and hypokalaemic alkalosis.

All patients need education on the need for steroid cover of any stress and should carry a steroid card or Medic-Alert bracelet. Hydrocortisone, 100 mg 8-hourly intramuscular, is required in patients undergoing surgery until they can take their medication normally.

## PHAEOCHROMOCYTOMA

### Presentation

The main symptoms are intermittent headache, sweating and palpitations, each found in about two thirds of patients. Less commonly the patient may have noticed tremor, anorexia, nausea, and facial pallor or flushing. Episodic attacks with complete interim normality are suggestive features. Weight loss and constipation are also found.

### Examination

Persistent hypertension is found in 65 per cent of patients but is paroxysmal in 30 per cent. There may be tachycardia, tremor and sweating, all of which can confuse the picture with thyrotoxicosis.

Special features to be sought are the presence of neurofibromas and café-au-lait spots, facial haemangiomas and thyroid tumours, because of the association of phaeochromocytomas with neurofibromatosis, the Sturge–Weber syndrome and medullary carcinoma of the thyroid.

### Investigation

The mainstay of diagnosis is demonstration of excess catecholamine excretion, either by measuring the metabolites vanillylmandelic acid and metanephrines in the urine or, better still, plasma catecholamines. Antihypertensive drugs, in particular vasodilators and methyldopa, can affect the interpretation of plasma catecholamine assays. Samples should be taken after the patient has lain flat for an hour. Localizing the tumour, which is extra-adrenal in 10 per cent of cases, and malignant in another 10 per cent, is probably best done initially with abdominal CT scanning. If this fails, whole-body CT scanning together with $^{131}$I-MIBG (metaiodobenzylguanidine) radionuclide localization of the tumour should be considered.

### Treatment

The treatment for phaeochromocytoma is excision. Before surgery, careful control of hypertension is essential and is best achieved with phenoxybenzamine, 20 mg daily, given in one or two doses, and propranolol, 40 mg twice a day. Never give a β-blocker alone because this may worsen hypertension. These initial doses should be increased as indicated but remember that phenoxybenzamine has a long half-life and may accumulate. Acute hypertensive crises can be dealt with using intravenous bolus injections of phentolamine, 2 to 5 mg (duration of action, 5 min) and may require several doses. This can also be given by an intravenous infusion at 1 mg/min. Sodium nitroprusside by infusion is an alternative.

Preoperative management requires specialist consultation between physician, anaesthetist and surgeon, and the ideal regimen is as yet unclear. Complete α-adrenergic blockade may prevent hypertensive crises during surgery but has the disadvantage of sometimes profound hypotension after tumour removal. A reasonable approach is to continue propranolol but stop phenoxybenzamine 12 to 18 h before surgery.

## PRIMARY HYPERPARATHYROIDISM

### Presentation

This has an annual incidence of 26 for 100 000 and is twice as common in women, usually presenting between the ages of 40 to 60 years. Many cases are discovered when the calcium is checked as part of a biochemical screen and symptoms, if any, are only correctly identified in retrospect. Renal calculi and bone aches are common presentations. If the hypercalcaemia is severe, the patient may complain of anorexia, nausea, constipation, thirst and polyuria. A proximal myopathy may cause muscle weakness but general fatigue is more common. The diagnosis should also be considered if a patient presents with peptic ulceration (occurring in 10 per cent of primary hyperparathyroidism) or acute pancreatitis.

### Examination

Corneal calcification is unusual in the absence of renal failure but should be sought by examining the medial and lateral junctions between the cornea and the sclera. It forms a thin white line just inside the cornea, best detected using an oblique beam of light from a torch, or better still using a slit lamp. Very rarely, giant cell granulomas ('brown tumours') in the jaw may be found, or the parathyroid tumour may be palpable.

### Investigation

Diagnosis depends on finding a high serum calcium with a high or normal level of parathyroid hormone. Serum calcium should be measured fasting, corrected for albumin level and repeated several times. Renal function should also be checked.

Localization of a parathyroid adenoma can be difficult. Selective venous sampling for parathyroid hormone levels may be of help but requires expert radiology. CT scanning or radionuclide scanning with $^{75}$Se-methionine may also be used.

### Treatment

In young patients with primary hyperparathyroidism, and in any patient with hypercalcaemia persistently greater than 2.8 mmol/l, surgery is indicated. Difficulties may be encountered if the cause is the rare diffuse hyperplasia rather than a single adenoma or if the tumour is mediastinal (5 per cent of cases). Multiple tumours must also be excluded.

Optimum management of an elderly asymptomatic patient, in whom the hypercalcaemia may be an incidental finding, is less clear. Provided the calcium is maintained at a reasonable level (<2.8 mmol/l), there seems little point in immediate surgery because dietary measures to lower calcium or maintain a high fluid intake in these patients are often all that is required.

Severe hypercalcaemia (>4 mmol/l) is usually the result of a malignancy (80 per cent of cases) but hyperparathyroidism can also present in this way. Emergency management in all cases is by intravenous fluids (>6 l daily) with careful monitoring, and other treatments are not indicated unless this fails. Hypokalaemia is often an avoidable problem if properly anticipated. Frusemide does not offer any extra advantage if sufficient fluid is given, If absolutely uncontrollable with fluids only, intravenous neutral phosphate (100 mmol over 6 h) may be tried but is hazardous. Mithramycin (25 µg/kg as an intravenous bolus) is also effective but has a delayed action (longer than 24 h). Biphosphonates such as pamidronate given by intravenous infusion have been a major recent innovation in the treatment of severe hypercalcaemia.

## HYPOPARATHYROIDISM

### Presentation

Idiopathic hypoparathyroidism, sometimes the result of autoimmunity, is much less common than the iatrogenic form resulting from thyroid or parathyroid surgery or radical removal of oesophageal or laryngeal carcinoma. Presentation is usually with paraesthesiae and muscle cramps. Chvostek's sign (hemi-facial twitching on percussing the facial nerve) and Trousseau's sign (carpal spasm after occluding circulation to the arm) may be positive and carpopedal spasm may occur as a spontaneous manifestation of the latter. Cataracts can result from prolonged hypocalcaemia.

### Investigation and treatment

Hypocalcaemia is the cardinal feature, usually with hyperphosphataemia, and the history of neck surgery will usually indicate the diagnosis. The hypocalcaemia of osteomalacia can be diagnosed by history, the low or normal serum phosphate and the raised alkaline phosphatase. Chronic renal failure should also be excluded.

Treatment is with 1 alpha-hydroxycholecalciferol (1αOHCC), 1 to 2 μg daily. The continued need for this in postsurgical patients should be assessed at intervals, although in many treatment needs to be lifelong. Emergency treatment of severe hypocalcaemia is slow intravenous injection of 10 to 20 ml of 10 per cent calcium gluconate; continuous intravenous infusion may be required in some cases and much larger doses than normal of 1αOHCC can be needed. Persistent hypocalcaemia may indicate concurrent hypomagnesaemia and levels should be repeatedly checked in these patients. Low magnesium can be corrected orally (10–20 ml of 40 per cent $MgSO_4$) or parenterally (5–10 ml of 50 per cent $MgSO_4$ intramuscularly or diluted in a litre of saline intravenously).

## Further reading and reference works

Aron D. C., Tyrrell J. B., Fitzgerald P. A., Findling J. W., Forsham P. H. (1981). Cushings disease; problems in diagnosis. *Medicine*, **60**, 25–35.

Beardwell C., Robertson G. L., eds. (1981). *The Pituitary*. Guildford: Butterworths.

Becker K. L., ed. (1990). *Principles and Practice of Endocrinology and Metabolism*. Philadelphia: J. B. Lippincott.

Belchetz P. E., ed. (1984). *Management of Pituitary Disease*. London: Chapman and Hall.

Bloom A., Ireland J. (1980). *A Colour Atlas of Diabetes*. London: Wolfe Medical.

De Visscher M., ed. (1981). *The Thyroid Gland*. New York: Raven Press.

Grossman A., Besser G. M. (1985). Prolactinomas. *Br. Med. J.*, **290**, 182–4.

Hall R., Evered D., Greene R. (1979). *A Colour Atlas of Endocrinology*. London: Wolfe Medical.

Hall R., Anderson J., Smart G. A., Besser M. (1980). *Fundamentals of Clinical Endocrinology*, 3rd edn. Tunbridge Wells: Pitman Medical.

Ingbar S. H., Braverman L. E., eds. (1986). *Werner's The Thyroid*, 5th edn. Philadelphia: J. B. Lippincott.

Krieger D. T. (1982). *Cushing's Syndrome*. Monographs on Endocrinology 22. Berlin: Springer Verlag.

Marble A., Krall L. P., Bradley R. F., Christlieb A. R., Soeldner J. S., eds. (1985). *Joslin's Diabetes Mellitus*, 12th edn. Philadelphia: Lea and Febiger.

Scanlon M. F., ed. (1983). *Neuroendocrinology*. Clinics in Endocrinology and Metabolism 12:3. London: W. B. Saunders.

Skyler J. S., Cahill G. F., eds. (1981). *Diabetes Mellitus*. New York: Yorke Medical Books.

Van der Spuy Z. M., Jacobs H. S. (1984). Management of endocrine disorders in pregnancy. *Postgrad. Med. J.*, **60**, 245–52 and 312–20.

Watkins P. J., ed. (1986). *Long Term Complications of Diabetes*. Clinics in Endocrinology and Metabolism 15: 4. London: W. B. Saunders.

Wilson J. D., Foster D. W. (1985). *Williams Textbook of Endocrinology*, 7th edn. Philadelphia: W. B. Saunders.

# 10

# RENAL MEDICINE

## John Isaacs and Leszek Borysiewicz

Renal disease is often associated with pathology in other organ systems. This may be a complication of the renal disease itself or an accompanying feature of a multisystem illness. In the space of one chapter, it is impossible to consider all the processes that result in renal impairment or the detailed pathophysiology of renal failure. Therefore we have taken a clinical approach to the diagnosis and management of common renal problems presenting in the context of general medicine. For a more detailed consideration of individual problems the reader is referred to a number of texts in renal medicine (see Further Reading).

## ASSESSMENT STRUCTURE

Circumstances inevitably will dictate the initial assessment of a renal patient, who could be critically ill or sitting in an outpatient consulting room. Obviously it is essential to confirm the presence of renal failure, which largely rests on a combination of simple blood chemistry and urine analysis. In broad terms the questions that require early attention include the duration of renal impairment (acute or chronic) and its aetiology, with particular emphasis on reversible factors and the presence of life-threatening complications. Furthermore, if the renal impairment is irreversible, a long-term plan of management must be formulated to enable early recognition of complications and determine the best form of replacement therapy.

## ACUTE RENAL FAILURE

Acute renal failure is operationally defined as a sudden reduction in the glomerular filtration rate (GFR), often but not invariably presenting with oliguria (urine output <400 ml/day in the adult). Classically, the causes of acute renal failure are subdivided into prerenal, renal and postrenal (Table 10.1). The commonest cause is loss of intravascular volume resulting in reduced renal blood flow, ultimately causing ischaemic damage to tubular cells—'acute tubular necrosis'. However, there are a number of other causes, some of which require immediate and specific therapeutic intervention (e.g., relief of urinary tract obstruction) and must be systematically excluded. Once established, acute tubular necrosis is a self-limiting condition, but if the circumstances leading to intravascular depletion are corrected at an early stage, it may be prevented altogether. Therefore the first question often posed by a patient with oliguria is whether renal hypoperfusion is present and if so is acute tubular necrosis already established?

Clinical examination of patients for signs of salt and water depletion is important. The classical signs of reduced peripheral perfusion—decreased skin turgor, tachycardia, (postural) hypotension and reduced central venous pressure—appear late and thus represent severe depletion. Other important information may be available in individual cases, such as daily weight measurements and fluid balance charts. Both the quantity and the nature of fluid loss are important, as a patient with severe burns or haemorrhage requires different replacement to one with intestinal fistulas or diabetic ketoacidosis.

Examination of the urine, both chemically and microscopically, is mandatory. The normal response to dehydration is a reduction in volume, increased osmolarity and urea concentration, and reduced sodium concentration ($[Na^+]$). When renal damage has occurred the $[Na^+]$ is increased with a fall in the osmolarity and urea concentra-

**Table 10.1 Classification of common causes of acute renal failure**

| Prerenal | Renal | Postrenal |
|---|---|---|
| Inadequate renal perfusion secondary to:<br>(a) loss of circulating volume:<br>    (i) haemorrhage;<br>    (ii) burns;<br>    (iii) gastrointestinal losses;<br>    (iv) polyuria, e.g., diabetic ketoacidosis<br>(b) hypotension:<br>    (i) septicaemia;<br>    (ii) pancreatitis;<br>    (iii) cardiogenic shock;<br>    (iv) congestive cardiac failure | Parenchymal damage:<br>(a) acute tubular necrosis—<br>    (i) inadequate renal perfusion;<br>    (ii) drugs, e.g., gentamicin, X-ray contrast;<br>    (iii) heavy metals, e.g., lead;<br>    (iv) pigmenturia, e.g., haemolysis, rhabdomyolysis;<br>    (v) Bence-Jones protein<br>(b) acute cortical necrosis<br>(c) acute glomerulonephritis<br>(d) interstitial nephritis<br>(e) crystalluria, e.g., uric acid<br>(f) 'vascular', e.g., arterial or venous thrombosis, vasculitis, disseminated intravascular coagulation | Obstruction to urine flow:<br>(a) ureteric—<br>    (i) calculi;<br>    (ii) blood clots;<br>    (iii) tumour;<br>    (iv) retroperitoneal fibrosis<br>(b) Bladder outlet—<br>    (i) prostatic hypertrophy;<br>    (ii) pelvic tumour;<br>    (iii) posterior urethral valves |

tion, together with the appearance of proteinuria and casts (Table 10.2).

Management of 'prerenal uraemia' consists of appropriate fluid replacement (crystalloid and/or colloid), often monitoring central venous pressure. Even if acute tubular necrosis appears likely, the possibility of 'incipient acute tubular necrosis' should be considered—a state between intravascular volume depletion and the development of acute tubular necrosis itself. Different measures have been employed in this situation, with the common aim of increasing renal blood flow to prevent the development of acute tubular necrosis. Mannitol infusion is probably the best studied in experimental models and 20 to 30 g intrave-

**Table 10.2 The urine in acute renal failure***

| | Prerenal uraemia | Established acute tubular necrosis |
|---|---|---|
| [Na$^+$] | <10 mmol/l | >20 mmol/l |
| urine/plasma [urea] | >10 | < 4 |
| urine/plasma osmolarity | >1.2 | <1.2 |

The fractional sodium excretion (FE$_{Na}$) is calculated as:

$$\frac{\text{urine/plasma [Na}^+\text{]}}{\text{urine/plasma [creatinine]}}$$

A value of less than 1 suggests prerenal uraemia, and greater than 1, acute tubular necrosis.

* The prior administration of diuretics invalidates these guidelines.

nously is a suggested dose in humans. However, there are doubts concerning its efficacy, and with the attendant risks of pulmonary oedema, haemolysis and cerebral dehydration, care should be exercised, particularly in the presence of continued oliguria. High-dose frusemide (250–500 mg in an infusion over 15–20 min) has been used and may increase urine volume but may cause nerve deafness especially if administered rapidly. Dopamine at low doses (1 μg/kg/min) produces renal vasodilation and may also be used to increase urine output. The relative efficacies of these different treatments await assessment in clinical trials.

The biochemical changes associated with acute renal failure are similar to those of chronic renal failure, particularly the increased creatinine and urea. However, due in part to the acute nature of the changes, certain metabolic complications require immediate attention:

(1) *Hyperkalaemia.* Hyperkalaemia frequently accompanies acute renal failure and requires immediate attention because of direct cardiac effects, often exacerbated because of a concurrent low plasma ionized calcium ([Ca$^{2+}$]). This is a particular problem when failure occurs with rhabdomyolysis or hypercatabolism, such as with burns or sepsis. A plasma potassium ([K$^+$]) greater than 6.5 to 7 mmol/l is considered dangerous but there is no precise relationship between the [K$^+$] and arrhythmias. The characteristic ECG changes of peaked T waves, disappearance of P waves,

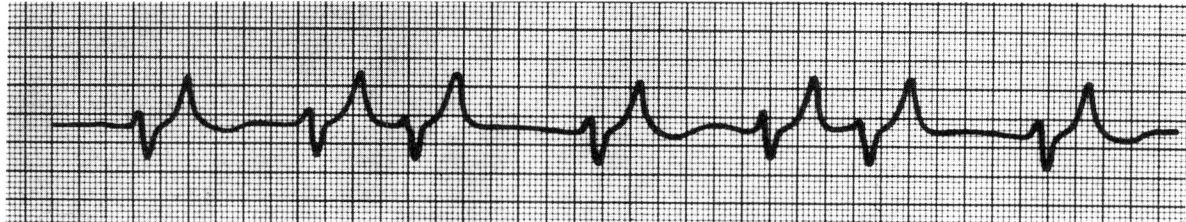

*Figure 10.1* ECG (lead II), from a patient with acute renal failure, showing the characteristic changes of hyperkalaemia. Note the peaked T waves, widened QRS complexes and reduced P waves.

widened QRS complexes and slurring of ST segments (Fig. 10.1) must be looked for.

Significant hyperkalaemia is an indication for dialysis, but as this may take time to institute, temporizing measures are often required:

(a) stop further $K^+$ intake, e.g., stored blood; do not use potassium-sparing diuretics in renal failure;

(b) calcium—10 per cent calcium gluconate can be given intravenously, particularly in the presence of ECG changes reflecting hyperkalaemia;

(c) glucose and insulin—50 g glucose with 20 u of Actrapid insulin administered intravenously accelerates intracellular uptake of $K^+$; this acts within 30 min and may cause the $K^+$ to fall by 1 mmol/l; the effect may be maintained by constant infusion (500 ml of 20 per cent dextrose and 25 iu Actrapid insulin over 2 h), whilst monitoring blood glucose;

(d) sodium bicarbonate—this will also promote intracellular transport of $K^+$ especially in the presence of acidosis; however the possibility of sodium overload and precipitation of tetany by further lowering the ionized $[Ca^{2+}]$ must be considered;

(e) ion exchange resins—30 g calcium resonium administered orally will enhance gastrointestinal loss but works only slowly (5–24 h); this is more suited to long-term control as in chronic failure rather than the management of hyperkalaemia of acute failure.

(2) *Hypocalcaemia*—corrected as indicated above.

Having confirmed the presence of acute renal failure and dealt with life-threatening metabolic abnormalities, further investigation should be directed towards establishing an aetiology: in particular a history suggestive of multisystem disease, and drug or toxin ingestion. As soon as practicable, investigations should be made (Table 10.3) to exclude a number of possible diagnoses.

The possibility of underlying chronic failure must not be forgotten. Often this is difficult to establish clinically—patients may complain of

**Table 10.3 Screening investigations in acute renal failure**

*Haematology*
Full blood count, including differential white cell count and platelets
ESR
Coagulation screen

*Biochemistry*
Liver function tests, calcium and phosphate
Uric acid
Creatine phosphokinase (CPK)
Glucose
Serum protein electrophoresis
C-reactive protein

*Immunology/serology*
Immunoglobulins
Antinuclear antibodies (including double-stranded DNA)
Rheumatoid factor
Anti-glomerular basement membrane antibody
Anti-neutrophil cytoplasmic antibody
Complement C3, C4
Cryoglobulins
HBsAg
Wassermann reaction
Antistreptolysin O titre

*Urine*
Bence-Jones protein
Bacteriology

*Miscellaneous*
Chest X-ray
Echocardiogram
Renal ultrasonography

pruritus and pigmentation, or have a history of hypertension, anaemia or bone disease but these features usually appear late in the course of chronic failure. Imaging may provide an indication of longstanding renal impairment by demonstrating reduced renal size or anatomical abnormalities, and also often excludes obstruction.

Acute tubular necrosis is the most common cause of acute renal failure but it is rarely confirmed histologically and is managed conservatively in view of its self-limiting course. Therefore it is a diagnosis of exclusion after considering the following possibilities:

(1) *Renal obstruction.* In the context of acute failure the most important causes are tumours, particularly of cervix, bladder, rectum and prostate, retroperitoneal fibrosis and obstruction of a single kidney, for example by calculi. The most effective screening test is ultrasound examination to show a dilated pelvicalyceal system (Fig. 10.2). Together with CT scans and retrograde and antegrade urography (often combined with temporary percutaneous drainage of an obstructed pelvicalyceal system), an accurate anatomical and aetiological diagnosis can often be made. Renal obstruction of longer than a few weeks' standing is associated with irreversible parenchymal damage. The urine proximal to the obstruction may be infected even if the urine distally is sterile on culture. Obstruction should be relieved as soon as possible under antibiotic cover (e.g., amoxycillin or aminoglycosides) and a sample of urine sent for bacteriological investigation. After the relief of obstruction there is a profound diuresis, which may persist for several weeks, requiring careful monitoring and replacement of sodium, potassium and water.

(2) *Acute glomerulonephritis.* Rapidly progressive glomerulonephritis may result in loss of renal function over two to three weeks. This may occur in association with vasculitis as in polyarteritis nodosa, systemic lupus erythematosus (SLE), Wegener's granulomatosis and cryoglobulinaemia. Other diagnoses include antiglomerular basement membrane (GBM) disease (Goodpasture's syndrome) and idiopathic crescentic nephritis. Rapid diagnosis of these conditions is imperative as specific immunosuppressive therapy may limit renal damage. In all cases, pulmonary symptoms, particularly haemoptysis, and

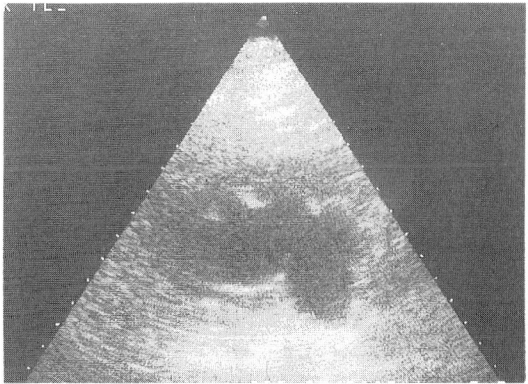

*Figure 10.2*  Renal ultrasound of kidneys from a patient with acute renal failure and bilateral ureteric obstruction secondary to carcinoma of bladder. Note the dilated pelvicalyceal system and relatively well preserved cortex indicating acute obstruction.

signs of multisystem involvement including cutaneous and retinal vasculitis, arthropathy, neuropathy and myopathy should be sought. This should be followed by appropriate serological investigations (see Table 10.3) such as anti-GBM antibodies, anti-DNA antibodies and complement levels, and early renal biopsy (Fig. 10.3).

(3) *Acute interstitial nephritis.* Acute renal failure following the ingestion of drugs, particularly non-steroidal anti-inflammatory agents, diuretics and antibiotics (e.g., penicillins, cephalosporins, sulphonamides and aminoglycosides), has been associated with tubular atrophy and interstitial infiltration with mononuclear cells and eosinophils. The duration of exposure to the agent has varied from days to months; in addition to the oliguria, proteinuria may occur. This is generally mild but may exceed 2 g/24 h in interstitial nephritis associated with some non-steroidal anti-inflammatory drugs. Associated findings have included pyrexia, flank pain, skin rash, arthralgia, abnormalities of liver function, eosinophilia and eosinophiluria. Withdrawal of the drug is often associated with recovery of renal function which may be accelerated by treatment with prednisolone. This diagnosis is not restricted to drug reactions, as it has been reported in association with a number of infections and sarcoidosis.

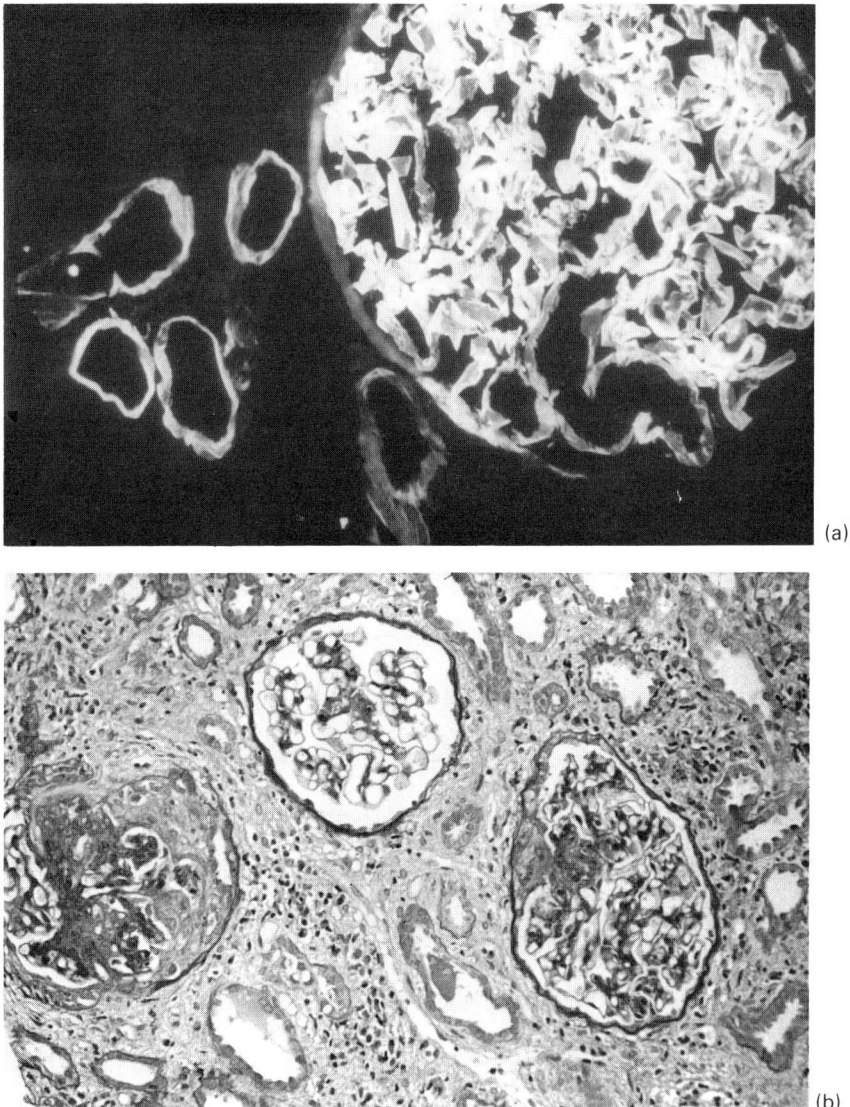

*Figure 10.3* Renal biopsies from patients with acute renal failure secondary to acute glomerulonephritis. (a) Linear staining of the glomerular basement membrane with antihuman IgG in a case of Goodpasture's syndrome ($\times$ 200). (b) Acute necrotizing glomerulonephritis in a patient with Wegener's granulomatosis. Note the infiltrate with mononuclear cells, and crescent formation ($\times$ 200). (Photographs courtesy of Dr C. M. Lockwood.)

(4) *Acute cortical necrosis.* This occurs in association with acute renal failure especially during pregnancy; it may follow eclampsia, uterine haemorrhage and septic abortion. The diagnosis should be considered in those with no recovery of renal function four weeks after the diagnosis of 'acute tubular necrosis'. There is a patchy necrosis of the renal cortex involving glomeruli and tubules. Renal biopsy or angiography showing narrowing of interlobular vessels is often diagnostic. Recovery of some renal function occurs in about half the patients but with severe residual impairment and associated hypertension.

## Complications and management of acute tubular necrosis

The precise aetiology and pathophysiology of acute tubular necrosis remain unknown. The onset of oliguria is associated with profound intrarenal vasoconstriction, which results in reduced filtration, and this may account for ischaemic damage to tubular cells. However, the mechanisms by which this ischaemic insult is maintained, to explain prolonged reduced renal function are unknown. Few of the patient's symptoms relate directly to renal impairment but rather to the circumstances that precipitated hypovolaemia. Symptoms and signs of 'uraemia' (see below) may be present, notably muscle cramps and a flapping tremor. Many of the recognized complications of renal failure, such as pericarditis, occur less frequently than in chronic renal failure but should nevertheless be looked for as they require immediate attention.

Depending on the clinical situation a decision must be made as to conservative management or dialysis. In either situation attention must be paid to a number of aspects:

(1) *Fluid balance.* Particular care must be taken with fluid balance, especially prior to the implementation of dialysis. Insensible loss in the average adult is estimated at 500 ml in temperate climates, although this may change dramatically, for example in association with pyrexia. Classically the daily fluid intake of adult oliguric patients with acute renal failure is 500 ml plus the previous day's urine output. However, this must be carefully controlled by strict monitoring of fluid balance, daily weights and postural blood pressure recordings.

(2) *Electrolyte balance.* Retention of $Na^+$ is often the case, thus a low dietary $Na^+$ intake (20 mmol/day) is recommended. However, in polyuric acute renal failure, considerable $Na^+$ loss may occur and the 24-h urinary $Na^+$ loss should be monitored and replaced as required. Dietary $K^+$ should also be restricted (<40 mmol/day).

(3) *Diet.* The dietary requirement in patients with acute renal failure managed conservatively is between 8400 and 16 800 J/day with 40 g of protein for the 'average 70 kg man'. This must be provided in the context of fluid restriction, if necessary by supplemental enteral or parenteral nutrition. Once dialysis is instituted the protein intake is increased, particularly to compensate for the protein loss associated with peritoneal dialysis. Furthermore, in hypercatabolic states, nitrogen intake must be increased. The extra fluid volume that this necessitates is removed by additional haemodialysis or haemofiltration.

(4) *Infection and gastrointestinal haemorrhage.* These are major reversible factors influencing the mortality associated with acute renal failure. Infections must be rapidly identified and treated with appropriate antibiotics and risk factors increasing susceptibility to infection, such as intravenous cannulas and urethral catheterization, reduced to a minimum. Ranitidine, 150 mg/day, or cimetidine, 200 mg twice daily, are often administered prophylactically to reduce the risk of gastrointestinal haemorrhage but there is little evidence of their efficacy.

In most instances there is little to choose between either haemo- or peritoneal dialysis for acute renal failure and for practical details the reader is referred to a separate review (see Oliver and Wing in 'Further Reading'). Haemodialysis is certainly preferred if there is hypercatabolism or the possibility of intra-abdominal injury. Furthermore there is less protein loss and a reduced risk of infection compared with peritoneal dialysis. However, peritoneal dialysis is more widely available, especially in non-specialist units, and is cheaper.

The usual outcome of acute failure due to tubular necrosis is recovery, though the prognosis is less good in certain clinical settings. As might be anticipated, mortality is higher in elderly patients or when acute renal failure occurs in cases of burns or trauma. In these situations the excess mortality is often influenced by concurrent problems. Hyperkalaemia is now uncommon as a cause of death and probably the major potentially reversible factors include infection and gastrointestinal haemorrhage, as discussed above. In patients who recover from acute tubular necrosis the GFR is rapidly returned to between 70 and 80 per cent of normal, although defects of tubular concentration may be detected for some time.

## CHRONIC RENAL FAILURE

There is a large functional reserve of kidney tissue, therefore slowly progressive disease processes often present only when end-stage renal failure is reached. Symptoms related to chronic failure are present when greater than 75 per cent of functional renal tissue is lost. Table 10.4, adapted from figures supplied to the European Dialysis and Transplantation Association, indicates the most frequent causes of chronic renal failure. However, certain factors have to be remembered in interpreting these data. Firstly, they relate only to chronic renal failure in industrialized countries and are probably very different in developing countries. Secondly, these data are for treated patients on long-term replacement therapy, skewed by excluding data on those rejected from programmes for management by lack of facilities (usually the very young and elderly) and they probably underrepresent those with multisystem diseases, such as diabetes and myeloma. Finally, up to one third of patients present in end-stage renal failure, making accurate diagnosis difficult, and conditions such as 'glomerulonephritis' do not imply that all these patients have biopsy-proven glomerulonephritis as a cause of chronic failure.

**Table 10.4 Common causes of chronic renal failure**

Glomerulonephritis
Pyelonephritis
Polycystic kidney disease
Diabetic nephropathy
Hypertensive nephrosclerosis
Analgesic nephropathy
Hereditary nephropathy

Patients present with chronic renal failure late but with entirely nonspecific symptoms. The commonest are general malaise, increasing tiredness and dyspnoea, although they are often preceded by nocturia. Specific enquiries, examination and investigations often reveal other features:

(1) *Gastrointestinal.* Anorexia with early morning nausea and vomiting are relatively common. Hiccups, due to a direct central effect, and gastrointestinal bleeding, exacerbated by the associated uraemic bleeding diathesis, may be late features.
(2) *Nervous system.* Patients will admit to a gradual deterioration in their mental ability, and work performance may have markedly deteriorated. Sleep disturbance, made worse by nocturia, is again common. This may be accompanied by the distressing symptom of 'restless legs' at night, as well as peripheral neuropathy.

(3) *Respiratory and cardiovascular.* Dyspnoea on exertion is frequently a late feature associated with cardiac failure secondary to hypertension and fluid overload. In addition, some patients develop bilateral dense opacities radiating from the lung hilum on chest X-ray with normal pulmonary artery pressures—'uraemic lung'.
(4) *Dermatological.* Pruritus is a particularly troublesome feature in end-stage disease and may be a consequence of hyperparathyroidism and uraemia. Symptomatic relief is provided by a reduced protein diet, cholestyramine, 5 g twice a day, and/or antihistamines, but this is temporary and dialysis is required.

## Investigation and management

As far as possible the underlying cause of renal failure should be established. This is important as certain forms of chronic impairment, such as analgesic nephropathy, may be retarded even at late stages. It also alerts to particular reversible conditions should renal function suddenly deteriorate during conservative management, and helps plan the most appropriate replacement therapy.

When following patients with chronic renal impairment, monitoring the rate of deterioration by repeated measurement of plasma creatinine is important. Creatinine is produced from muscle, therefore plasma creatinine concentration is dependent on body size. Until the GFR falls below 30 ml/min, the plasma creatinine is only marginally elevated but as the GFR declines further, the plasma creatinine increases in a curvilinear fashion. The rate of decline of renal function in an individual patient can be monitored with some precision by a plot of 1/[plasma creatinine] against time (Fig. 10.4). Once the GFR falls much below 20 ml/min there is often an inexorable decline in renal function. The mechanism for this is unknown, although the favoured explanation is damage to surviving nephrons caused by the hyperperfusion consequent upon reduced renal mass. This cannot be retarded by any therapeutic measure available to date, although studies are currently in progress into possible beneficial effects associated with the use of angiotensin converting enzyme inhibitors and lipid-lowering agents (see Further Reading). Monitoring the 1/creatinine plot for individual patients allows the progression to end-stage disease to be predicted

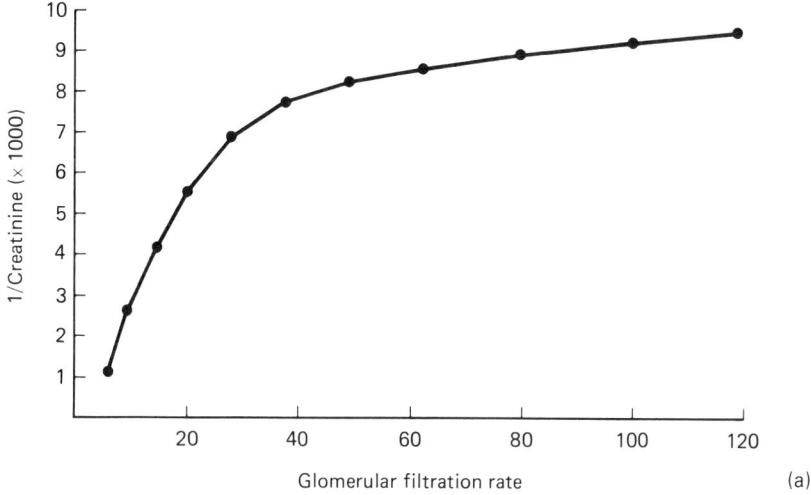

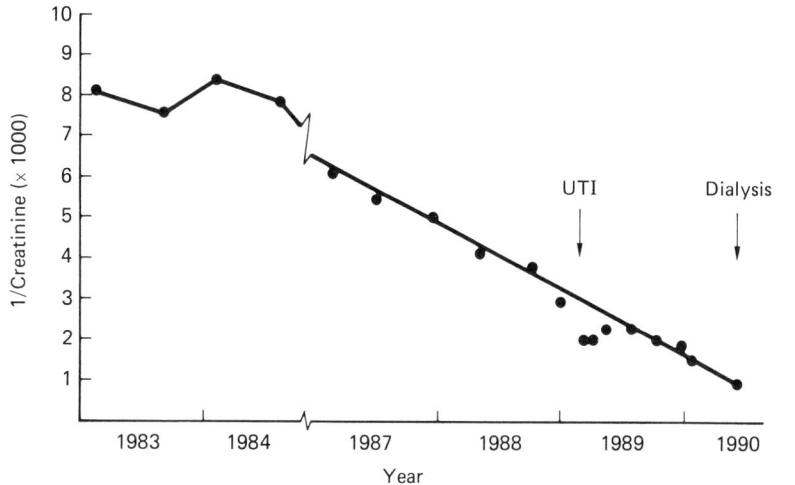

*Figure 10.4* (a) Plot of the reciprocal of plasma creatinine *vs.* GFR (measured as creatinine clearance). (b) Sequential plot of 1/creatinine in a patient with chronic renal failure secondary to Wegener's granulomatosis. Note the deviation from the predicted course at the time of a urinary tract infection (UTI). Dialysis was instituted during 1990

to a greater or lesser extent and any sudden deterioration of function from the predicted slope should initiate a search for possible reversible factors (Table 10.5).

### Drugs in renal failure

One of the major, preventable causes of sudden deterioration of renal function is the use of nephrotoxic drugs (Table 10.6). The reduced GFR blocks the excretion of a number of commonly used agents so that toxic levels may be readily

**Table 10.5 Reversible factors in chronic renal failure**

Uncontrolled hypertension
Dehydration
Nephrotoxic drugs
Infection, especially urinary
Elevated [calcium] × [phosphate] solubility product
Urinary tract obstruction
Cardiac failure

reached with 'normal' dosage regimens. A number of drugs are best avoided in moderate to severe renal impairment and the safest agents are those with a short half-life and an extrarenal route of excretion. Radiocontrast media may induce acute tubular necrosis in patients with reduced renal function, especially secondary to diabetes and myeloma.

### Conservative management of chronic renal failure

(1) *Dietary control.* Dietary management of patients with chronic failure is currently the subject of some controversy. An adequate calorie intake must be provided, but the influence of dietary protein upon the rate of deterioration of renal function is unknown. The original Giovenetti (20 g/day) diet was an effective means of reducing symptoms of uraemia before the availability of replacement therapy and a restriction of dietary protein is still used to control symptoms of chronic renal failure. However, it has been noted that reduced protein diets may also slow the rate

**Table 10.6 Drug therapy in chronic renal failure**

| Category | Normal dose | Reduced dose, monitor where possible | Avoid |
|---|---|---|---|
| Antibiotics | Erythromycin<br>Isoniazid<br>Rifampicin<br>Sulphonamides<br>(need high fluid<br>throughput) | Amphotericin<br>Cephalosporins<br>Doxycycline<br>Ethambutol<br>Metronidazole<br>Penicillins<br>Aminoglycosides ⎫ monitor<br>Vancomycin ⎭ levels | Tetracyclines |
| Respiratory | Salbutamol<br>Terbutaline<br>Theophylline | | |
| Cardiovascular system | Hydralazine<br>Labetalol<br>Metoprolol<br>Minoxidil<br>Nifedipine<br>Prazosin | Atenolol<br>Captopril<br>Digoxin (monitor)<br>Enalapril | Thiazides (ineffective)<br>$K^+$-sparing diuretics |
| Gastrointestinal | Calcium<br>carbonate | Aluminium-containing antacids<br>Cimetidine<br>Metoclopramide<br>Ranitidine | Carbenoxolone<br>Magnesium-containing antacids |
| Central nervous system | Carbamazepine<br>Chlorpromazine<br>Diazepam<br>Phenytoin<br>Sodium<br>valproate<br>Temazepam | Most other benzodiazepines | Lithium |
| Diabetes | Tolbutamide | Insulin | Chlorpropramide<br>Glibenclamide |
| Analgesics<br>+ gout | Sulindac | Allopurinol<br>Colchicine | Penicillamine<br>Probenecid<br>Avoid *NSAIDs if possible—<br>sulindac seems to cause least<br>inhibition of renal<br>prostaglandin synthesis |

* Non-steroidal anti-inflammatory drugs.

of deterioration of GFR, possibly by reducing hyperperfusion of 'normal' nephrons in the damaged kidney. This is being investigated in a number of trials and currently there is no consensus as to the role of dietary protein restriction.

(2) *Fluid and electrolytes.* The requirements in this instance vary with the underlying aetiology of the failure. In most cases, fluid retention does not become a major problem until end-stage failure is reached. Fluid retention may be overcome temporarily by the use of loop diuretics, such as frusemide in large doses. Sodium retention is often associated with hypertension (see below) and in most cases dietary sodium restriction to 40 mmol/day is instituted as end-stage disease approaches. However, in patients where the underlying process leading to renal impairment results in predominant tubular damage—interstitial nephropathy, pyelonephritis, analgesic nephropathy—a salt-losing state may result. Inability to conserve salt and water results in postural hypotension, though hypertension may supervene late in the disease process. The use of loop diuretics is best avoided because of the danger of precipitating hypovolaemia. Moreover, salt supplements in the form of sodium bicarbonate or slow-release $Na^+$, monitored by measuring sodium balance and postural blood pressure, are frequently required.

Plasma potassium does not rise until end-stage disease and dietary restriction to 40 mmol/day is usually adequate. However, if plasma levels rise in spite of this, control can be retained temporarily by using ion exchange resins (see above).

(3) *Hypertension.* The control of blood pressure is important in preserving renal function in chronic renal failure and in reducing risk factors for cerebrovascular events. Control of blood pressure should be as for adult patients with essential hypertension—resting systolic BP <160 mmHg and diastolic BP <90 mmHg. This can normally be achieved with a combination of β-blockers and vasodilators, after suitable dosage adjustments for the degree of renal impairment. As discussed previously, care must be taken if the patient has a salt-losing nephropathy, or autonomic neuropathy, as in diabetic patients.

(4) *Other metabolic abnormalities.* There is a persistent metabolic acidosis, which like many of the complications of chronic renal failure is probably multifactorial in aetiology. There is impaired reabsorption of bicarbonate in the proximal tubules and reduced ammoniagenesis, and excess $H^+$ ions are buffered in bone tissue. The acidosis is often asymptomatic until end-stage disease, but can be corrected by sodium bicarbonate if required.

Numerous endocrine abnormalities have been documented, including a prolonged insulin half-life in patients with diabetes, resulting in reduced insulin requirements as renal failure progresses in these patients. In addition there is peripheral insulin resistance, producing a diabetic-like glucose tolerance test in chronic failure. Thyroid function is reduced but prolactin and gastrin secretion are enhanced. Patients with chronic renal failure often have a hypertriglyceridaemia which may be related to the high frequency of vascular events in this group.

### Replacement therapy

It is beyond the scope of this chapter to consider the detailed long-term management of patients by dialysis and transplantation, and the reader is referred to reviews in 'Further Reading'.

### Management of complications of chronic renal failure

In addition to the metabolic disturbances described above, progressive deterioration of renal function results in the development of a normochromic normocytic anaemia and bone disease.

### Anaemia of chronic renal failure

In patients with chronic renal failure there are many possible causes for anaemia in addition to deficiency of erythropoietin. Blood loss and loss of iron stores has to be excluded, together with folate deficiency, especially if the patient is on maintenance dialysis. In these circumstances prophylactic ferrous sulphate (250 mg/day) and folate (5 mg/day)—often combined in the form of a water-soluble multivitamin preparation—may be given.

Erythropoietin, secreted by the kidney to stimulate red cell production by the marrow, gradually falls as the functional renal mass is reduced. This results in a normochromic normocytic anaemia of increasing severity in most cases. In certain cases, e.g., polycystic kidney disease, production of erythropoietin may be maintained and this characteristic anaemia does not occur. The severity of the anaemia is partially offset by the shift of the oxygen dissociation curve to the left, possibly as a result of the concurrent acidosis. The recent introduction of recombinant erythropoietin has revolutionized the management of the anaemia of chronic renal failure (see further reading).

### Renal bone disease

Several factors, some of them still not clearly identified, combine to induce the bone disease common to end-stage renal failure regardless of underlying aetiology. Phosphate retention may occur early in the course of renal failure, resulting in increased secretion of parathyroid hormone (PTH). This is linked to a reduced circulating level of 1,25 dihydroxycholecalciferol, probably a consequence of increased circulating PTH and damage to renal cells, the major site of the 1-hydroxylation step. This results in the characteristic changes of a raised serum phosphate ($[PO_4^{2-}]$), low $[Ca^{2+}]$ and raised PTH (secondary hyperparathyroidism). This state is often held responsible for osteitis fibrosa—characterized by subperiosteal erosions commonly seen in X-rays of the hand (Fig. 10.5). The reduced 1,25 dihydroxy-cholecalciferol results in features suggestive of an osteomalacic element to the disease, sometimes with Looser's zones on X-rays of the pelvis and acromion. In addition, ectopic soft-tissue calcification, e.g., at the sclero-conjunctival junction, may occur. A number of other factors, such as metabolic acidosis, may also contribute to this overall picture.

Treatment is currently empirical. An elevated $[PO_4^{2-}]$ can reduce GFR (Table 10.5), and thus control of dietary $[PO_4^{2-}]$ by use of binders such as calcium carbonate or aluminium hydroxide may retard the development of end-stage disease. Aluminium itself may accumulate in renal failure, resulting in bone damage, dementia and anaemia (which is resistant to therapy with erythropoietin). Therefore aluminium-containing compounds are best avoided. 1-Hydroxycholecalciferol (0.25–1.0 µg daily) can also be administered, with frequent monitoring of $[Ca^{2+}]$ to avoid hypercalcaemic damage to the kidneys and other organs. In addition, a sustained increase in $[Ca^{2+}]$ should

alert to the possible development of tertiary hyperparathyroidism. Parathyroidectomy may be required to control worsening osteitis fibrosa and persistent hypercalcaemia.

## GLOMERULONEPHRITIS

The commonest cause of chronic renal failure is glomerulonephritis (see Table 10.4), and this broad diagnosis is a heading for a number of inflammatory conditions that affect glomeruli. The aetiology in the majority of histologically identifiable categories remains unknown. It is beyond the scope of this chapter to consider individual conditions in detail but the major correlations between histological appearances, clinical presentation and prognosis are shown in Table 10.7.

## PROTEINURIA AND THE NEPHROTIC SYNDROME

### Asymptomatic proteinuria

One of the most common problems requiring further investigation is the detection of asymptomatic and symptomatic proteinuria. Even if the patient is asymptomatic, one must decide whether this finding is indicative of underlying renal disease and what is the likely prognosis? The glomerular basement membrane is an effective filtration barrier by means of:

(1) *Size*. There is a reduction in filtration with increasing size: small proteins, e.g., Bence-Jones proteins, are easily passed, as are small amounts of albumin, but larger proteins rarely enter the glomerular filtrate.

(2) *Charge*. In addition to the size barrier there is a preponderance of polyanionic aminoglycans and glycoproteins in the basement membrane and these prevent the loss of negatively charged molecules more readily than positively charged ones. This mechanism may be markedly impaired in minimal change nephrotic syndrome in children.

If proteins pass through into the filtrate, epithelial cells can remove this filtered load. In significant proteinuria there is a breakdown of the normal filtration barrier and the ability of epithelial cells to reabsorb protein is exceeded. In normal urine about 150 mg/24 h of proteinuria

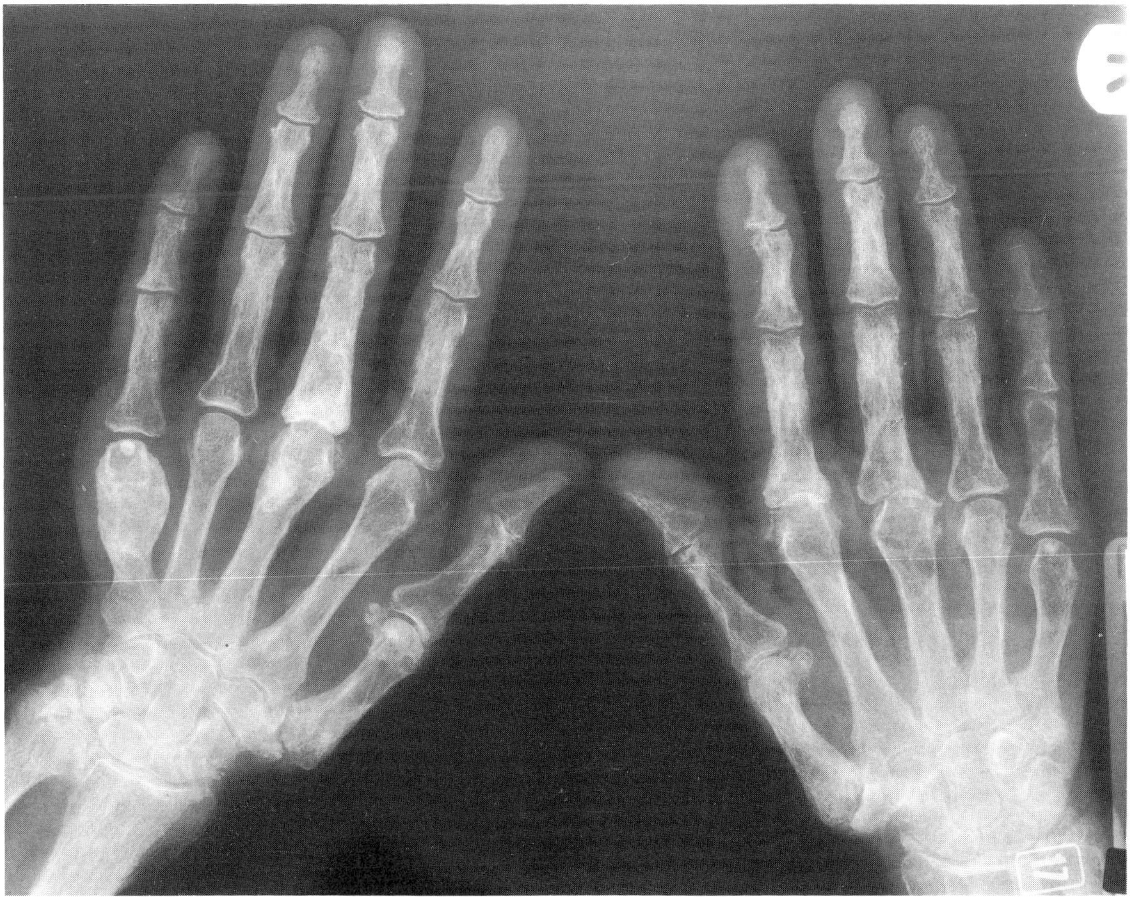

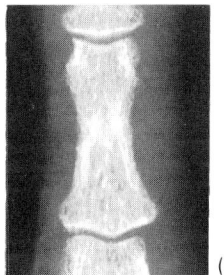

*Figure 10.5* (a) Hand and (b) middle phalanx X-ray of a patient on chronic haemodialysis showing subperiosteal erosions indicative of secondary hyperparathyroidism.

may be detected—made up of albumin and secreted tubular glycoproteins such as Tamm–Horsfall protein.

Proteinuria may arise without serious underlying renal disease, and can often be detected after strenuous exercise, at high altitudes and during febrile episodes. Orthostatic proteinuria occurs most commonly in young men and may result in asymptomatic proteinuria of up to 2 g/day, i.e., this is *not* a cause of nephrotic syndrome. The aetiology of this condition is unknown, but proteinuria is only detected when the patient is upright and is probably related to increased renal blood flow and filtration in the upright position. Histological studies of such patients have revealed minor glomerular abnormalities, which on follow-up have resulted in little or no loss of renal function.

Having excluded the above possibilities, the source of the proteinuria should be considered.

Symptomatic proteinuria, presenting as the nephrotic syndrome, is invariably due to increased glomerular permeability from underlying glomerulopathy (see Table 10.7). However, low levels of proteinuria may result from inflammation of the

**Table 10.7 Glomerulonephritis—a classification and common clinical presentations**

| Histology | Common clinical presentation | Serum complement (C3) | Associations | Prognosis |
|---|---|---|---|---|
| Minimal change | Nephrotic syndrome | Normal | Lymphoma in adults; non-steroidal anti-inflammatory drugs | Good. Usually responds to steroid therapy |
| Membranous | Nephrotic syndrome | Normal | Tumours, especially gastrointestinal, drugs (gold, penicillamine, captopril), hepatitis B, malaria | Variable: slow decline in renal function in 30% of patients |
| Focal, segmental glomerulosclerosis | Proteinuria, nephrotic syndrome | Normal | Heroin abuse; may initially be misdiagnosed as minimal change | Proteinuria may be steroid dependent; renal function may slowly deteriorate |
| Mesangial IgA disease | Haematuria + proteinuria Nephrotic syndrome | Normal (serum IgA may be elevated) | May follow upper respiratory infection; this histological picture is seen in Henoch–Schönlein purpura | Variable: 25% develop end-stage renal disease |
| Mesangiocapillary type I | Haematuria + proteinuria → Nephrotic syndrome | ↓ | Shunts for hydrocephalus; sickle cell disease | Progression to end-stage renal failure likely |
| Mesangiocapillary type II | Haematuria + proteinuria Nephrotic syndrome | ↓ (C3 nephritic factor may be present in serum) | Partial lipodystrophy | Progression to end-stage renal failure likely |
| Acute exudative | Haematuria + proteinuria Acute renal failure | ↓ | Follows acute streprococcal infection of throat or skin | Most cases resolve |
| Crescentic | Acute renal failure (rapidly progressive glomerulonephritis) | Depends upon aetiology | Systemic vasculitis, e.g. systemic lupus erythematosus, Wegener's granulomatosis, cryoglobulinaemia, subacute bacterial endocarditis | Progressive unless immunosuppressive treatment instituted early |
| Anti-glomerular basement membrane disease | Acute renal failure | Normal | Lung haemorrhage in Goodpasture's syndrome | Progressive unless immunosuppressive treatment instituted early |
| Focal proliferative glomerulonephritis | Haematuria, proteinuria, renal impairment | Depends upon aetiology | Systemic lupus erythematosus, subacute bacterial endocarditis, shunts for hydrocephalus, polyarteritis nodosa | Progressive unless underlying condition treated |

urinary tract, such as that associated with infection, increased losses secondary to tubular damage, or the presence of unusual plasma proteins, e.g., Bence-Jones proteinuria.

## Nephrotic syndrome

This is operationally defined as hypoalbuminaemia with oedema in the presence of heavy ($>5$ g/day) proteinuria. Oedema is unlikely to be present until the serum albumin falls below 30 g/l. The reduction in albumin has occurred in the face of maximum rates of production by the liver, often resulting in loss of muscle mass, which may only be evident once oedema has been treated. Proteinuria may be selective for the passage of small molecular-weight proteins, such as albumin, or non-selective. Selectivity is clinically assessed by comparing clearances of a low molecular-weight protein, such as transferrin, with a high molecular weight protein, such as IgG. The presence of a selective proteinuria implies minimal change glomerulonephritis but in adults, selectivity may be periodically observed in other conditions such as amyloidosis.

The reduction in plasma oncotic pressure results in increased interstitial fluid, detected as oedema—pedal oedema on standing or periorbital on lying. Furthermore, there is a positive $Na^+$ balance, although plasma $[Na^+]$ and $[K^+]$ may be reduced as a result of 'secondary hyperaldosteronism'. There is an increase in total cholesterol with increased production of very low density lipoprotein (VLDL) and low density lipoprotein (LDL) by the liver. This is a direct consequence of hypoalbuminaemia, as treating this alone restores the lipid abnormality. Excess lipid may spill over into the urine and 'fat bodies' can sometimes be detected in the urinary sediment.

### Diagnosis

The aim of recognizing the underlying glomerulonephritis causing the nephrotic syndrome (see Table 10.7) is to identify those individuals with minimal change nephritis, as regardless of age they may respond to steroid therapy. The frequency of minimal change nephrotic syndrome is age-dependent—in children under 5 years the majority have this condition and a therapeutic trial of high-dose steroid therapy is indicated (see below). However, in adults the frequency of minimal change nephritis is much smaller ($<5$ per

cent) and thus renal biopsy is indicated in nearly all cases. The detection of minimal change nephritis in adults should alert to the possibility of an underlying lymphoma.

### Complications

Complications arising in patients with nephrotic syndrome are related both to the nature of the nephritis and its treatment:

(1) *Infection.* There is a higher incidence of infection, particularly chest infection. The possibility of infection must always be borne in mind, particularly as treatment with steroids may mask the usual symptoms and signs. Pneumococcal peritonitis may present acutely with abdominal pain, rebound tenderness and pyrexia. However, abdominal pain may also be a direct result of oedema.

(2) *Venous thrombosis.* There is an increased frequency of deep venous thrombosis in leg veins, possibly as a result of the increased plasma viscosity and inactivity in the presence of gross oedema. However, renal vein thrombosis, previously thought to be a cause of heavy proteinuria, is now recognized as a specific complication of nephrotic syndrome, particularly with mesangiocapillary and membranous nephritis. The difficulty is that the classical features of renal vein thrombosis—haematuria with red cell casts and an increase in proteinuria—may be absent, and the patient may present with pulmonary embolism. Thus anticoagulant therapy may be instituted prophylactically.

(3) *Precipitation of acute tubular necrosis.* The reduced GFR consequent on a low circulating volume may be compromised further by the injudicious use of loop diuretics, thus precipitating acute tubular necrosis.

### Treatment and prognosis

#### Drug therapy

The primary aim of management of the nephrotic syndrome is to identify the nature of the glomerular lesion, treat the underlying cause if possible, e.g., chronic infection in amyloidosis, or to arrest the protein leak. This latter is only readily achieved in minimal change glomerulonephritis, which will respond to between 60 and 100 mg/day of prednisolone for six to eight weeks, reducing to alternate-day therapy, then tailing the dose down over six months, observing for possible recurrence of proteinuria. A small proportion of patients will relapse within this period, and others will have a recurrence after ending the treatment. In such cases, chlorambucil or cyclophosphamide may be used to halt protein loss, at the risk of azoospermia, haemorrhagic cystitis and bone marrow suppression. In some individuals the proteinuria remains steroid responsive, but dose reduction results in rapid recurrence. Such patients may remain steroid dependent and in some instances repeat renal biopsy indicates the development of a focal segmental glomerulosclerosis, missed by sampling error on the first biopsy. Steroids and other immunosuppressive agents may have a role to play in arresting the proteinuria associated with membranous glomerulonephritis but the evidence supporting a beneficial effect on the progression of renal impairment is anecdotal.

In patients without a steroid-responsive lesion, some reduction of proteinuria may be obtained with indomethacin. This is only possible where protein loss is very high and GFR is relatively normal, as the reduction in proteinuria is at the expense of a reduction in GFR. Where the renal lesion is progressive there is a decline in the degree of proteinuria as renal function deteriorates.

### Dietary measures

A high protein diet (100 g/day) must be provided to reduce tissue catabolism and a low $Na^+$ (40 mmol/day) diet reduces salt retention.

### Diuretic therapy

The danger of diuretic therapy is the precipitation of acute tubular necrosis by further exacerbating the hypovolaemic state of nephrotic patients. Diuresis should be relatively slow; treatment with thiazide diuretics in conjunction with spironolactone is often adequate. If necessary, loop diuretics should be gradually increased from low doses, using the recording of daily weights and postural blood pressure as a guide to dosage.

### Plasma expanders

These are indicated where there is severe oedema and a failure to obtain an adequate diuresis with diuretics alone.

### Antibiotic prophylaxis

This should not be used but prompt treatment of any infection with appropriate antibiotics is required.

## URINARY TRACT INFECTION

### Lower urinary tract infection

Urinary tract infection is the commonest renal problem encountered in general practice, accounting for about 12 per 1000 consultations, and the majority of these cases are due to lower urinary tract infection. Infection may be asymptomatic or associated with frequency, dysuria and occasionally haematuria or the passage of foul-smelling urine. The first presentation of lower urinary tract infection may be Gram-negative septicaemia and this accounts for 20 to 30 per cent of all cases of Gram-negative septicaemia, particularly in elderly patients.

The common pathogens encountered are *Escherichia coli*, micrococci, *Proteus mirabilis* and *Staphylococcus saprophyticus*. Less common pathogens may also be isolated, often in association with an underlying renal abnormality. Infection with *E. coli* in women occurs probably by faecal contamination, particularly in association with intercourse ('honeymoon cystitis').

Diagnosis is dependent upon obtaining a significant culture of microorganisms in a midstream urine specimen. These cultures must be carefully collected and stored at 4°C if not set up on a dip-slide culture immediately. A bacterial count of more than $10^5$ colonies/ml has an 85 per cent probability of representing a true pathogen. However, this is only a relative finding: thus it must be remembered that a pure culture of one organism may be significant at lower counts, and lower colony counts may also be significant in partially treated infections. Furthermore, some fastidious organisms, such as streptococci or mycoplasmas, may be difficult to isolate or require special culture conditions other than the commonly employed MacConkey's agar.

Infection is accompanied by pyuria but it is important to remember that sterile pyuria can also occur (renal tuberculosis must be excluded in such cases), and infection may occur in the absence of pyuria. If there is continuing difficulty in isolating an organism, suprapubic aspiration may be performed. Firstly, a diuresis is induced with 20 mg frusemide or several glasses of water, and then a fine needle is inserted in the midline 2.5 cm above the symphysis pubis, *when the bladder is palpable*. Any organism isolated from such a specimen is significant and the previously discussed quantitative cultures are unnecessary.

### Treatment

In most cases, treatment of symptoms has to be instituted before the results of culture and sensitivity tests are available, therefore the sensitivity of the locally prevalent organisms should be known. However, treatment with co-trimoxazole (2 tabs, twice a day), trimethoprim (200 mg, twice a day) or ampicillin (250 mg, four times a day) for seven days is often adequate. Alternatively, single high-dose treatment has been used successfully (amoxycillin, 3 g). Symptoms will usually subside within one to two days but if they persist for longer, then the culture results should be available and a different antibiotic, to which the organism is susceptible, can be prescribed. There is no place for higher dose treatment with the first agent selected, provided that a therapeutic dose was used in the first instance. Several important questions arise in the further management of such patients:

(1) *Treatment of relapse/reinfection*. Arbitrarily these two are separated by the former occurring within six weeks and the latter after this time. Relapsing infections are common, and may be due to poor antibiotic selection, inadequate therapy (try high-dose treatment) or an underlying abnormality, especially renal calculi. Symptoms may persist in the absence of obvious precipitants however, and long-term treatment with a single night-time dose of co-trimoxazole or a cephalosporin for 12 months may be required to block nocturnal replication of bacteria.

In the case of repeated reinfection, having excluded an underlying anatomical abnormality, a high fluid intake and either long-term therapy as outlined above or repeated courses of antibiotics at the first onset of symptoms may be worth trying.

(2) *Radiological investigation*. In most instances, lower urinary tract infections in males are associated with an anatomical abnormality, which may require further therapy. In child-ren, radiological abnormalities in both sexes are frequent, but in adult women investigation is only required if frequent relapse or reinfection occurs.

(3) *Asymptomatic bacteriuria*. Asymptomatic infections are common particularly in girls (1–2 per cent) and adult women (3–5 per cent); they are uncommon in boys (0.05 per cent). An increase in these in adult women is particularly associated with parity, and during pregnancy the frequency of asymptomatic bacteriuria is high (30 per cent) and may be followed by symptomatic infection later. Among children, particularly in boys, there is a high prevalence of structural abnormality especially reflux. Screening for asymptomatic infection is not routine but should be considered in pregnancy and in those with other renal dysfunction or on immunosuppressive therapy.

(4) *Acute urethral syndrome*. Approximately half of women presenting with symptoms of cystitis have negative bacterial cultures. Symptoms may be related to sexual intercourse and repeated episodes of pain and frequency may occur. In these circumstances, repeated cultures looking for fastidious organisms and a careful search for vaginal pathogens, including chlamydia and gonococci, should be made. In about half of such cases a pathogen will be identified and appropriate antibacterial therapy can be instituted. However, in the absence of confirmation, antibiotics are avoided except for a trial of postcoital antibiotics in cases associated with sexual intercourse.

### Upper urinary tract infection

#### Acute pyelonephritis

The usual presentation is fever (often with rigors) associated with loin pain, but this clinical presentation may also be associated with lower urinary tract infection. The usual organisms are *E. coli* and *Proteus* and it is likely that in most instances the infection ascends the urinary tract to involve the pelvis and parenchyma of the kidney. Infection may be associated with the development of a perirenal abscess. Conditions predisposing to ascending infection include diabetes, pregnancy and urinary obstruction. In pregnancy the treatment of associated asymptomatic bacteriuria may prevent the development of later pyelonephritis. Blood and urine are taken for culture and treatment is started with amoxycillin or trimethoprim on the assumption that the likeliest pathogen is *E. coli*. The fever should resolve within 48 h with an effective antibiotic and failure should be managed as described for lower urinary tract infection. In particular a careful check must be made to exclude obstruction or the development of an abscess, for which surgery may be required.

### 'Chronic pyelonephritis'

This is a common cause of end-stage renal failure (Table 10.4), yet the exact aetiology is unknown. It is probably a form of interstitial nephritis associated with chronic or recurrent renal infection, resulting in loss of renal function. Renal damage occurs by scarring associated with vesico-ureteric reflux. Back pressure secondary to reflux may cause the scars and these can be secondarily infected. These scars and recurrent urinary infections may remain asymptomatic, with the patient presenting with features suggestive of chronic renal failure. Diagnosis is radiological, with the coincident presence of cortical scars in the same position as a dilated calyx.

Treatment is aimed at preventing infections in children identified with renal scars and reflux. The latter condition tends to clear spontaneously usually at about 4 years of age, and the role of surgical correction remains unknown. In adults with such scars, symptomatic infection or obstruction should be promptly treated. However, unless there is significant renal impairment at the time of diagnosis, progression to renal failure in adults is uncommon.

Other conditions presenting with loin pain include obstruction (especially due to renal calculi), analgesic nephropathy and loin pain–haematuria syndrome. Phenacetin, the commonest cause of analgesic nephropathy, is no longer available in the UK; however, other non-steroidal anti-inflammatory agents have been implicated. Presentation is often nonspecific, ranging from hypertension to urinary infection or papillary necrosis. Diagnosis is radiological. Both kidneys may be affected by scarring, with no focal areas of hypertrophy (often seen in cases of reflux nephropathy) and features of papillary necrosis may be evident.

## RENAL TUBULAR DISORDERS

### Renal tubular acidosis

Renal tubular acidosis (RTA) may occur in several forms of which two are relatively well defined:

(1) *Proximal (type II)*. The proximal tubule is the main site of reabsorption of filtered bicarbonate. In proximal tubular acidosis this mechanism is disrupted, thus there is a net loss of filtered bicarbonate resulting in a failure to acidify the urine. However, in cases where there is systemic acidosis, such that filtered bicarbonate is reduced, the urine may then be acidified.

Proximal renal tubular acidosis usually occurs as part of Fanconi's syndrome (see below) and the differential features from distal RTA are summarized in Table 10.8. Treatment is with bicarbonate replacement—large doses of sodium bicarbonate with $K^+$ supplements. The bicarbonate requirement may be significantly reduced by concomitant administration of thiazide diuretics, although this also results in an increased requirement for $K^+$.

(2) *Distal (type I)*. In contrast there is little bicarbonate loss in the urine in distal tubular acidosis, and there is no fall in the urine pH with acidosis. The mechanism of this form of acidosis is unclear and both back-diffusion and failure of $H^+$ secretion in the distal tubule may be important. There are numerous causes of distal renal tubular acidosis (Table 10.8). Nephrocalcinosis commonly occurs, and patients also have rickets or osteomalacia, which responds to correction of the acidosis. Renal function is well preserved but secondary damage by renal calculi and nephrocalcinosis may result in renal impairment. The acidosis may be corrected with relatively low-dose sodium bicarbonate, often equivalent to the total endogenous acid production at 1 mmol/kg/day. Potassium supplements are also required.

### Proximal tubular disorders

Defects of proximal renal tubular function affect many of the functions of the proximal tubule as summarized in Fanconi's syndrome—proximal tubular acidosis, hyperphosphaturia, glycosuria and generalized aminoaciduria. The commonest causes are outlined in Table 10.9. Specific amino-

**Table 10.8 Renal tubular acidosis**

|  | Type I (distal) | Type II (proximal) |
| --- | --- | --- |
| Site of defect | Distal tubule | Proximal tubule |
| Renal calculi | ++ | Rare |
| Minimum urine pH | >6.0 | <5.4 |
| Bicarbonate requirement | Low | High |
| Nephrocalcinosis and bone disease | Common | Rare |
| Prognosis | Related to degree of nephrocalcinosis | Invariably good |
| Secondary associations | Hyperparathyroidism | Fanconi's syndrome |
|  | Hyperthyroidism | Cystinosis |
|  | Amphotericin toxicity | Malnutrition |
|  | Vitamin D toxicity |  |
|  | Malnutrition |  |
|  | Hypergammaglobulinaemia |  |

acidurias occur with selective transport defects, e.g., Hartnup disease (with a selective loss of neutral amino acids) or cystinuria (with loss of cystine, lysine and arginine, and the formation of renal stones).

Defects of phosphate excretion, such as X-linked hypophosphataemic rickets, pseudohypoparathyroidism and vitamin D-dependent rickets, are discussed elsewhere.

## Distal tubular disorders

In addition to distal tubular acidosis, distal tubular abnormalities may result in a failure of renal

**Table 10.9 Causes of Fanconi's syndrome**

*Inherited*
Primary
Secondary:
  cystinosis
  Wilson's disease
  tyrosinosis
  galactosaemia

*Acquired*
Toxins:
  lead
  zinc
  mercury
  expired tetracyclines
Deficiency states:
  vitamin D
Primary hyperparathyroidism
Renal disease:
  acute tubular necrosis
  hypokalaemia
  multiple myeloma
  transplant rejection
Malignant disease

concentrating mechanisms. Numerous diseases may affect renal papillae and medullary function more severely than GFR, e.g., medullary cystic disease, polycystic disease and myeloma.

Hypercalcaemia of any cause is often associated with polyuria, which resolves rapidly on correcting the hypercalcaemia. Hypokalaemia can produce defects in the medullary concentrating mechanism, as can sickle cell disease, presumably by sickling induced by the hyperosmolarity of the renal medulla. Nephrogenic diabetes insipidus—a failure of the collecting ducts to respond to the effect of ADH—may occur in an inherited form, often detected in infancy as failure to thrive accompanied by polyuria, polydipsia and hypernatraemia that is high enough to precipitate convulsions. Treatment is with diluted feeds and thiazide diuretics, which may paradoxically reduce urine volume. Acquired nephrogenic diabetes insipidus is frequently drug related. Lithium and demeclocycline make the collecting duct resistant to antidiuretic hormone, whereas colchicine, vinblastine, dextropropoxyphene and amphotericin may damage tubular cells so that they fail to respond to the hormone.

## RENAL DYSFUNCTION IN SYSTEMIC DISEASE

The kidney is affected in a number of systemic diseases which are not dealt with in this chapter but are described elsewhere, including diabetes mellitus (p. 230), multiple myeloma (p. 151), systemic lupus erythematosus (p. 218), systemic sclerosis (p. 198) and polyarteritis nodosa (p. 200).

## Further reading

Adamson J. W. et al. (1990). Treatment of the anaemia of chronic renal disease with recombinant human erythropoietin. *Annu. Rev. Med.*, **41**, 349–60.

Asscher A. W. (1980). *The Challenge of Urinary Tract Infections*. London: Academic Press.

Brenner B. M., Rector F. C., eds. (1986). *The Kidney*, 3rd ed. Philadelphia: W.B. Saunders.

de Wardner H. (1985). *The Kidney – An Outline of Normal and Abnormal Function*. Edinburgh: Churchill Livingstone.

Herbert L. A. *et al.* (1990). On the natural tendency to progressive loss of remaining kidney function in patients with impaired renal function. *Med. Clin. of North America*, **74**, 1011–24.

Klahr S., Schreiner G., Ichikawa I. (1988). The progression of renal disease. *N. Engl. J. Med.*, **318**, 1657–69.

Klahr S. (1990). Potential factors responsible for the progression of renal failure. An overview. *Contrib. Nephrol.*, **77**, 77–85.

Marsh F. P. (1985). *Postgraduate Nephrology*. London: Heinemann.

Meyers B. D., Moran S. M. (1986). Haemodynamically mediated acute renal failure. *N. Engl. J. Med.*, **314**, 97–105.

Oliver D. O., Wing A. J. (1987). Chronic renal failure, dialysis and transplantation. In *Oxford Textbook of Medicine*, 2nd edn (Weatherall D. J., Ledingham J. G. G., Warrell D. A., eds.) Oxford: Oxford University Press, pp. 18.134–18.156.

Opsahl J. A. *et al.* (1990). Angiotensin-converting enzyme inhibitors in chronic renal failure. *Drugs 39 suppl* **2**, 23–32.

Pusey C. D., Lockwood C. M. (1984). Plasma exchange for glomerular disease. In *Nephrology* (Robinson R., ed) New York: Springer-Verlag, pp. 1474–85.

Pusey C. D., Saltissi S., Bloodworth L., Rainford D. J., Christie J. (1983). Drug associated acute interstitial nephritis: clinical and pathological features, and the response to high dose steroid therapy. *Quarterly J. Med.*, **52**, 194–211.

Winearls C. G., Oliver D. O., Pippard M. J., Reid C., Downing M. R., Cotes P. M. (1986). Effect of human erythropoietin derived from recombinant DNA on the anaemia of patients maintained by chronic haemodialysis. *Lancet* **ii**, 1175–8.

## ACKNOWLEDGEMENT

The authors are grateful to Dr D. Oliviera for critical reading of the manuscript.

# 11

# GASTROENTEROLOGY

Humphrey Hodgson

Gastroenterological problems are extremely common. Data from the Hospital Inpatient Enquiry show that about 10 per cent of a district hospital's beds is occupied at any one time by patients with gastrointestinal or liver diseases. Yet for each patient admitted to hospital with such complaints, many more are assessed, diagnosed and treated as outpatients. The disease processes encompass the entire range of pathology—neoplastic, infectious, inflammatory, immunological, biochemical and congenital conditions, and disorders of unknown cause. In about one third of outpatients presenting with gastrointestinal symptoms, it is thought that no structural, infective or biochemical disorder is present; such patients are labelled as having 'functional disorders', and in these psychological or social factors may be primarily responsible.

## APPROACH TO THE PATIENT

In the assessment of gastroenterological disorders, there are a number of cardinal symptoms that may immediately focus the attention of the clinician upon one particular intra-abdominal organ, and dictate the most effective and economical means of investigation. This is usually successful, but too blinkered an approach will eventually catch the clinician out: disease processes outside the abdomen may present with abdominal symptoms—for example, pain from a congested liver may be a presenting feature of cardiac disease, and brain tumours with raised intracranial pressure may cause vomiting. Previous chapters have emphasized the importance of considering the patient as a whole.

The approach to the patient with gastrointestinal disease will nonetheless be considered here in terms of these primary complaints, followed by the physical examination and special investigations appropriate for each symptom complex. The last portion of the chapter deals with the investigation of liver disease.

## PRESENTING COMPLAINTS

### Difficulty in swallowing

Difficulty in swallowing (dysphagia) covers a number of sensations that the patient may describe. These include:
(1) *Difficulty in starting the swallow*—this results usually from neurological or muscular diseases, such as bulbar and pseudobulbar palsy, motor neurone disease and myasthenia gravis. Associated symptoms include drooling due to difficulty in swallowing saliva, or spillage of saliva into the bronchi and resultant aspiration pneumonia.
(2) *Food sticking after swallowing has started.* This suggests the presence of a structural lesion in the oesophagus. Many patients turn out to be able to localize accurately where the food is sticking by pointing at the appropriate level on the sternum, but others localize sticking either to the upper or lower end of the oesophagus, irrespective of the site of narrowing. The nature of material that elicits the symptom should be clarified. Progressive dysphagia, first for solids and then for sloppy and liquid foods, is a sinister sign strongly suggestive of cancer of the oesophagus, although it can also occur with peptic strictures from recurrent oesophagitis due to acid reflux. Such patients will often have a long history of heartburn (see below). Non-progressive dysphagia may represent a benign structural lesion, such as mucosal web in the upper

oesophagus or a benign 'ring' in the lower oesophagus. Food sticking intermittently, both solids and liquids, suggests disordered motility of the oesophagus, commonly either achalasia or oesophageal spasm. Oesophageal spasm is a painful condition, with incoordinated contractions resulting in pain and dysphagia. In achalasia the normal relaxation of the lower oesophageal sphincter after swallowing does not occur, so that the oesophagus may dilate to form a food–fluid-filled bag, until the pressure of gravity—often some hours after a meal—opens the sphincter and lets the oesophagus empty.

With any cause of oesophageal obstruction, regurgitation of food and liquid into the mouth may occur. The fluid is usually bland rather than bitter as it does not contain gastric acid. Nocturnal regurgitation may be associated with choking, aspiration and repeated episodes of pneumonia.

(3) 'A lump in the throat' (globus hystericus). Some patients, particularly highly anxious individuals at times of stress, complain of a sensation of a lump in the throat, without having eaten or drunk, unrelieved by initiation of swallowing, or associated with a temporary inability to swallow. This is a temporary functional disorder associated with anxiety.

### Loss of appetite

This is a highly nonspecific symptom. When it is associated with other features of anxiety or depression, it may be functional, but in particular when associated with weight loss it suggests significant organic disease. A maintained appetite in the context of other abdominal symptoms is a reassuring sign that suggests serious disease is less likely to be found.

### Nausea and vomiting

Nausea with vomiting is a nonspecific symptom. In young men, morning nausea, particularly if associated with retching without production of vomitus, is strongly suggestive of alcoholism. In young women, morning nausea suggests pregnancy. Nausea may also be a concomitant of abdominal pains, particularly those that reflect spasm of smooth muscle in a hollow organ—for example,

the biliary tract when it is obstructed or the colon in functional bowel disease.

Vomiting is a much more significant disturbance, involving reverse peristalsis of the stomach and expulsion of the gastric contents. It is rare as a purely functional disorder, although in a few patients the diagnosis of 'hysterical vomiting' is finally made. Severe family stress usully underlies this condition. More often, vomiting reflects organic disease affecting the stomach, duodenum or small intestine. When short-lived and associated with fever or diarrhoea, food poisoning due to bacteria or their toxins or viral gastroenteritis are usually the cause. When present over more than a few days, vomiting needs further investigation. It may be associated with severe pain as discussed in the next section. In the absence of pain apart from that involved in the process of vomiting, persistent vomiting suggests obstruction to the outflow tract of the stomach, as seen with antral carcinoma or narrowing due to longstanding duodenal ulceration.

The nature of the vomitus may be significant. Vomitus in which food ingested many hours before can be recognized suggests obstruction of the gastric outlet as the stomach usually empties within four to six hours of eating. Vomiting of blood is discussed below. Vomiting should be distinguished from regurgitation, when food returns to the mouth from the oesophagus without reverse peristalsis. Another well described but not particularly common symptom, distinct from either vomiting or regurgitation, is the sensation of waterbrash, in which the mouth fills with salty water—excess saliva—a phenomenon sometimes found as a symptom of peptic ulceration.

Both nausea and vomiting can reflect events elsewhere in the body, including raised intracranial pressure, severe metabolic complications, such as renal failure or diabetic ketoacidosis, or side-effects of drugs. Prolonged and persistent vomiting, as seen with obstruction of the gastric outlet, can induce metabolic changes, classically a hypokalaemic alkalosis, and secondary potassium loss from the kidney—and these should be sought.

### Pain

Abdominal pain is the most common reason for referral to a gastroenterologist. Classical symptom complexes implicating one particular organ can often be recognized, but some pains are poorly localized and characterized. The site and radiation of the pain should be defined, and its duration (minutes or hours), its character (sharp, dull, intermittent), its periodicity (how many days a week?; every day for some weeks and then not at all for some months?), its timing and relationship to eating, defecation and sleep. Relieving and precipitating factors should be elucidated. Associated symptoms, such as nausea, vomiting, and weight loss, should be established. The major patterns of pain are as follows:

(1) *Heartburn* (pyrosis). This term should be reserved for the sensations that may occur when gastric acid refluxes into oesophagus. Patients may use the term to describe other abdominal sensations, so the precise meaning should be elucidated. Heartburn is a raw, burning sensation, felt retrosternally, lasting for some minutes. It may start in the epigastrium and travel up to the back of the throat. It is commonly precipitated by large meals, alcohol, stooping and lying flat in bed at night; it is rapidly relieved by drinking milk. Most people experience it at some time as a minor inconvenience, but persistent or severe heartburn suggests repeated reflux of acid into the oesophagus and resultant oesophagitis. When this is severe, dysphagia may result. Reflux is often but not invariably associated with hiatus hernia, although the latter is extremely common and often asymptomatic. A long history of heartburn may eventually be complicated by dysphagia for solids as stricture formation occurs.

(2) *Dyspepsia.* Epigastric pain altered by food is the classical symptom of peptic ulceration. It was once believed that ulcers in different sites could be clinically differentiated by their history, but the ability now to distinguish accurately by investigation (e.g., endoscopy) between duodenal and gastric ulceration, duodenitis and gastritis, has shown that the symptoms of these all overlap. Frequently a history of epigastric discomfort related to food is associated with negative findings on further investigation, particularly in anxious individuals. The classical history of duodenal ulcer is of epigastric pain, relieved by food, brought on by hunger. The pain may remain epigastric or radiate through to the back, particularly if the ulcer is situated posteriorly in the duodenum. Antacids relieve the symptoms, usually within minutes. The pain often awakens the patient in the early hours of the morning.

Symptoms may come in bouts, troubling the patients daily for several weeks and then remitting for months or years. Associated nausea and sometimes vomiting occur, particularly with gastric ulcers and those in the prepyloric area. Ulcers in the stomach and gastritis are classically, but not exclusively, associated with exacerbation on eating. In establishing a diagnosis of a duodenal ulcer, a family history provides strong collateral evidence.

(3) *Gall bladder and biliary pain.* Pain from the biliary tract may reflect either spasm of smooth muscle or acute inflammation. The first is due to obstruction of the common bile duct or the neck of the gall bladder, usually by a gallstone. The full-blown syndrome of biliary colic is unmistakable. There is severe pain in the right upper quadrant, radiating laterally to the back. Like other colicky pains it comes in waves, but usually superimposed upon a chronic, severe discomfort. The pain may last several hours; nausea and severe vomiting, presumably as a reflex, are common. Patients classically roam around and shift about to find a comfortable position. The pain from an inflamed gallbladder is in a similar site, with a greater tendency to radiate to the shoulder. Much more difficult to analyse are the minor degrees of discomfort attributed to the contraction, after eating, of a diseased gall bladder containing stones. Mild pain in the right upper quadrant or epigastric pain, excessive belching, or merely nausea and abdominal discomfort are all attributed to gallstones, usually when these symptoms occur half an hour to two hours after meals, particularly if the meal is fatty. The problem is that gallstones are extremely common even in the absence of symptoms (15–30 per cent of the adult population) and minor 'flatulent dyspepsia' is a thin basis on which to advocate cholecystectomy.

(4) *Pancreatic pain.* Chronic inflammation of the pancreas—most commonly a consequence of alcoholism—can present with severe pain in the back just below the shoulder blades, brought about by eating or alcohol, and which may be mildly relieved by leaning forward. Whilst this pattern is readily recognizable, such a history is also compatible with duodenal ulceration; furthermore, much chronic pancreatitic pain is extremely ill-defined. The

symptoms attributed to chronic pancreatitis are highly variable, and poorly-defined dyspepsia affecting the epigastrium or right or left side of the upper abdomen, with an indefinite relationship to food, may also reflect this condition. Under these conditions the clinician may forget to consider the possibility of pancreatic pain. Cancer of the pancreas may be painless, but extension of the tumour outside the normal confines of the gland can initiate the typical, unremitting central back pain.

(5) *Intestinal pain.* The normal peristaltic movements of the intestine are usually painless, although patients may be aware of gurglings and movements within the abdomen. Short-lived, acute episodes of painful peristalsis—intestinal colic—are part of everyone's experience, usually due to acute gastroenteritis. However, the development of repeated or persistent episodes of painful peristalsis usually indicates some degree of intestinal narrowing or obstruction, most commonly due to adhesions from previous surgery or tumours. The symptom complex includes intermittent sharp exacerbations of pain, doubling the patient up if severe, and associated gurglings and churnings and sometimes distension of the abdomen. Colic of the small intestine is characteristically poorly localized, but predominantly central and above the umbilicus, whereas colonic colic is in the abdomen and the hypogastrium.

Inflammation of the intestine can also be painful, and transmural inflammation with secondary inflammation of the parietal peritoneum, such as occurs in appendicitis, leads to well-localized, constant pain over the inflamed peritoneum, worse on movement or prodding. Diffuse chronic inflammation, such as in Crohn's disease, is usually not painful in the small intestine unless it is associated with narrowing and thus colic. Diffuse chronic inflammation of the colon, however, such as in ulcerative colitis or colonic Crohn's disease, even in the absence of any obstruction, is often associated with cramping pains in the lower abdomen and a desire to defecate, relieved when the bowels are opened.

(6) *Severe acute abdominal pain.* There are a number of rarer causes of abdominal pain that should be considered in addition to the classical surgical emergencies. The pain of coronary artery insufficiency, either as angina or when myocardial infarction has occurred, can predominantly be felt epigastrically. Aortic disease, due either to dissection or dilatation of an aneurysm, may present with either back or epigastric pain. Intestinal ischaemia, due to narrowing of at least two of the major arteries supplying the gut, can cause recurrent epigastric pain of a non-colicky nature, coming on between 10 minutes and half an hour after eating and lasting for up to two hours. It is a characteristic of intestinal angina due to gut ischaemia that patients lose weight and avoid eating as they do not wish to bring the pain on.

## Bleeding

Bleeding from the gut varies from the acute and life-threatening to the chronic and trivial. Most acute bleeding comes from the upper gastrointestinal tract, but may present either with haematemesis and melaena, or with just melaena. The source of upper gastrointestinal haemorrhage may be the oesophagus, stomach or duodenum, but only very rarely the biliary tract, pancreas or upper jejunum.

Oesophageal bleeding may reflect oesophageal varices associated with portal hypertension, or oesophageal ulceration due to either oesophagitis or more rarely tumour. Oesophageal bleeding can be of bright-red blood if immediately vomited, or of altered blood if the blood has first trickled into the stomach before vomiting. Relatively slow oesophageal bleeding can present only with melaena.

The other common sources of upper gastrointestinal haemorrhage are duodenal and gastric ulceration and gastric erosions, the latter often associated with the ingestion of aspirin or alcohol. The possibility of a Mallory–Weiss tear, a mucosal slit at the oesophago-gastric junction brought on by vomiting, should be recognizable from the classic history of retching or vomiting without associated haemorrhage, followed by a gastrointestinal bleed. This again is usually associated with alcoholic binges. Apart from this story and the importance of drug ingestion, the historical features of whether or not pain is present at the time of haemorrhage, whether or not previous dyspepsia has occurred, etc., are often misleading in assessing the probable cause of haemorrhage, and further investigation is required.

Whilst upper gastrointestinal haemorrhage is

often a medical emergency, haemorrhage from the lower gastrointestinal tract is rarely so. Bleeding from haemorrhoids is the commonest, usually causing bright-red bleeding, often with blood only seen on the toilet paper after defecation. It is, however, dangerous to assume that haemorrhoids are the source of lower gastrointestinal bleeding because cancers, polyps, diverticular disease and vascular malformations can all cause rectal bleeding. Bleeding can also be a prominent symptom of inflammatory colitis, in which case it will be associated with diarrhoea. Bleeding from the distal colon—predominantly the left side of the colon—is usually fairly bright-red, but from the caecum it is plum-coloured or darker. Bleeding from polyps and caecal carcinomas can of course be occult.

## Abnormal bowel habit

There is a wide variation in normal bowel habit from the passage of two to three loose stools daily to the passage of hard motions every second or third day. Thus change in a pre-existing pattern is more likely to be of importance than any long-standing deviation from what the patient (or the doctor) regards as the hypothetical norm.

(1) *Constipation* is the term used to describe the infrequent passage of stools, which due to their long sojourn in the colon tend to become particularly dehydrated and hard. 'Trivial' causes of constipation include prolonged immobility, diminished food intake and medication with constipating agents. Much constipation associated with epigastric pain is due to the ingestion of calcium- or aluminium-containing antacids. Constipation requires further investigation when it is of recent origin, or when it is associated with colicky abdominal pain. Absolute constipation, followed by abdominal distension, are cardinal features of intestinal obstruction. Hypercalcaemia and myxoedema can present with relative constipation.

(2) *Diarrhoea.* The term diarrhoea requires careful definition, as it may be used to describe a variety of states from a moderate frequency of formed but scanty stools to massive volumes of liquid stool. Many patients with the 'diarrhoeic' form of the irritable bowel syndrome (see below) have two to three loose motions in the morning, usually after food, but the total mass of stool remains normal. Diarrhoea that

wakes a patient at night is usually a significant factor, and the passage of blood and mucus are obviously abnormal. The passage of colonic mucus alone, however, need not indicate pathology. Although much has been made of the descriptions of pale, floating, or foul-smelling stools as indicators of steatorrhoea, this is often unreliable. The observation of oil floating rainbow-like on the surface of the stools or lavatory-pan water is, however, significant; it usually implies severe steatorrhoea of the degree only commonly associated with pancreatic insufficiency or extensive resection of the small gut. The symptom of tenesmus—incomplete evacuation of the bowel—is a useful pointer, which should be inquired about, as it suggests rectal involvement due to colitis or rarely a rectal mass. Inflammatory colitis, or ischaemic change in the colon, is often associated with crampy colonic colic, but disease of the small intestine can also cause colonic colic as excess fluid enters the colon. Under normal conditions less than 1.25 l of intestinal fluid leaves the small gut to enter the colon, which usually reduces the volume to less than 300 g. Liquid stool volumes of over 1.5 g/day or more are therefore strongly suggestive of disease of the small gut.

## Weight loss

In combination with other gastrointestinal symptoms, weight loss is obviously an important feature, but again anxiety, and other systemic conditions, such as thyrotoxicosis, tuberculosis and diabetes, should be considered.

## Other gastrointestinal symptoms

There is a variety of other less well-defined gastrointestinal complaints. These include abdominal distension, particularly after meals, which may often affect the upper rather than the lower part of the abdomen. This is one classical manifestation of functional bowel disease, and has recently been attributed to delay in emptying of the small intestine into the caecum. Other manifestations of the irritable bowel syndrome include alternating constipation and diarrhoea, colicky colon pain, and intermittent discomfort in the right upper quadrant, left upper quadrant, or left lower quadrant of the abdomen. The presence of longstanding symptoms and otherwise good health, an onset dating back many years, or alternatively a history of an acute attack of gastroenteritis following which things never returned to normal, are suggestive clinical features in the diagnosis of the irritable bowel syndrome.

## PHYSICAL EXAMINATION

The historical features outlined above will have suggested a short differential diagnosis, and in many patients with gastrointestinal disease no abnormal physical findings will be demonstrable. Nonetheless, a physical examination, which should not be confined only to the abdomen, should be made. Aspects of the general physical examination that may provide useful clues to gastroenterological and hepatic conditions are shown in Table 11.1.

### Abdominal examination

The general principles of physical examination are covered elsewhere but the following features have particular relevance to the gastroenterologist.

### Liver

An enlarged, tender liver may be inflamed, congested or the site of an abscess or tumour. The patency of the hepatic venous drainage can be checked by showing elevation of the jugular venous pressure on pressing over the liver. Although a crude physical sign, there is a good correlation between the finding of a fibrous, hard liver and cirrhosis. Rapid changes in liver size may indicate mobilization of fat, and in alcoholic patients the liver may diminish in size rapidly on abstention from alcohol. A hepatic bruit may be heard in alcoholic hepatitis or in patients with tumours.

### Spleen

Palpating the spleen can be difficult: rotating the patient on to the right side, a helping examiner's hand in the left flank, and deep inspiration may all help the examining fingers.

### Ascites

Whilst gross ascites is easy to detect, one may be misled into diagnosing ascites in gross obesity as

**Table 11.1 Physical signs of gastrointestinal disease**

| | |
|---|---|
| *Hands* | |
| Liver palms | Acute or chronic liver disease |
| Clubbing | Cirrhosis, Crohn's disease |
| Leuconychia | Liver disease, protein-losing enteropathy |
| Dupuytren's contracture | Alcoholism |
| *Skin* | |
| Spider naevi | Cirrhosis or hepatitis |
| White spots | Chronic liver disease |
| Pigmentation | Haemochromatosis, internal malignancy, malabsorption |
| Blisters, depigmentation | Porphyria cutanea tarda |
| *Eyes* | |
| Coloration | Jaundice |
| Episcleritis/iritis | Inflammatory bowel disease |
| Retinal appearances | Pseudoxanthoma elasticum |
| *Venous pressure* | Hepatic pain in congestive cardiac failure— cardiological causes of ascites or protein-losing enteropathy |
| *Lymphadenopathy* | Carcinoma of the stomach and other malignancies |
| *Cyanosis* | Severe liver disease |
| *Anaemia* | Acute and chronic gastrointestinal blood loss |
| *Cardiac disease and peripheral pulses* | Intestinal angina, ischaemic gut disease, mesenteric emboli |
| *Gynaecomastia* | Chronic liver disease |
| *Peripheral neuropathy* | Alcoholism, amyloidosis, porphyria |
| *Encephalopathy* | Liver disease |

fat is liquid at room temperature. Minor degrees of ascites can be difficult to detect.

### Abdominal bruits

Bruits in the epigastrium are not necessarily pathological as the superior mesenteric artery may often be stretched over the pancreas. Nonetheless, they should lead to consideration of a diagnosis of intestinal ischaemia or a pancreatic tumour.

### Hernial orifices, scars

These are relevant in the context of colicky abdominal pain.

## INVESTIGATIONS

The particular gastroenterological relevance of the routine blood tests is as follows.

### Haemoglobin

A low haemoglobin is strongly suggestive of acute or chronic gastrointestinal bleeding; in the latter an iron deficiency pattern should be recognizable. However, patients with Crohn's disease or other inflammatory conditions may have a normochromic normocytic anaemia, and malabsorption may result in microcytic, normocytic or macrocytic anaemia, depending on the precise deficiencies present. Any anaemia should be pursued by investigation of the serum iron and total iron-binding capacity, red cell and serum folate, and vitamin $B_{12}$ level. The vitamin $B_{12}$ level in serum is a useful 'function test' in gastroenterology. Normal gastric function is required for production of intrinsic factor, and normal function of the terminal ileum for absorption of vitamin $B_{12}$. In some patients with pancreatic insufficiency, vitamin $B_{12}$ deficiency may occur because pancreatic enzymes are required to digest nonspecific vitamin $B_{12}$-binding factors produced by the stomach.

### Urea and electrolytes

Watery diarrhoea may be associated with a hypokalaemic alkalosis, and profoundly low potassium levels may occur with endocrine tumour-associated secretory diarrhoea, with the ingestion of laxatives, and with the presence of a villous adenoma in the colon weeping a potassium-rich fluid. A marked elevation in blood urea in comparison with creatinine may indicate prerenal problems, as seen in dehydration, or reflect breakdown of blood in the gut after gastrointestinal bleeding.

### Biochemical profile

The liver function tests are discussed later. A low serum albumin suggests severe liver disease or a protein-losing enteropathy associated with diffuse mucosal inflammation. This will be linked with a low serum calcium, but the correlation between the two should be checked. Hypocalcaemia may occur in malabsorption, and hypercalcaemia suggests primary hyperparathyroidism, often a feature of multiple endocrine adenomatosis and relevant to syndromes such as the Zollinger–Ellison and the watery diarrhoea and hyperkalaemia syndrome.

### Acute phase reactants

C-reactive protein and serum orosomucoid (now often measured as $\alpha_1$ acid glycoprotein) are markers of acute inflammation, often used to monitor acute inflammation in the gut. They may be abnormal when the ESR is normal.

## SPECIAL INVESTIGATIONS

Special investigations in the gastrointestinal tract normally involve two phases—the demonstration of structure of the organ, followed if need be by some function testing. This section briefly outlines the investigations appropriate to each organ when one of the cardinal symptoms referred to above appears to be responsible for the patient's condition.

### Oesophagus

#### Barium swallow

In non-urgent cases, the barium swallow is the appropriate first investigation for oesophageal disease. It is to be preferred to endoscopy, as on occasions unsuspected diverticula or strictures may render endoscopy hazardous. A barium swallow is a dynamic investigation, and the radiologist who performs it gains more information than the physician who reviews the film afterwards. It will provide evidence of major anatomical abnormalities—strictures, tumours, diverticula—and of extrinsic compressive lesions, such as lymph nodes, the left atrium in the presence of cardiac disease or an unfolded aorta. Even in the absence of hiatus hernia, the presence of gastrointestinal reflux should be sought by the radiologist, placing the patient in the head-down position. Diffuse mucosal irregularity may suggest inflammation, and if particularly severe and extensive, be a clue to the diagnosis of oesophageal candidiasis. Oesophageal varices may be prominent, but if small can be missed by the radiologist: if a 'reverse Valsalva manoeuvre'—inspiration against a closed glottis—is performed, previously trivial oesophageal varices may be more easily seen. The radiologist has the opportunity to observe whether or not peristalsis is normally present, its absence being an early sign of diffuse diseases such as scleroderma. Marked abnormalities of oesophageal motility, such as the 'corkscrew' oesophagus of diffuse oesophageal spasm, may also be seen. Barium swallow is in particular better than endoscopy for illustrating events at the upper end of the oesophagus, such as incoordinated contraction of the cricopharyngeal muscle.

### Endoscopy

Endoscopic investigation of the oesophagus is most productive in demonstrating structural lesions, such as tumours and peptic strictures, and the presence or absence of oesophagitis. The procedure will demonstrate whether or not there is a hiatus hernia. When there is only mild oesophagitis present endoscopically (reddening of the mucosa), there is a poor correlation with the findings of histological studies that look for inflammation in the squamous lining of the lower oesophagus. In the presence of severe ulceration, and in particular when an underlying neoplasm is suspected, endoscopic biopsies may be disappointing as the relatively small samples may only show superficial exudate and necrotic tissue. The addition of cytological sampling, and a repeat biopsy, may be necessary.

### Motility studies

Motility studies are mainly used for the investigation of non-progressive, intermittent dysphagia and intermittent oesophageal pain, and to confirm the diagnosis of achalasia when the appearances of the oesophagus on the barium swallow have not yet progressed to the classical ones of a dilated oesophagus tapering down to a narrowed, hyperactive sphincter. Such studies involve pressure recording from three open perfused catheters situated at intervals down the oesophagus, so that the presence or absence, progression and amplitude of peristaltic waves, and the modulation of sphincter pressures, can be analysed.

### Oesophageal pH monitoring test and Bernstein test

Rarely, the gastroenterologist will feel the need to monitor the oesophageal pH or alternatively make a Bernstein test. Ambulatory monitoring of oesophageal pH, involving an indwelling naso-oesophageal pH meter probe attached to a 24-h recording tape, may be useful in elucidating the cause of chest pain, but is of more value as a research tool for investigating the effect of drugs in reducing the incidence of episodes of reflux oesophagitis. The Bernstein test, trickling normal saline or dilute hydrochloric acid over the lower oesophagus, is a means of correlating obscure chest pain with the presence of acid in the oesophagus.

### Stomach and duodenum

Over the past 10 years the barium meal has been replaced by upper gastrointestinal endoscopy as the investigation of choice for the anatomy of the stomach and duodenum. However, the barium meal maintains some advantages. It is less unpleasant for the patient, less demanding on the physician's time (though more on the radiologist's!) and may remain a suitable technique for the very frail and for patients with severe rheumatoid disease affecting the neck, in whom endoscopy should be avoided if possible. The recent introduction of double-contrast barium meals, using both air and barium, goes some way in skilled hands to correcting one of the major deficiencies of barium radiography—the inability to visualize clearly mucosal lesions. Apart from the advantages outlined above, however, the only major advantage of a barium meal over endoscopy is that it may be superior in demonstrating whether the stomach is mobile or not; an immobile stomach may suggest the presence of an infiltrating, linitus plastica form of cancer.

Most patients who require investigation of the upper intestine will be submitted to endoscopy. Radiologically invisible lesions, such as duodenitis, gastritis and Mallory–Weiss tears, will become apparent. The parts immediately below the gastro-oesophageal junction and the first part of the duodenum just over the lip of the pylorus are relatively blind areas in which inexperienced endoscopists may miss lesions. As in the oesophagus, biopsies of ulcerated areas may be disappointing, and in some series the endoscopic appearances of gastric ulcers have given a far better indication of the presence or absence of malignancy than changes found in the biopsy.

Antral *Helicobacter pylori* infection, associated with duodenal ulcer, can be diagnosed on histology, or by detecting its urease enzyme chemically. The value of gastric function tests now appears limited. The demonstration of a grossly elevated basal as well as pentagastrin-stimulated acid output may be of value in assessing patients who may have gastrin-producing tumours—the Zollinger–Ellison syndrome. The completeness of a previously performed surgical vagotomy can be checked by assessing basal acid output or by an insulin test. The serum gastrin is typically elevated in patients with Zollinger–Ellison syndrome, but it is also raised in achlorhydria and thus some of the highest levels are seen amongst patients with pernicious anaemia. Elevations of serum gastrin also occur in patients taking H$_2$-antagonists, and after gastric surgery or vagotomy, and these may lead to diagnostic confusion.

### Gall bladder and biliary tree

In investigating the gall bladder, unless there is a serious mass lesion present (such as a carcinoma, empyema or mucocele), the main object is to demonstrate gallstones. These are only radio-paque in about 10 per cent of cases, and thus plain abdominal radiographs are of limited value, although they may show evidence suggestive of disease if air is visible within the biliary tract. The most easily made screening test for gallstones is at present ultrasonography of the gall bladder, per-formed during fasting, in which gallstones and their position in the biliary tree or common bile duct should be clear from their echodensity and the acoustic shadow they cast behind them. Very small stones and 'biliary sludge' may be missed. Ultrasonography is of major value in defining the size, and the presence or absence of dilatation, of the common bile duct and intrahepatic bile ducts.

Oral cholecystography has become less fashion-able for identifying gallstones, although its sensiti-vity is probably the same as that of ultrasound. However, it requires a control film and the ad-ministration of an oral dye, and if the gall bladder is diseased no image may be obtained. Very small cholesterol gallstones may only be visualized on the erect film of the gall bladder, where they may form a straight line of floating stones held in the density gradient that the radiopaque dye has created within the gall bladder. A cholecystogram also allows more accurate measurement of the size of the stones, together with an assessment of whether the gall bladder still contracts or not, and this information is important if medical dissolution of the stones with oral bile acid is being con-sidered. Intravenous cholangiography as a means of imaging the gall bladder and common bile

duct when single-dose and double-dose oral cholecystography have failed has now largely gone out of fashion. The risk of anaphylactic reactions to this contrast medium is greater than with other radiological media, and the films are often not of good quality. Further investigation of the biliary tree is discussed later in the context of the jaundiced patient.

### Other intra-abdominal organs

Plain abdominal X-ray of the pancreas is fre-quently a rewarding investigation. Diffuse pan-creatic calcification makes the diagnosis of chronic pancreatitis, although the aetiology will require further study. Ultrasonography is of value in good hands for investigating pancreatic disease, although the retroperitoneal position of the organ, and the confounding issues of overlying fat, gas, and bowel, may make interpretation difficult. Ultrasound, however, may be useful for finding mass lesions such as carcinomas, and for identify-ing complications of acute and chronic pancreati-tis, such as pseudocysts and abscesses. It is particu-larly important to be aware of the presence of a pseudocyst, as this is taken as a contraindication to subsequent endoscopic pancreatography because of the risk of causing infection. Ultrasonography may also show dilated intrapancreatic ducts and intrapancreatic stones in chronic pancreatitis. In the majority of cases of non-calcific chronic pan-creatitis, however, an ultrasound scan will be inadequate to define the presence of pancreatic abnormality and further investigations will be required.

CT scanning has a similar scope to that of ultrasound for the pancreas, being useful if defi-nite lesions such as cancers or cysts are identified, but liable to miss minor or moderate disease. If the loops of the upper gut are poorly opacified by oral contrast, highly misleading information can be gained from the CT scan.

In recent years, as the technique has become more widely available, physicians have tended to proceed earlier to endoscopic pancreatography, injecting dye through the ampulla of Vater in order to show a dilated or strictured main pancrea-tic duct, with a paucity of side branches, which may be ectatic. Intrapancreatic stones may also be seen. As with much of pancreatic disease, this is a very helpful test for a definite chronic pancreatitis but there is a large 'grey area' of 'minimal change' pancreatitis in which only minor dilatation at the orifices of the side ducts or a slight paucity of the side ducts may be seen.

Tests of pancreatic function are the alternative, the purpose being to show the presence of chronic pancreatic disease. The presence of frank pancreatic insufficiency with steatorrhoea does not occur until about 90 per cent of the exocrine function of the gland has been destroyed. Similarly, pancreatic function tests of definite abnormality are relatively easy to obtain in obvious or chronic calcific pancreatitis but are often borderline in those patients who are diagnostic problems. The most widely used pancreatic function test is duodenal intubation followed by the administration of a Lundh test meal consisting, for example, of a mixture of corn oil, skimmed milk and dextrose, and then by serial collection of pancreatic juice for analysis of bicarbonate and enzyme concentrations. The classical finding in chronic pancreatitis is a normal volume of pancreatic fluid with a low concentration of enzyme and bicarbonate. (This contrasts with the classical findings in cancer of the pancreas, where a small volume of normal-quality juice is obtained.) Alternative intubation techniques involve the intravenous administration of the hormone secretin–pancreozymin to cause pancreatic secretion.

In recent years there has been a tendency to seek tubeless alternatives to tests of pancreatic function. These include the administration of para-amino benzoic acid (PABA) linked via a trypsin-sensitive bond to a carrier. In the presence of normal trypsin activity, a substantial amount of PABA is liberated in the upper intestine and can be quantified in the urine. A normal result in such a test implies, in addition, a normal hepatic and renal function, and modifications of this test have been introduced in which a small tracer amount of labelled PABA in the free form is added, so that abnormalities in liver and kidney function can be corrected for.

An alternative but similar test is the fluorescein dilaurate test, in which a diester conjugated with fluorescein is given by mouth. Pancreatic enzymes will release fluorescein, which can be quantitated in the urine.

## Investigation of diarrhoea and malabsorption

In the majority of cases, the historical features already outlined will have suggested whether diarrhoea is colonic or small intestinal in origin.

However, initial clinical examination should include sigmoidoscopy. Sigmoidoscopic examination can be performed in outpatients without preparation in the majority of cases, and inspection of the lower 15 cm of the rectal mucosa is straightforward and useful for excluding diffuse mucosal lesions, such as ulcerative colitis. Crohn's disease and ischaemic colitis may be patchy so colonic inflammation cannot, therefore, be excluded by sigmoidoscopy. The normal colonic mucosa is pale, with clearly defined blood vessels coursing in its surface. However, minor degrees of oedema, with some obliteration of this vascular pattern, are still within the normal range. Physicians differ about the interpretation of many sigmoidoscopic appearances, such as 'granularity', but the presence of spontaneous bleeding, contact bleeding, ulceration and pus are reproducible findings. In some cases of inflammatory bowel disease, histological abnormalities and granuloma may be present in a macroscopically normal mucosa, and a rectal biopsy (taken within 12 cm of the anal margin and on the posterior wall for maximum safety) is therefore recommended.

Stool culture and microscopy should not be neglected in chronic diarrhoea. Giardiasis may be diagnosed in this way, often dating back some months to travel overseas. However, for this diagnosis to be firmly excluded, inspection of duodenal juice is required. If a colitis is demonstrated, culture should include the special conditions for growing *Campylobacter* and recognizing *Clostridium difficile* (responsible for pseudomembranous colitis), in addition to the routine investigations.

An anatomical approach to diagnosis is used for patients in whom a small intestinal cause for diarrhoea is suspected on the basis of indefinite clinical signs of steatorrhoea, blood tests suggesting hematinic or other deficiency and normal sigmoidoscopic appearances. The function tests beloved of gastroenterology textbooks 20 years ago are now rarely called for. The physician should proceed to demonstrate the anatomy and histological appearances of the small intestinal mucosa. Barium studies of the small intestine should be carried out separately and not combined with barium swallow and meal. The routine small bowel follow-through is time consuming but in skilled hands gives good pictures of the intestine, with the normal feathery pattern of the jejunum giving way to a smoother, toothpaste-like appearance in the ileum. In recent years, radiologists have moved to the use of intubated small-bowel enemas, pouring dilute barium into the small intestine via a tube placed in the duodenum. This dilates the intestine a little, somewhat effaces the feathery pattern of the upper small intestine, but has advantages both in speed and in the ability to see through overlapping loops.

Whilst a malabsorption pattern on the barium examination of the small intestine is a useful feature, it does not exclude diffuse mucosal disease. Coeliac disease in particular, the most common diffuse malabsorptive condition in the West, can occur with normal appearances. Some specific patterns of malabsorption may be recognized—the regular, pallisaded appearance of lymphangiectasia, multiple jejunal diverticula, the broad-barred pattern of Whipple's disease, and local areas of inflammation from radiation injury or, most commonly, Crohn's disease in the terminal ileum.

To confirm the presence of diffuse mucosal disease histologically and to identify its specific cause, or to exclude this possibility despite a radiographically normal jejunal mucosa, a biopsy of the small intestine should be obtained. Most effectively this is done with a Crosby capsule, advancing this under fluoroscopic visualization until it lies just within the jejunum past the ligament of Treitz and obtaining a biopsy by suction. Jejunal juice should be taken at the same time and examined by microscope immediately for mobile parasites such as *Giardia*. This type of biopsy should not be performed in the presence of jejunal diverticula as these thin-walled structures can be perforated by the capsule. Such a biopsy would not be required having demonstrated the presence of jejunal diverticula as bacterial overgrowth would then be the probable cause of malabsorption; however, obviating the risk of perforating an unsuspected diverticulum is the major reason for advocating radiography before biopsy.

An alternative to jejunal biopsy by capsule is multiple duodenal biopsies at endoscopy; this avoids the risks of taking biopsies of diverticula. However, the normal appearances of the duodenum are variable, and in otherwise normal individuals, finger-like villi, characteristic of the jejunum, may not always be found. If they are found, however, a duodenal biopsy obtained at endoscopy is an effective means of excluding diffuse mucosal lesions such as coeliac disease and Whipple's disease. The presence of a structurally

normal small intestine, both radiologically and on biopsy, in the presence of malabsorption, will focus attention on the pancreas as a cause.

When using this scheme, the value of function tests of the small intestine—xylose absorption tests for carbohydrate absorption, 3- or 5-day faecal fat collections for fat absorption, and Schilling tests to assess ileal function—is fairly limited, but they retain some role.

A recently advocated test, which has yet to find its place, is the use of the SeHCat absorption. This measures the absorption of a selenium-labelled bile acid, given by mouth and followed by whole-body counting. Absorption of bile acids is a specific function of the ileum, and diminished retention of SeHCat is therefore a marker for ileal disease. As the radiological appearances of the terminal ileum are sometimes difficult to categorize as definitely normal or abnormal, this test may well prove to be of value in confirming minor abnormalities that are not clear radiologically, and thus help in the diagnosis of early Crohn's disease affecting the ileum. Other tests are, however, being introduced for the detection of minor degrees of inflammatory change in the small intestine, such as the use of labelled leucocyte scans, which in specialized centres often produce excellent results, showing localization of radioactivity over inflamed areas.

There are two other groups of functional tests that are of considerable clinical use. The first is for the diagnosis of carbohydrate malabsorption. Lactose malabsorption, due to deficiency of the disaccharidase lactase in the small intestinal enterocyte, is a relatively common cause of diarrhoea. The undigested carbohydrate enters the colon, where it is fermented by bacteria; this produces gas and osmotically active small molecules, resulting in diarrhoea. Lactase deficiency can explain the onset of diarrhoea when patients put themselves on a bland, milk-based diet. In the Northern European caucasian peoples, lactase is maintained in the majority of adults throughout their life, but in other races lactase disappears shortly after weaning. The condition may be diagnosed by a lactose tolerance test—administering 50 to 100 g of lactose and measuring an elevation in the blood glucose as the split monosaccharide is absorbed. Of much more value in making the diagnosis is to establish whether such a lactose load ushers in the symptoms of which the patient is complaining. An alternative approach is to use a hydrogen breath analyser: lactose is given and the increase in breath hydrogen measured as this gas is generated by bacterial degradation of the carbohydrate.

Another breath test of value in the diagnosis of bacterial overgrowth in the small intestine is based on the ability of bacteria to deconjugate bile salts. If the radioactive $^{14}$C-labelled bile acid, glycocholic acid, is administered by mouth, then usually only a very small proportion of radioactive $CO_2$ appears in the breath, the majority of the bile salt being absorbed intact in the terminal ileum. In the presence of bacterial overgrowth in the upper small intestine, there is a rapid rise in exhaled radioactive $CO_2$ due to bacterial degradation of the bile acid. Similarly, ileal resection will lead to a rise in exhaled radioactive $CO_2$. Bacterial overgrowth is a not uncommon cause of diarrhoea, particularly in the elderly. It is almost always on the basis of some physiological abnormality, such as achlorhydria associated with old age or pernicious anaemia, or anatomical abnormalities such as previous gastric surgery, the formation of blind loops, jejunal diverticula, etc. Simple intubation techniques, followed by culture, are poor tools for diagnosing bacterial overgrowth, as without sophisticated quantitative techniques the significance of bacterial cultures from the upper gut is difficult to assess.

The investigation of the colon, in the context of altered bowel habit, is much more straightforward than that of the small intestine. After sigmoidoscopy, barium enema should be performed. It is advisable not to do this within 24 h of a rectal biopsy because of the possibility of perforating the colon or of barium tracking submucosally, though this has undoubtedly been overemphasized as a risk. Clinicians should insist on double-contrast barium enemas, as the combination of air and contrast medium is substantially more discriminating than the old-fashioned, single-contrast barium enema. It is inadvisable to perform a barium enema in the context of an acute colitis, and it is indeed normally unnecessary to do so. In acute colitis, the plain abdominal film is extremely useful, showing not only the presence or absence of dilatation but, from inspection of the gas shadows within the colon, the absence of haustration and the presence of mucosal oedema. Flexible colonoscopy is a major advance and has led to the ability to diagnose mucosal lesions of inflammation lying away from the rectum (notably Crohn's disease involving the colon patchily), and more importantly the ability to assess and remove small neoplastic lesions. Polyps can be biopsied,

snared and removed *in toto*. Dubious lesions seen on barium enema can be elucidated, and the difficult area of the narrowed sigmoid colon in the presence of diverticular disease, a common lurking ground for carcinoma, can be directly inspected.

### Gastrointestinal bleeding

The diagnostic approach in the majority of cases of gastrointestinal bleeding is straightforward. Most acute bleeding, whether melaena or haematemesis and melaena, comes from the upper gastrointestinal tract, and urgent endoscopy is often recommended. Disappointingly, there has been little proof that the complications and inconvenience of urgent endoscopy produce better results than endoscopy 'next morning'. However, this picture may be altered by the potential of interventional endoscopy using laser therapy or other means of stopping bleeding, particularly of ulcers, which have prognostic signs of rebleeding such as visible vessels.

The main problem with acute endoscopy of the upper intestine during bleeding is the complication of blood obscuring vision. It is more sensible to wash extensive blood clot off with water jets in order to confirm the diagnosis rather than leave the problem unresolved, despite the small risk of restarting bleeding that this involves. There is a tendency for gastric erosions to appear during the acute stress of bleeding, and this has been put forward as an additional reason for performing early endoscopy. The upper gastrointestinal endoscopy should be as complete as possible under the circumstances, because there may be multiple lesions, and the mere presence of oesophageal varices should not be taken as evidence that they have bled. When the source of upper gastrointestinal bleeding is elusive, the possibility should be considered of bleeding from the biliary tract or liver, or even more rarely from the pancreas. Under these circumstances, angiography may be required to prove the diagnosis.

Lower gastrointestinal bleeding is much more rarely a serious or life-threatening condition. In contrast to the upper gastrointestinal tract, urgent endoscopy is often unsatisfactory, and in an unprepared colon in the presence of bleeding it is frequently difficult to identify the source of bleeding at colonoscopy. A period of conservative management, followed by colonoscopy after preparation, is usually more productive. It is unwise, however, to perform a barium enema where there is serious colonic bleeding, as two of the major sources of this type of haemorrhage—angiodysplasia and bleeding from blood vessels in diverticula—will either not be seen or not be proven to be relevant by barium enema, and the performance of contrast barium studies will prevent the use of angiography for a few days. Recurrent colonic bleeding, or severe gastrointestinal bleeding undiagnosed by other modalities, can usually be identified by visceral angiography.

## LIVER DISEASE

Liver disease presents with jaundice, with other clinical findings such as hepatomegaly, splenomegaly, ascites, bleeding varices or encephalopathy, or by the coincidental finding of abnormal liver function tests. The salient historical points to be elucidated are the same whether the clinical context is suspected acute or chronic liver disease, and here will be largely discussed in the context of the recent onset of jaundice.

Unlike much else in gastroenterology, the investigation of jaundice is logical and an organic disease is always present. The several hundred causes of jaundice can be fitted into the well-established physiological framework—prehepatic jaundice due to excess bilirubin production or decreased bilirubin uptake into the liver; hepatic jaundice due to parenchymal liver disease; and posthepatic jaundice due to failure to excrete bile. The latter may reflect disease in the macroscopic biliary apparatus—classical surgical jaundice—or within the liver substance due to conditions affecting the biliary canaliculi.

### History

In taking the history of a patient with a recent onset of jaundice, the presence or absence of associated symptoms is the main concern. Viral hepatitis is suggested by a few days malaise preceding the onset of jaundice, often associated with mild fever and diarrhoea. There may be some pain: the pain of hepatitis is due to a swollen liver, is localized in the right upper quadrant of the abdomen, and is usually not very prominent, but it can occasionally be surprisingly severe. Fevers with hepatitis are usually not marked but on occasion can reach over 38.5°C. In clinical hepatitis, there are classical serial changes in urine and stool colour, the urine becoming dark before the onset of jaundice but the stool often not becoming pale until jaundice occurs. The onset of pale stools indicates intrahepatic cholestasis; this may be a particularly prolonged feature in a few patients with hepatitis and has been identified as particularly common in some patients with non-A non-B hepatitis. Many patients with hepatitis itch, but as this too is a manifestation of cholestasis and is associated with bile salt deposition in the skin, it usually comes on after the onset of clinical jaundice. This is in contrast to the symptoms of many patients with obstructive jaundice, particularly when of insidious onset, in whom itching may be an early feature. Some patients, notably with hepatitis B, may develop an urticarial rash and joint pains during the week or two before the onset of hepatitis.

Hepatitis may be easy to recognize when it presents with 'flu-like symptoms. However, some patients with hepatitis really remain remarkably well and their very high levels of serum transaminases on blood testing may come as a surprise. Patients with obstructive jaundice due to gallstones usually differ from the patient with hepatitis by the presence of severe pain, which may be complicated by rigors if cholangitis supervenes. This, however, is only the classical pattern, and may not invariably be present. In elderly patients in particular, jaundice due to gallstones may be painless, and indeed cholangitis due to stones in the common bile duct may occur in the absence of both jaundice and pain. Obstructive jaundice due to pancreatic carcinoma is typically painless, but may be associated with back pain if the tumour is extending out of the head of the pancreas.

Increasingly the social history of patients presenting with jaundice is of importance. Homosexuals and drug addicts are particularly at risk for hepatitis B, and drug addicts for non-A non-B hepatitis. Haemophiliacs and other recipients of blood and blood products are also at risk from these agents. Many cases of hepatitis are attributed to drugs, and a full drug history is mandatory. An alcohol history is also important; most people lie about their alcohol intake.

### Physical examination

In examining a patient with jaundice, the main clinical priorities are to decide whether or not chronic liver disease is present, and whether there is hepatic failure.

Stigmata of chronic liver disease include erythematous palms, white nails, white spots on the skin, multiple spider naevi and pigmentation. However, acute liver disease can be associated with a few spider naevi. The liver is of variable size in hepatitis, although a very small liver, or a rapid diminution in its size over 24 to 48 h in hepatitis, is a poor prognostic sign. Splenomegaly in the clinical context of hepatitis suggests either chronicity or infection with Epstein–Barr virus. It is unwise to make the diagnosis of obstructive jaundice in the absence of a palpable liver, although this can be the case when gallstone obstruction complicates cirrhosis. Alcoholics frequently present with large, fat-laden livers, usually in the absence of jaundice. There may be a rapid diminution in liver size as fat is mobilized following abstention from alcohol.

Ascites may complicate acute or chronic liver disease, but much more commonly the latter. In the insidious development of ascites, cardiac and renal causes should be excluded by assessing the jugular venous pressure and the urine for protein. Hepatic venous obstruction is classically associated with a tender, painful liver with jaundice and ascites, and an absent hepatojugular reflux on pressing over the liver. The assessment of the patient with ascites should involve sampling the ascitic fluid and measuring its protein concentration, cell count and possibly its pH, as well as culture and cytological examination. Spontaneous bacterial peritonitis relatively frequently complicates pre-existing cirrhosis, and an early clue to its presence will be a high polymorphonuclear leucocyte count (greater than 300).

### Special investigations

#### Biochemical tests

With the ready availability of blood chemical estimations, less reliance is placed on the finding of urobilinogen and bilirubin in the urine. The presence of urobilinogen in excess without bilirubin in the urine makes the diagnosis of 'acholuric jaundice', which is a prehepatic jaundice due to overproduction of bilirubin or decreased uptake, most commonly haemolysis.

The routine biochemical estimations commonly performed are of bilirubin, alkaline phosphatase and hepatocellular enzyme such as aspartate aminotransferase (SGOT). An elevated bilirubin in the absence of an elevated alkaline phosphatase or SGOT suggests either haemolysis or Gilbert's syndrome, a benign familial deficiency in the mechanism for conjugating bilirubin within the liver cell. Isolated elevation of bilirubin may also be found in thyrotoxicosis, cardiac failure, or after viral hepatitis, but these are not specific findings.

In the presence of jaundice, the relationship between any elevation in levels of alkaline phosphatase and aminotransferase provides the major clue to whether the jaundice is hepatocellular or due to 'posthepatic' causes—i.e., surgical obstructive jaundice or intrahepatic cholestasis. Classically in a posthepatic jaundice, the alkaline phosphatase is greater than 2.5 times the upper limit of normal, with only a minor elevation of hepatocellular enzymes—no more than 2 to 3 times normal. This contrasts with the finding in patients with hepatocellular jaundice, such as viral hepatitis, in whom the aminotransferase may be 3 to 30 times normal, with only modest elevations of the alkaline phosphatase, usually less than 3 times normal.

There are, of course, exceptions to this. With prolonged viral hepatitis, intrahepatic cholestasis may occur, with a marked elevation of the alkaline phosphatase at the time that the major damage to liver cells has passed and the transaminase levels are no longer dramatically elevated. Conversely, with prolonged obstruction, secondary hepatocellular damage may lead to greater elevations of the transaminase levels. For these reasons the liver function tests obtained earliest in the course of jaundice are usually the most discriminating. Alcoholic hepatitis may be associated with only minor elevations of SGOT. Many people assay the gamma glutamyl transpeptidase (GGT) as a screen for the presence of alcoholism. Enzyme induction from any cause, such as anti-epileptic treatment, also raises the level of this enzyme.

#### Viral serology

The ability to identify hepatitis A and hepatitis B by serology has increased the confidence with which acute and chronic viral liver disease can be diagnosed. The virus of hepatitis A usually disappears from the faeces at the time jaundice appears and is thus of little use diagnostically in the individual patient. However, antibody titres for antihepatitis A are of value. In a recently jaundiced patient, the presence of antihepatitis A antibody of the IgM class strongly indicates that the current hepatitis is due to this virus. Detection of IgG antibody merely indicates past infection, which is extremely common.

In the majority of patients infected with hepatitis B, the virus is detectable in the blood, in the form of hepatitis B surface antigen (HBsAg). In an acute uncomplicated viral hepatitis of type B, from which the patient makes a complete recovery, HBsAg is detected from a few weeks before the onset of jaundice until up to six months after, although the majority of patients will have cleared the virus within three months. Failure to do so indicates the presence of chronic carriage and probably chronic liver disease. During uncomplicated acute virus hepatitis, patients develop antibody to the surface coat of the virus (hepatitis B surface antibody) and the core of the virus (hepatitis B core antibody). The surface antibody remains lifelong and is protective.

Interpretation of hepatitis B markers in the presence of chronic liver disease is a great deal more complex. The majority of patients with hepatitis B-associated chronic liver disease carry HBsAg in their blood, but there are a few in which insufficient viral coat protein is exported from the liver into the blood, and in these patients the detection of circulating antibody to hepatitis B core can indicate the persisting presence of virus in the liver. Patients with hepatitis B in the blood chronically can be subdivided into those with e antigen or with e antibody. The e antigen is associated with the presence of full viral particles in the blood, capable of replicating when introduced into another liver cell, and is therefore a marker for highly infectious blood.

There is now a marker for one form of non-A non-B hepatitis. NANB hepatitis currently causes about one third of acute hepatitis in hospitals in the UK. A minority of patients with hepatitis is experiencing infection with cytomegalovirus, Epstein–Barr virus or very rarely herpes virus. The identification of antibodies to hepatitis C, which is strongly associated with post-transfusion hepatitis, is an important marker in chronic liver disease. It takes some months for antihepatitis C to appear after infection, so the test is of less use in acute hepatitis.

The detection of autoantibodies is valuable in the diagnosis of chronic liver disease, and particularly in those patients with apparent acute viral hepatitis but with no serological markers who do not make a rapid recovery. Some 70 to 80 per cent of patients with autoimmune chronic active hepatitis have high levels of smooth muscle antibodies, with smaller proportions having antinuclear factor and antimitochondrial antibodies. Low titres of smooth muscle antibody are commonly found during acute liver damage of any sort.

Serum immunoglobulins become elevated in liver disease of any sort, but the greatest rises are found in chronic liver disease, with typical patterns of a high IgG in autoimmune chronic active hepatitis, a high IgM in primary biliary cirrhosis, and a high IgA in alcoholic cirrhosis. There is, however, a great deal of overlap in these patterns.

Other relevant investigations in chronic liver disease include the alphafetoprotein as a marker of primary hepatocellular cancer. Modest elevations of alphafetoprotein also occur during regeneration of the liver. Serum iron and ferritin, serum and urinary copper and caeruloplasmin, are important screening tests, particularly if there is a family history of liver disease. The possibility of diagnosing treatable lesions, such as haemochromatosis and Wilson's disease, and autoimmune chronic active hepatitis, is one of the main justifications for taking liver biopsies in chronic disease, as there are specific therapies available for these.

### Imaging of the liver and biliary tree

Clearly not every patient with jaundice or liver disease requires invasive investigation and histological examination of the liver. Cases of apparent acute uncomplicated viral hepatitis, the otherwise fit HBsAg carrier, and the minor abnormalities in liver function tests of the exuberant social drinker can be managed without histological investigation. Once, however, matters are not straightforward and there is no spontaneous improvement, then further investigations should be made.

This is best illustrated by the approach to a patient with cholestatic liver function tests, who is not improving and has had jaundice for some weeks. This is the classical dilemma of whether such a patient has surgical obstructive jaundice, which will not get better without an operation, or cholestatic viral hepatitis, which will eventually improve and may be adversely affected by laparotomy. In brief, the necessary approach involves ultrasonography of the liver to see whether there is evidence of obstruction, and if there, the delineation of the biliary tree by cholangiography before surgery. If, however, there is no evidence of obstruction, a liver biopsy should be taken.

## Ultrasonography

This has replaced other modalities as the first imaging procedure of the liver. It can show the presence of dilated intrahepatic, common hepatic, and common bile ducts in patients with low biliary obstruction; and it can frequently define the nature of the obstruction (an enlarged pancreatic head in pancreatic carcinoma, gallstones within the common bile duct in cholelithiasis). It may detect the level of obstruction in the biliary tree. Other space-occupying lesions, such as cysts or metastatic deposits, can be detected. Other information such as the presence of splenomegaly, patency of the portal vein and hepatic venous drainage can be determined.

Similar information can be obtained by CT scanning. The routine isotope scan of the liver has now much less place in the investigation of liver disease, and very little to offer in the investigation of suspected obstructive jaundice. It may be still of value for identifying space-occupying lesions in the liver. All these modalities—ultrasound, CT and liver scan—are claimed to be of value in showing diffuse parenchymal disease—fatty infiltration, cirrhosis, etc. While these can be helpful they are not an accurate means of either diagnosing or excluding these conditions.

## Cholangiography

If ultrasonography shows the presence of dilated ducts, these should be further delineated before surgery unless the appearances are entirely unequivocal. There is a choice of two techniques: percutaneous cholangiography using a 'skinny needle' or endoscopic retrograde cholangiography.

Percutaneous cholangiography, since the introduction of the flexible 'skinny needle', is straightforward, safe and easy to perform. The patient should be pretreated with antibiotics to lessen the risk of inducing cholangitis and septicaemia, and clotting and platelet studies should be done as outlined under 'Liver biopsy' below. The needle is introduced, usually laterally, into the liver, and dye injected, which will visualize the biliary system as far down as the level of obstruction. Percutaneous cholangiography should always be possible in the presence of dilated ducts. The alternative approach, endoscopic cholangiography, requires much more expertise as the endoscopist must cannulate the ampulla of Vater using a side-viewing endoscope. This too has a risk of inducing cholangitis in an obstructed system and should, also, be covered with antibiotics. It has the advantages of displaying both the lower end of the common bile duct and the pancreatic duct, and may therefore give further evidence about the aetiology of lower obstruction. It also provides direct visualization of the ampulla of Vater, allowing the diagnosis of ampullary carcinoma to be made. In recent years it has developed therapeutic possibilities, with the extraction of common duct stones and sphincterotomy now being feasible. However, even in the most skilled hands, cannulation of the biliary tree is not always possible.

## Liver biopsy

In the cholestatic patient in whom dilated bile ducts have ben excluded, liver biopsy should be performed. Routine liver biopsy is safe provided the prothrombin time is not prolonged more than 3 to 4 s over the control, and provided the platelet count is greater than 80 000. In the setting of cholestasis, medical causes include viral and drug-induced hepatitis, primary biliary cirrhosis, and bilirubin transport defects such as the Dubin–Johnson syndrome. However, despite the absence of dilated ducts on ultrasonography, it is still possible that liver biopsy may reveal disease of the large duct, with oedema and a polymorphonuclear infiltrate in the portal tracts suggesting that obstruction is present. Under these circumstances the bile duct should then be imaged by either percutaneous cholangiography or endoscopic cholangiography. Without dilated bile ducts, the success rate of percutaneous cholangiography is of the order of 70 to 80 per cent in visualizing the intrahepatic bile ducts. The circumstances under which large-duct obstruction is missed by ultrasound include those of non-distensible bile ducts, such as are found in sclerosing cholangitis after repeated ascending cholangitis, or those of a diffuse cholangiocarcinoma or of a very recent onset of jaundice.

In the diagnosis of chronic liver disease, the ability to take a liver biopsy is more likely to be jeopardized by clotting deficiencies, the presence of severe ascites (which may make tearing of the liver capsule during the procedure more likely), or thrombocytopenia. Alternative approaches to liver biopsy include the transvenous route, passing a biotome via the jugular into the hepatic vein, or performing a percutaneous biopsy via a flexible sheath and plugging the entry route into the liver with absorbable foam. In the context of space-occupying lesions in the liver, particularly in the diagnosis of potential metastases, ultrasound- or CT-guided biopsy are now proving useful.

## Further reading

Nolan D. J. (1981). Barium examination of the small intestine. Progress report. *Gut*, **22**, 682–94.

Foley W. D., Stewart E. T., Lawson T. L., Geenan J., Loguidice J., Maher L., Unger G. F. (1980). Computed tomography, ultrasonography and endoscopic retrograde cholangiopancreography in the diagnosis of pancreatic disease: a comparative study. *Gastroint. Radiol.*, **5**, 29–35.

Braganza J. M. (1982). Does your patient have pancreatic disease? *J. Roy. Coll. Phys. London*, **16**, 13–22.

Turnberg L. A. (1979). The pathophysiology of diarrhoea. *Clin. Gastroenterol.*, **8**, 551–68.

Manning A. P., Thompson W. G., Heaton K. W., Morris A. F. (1978). Towards positive diagnosis of the irritable bowel. *Br. Med. J.*, **2**, 653–4.

Hirschowitz B. (1983). Natural history of duodenal ulceration. *Gastroenterol.*, **85**, 967–70.

Scott B. B., Losowsky M. S. (1977). The definition and diagnosis of coeliac disease. *J. Roy. Coll. Phys. London*, **11**, 405–12.

Sherlock S. (1985). *Diseases of the liver and biliary system*, 7th edn. Oxford: Blackwell Scientific.

Wright R., Alberti K. G. M. M., Karran S., Millward-Sadler G. H., eds. (1985). *Liver and biliary disease*, 2nd edn. London: W. B. Saunders.

Bouchier I. A. D., Allan R. A., Hodgson H. J. F., Keightley M., eds. (1984). *Textbook of Gastroenterology*. London: Baillière Tindall.

# 12

# OPHTHALMOLOGY

David J. Spalton

## INTRODUCTION

In the majority of patients a simple clinical examination of the eye can produce a working diagnosis for safe management of ophthalmic conditions. A torch and ophthalmoscope are necessary but sophisticated ophthalmic equipment is not essential providing the non-specialist is aware of when to refer patients to an ophthalmologist. The torch should provide a solid, focused beam of bright light. A household torch with a 'hollow' central beam is not adequate as the centre of the beam is not filled in at close working distances. The disposable pocket torches often handed out by pharmaceutical companies are ideal and sometimes they can be fitted with a blue filter to show up fluorescent staining, which is a bonus. It is well worth having an ophthalmoscope of one's own because one then gets used to using a certain type of instrument, its availability leads to more frequent use, and there is an incentive to keep the batteries fresh and the light bright. There are many types of ophthalmoscope available but the main characteristics required in choosing one are robustness and a halogen light bulb. More expensive models have more focusing lenses and many gimmicks, such as graticules, but the only addition of any potential value is a green 'red-free' filter, which some people find useful to show up detail of the retinal blood vessels and nerve fibres. The importance of a good bright light source cannot be overemphasized.

## EXAMINATION OF THE EYE

It is necessary to have a routine for ophthalmic examination. This leads to a logical approach, which in fact shortens the time required and prevents significant findings being overlooked. Ophthalmology is a highly visual specialty where the signs and diagnosis are usually apparent for all to see and the ophthalmologist only exercises superior diagnostic skills by knowing how to use the equipment, knowledge of the variations of the normal eye and an appreciation of what pathology to look for. History taking, although important, is perhaps more limited in ophthalmology as the symptoms are frequently restricted.

The most important question to ask any patient with an ocular problem is whether or not they have lost vision, as this immediately separates those with serious disease from those in a potentially less severe group. Sudden visual loss is frequently a reflection of vascular pathology, for example, a retinal arterial or venous occlusion, and is often untreatable but one must always be wary of the patient with progressive visual loss as this frequently implies ocular or neuro-ophthalmic disease, which can be reversed or halted.

### Visual acuity

This is usually tested at a distance of 6 m or 20 ft to prevent the effects of accommodation or presbyopia from interfering. The Snellen chart is the accepted clinical measure, and this test should ideally be done with a properly illuminated chart rather than a printed cardboard sheet. However, a useful clinical test in non-specialist practice is simply to ask the patient to hold a hand over each eye in turn and to ask whether or not he or she sees as well as normally with each eye. Normal acuity is denoted as '6/6' (or 20/20 in the USA) and this means that the patient has the theoretically best acuity by being able to see at 6 m a letter the size of each component of which subtends one minute of arc at the nodal point of the eye. Whilst this is theoretically the best or 'normal' acuity that an eye can have, young people with normal eyes should see '6/5', which is better than 'normal'. In middle age the 'normal' acuity is 6/6 and this falls with further ageing because of lens opacities and loss of retinal function. A visual acuity of 6/18 implies that the patient sees at 6 m the size of letter that a normal person sees at 18 m. The top letter on the chart is denoted accordingly as 6/60, i.e., a person with normal acuity would be able to see a letter of this size at 60 m. Poorer vision than this is recorded in descending order as counting fingers, hand movements or perception of light.

The patient's acuity is recorded with their distance spectacles if he or she has a refractive error. A patient may not see normally with spectacles, either because they are wrong or simply out of date, or because there is also some ocular pathology present. Simple refractive errors can be rapidly corrected by getting the patient to read the chart through a 'pin-hole aperture'. This eliminates moderate refractive errors in the same way as a pin-hole camera produces a sharp image without lenses. Thus, if a patient sees 6/18 with spectacles and improves to 6/6 with a pin-hole, the implication is that the poor acuity can be attributed to the spectacles and that he or she needs another refraction. However, a patient who sees 6/18 with spectacles but improves to 6/12 with a pin-hole test requires new spectacles to improve sight but also has some ocular pathology contributing to the poor vision. By using both eyes, the patient normally has better acuity than on seeing with either eye individually. To hold a normal driving licence in Britian an acuity of 6/12 or better is required (equivalent to reading a car number plate at 25 yards).

Assessment of near vision is necessary but less helpful in the clinical examination because factors of magnification and presbyopia become important. It is tested by using reading spectacles when necessary (most patients over 45 years are presbyopic and require some reading aid) with a card printed in types of decreasing size. Reading type size N5 should be easily obtained by a healthy eye and N8 is equivalent to newsprint. Near vision is extremely important as most of us require to be able to do close work. Due to the magnification effects, an eye with 6/18 vision may well be able to manage N5; alternatively an eye with macular pathology may do far worse than expected. This problem must be borne in mind in the bedside diagnosis of patients when near vision is sometimes used to assess visual function.

## Colour vision

Loss of colour sensation is an important feature of disease of the optic nerve, chiasm or tract (the anterior visual pathway) and is a useful means of separating the types of loss of vision caused by macular or retrobulbar pathology. There are many sophisticated ways of assessing colour vision but from the clinical point of view all that is necessary is to ask the patient to view the Ishihara plates and read out the numbers. British caucasian males have a high incidence of congenital red/green colour blindness but they will frequently be aware of this if it is severe and this congenital loss is symmetrical and equal in both eyes. Patients with neuro-ophthalmic defects, such as optic neuritis or chiasmal compression, may have great difficulty in reading the plates. This degree of difficulty depends on the extent of the damage. With severe defects they may not be able to read any plate, with less severe defects they may miss or confuse some plates, and with more subtle, asymmetrical defects the colours of the numbers just look brighter or better with the better eye. There is no advantage in recording the findings for each plate individually but the number of plates seen correctly can be recorded, e.g., right eye: 6 out of 17 plates seen correctly. Loss of colour sensation is useful both from the initial diagnostic point of view and also in the follow-up of the patient, when progressive deterioration or improvement may be found. Subtleties in the pattern of colour defect can have some diagnostic significance, for example, red–green (in nerve diseases) or blue–yellow defects (with optic retinal diseases) but these are outside the realms of normal clinical practice.

## Pupils

Examination of the pupil might be thought of as rather limited. The pupil can, of course, only do two things—contract or dilate. But pupillary examination can provide objective evidence of visual pathology and for this reason the relative afferent pupillary defect (RAPD) has been called the most important sign in ophthalmology. Objective signs in ophthalmology are unusual as most of the examination is subjective, e.g., visual acuity or fields, and the only objective evidence of disease of the retrobulbar visual pathways may be an RAPD or optic atrophy.

Pupils should be examined in a darkened room with a bright torch and the patient focusing in the distance so that accommodation is controlled. Both pupils should be examined for equality of size: the finding of anisocoria should immediately prompt the examiner to look at the eyelids for ptosis (for Horner's syndrome, IIIrd nerve palsy). Both pupils are then checked individually to see if they react to light. (Beware of patients using eyedrops or systemic drugs that affect the pupil.) After this the torch is swung between the two eyes and the contraction and dilatation of each pupil is observed to assess the pupillary tone. Normally both pupils have equal tone. With asymmetrical lesions of the anterior visual pathway the input of light on the IIIrd nerve nucleus in the midbrain will vary. For example, if a patient has a lesion such as demyelination of the optic nerve on the right side, shining the light in the left eye will produce a brisk constriction of both pupils by the direct and consensual reflexes mediated through the optic nerve, chiasm, optic tract Edinger–Westphal nucleus in the midbrain to each IIIrd nerve. When the light is rapidly transferred to the right eye, however, less stimulation of the Edinger–Westphal nucleus is produced because some of the optic nerve fibres are lost or malfunctioning. Tone is removed from the IIIrd nerves which provide the efferent pathway and both pupils are seen to dilate. With practice, subtle defects in loss of pupillary control can be detected, which can be confirmed by finding the fellow signs of poor acuity and colour vision, changes in the optic disc and visual field defect.

An RAPD can be produced both by ocular or retrobulbar pathology but if an ocular defect is responsible it is always obvious to the examiner. Cataracts do not produce an RAPD as they merely scatter light but a significant vitreous haemorrhage will absorb light and do so. To produce an RAPD about 25 per cent of the retina must be affected, e.g., by retinal detachment or vascular occlusion, which will be readily apparent to the examiner. An RAPD, therefore, in the absence of obvious retinal pathology implies that a lesion of the anterior visual pathway (optic nerve, chiasm and optic tract) must be sought. The pupillary fibres leave the optic tract to pass to the midbrain: lesions of the optic radiation and visual cortex cannot produce an RAPD.

Pupillary size is controlled by an efferent (IIIrd nerve) system and by the anatomy or pathology of the iris. Sectioning of or damage to an optic nerve (or lesions of the afferent visual pathway) will not produce a difference in pupillary diameter.

## Ocular movements

An analysis of diplopia, particularly vertical diplopia, is usually beyond the realms of the non-specialist and such patients are best referred to an ophthalmologist for accurate diagnosis and measurement of the underlying abnormality. This should not preclude, however, simple observation of the range of ocular movements. It is important to be sure that the patient has true diplopia in contrast to monocular diplopia or blurring by confirming that the double vision is corrected by covering one eye. If diplopia is present it should be noted whether it is horizontal (i.e., due to pathology of the lateral or medial recti) or vertical (superior or inferior recti, or obliques). Patients often find it difficult to describe their diplopia accurately and sometimes it is easier to get them to demonstrate it by asking them to hold their head straight and follow with their eyes a light that is moved to the extremes of horizontal, vertical and oblique gaze, and then to tell the examiner when it becomes double. Special attention should be paid to the extremes of horizontal gaze and to looking up and down from the horizontal position. Patients with diplopia often adopt an associated head posture in an attempt to control their symptoms.

Diplopia that cannot be explained on a neurological basis will suggest that myasthenia gravis, thyroid eye disease, ocular myopathy or orbital trauma or tumours should be excluded. Myasthenia gravis and ocular myopathy are usually associated with weakness of the orbicularis oculi muscle as well.

Another aspect of ocular motility is to assess supranuclear control of the IIIrd, IVth and VIth nerves. There are four basic systems—saccadic fixational movements, pursuit or following movements and vestibular input, which is concerned with coordinating ocular with head and neck posture, as well as convergence. By definition, supranuclear control of gaze is conjugate (moving both eyes as a yoked pair). Saccades are rapid movements concerned with refixation of the eyes to another object of visual regard. They are generated by the contralateral premotor frontal cortex, i.e., a saccade to the right is originated in the left cortex. Pursuit movements probably originate in the ipsilateral occipitoparietal lobes. They control following movements of the eyes, keeping the foveas fixed on the object of regard. Vestibular movements originate in the inner ear and are transmitted by the VIIIth nerve to the vestibular nuclei in the pons. Little is known about the mechanism of vergence control. All types of supranuclear inputs are passed to the parapontine reticular formation in the pons at the level of the VIth nucleus, which integrates them and coordinates the IIIrd, IVth, and VIth nuclei through the tract known as the medial longitudinal fasciculus. Lesions of this tract are common and are known as internuclear ophthalmoplegias. This is a paralysis of the adducting eye on lateral gaze with nystagmus of the abducting eye, usually with preservation of convergence. Bilateral internuclear ophthalmoplegia is a common finding in multiple sclerosis; unilateral lesions usually indicate vascular pontine disease. Conjugate eye movements are normally tested in both the horizontal and vertical meridians: basically, lesions producing horizontal defects are localized to the pons whilst vertical gaze is controlled by structures in the upper midbrain. Optokinetic nystagmus (elicited by looking at the stripes on a rotating drum) is used to test the integration of saccadic and pursuit movements.

Nystagmus is a complicated and difficult subject, even for those interested in the condition. It should be elicited by examining the eyes in the primary position of gaze, and then at 30° of lateral and vertical gaze. Instability of fixation should be noted and the 'wave form' observed. Simply nystagmus must be divided into congenital and acquired types: the most common types of acquired nystagmus are gaze-evoked or vestibular. There are, however, many other different types of oscillatory ocular movements.

## Ophthalmoscopy

It is often easier to check the fundi before the visual fields as, frequently, fundoscopy will confirm the examiner's suspicions and suggest the field defect that should be sought. However, if fields are to be charted properly this is best done without pupillary dilatation.

Fundoscopy requires dilatation of the pupils. In young, otherwise healthy eyes the optic disc can usually be visualized easily but to examine the fundus or macula more adequately or to see the optic discs properly it is essential to dilate the pupils. This requires a short-acting mydriatic, such as eye-drops of tropicamide (Mydriacil) or cyclopentolate (Mydrilate). Physicians are often over-wary of producing an attack of angle-closure glaucoma by dilating the pupils. It must be emphasized this is very rare and is usually only seen in the elderly patient who is substantially predisposed to acute glaucoma. Providing that patients are warned that if they get pain and redness or blurred vision in the next few hours they should seek medical advice, pupillary dilatation is safe and the advantages of accurate diagnosis far outweigh the minimal risks involved. In my own department, where 55000 patients are seen each year and where a substantial proportion of these will be given dilating drops, in only two or three patients a year will an attack of acute glaucoma be induced. Patients will, however, find that dilating their pupils blurs their vision because accommodation is paralysed until the drops wear off over four to five hours.

To get a good view of the fundus with a direct ophthalmoscope one must get as close to the patient as possible, using the right eye to look at the patient's right eye and vice versa. It is a good idea to raise the patient's upper lid with the thumb and get so close that the examiner's nose is in contact with this thumb as this gives the widest possible view. It is impossible accurately to 'preset' the focus on the ophthalmoscope as both the refraction and accommodation of the examiner's eye and the patient's eye will vary. Instead the examiner should focus on the red reflex from 15 to 20 cm (6–8 in) away, with the patient fixing their gaze in the distance and just above the horizon. Opacities such as cataract in the visual media will appear dark against this reflex. On rapidly moving close to the patient, the retina will be seen and a blood vessel located. This is then brought into focus by spinning the focusing lenses, and the vessels can be followed back to the optic disc. After observing the disc the vessels are followed out into their quadrants and the macula viewed by getting the patient to look straight into the light.

In very highly myopic patients the fundus is difficult to visualize and these patients are best examined by looking with the ophthalmoscope through their spectacles.

By using an ordinary direct ophthalmoscope the non-specialist can examine the optic disc, posterior pole of the eye and equatorial retina in detail. An ophthalmologist will get a better overall view using an indirect ophthalmoscope, which produces a less magnified but larger field of view and allows the peripheral retina to be observed completely. It also enables the ophthalmologist to see through moderate amounts of cateract or vitreous opacity. Examination of the fundus is aided by colour photography to record physical signs and fluorescein angiography to demonstrate the vascular circulation in the eye and the blood–retinal barriers.

## Visual fields

Diagnostic visual fields are easily performed by confrontation techniques but specialist equipment is necessary to plot the fields for sequential follow-up. From a diagnostic and localizing point of view it is the pattern of field loss that is important and this should correlate with the other physical signs. Retinal lesions lead to uniocular defects by interfering with the retinal ganglion cells and their fibres to produce the typical inverted mirror-image of the fundus pathology. Thus, occlusion of a superior, temporal branch artery can be expected to produce an inferior, nasal field defect. Constriction of the field will be seen with retinal dystrophies—for example, retinitis pigmentosa—or with disease of the optic disc, such as severe glaucoma or longstanding papilloedema. Hysterical patients also tend to have constricted, telescopic visual fields. Interruption of a bundle of nerve fibres will produce an 'arcuate' pattern of field defect, i.e., an inverted, mirror-image pattern arching out from the optic disc or retinal lesion, as in early glaucoma.

Ischaemic infarction of the optic disc produces an inferior altitudinal defect, i.e., a field defect inferiorly that passes horizontally through fixation. Lesions of the optic nerve from whatever cause produce a central scotoma, chiasmal lesions a bitemporal hemianopia and all retrochiasmal lesions a homonymous hemianopia. Visual acuity is lost with lesions of the optic disc, nerve and chiasm but with all homonymous lesions the acuity should be normal (6/6) unless there is other ocular pathology because the macula is represented bilaterally in the occipital cortex.

A red pin is the best target for confrontation field testing. This is probably because the visual pathways behind the globe are basically concerned with macular function (60 per cent of optic nerve fibres subserve the central 30° of field) and colour sensitivity is derived from cones in the macular area. Neurological defects respect the midline and do not encroach from the periphery. Thus an early bitemporal defect will present as desaturation of red in the central temporal field adjacent to

fixation and the patient will notice a sudden jump of increased colour perception as the target crosses the midline to the nasal field. Temporal and hemianopic defects start centrally and progress outwards: they do not first affect the outer most temporal field and creep in, neither do they ever slope across the vertical meridian.

Central scotomas are often difficult to identify as they are usually partial. With a unilateral defect it is often easiest to ask patients to compare the redness of the target pin in each eye individually and in the affected eye, to start with the red target centrally and move it peripherally until they notice a change in increased redness. With this technique even very subtle scotomas to red can be plotted. Central scotomas are usually associated with poor visual acuity.

Any technique of field testing requires the patient to be able to cooperate and maintain fixation. It is often very tempting for the patient to follow or search for the target and consequently this produces gross artifacts. Fixation is best controlled by direct observation during testing. Another point to watch is that the fellow eye is properly occluded with the palm of the hand. Patients with poor vision in the affected eye often tend to peep through the fingers covering the occluded eye.

## VASCULAR RETINOPATHIES

### Introduction

Vascular retinopathies usually produce sudden visual loss in eyes that are white and externally appear normal. They occur most commonly in elderly people and the diagnosis is made from interpreting the appearances of the fundus through a dilated pupil. The most important aspect of the diagnosis lies in the detection and investigation of underlying systemic vascular disease.

### Retinal embolization

Retinal emboli may produce transient or permanent unilateral visual loss, which may be partial or complete depending on where within the vascular tree the blockage occurs. Amaurosis fugax is the name given to transient visual loss caused by the passage of emboli through the retinal circulation. The patient typically experiences a unilateral attack of visual loss; this comes on suddenly over a few seconds as a greying out and complete loss of vision that lasts from a few minutes to two to four hours, there is then complete and rapid visual recovery over one to two minutes as the obstruction fragments or passes. Patients may get repeated attacks, sometimes associated with evidence of transient neurological deficit. Visual loss is usually complete but on occasions it may have an altitudinal character like a curtain coming up or down if only one retinal branch artery is affected. It is particularly important to try to get the patient to ascertain that the attack has been completely unilateral by covering each eye during an attack. This is because it is easy to confuse the changes of hemianopic temporal field loss that come from contralateral cortical ischaemia due to posterior cerebral artery disease with those of unilateral visual loss. Transient cortical ischaemia produces, of course, a homonymous hemianopia; it is often associated with zig-zag flashing lights and sometimes tinnitus, vertigo or neurological deficit from involvement of the brainstem due to occlusion of the basilar artery or its branches. In young people or others with a relevant history, migraine must be considered in its various forms.

Retinal emboli are commonly of three types—platelet–fibrin, cholesterol or calcific: the first two types usually originate from atheromatous plaques, commonly at the bifurcation of the common carotid artery, and the third type from mitral or aortic valve disease. The platelet–fibrin emboli can sometimes be seen in the retinal arteries as a porridge-like substance slowly passing through the retinal circulation during the attack. Cholesterol crystals are seen as a yellow refractile crystal, usually at a bifurcation, and can persist for a long time in the retinal circulation (Plate 12.1). As they have a planar shape they do not necessarily cause vascular occlusion. Calcific emboli are less common. They have a globular white shiny appearance and they tend to lie in the vicinity of the optic disc, usually producing complete vascular occlusion.

The importance of retinal embolization or amaurosis fugax lies in the appreciation that such patients carry a significantly increased risk of suffering a major cerebral vascular occlusion and that prophylactic treatment may prevent this. Patients should be investigated for hypertension and underlying vascular disease, such as diabetes or polycythaemia. Smoking should be stopped. Patients who may be suitable for carotid endarter-

ectomy require digital subtraction angiography to delineate carotid atheroma with a view to surgery as well as echocardiography to exclude cardiac valvular pathology. In young patients, other causes of amaurosis fugax include mitral valve prolapse, cardiac disease, arteritis, hyperlipidaemia or hyperaggregation of platelets. In the majority of younger patients the symptoms are benign and permanent neurological deficit is rare. In the elderly who are not candidates for surgery, low-dose aspirin is probably the most satisfactory prophylaxis (provided they have no peptic ulceration).

## Central retinal artery occlusion

The patient notices sudden visual loss that is usually virtually complete, although sometimes a bit of peripheral visual field may be spared through supply of the most peripheral and thinnest retina from the choroid, or the central retina from a spared cilioretinal artery (supplied from the choroidal circulation). Rarely, a cilioretinal artery can be of such size and distribution as to supply the central retinal area and therefore spare central vision and acuity. Sometimes, and rather surprisingly, a patient will only notice uniocular visual loss coincidentally some time after it has occurred.

The acute fundus signs are of cloudy white intracellular oedema affecting the posterior pole where the retina is thickest and becoming much less noticeable to the periphery where the retina is thinner. A 'cherry-red spot' is seen in the macula (Plate 12.2). Here the whiteness of the infarcted retina is contrasted against the normal and preserved vascular supply of the choroid seen through the 'window' of the macula, which is only a few cells thick. These appearances are easiest to see in pigmented eyes and disappear from within a few days to two to three weeks. Sometimes emboli can be seen within the retinal circulation but platelet–fibrin emboli can be difficult to differentiate from 'cattle trucking' of erythrocytes in the vessels due to vascular stasis. There may be mild swelling of the optic disc in the acute stage from stasis of retrograde axoplasmic flow.

Central retinal artery occlusion usually occurs in elderly people, either as a result of embolization or of local thrombosis within the artery. It is a relatively uncommon presentation of temporal arteritis but all patients require an ESR as an urgent procedure in the acute stages to exclude this diagnosis. In young patients an arteritis or collagen disease can produce central retinal artery occlusion.

If a patient is seen within hours of visual loss (less than 12–24 h), it is worth trying to produce visual recovery by assuming that the occlusion is embolic and by attempting to dislodge it by lowering the intraocular pressure with digital massage, intravenous acetazolamide or by draining aqueous humour. Such treatment is, however, rarely successful and the visual recovery is usually negligible. After the attack the patient requires investigation along the lines already described for those with amaurosis fugax.

## Branch retinal artery occlusion

This is virtually always embolic. The patient presents with acute visual loss in the sector of the visual field corresponding to the retinal occlusion. Small occlusions can frequently be asymptomatic. The physical signs are the same as those of central retinal artery occlusion but limited to the territory of the affected branch artery.

## Central retinal vein occlusion

The features of venous occlusion in the retina are haemorrhages throughout the territory of the affected vessel and, with central vein occlusion these extend to the equatorial retina. These may lie in the retinal nerve fibre layer (flame shaped) or deeper to this (blotch-like). Where there is severe retinal ischaemia the haemorrhages have a darker brown appearance and a larger, more diffuse appearance. Other signs of retinal venous occlusion are venous engorgement, cotton-wool spots (indicating microvascular ischaemia), retinal and macular oedema and closure of the capillary vascular bed. In some patients there may be swelling of the optic disc and, in really acute or severe cases, a certain amount of vitreous haemorrhage.

Central retinal vein occlusion, in common with other occlusive vascular disease, is normally seen in elderly people: the typical symptom is to awake in the morning with uniocular visual loss in an eye that had previously normal vision. The retinal appearances are unilateral but frequently signs of arteriosclerosis can be found in the fellow eye and sequential disease in this eye is not uncommon.

The occlusion occurs within the optic nerve behind the lamina cribrosa where the central retinal artery and vein share a common sheath. Arteriosclerotic changes here compromise the venous return by compressing the venous wall. Central retinal vein occlusion can vary from the mild to the severe (Plate 12.3). The milder changes resolve over several months with recovery of vision in the affected eye. In more severe cases, retinal ischaemia with structural damage precludes any recovery. Central vein occlusion has a well-known association with raised intraocular pressure and it is essential that all patients have this checked. The fellow eye may also be affected and appropriate treatment with drugs to lower the intraocular pressure may save this eye on which the patient relies for future vision. All patients require to be screened for underlying vascular disease, such as hypertension and diabetes. No treatment has been shown to improve the visual prognosis once central retinal vein occlusion has occurred and, in particular, anticoagulation is contraindicated as this can lead to disastrous vitreous haemorrhage.

Some patients with central vein occlusion suffer widespread closure of the retinal capillary bed at the time of initial occlusion. The precise reason for this is unknown but it is more common in severely affected eyes and less common in younger patients. These patients are likely to develop neovascular glaucoma and this typically starts to occur about three months after the occlusion. The aetiology, morphology and treatment of this condition have much in common with neovascularization in the diabetic eye with the exception that in central vein occlusion patients do not develop neovascularization of the retina or optic disc. Instead, neovascularization (or rubeosis) of the anterior surface of the iris occurs which is thought to be due to the secretion of a neovascularizing factor from the hypoxic retina. Rubeosis is initially seen as a fine network of vessels around the pupillary margin, which spreads to occlude the angle of the anterior chamber and obstruct the drainage of aqueous humour, eventually leading to glaucoma and a blind and painful eye. Retinal capillary closure can be demonstrated easily by fluorescein angiography and timely panretinal photocoagulation can prevent rubeosis and salvage whatever vision remains in the eye. In the resolving stages of central retinal vein occlusion collateral vessels frequently appear on the optic disc, shunting blood from the high pressure of the obstructed central retinal vein to the lower pressure of choroidal veins. These vessels can be confused with neovascularization of the optic disc but are easily differentiated clinically or by fluorescein angiography if necessary.

## Branch retinal vein occlusion

This is one of the commoner vascular retinopathies and is normally the result of occlusion of a temporal retinal vein at the site of an arterial crossing. Here the hypertrophic arterial wall compresses the underlying vein. The physical signs are no different from those of a central retinal vein occlusion with the exception that they are limited to the appropriate vascular territory (Plate 12.4). Branch retinal vein occlusion is most commonly seen in hypertensive patients. If the macula is affected the patient will present with blurred vision; otherwise the branch retinal vein occlusion may be asymptomatic.

When there is sufficient retinal ischaemia, neovascularization may occur, either at the junction of the adjacent healthy retina or on the optic disc, but rubeosis of the iris is exceptional. When neovascularization is severe it can be controlled by laser photocoagulation of the affected area. A few patients lose further vision after the acute stages from accumulating macular oedema or deposition of hard exudate and laser can be used to control this in appropriate cases.

## Hyperviscosity

Hyperviscosity syndromes produce a bilateral retinopathy of dilated retinal veins with scattered, blotchy haemorrhages in the posterior poles and peripheral fundus and occasionally cotton-wool spots. The retinopathy is usually mild, although severe cases with ocular ischaemia can occur. The most common causes are polycythaemia or Waldenström's macroglobulinaemia, and when looked at critically, the retinopathy is probably related more to other associated haematological changes, particularly thrombocytopenia, than to increased blood viscosity in its own right.

## Slow flow retinopathy

This is a bilateral or unilateral retinopathy of similar appearance to that associated with mild central retinal vein occlusion or hyperviscosity syndromes but with the differentiating feature of a very low pulse pressure in the central retinal artery. On ophthalmoscopy the artery is seen to collapse and pulsate with minimal pressure on the eye from the examiner's finger. The poor arterial perfusion is usually due to severe carotid atheroma or occasionally to arteritis, both leading to a reduced perfusion pressure across the retinal capillary bed. This can sometimes be so severe as to produce capillary closure and neovascularization. Patients present with symptoms similar to those of amaurosis fugax, complaining of recurrent attacks of blurred vision, which they often describe as having an additional bright 'watery' effect – they invariably have widespread vascular disease.

## Anaemia

Anaemic patients, from whatever cause, can develop a retinopathy with blotchy retinal haemorrhages. These occur most commonly in the peripheral retina and are usually asymptomatic. Roth's spots (haemorrhages with white centres) can sometimes be found in the equatorial retina: they are a sign of the anaemia and are not necessarily a feature of subacute bacterial endocarditis.

## Sickle cell retinopathy

Patients with sickle cell disease from various haemoglobinopathies may develop a retinopathy that reflects both their anaemia and the specific disease. Changes are found in the peripheral retina which will be missed unless the patient is examined with dilated pupils. In the equatorial retina, decreasing arterial calibre and relative hypoxia are said to produce sickling, leading to arterial occlusion. Examination shows sclerosis of peripheral arteries and veins with anastomotic channels between them. This produces hypoxia, and neovascularization of the retina may appear along the junction of normal and abnormal retina in a similar way to that in a diabetic eye. These peripheral fronds of neovascularization look like fronds of West Indian coral and by analogy are known as 'sea fans' (Plate 12.5). In common with neovascular tissue in the eye from other causes they may bleed to produce vitreous haemorrhage, fibrosis and retinal detachment. Sickle cell retinopathy, however, has a fairly good prognosis and a relatively benign natural history so that laser photocoagulation is only needed in special situations. Furthermore, photocoagulation of the peripheral retina carries the danger of making the retinopathy move centripetally with more risk to central vision.

## Hypertensive retinopathy

The eye has two sources of vascular supply—the retinal and choroidal circulation—and hypertensive changes can be seen in both. Some idea of the acuteness, severity and duration of hypertension can be obtained from the fundal appearances.

Longstanding hypertension produces compensatory changes in the retinal arteries, which are, by histological criteria, arterioles. The arterial wall becomes hyperplastic and thickened, leading to an increased light reflex from the wall and nipping of the underlying vein where it crosses under the artery. At this point both vessels share a common fascial sheath and the thickened arterial wall compresses the underlying vein; for this reason, hypertension is a common finding in retinal branch vein occlusions. Changes in the muscular layer of the artery lead to segments of focal narrowing and dilation in the artery as well as generalized constriction of the vessel (Plate 12.6). These changes are difficult to differentiate from the normal arteriosclerotic changes of ageing. 'Blind viewing' trials of retinal photographs have shown that the changes of essential hypertension cannot be accurately differentiated from those of arteriosclerosis without further clinical information: arteriovenous crossing would have a different significance in a 20-year-old compared to a 70-year-old patient.

More severe hypertension leads to a failure of autoregulation and transmission of the high arterial pressure to the retinal capillary bed. Fibrinoid necrosis can be found pathologically in the vessel wall and with this cotton-wool spots and haemorrhages are seen in the fundus, particularly in the posterior pole. Ischaemia of the small vessels in the disc produces swelling of the optic disc (Plate 12.7). The choroidal arterioles are said to be wider and shorter than the retinal vessels and, with acute hypertension, they allow the arterial pressure to be transmitted more directly to the choroidal capillary network, leading to breakdown of the outer blood–retina barrier to produce exudative retinal detachments or choroidal infarcts. Exudative retinal detachments may cause the patient to present with blurred vision but such extreme ocular pathology is rare, being seen, for example, in severe pre-eclamptic toxaemia. The retinal detachment settles rapidly with control of the blood pressure.

In the past, hypertensive retinopathy was classified into four groups of increasing severity. It has now been appreciated that groups 1 and 2 (silver wiring, copper wiring, attenuation and nipping) represent compensatory arterial changes; they cannot be differentiated easily from each other or from arteriosclerosis without recourse to further clinical information and are now grouped together as compensated hypertensive retinopathy. Stage 3 (cotton-wool spots, haemorrhages) and stage 4 (additional optic disc swelling) are an artificial separation and are now classified as accelerated hypertensive retinopathy. It is important not to confuse other focal retinal pathology, such as branch or central retinal vein occlusion, with hypertensive changes, although these are often found in hypertensive patients.

Swelling of the optic disc in hypertension is probably due to local ischaemic and hypoxic changes in the disc itself rather than raised intracranial pressure, although such severely ill patients may have coexisting hypertensive encephalopathy. With severe swelling it is particularly important to control the blood pressure slowly, as abrupt falls can lead to infarction of the disc and blindness. As the swelling of the disc resolves a macular star of lipid deposition frequently appears, most prominently on the nasal side of the macula. It may cause some blurring of vision before the lipid absorbs over several weeks, usually with visual recovery. Patients with renal failure with decompensated hypertensive retinopathy have a tendency to develop widespread deposition of hard exudates throughout the retina.

From the fundal appearance, therefore, the physician can determine whether the patient has compensated arterial changes, and by the degree and severity of these obtain some idea of the state of the vascular tree elsewhere in the body and the duration of the disease. Acute accelerated hypertension produces a retinopathy in which compensatory arterial changes have not had time to evolve. Other patients can be seen to have compensatory changes, indicating that the hypertension has decompensated after an acute on chronic course.

## Diabetic retinopathy

The major risk factor for diabetic retinopathy is duration of disease and the longer this is, the more likely it is that changes will be seen in the eye. There is also a difference between early- and late-onset diabetics: after 10 years of insulin-dependent diabetes about half of patients will show evidence of retinopathy whereas non-insulin dependent patients may reach this incidence after five years. Hypertension and renal failure may also influence the onset of retinopathy but not to the same extent as does duration. These conditions will also produce their own characteristic changes and it is not uncommon for diabetic patients to have a composite retinopathy that reflects this (i.e., both diabetic and hypertension changes in the same eye).

There is good eveidence to suggest that meticulous control of the diabetes retards the development of retinopathy but once retinopathy is established the influence of establishing good control is more complex. Patients with background retinopathy may initially deteriorate more than poorly controlled patients for one to two years before faring relatively better. With neovascularization, good control can lead to an initial deterioration of the retinopathy, probably through alterations in retinal blood flow. These changes are, however, of more interest to the ophthalmologist and it is sensible to advise all patients to maintain the best possible control of their diabetes. Other factors, such as hormonal influences, are also important in the pathogenesis of diabetic retinopathy. Retinopathy does not occur before puberty and it deteriorates substantially with pregnancy. All pregnant diabetics require careful ocular monitoring throughout pregnancy with treatment of retinopathy along the established lines; diabetic retinopathy is not an indication for abortion. After delivery the retinopathy tends to improve. Patients with optic atrophy, glaucoma, retinal atrophy, high myopia or vascular insufficiency of the eye may be protected from retinopathy, prob-ably because of the lower metabolic demands of the eye, and this can explain cases of highly asymmetrical ocular involvement.

The hallmark of diabetic retinopathy are micro-aneurysms, and whilst these can be found in other retinopathies, they never occur in the same profusion. The other early features are blot haemorrhages and areas of capillary closure. Hard exudation and cotton-wool spots appear later. The earliest changes in diabetic retinopathy are restricted to the capillary circulation and changes are not seen in the major retinal arteries and veins until later in the disease. The retinal changes of diabetes are unique, too, not being found in the microvascular bed of any other organ in the body.

The management of diabetic retinopathy has been greatly aided by classification (Fig. 12.1) and understanding of the types of retinopathy. Although a few patients may present with a retinopathy as the first sign of diabetes, retinopathy does not affect vision until the macula or vitreous is involved. (For this reason patients cannot be screened by visual acuity alone.) The earliest changes seen are microaneurysms and haemorrhages (dots and blots) with small areas of capillary closure and later hard exudates in the posterior pole of the eye. Frequently the earliest changes are found in the area temporal to the macula in the watershed between the superior and inferior temporal arteries. This early retinopathy is known as 'background' retinopathy and these patients have normal vision. From here, the retinopathy can deteriorate in two main ways (see Fig. 12.1). Most patients (70 per cent) lose vision from macular involvement as a result of deposition of hard exudate, macular oedema or ischaemic changes. This is known as a 'maculopathy' and whilst these patients may become legally blind (visual acuity less than 6/60) they still retain enough peripheral retina and navigating vision to

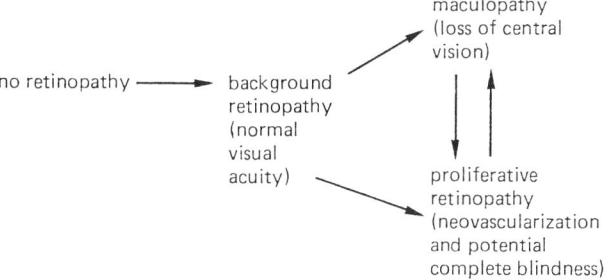

*Figure 12.1* Flow diagram of diabetic retinopathy.

lead independent lives (Plate 12.8). The other group are those that predominantly develop capillary closure and retinal hypoxia (Plate 12.9). This stimulates neovascularization, which occurs on the retina at the junction of healthy and abnormal tissue, on the optic disc and eventually on the iris, leading to neovascular glaucoma—this is normally a terminal event for the eye. Initially, the neovascularization lies flat on the retinal surface but changes occur in the vitreous gel, which contracts pulling the frond of neovascularization forwards and proliferating on the retrohyaloid surface. (The vessels do not actually penetrate the gel itself.) These vessels are fragile: they rupture with minor trauma, producing retinal or vitreous haemorrhage, and stimulate fibrosis with traction on the retina producing detachment. This is sometimes known as retinitis proliferans. This group of patients with neovascularization is classified as having a 'proliferative' or 'neovascular' retinopathy (Plate 12.10). This is an extremely serious complication as it leads to complete blindness; long-term studies have shown that an untreated patient with neovascularization has a 70 per cent chance of becoming completely blind in that eye over a 5-year period. Other signs of diabetic retinopathy are cotton-wool spots, which indicate microvascular ischaemia, and beading of retinal veins. Both of these are signs of retinal ischaemia, indicating that the patient should be followed more carefully, and some authorities subclassify these patients as having a 'preproliferative' retinopathy. Although the classification into maculopathy or proliferative retinopathy is helpful in managing patients, both types may coexist in the same eye.

All diabetic patients should have their eyes and corrected visual acuity checked annually and those with loss of acuity or neovascularization should be referred for treatment. Cataracts are, of course, more common in diabetes and eminently treatable by conventional surgery. Neovascularization is an absolute indication for panretinal photocoagulation. This involves treating the peripheral retina with approximately 2000 laser burns. The supposed rationale of the treatment is to convert hypoxic retina to ischaemic retina, so reducing its metabolic demand. After a successful panretinal photocoagulation, neovascularization regresses to inert fibrous tissue in a few weeks. The macula is not treated and visual acuity is retained but the patient may notice some constriction of the visual field and poor night vision. Maculopathy is more difficult to treat and only those with good acuity and focal areas of leakage and lipid deposition respond to treatment by destroying the focal areas of leakage with laser burns. To get full advantage from this, these patients should be referred before their acuity has fallen below 6/12; after this, permanent retinal damage occurs, which prevents visual improvement despite successful treatment of the retinopathy. Macular oedema and ischaemia may be treated by grid photocoagulation which may retard progressive visual loss. There is no longer any role for pituitary ablation (which was effective) in the treatment of retinopathy and no drugs have so far been shown to influence the outcome. Aldose reductase inhibitors, however, show potential and trials with these drugs are now commencing. Initial results though are discouraging. Vitreoretinal surgery can be worthwhile in carefully selected patients with visual loss from severe retinopathy with vitreous haemorrhage, retinal traction or detachment. This type of surgery is highly sophisticated and time consuming and may involve removing a cataractous lens as well as vitreous haemorrhage, and dissection of preretinal fibrosis with removal of membranes to flatten a retinal detachment—all in the same procedure.

## INFLAMMATORY EYE DISEASE

### Episcleritis

Episcleritis produces a localized area of redness on the surface of the globe. Patients usually complain of minor irritation and discomfort and may get frequent relapses. It responds well to topical steroids. Ocular complications are few and the prognosis good. It is rarely associated with systemic disease, although some patients may have bowel problems.

### Scleritis

This is a much more serious condition than episcleritis, being associated with serious ocular problems and systemic disease. It is commonly associated with collagen disorders, gout, herpes zoster ophthalmicus or local trauma. It can affect the anterior or posterior sclera, normally producing a localized area of redness of much more intensity than episcleritis, and is often extremely painful, which is a useful differentiating symptom.

Examination with a slit lamp shows that the sclera is thickened and oedematous and sometimes signs of scleral thinning are apparent, revealing the bluish-black appearance of the choroid through the thinned sclera. If necessary a drop of adrenaline 1:1000 applied topically will blanch the conjunctival and episcleral vessels revealing the scleritis more clearly. Posterior scleritis can be associated with severe pain, proptosis and limited ocular movement. Inflammation from the sclera may overspill to involve the cornea, iris or choroid, producing keratitis, iritis or choroiditis. Visual loss from cataract, glaucoma or retinal involvement is common and damage to the optic nerve can occur with posterior scleritis. Cases of scleritis require systemic non-steroidal anti-inflammatory drugs or steroids to control the ocular disease.

Scleromalacia perforans is a specific condition occurring in longstanding seropositive rheumatoid patients. The sclera becomes ischaemic from vasculitis, melts and absorbs in a white eye, without much pain or many inflammatory signs, revealing the bluish-black underlying choroid. Perforation of the globe is rare but vision is frequently lost from other ocular complications.

## Uveitis

The uveal tract consists of the iris, ciliary body and choroid lying in continuity with each other; apart from the specialized functions of the pupil and accommodation it is basically concerned with the nutrition of the eye. Uveitis can be divided into anterior, posterior or panuveitis, depending on which part of the eye is principally affected, but it is not surprising that a severe inflammation in one area may produce overspill inflammation in another, i.e., a choroiditis may show signs of anterior uveitis, or inflammation in the cornea or sclera may show signs of uveitis. Uveitis is also an important component of surgical or traumatic injury to the eye.

Anterior uveitis can be subdivided into acute or chronic types but this is not a rigid classification: an acute anterior uveitis can become chronic or a chronic anterior uveitis may have acute exacerbations. Redness, pain of an aching nature, photophobia and watery discharge are signs of acute anterior uveitis (iritis). Vision is blurred if the ocular media are obscured by inflammatory exudate.

Examination of the eye will show infection (redness) in the circumcorneal or limbal area, which is known as ciliary infection; in this region the conjunctival and intraocular circulations anastomose. Slit lamp examination shows signs of increased vascular permeability within the anterior chamber with leakage of protein (flare) and cells (leucocytes) in the aqueous humour. These may precipitate on the back of the cornea and are known as keratitic precipitates; adhesions form between the iris and anterior lens capsule (posterior synechiae). With acute anterior uveitis the visual prognosis is generally good but vision can sometimes be lost from glaucoma, cataract or macular oedema. Most patients can be treated adequately with topical steroids and atropine; subconjunctival steroid injections can be useful but systemic steroids are rarely needed.

Chronic anterior uveitis produces a white or whiter eye, fewer cells in the anterior chamber but more proteinaceous flare, and a more protracted clinical course, extending over at least three months. Many of these patients are said to have a granulomatous type of uveitis and by this is meant that the keratitic precipitates have a whitish, globular, 'mutton fat' appearance. Some of these patients may have an underlying 'granulomatous' disorder such as sarcoidosis, tuberculosis, toxoplasmosis or syphilis, but frequently no evidence of systemic disease can be found.

The systemic associations of acute anterior uveitis are numerous but in the absence of specific clinical indications the new, 'idiopathic' case requires a blood count and ESR, serology for syphilis and X-rays of the chest and sacroiliac joints. About half of patients with acute anterior uveitis will be HLA B27-positive. The most common associations in British practice of acute anterior uveitis are ankylosing spondylitis, sarcoidosis and Reiter's syndrome. Chronic anterior uveitis can also be associated with these diseases as well as with juvenile pauciarticular arthritis, which can present as an entirely white eye with visual loss from cataract, glaucoma or band keratopathy. Ocular problems are particularly common in girls with seronegative pauciarticular disease who are antinuclear antibody-positive and these children require regular screening for ocular complications.

Posterior uveitis is, if anything, an even more nebulous entity than anterior uveitis. Many cases have a nonspecific ocular appearance and no underlying systemic disease. The presenting symptoms are normally 'floaters' or blurred vision from cellular infiltration of the vitreous gel or macular oedema. The eye is white unless there is significant overspill inflammation into the anterior chamber. Examination shows a vitreous cellular infiltrate, sometimes with accumulations of cells in the gel, known as 'snowballs'. Depending on the type of posterior uveitis there may be additional signs of retinal vasculitis, infiltration over the pars plana, macular oedema, swelling of the optic disc or focal choroiditis. Patients lose vision from cataract, glaucoma or macular oedema and retinal destruction.

Toxoplasmosis can usually be diagnosed from the typical fundal appearances, which are areas of focal, pigmented scarring in one or both eyes, usually in the posterior pole. Toxoplasmosis cannot be diagnosed in the absence of these chorioretinal scars. It is almost always due to congenital transplacental infection; acquired ocular disease is rare. The scars remain asymptomatic and quiescent but may reactivate in young adults when a vitreous infiltrate with a fluffy whitish area of chorioretinitis will be seen around the lesion (Plate 12.11). Relapses may vary from mild to severe and may require treatment with systemic steroids and clindamycin to prevent or limit further retinal damage. Most patients have a limited number of relapses. The toxoplasma dye test is always postitive but the titres do not correspond with the severity of the ocular inflammation. Toxocariasis is much rarer than toxoplasmosis and is usually seen in children who have contact with puppies; strangely there is usually no history of associated visceral larva migrans. The ocular disease is unilateral with peripheral or central retinal granulomas being found, and a diagnosis can usually be made on the morphology of the ocular disease and confirmed by finding a positive test for *Toxocara* by enzyme-linked immunosorbent assay.

Pars planitis is one of the commonest causes of posterior uveitis and represents a morphological ocular syndrome. Systemic investigation is almost always unhelpful but a few patients can have associated sarcoidosis or multiple sclerosis. The disease affects one or both eyes in young adults. Systemic steroids are often required to control the disease, which eventually burns out after a protracted course with relapses and remissions over many years.

About a quarter of patients with sarcoidosis get ocular changes—either anterior uveitis, posterior uveitis or retinal vasculitis, and the ocular signs can produce relatively specific changes that can suggest the systemic diagnosis. As well as a vitreous cellular infiltrate, focal atrophy of areas of pigment epithelium may be seen, particularly in the inferior equatorial retina, and a focal periphlebitis of the smaller retinal veins is common, which can lead to venous occlusion and neovascularization. Similar retinal vascular changes can be seen associated with tuberculosis, particularly in people of Middle Eastern or Asiatic origin. Similar retinal vasculitis that is of idiopathic origin is sometimes known as 'Eales' disease' after the Birmingham ophthalmologist who first described the ocular changes.

Behçet's disease is associated with uveitis, which is the most serious aspect of the syndrome. It is important to inquire of all patients with uveitis whether they have suffered oral or genital ulceration. Other features of the disease are arthritis, skin lesions (erythema nodosum, pyogenic pustules), venous thrombosis and neurological involvement. The disease may produce anterior uveitis and a pronounced tendency to hypopyon but the most serious aspect is a severe posterior uveitis—usually in both eyes with retinal destruction from infiltrates, vasculitis, venous occlusions and neovascularization. Although the disease is usually recognized in people of Middle Eastern or Far Eastern origin it is being increasingly found in British caucasian patients, though often in a less dramatic and milder form. The diagnosis is made on clinical grounds but there is a high frequency of HLA B51 in patients with ocular disease and it has been surmised that a genetic susceptibility to the disease lies along the pathway of the old silk routes across Asia. Patients virtually always require systemic therapy to control their disease. Frequently, systemic steroids are insufficient and cytotoxic drugs such as azathioprine or chlorambucil are necessary. Cyclosporin A is effective but at the expense of serious side-effects if the drug is not carefully monitored.

## THYROID EYE DISEASE

Orbital involvement is common in patients with a history of thyroid disease. Usually the patient is thyrotoxic and the orbital signs start within the first two years after diagnosis, but thyroid eye disease can occur in hypothyroid and euthyroid patients and may precede the hormonal changes or occur many years later when the endocrine

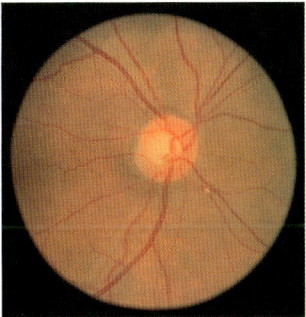

**Plate 12.1.** A cholesterol crystal impacted at the bifurcation of the inferior nasal branch retinal artery.

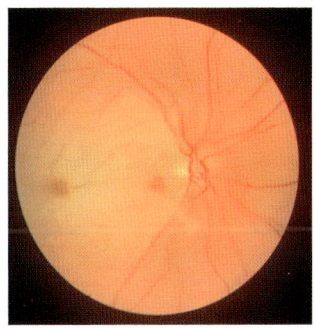

**Plate 12.2.** An acute central retinal artery occlusion showing a "cherry red" spot at the macula. No emboli can be seen in the retinal circulation.

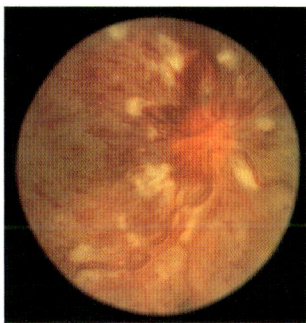

**Plate 12.3.** A central retinal vein occlusion with ischaemic changes. Note the swelling of the optic disc and the cotton wool spots.

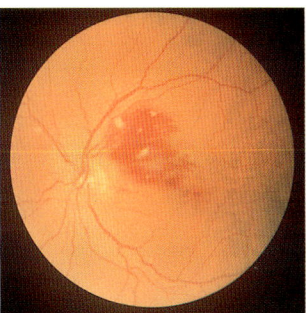

**Plate 12.4.** A branch retinal vein occlusion.

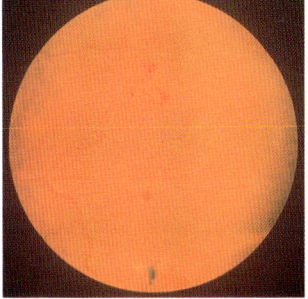

**Plate 12.5.** A view of the peripheral fundus in a patient with HbSC disease. There is avascularity of the peripheral retina and abnormal anastomoses between the arteries and veins. Note the early fronds of neovascularization at the junction between normal and abnormal retina.

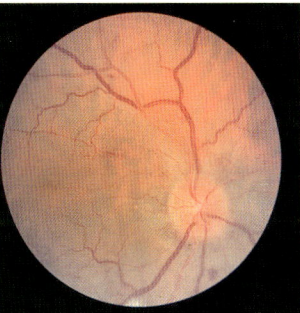

**Plate 12.6.** Hypertensive retinopathy. Retinal haemorrhages are present. Note the arteriovenous crossing changes and arterial attenuation which suggest that there has been time for compensatory changes to occur in the arteries.

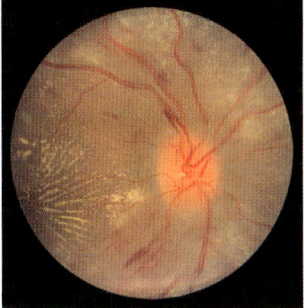

**Plate 12.7.** Acute malignant hypertension in the resolving phase. Note the macular star.

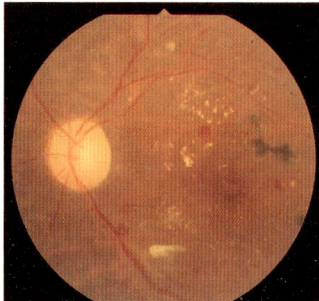

**Plate 12.8.** Diabetic maculopathy. The pigmented area temporal to the macula are previous laser burns.

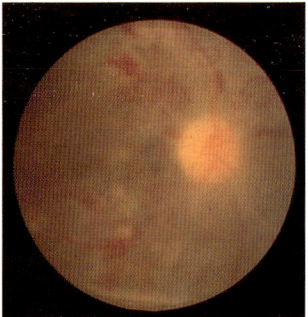 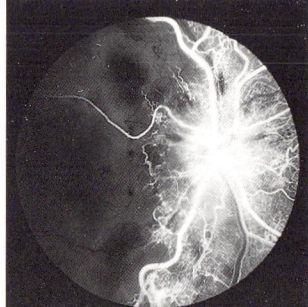

**Plate 12.9.** (a) and (b). Colour photograph and fluorescein angiogram in a patient with severe diabetic retinopathy. The fluorescein angiogram shows gross capillary closure temporal to the optic disc and although neovascularization is not apparent as yet its appearance is imminent.

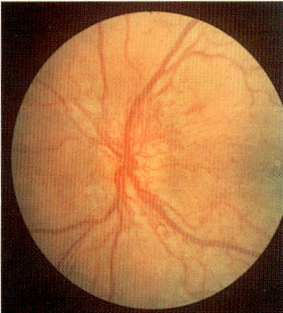 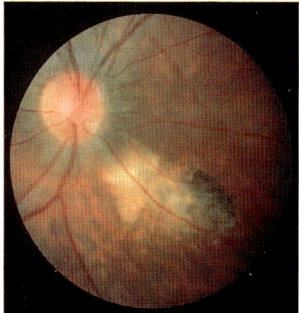 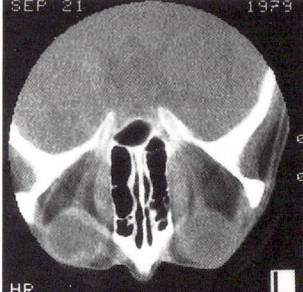

**Plate 12.10.** Neovascularization of the optic disc with proliferative diabetic retinopathy.

**Plate 12.11.** Toxoplasmic chorio-retinitis with reactivation (fluffy white area) adjacent to a previous congenital scar.

**Plate 12.12.** Orbital CT scan of a patient with thyroid eye disease.There is hypertrophy of the medial rectus muscle in each orbit.

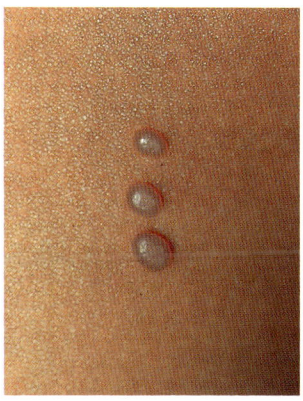

**Plate 13.1.** Skin coloured dome shaped umbilicated papules of Molluscum Contagiosum

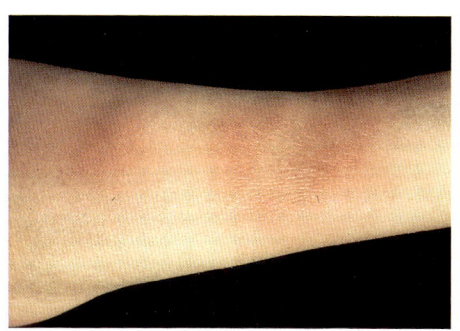

**Plate 13.2.** Erythema Nodusum

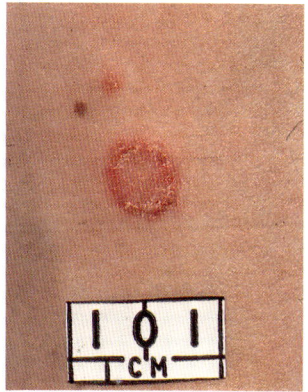

**Plate 13.3.** Tinea Corporis (with peripheral scale)

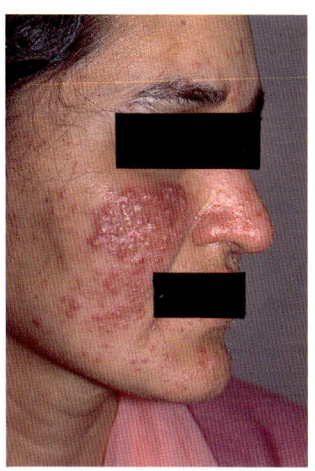

**Plate 13.4.** Acne Rosacea

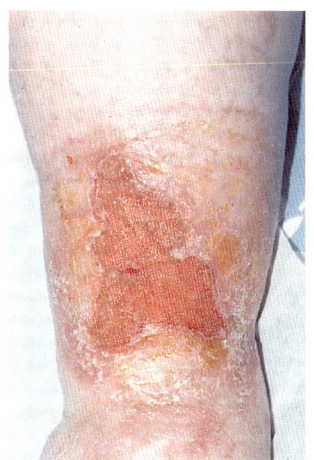

**Plate 13.5.** Chronic venous ulcer

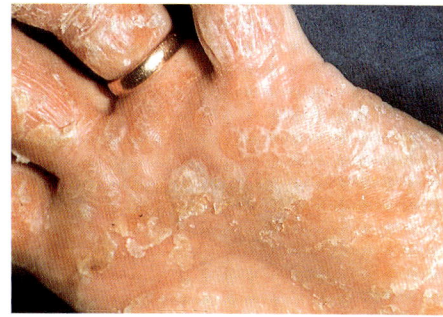

**Plate 13.6.** Acute vesicular hand eczema (Pompholyx)

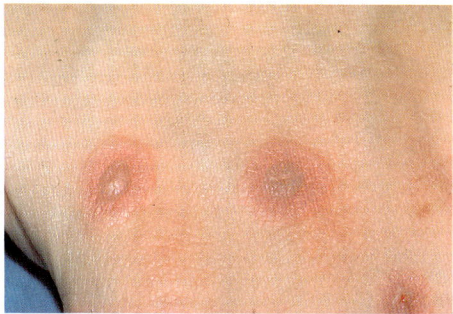

**Plate 13.7.** 'Target' lesions erythema multiforme showing concentric rings with central bulla

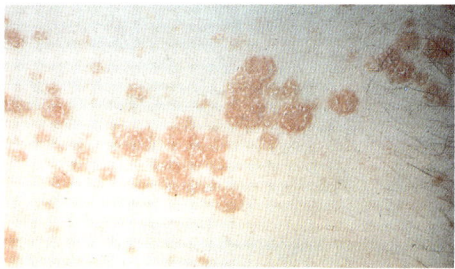

**Plate 13.8.** Small well-defined erythematous scaly plaques of psoriasis

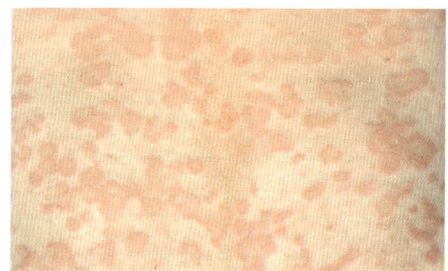

**Plate 13.9.** Acute urticaria

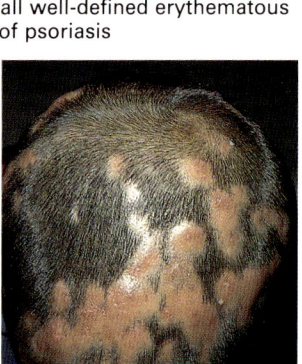

**Plate 13.10.** Patchy motheaten hair loss of scalp ringworm (Tinea Capitus)

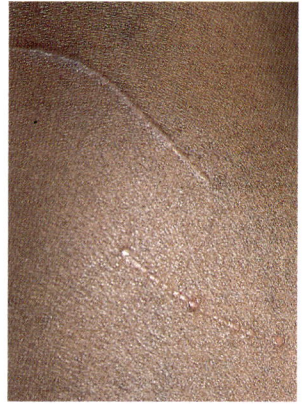

**Plate 13.11.** The appearance of skin lesions in lines of trauma (scratch marks). Lichen planus.

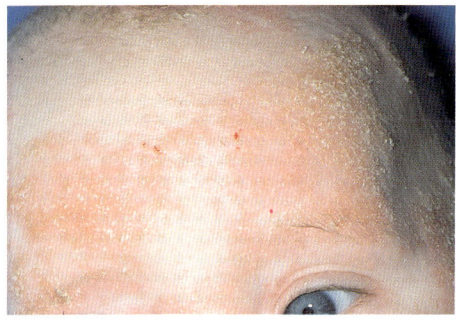

**Plate 13.12.** Atopic eczema. Crusted erythematous lesions

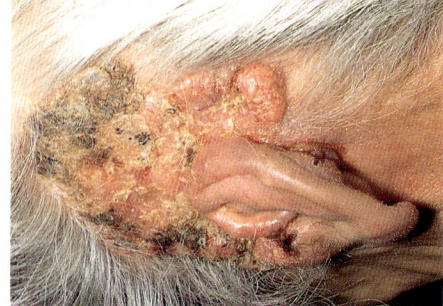

**Plate 13.13.** Basal cell carcinoma. Rolled edge to ulcer

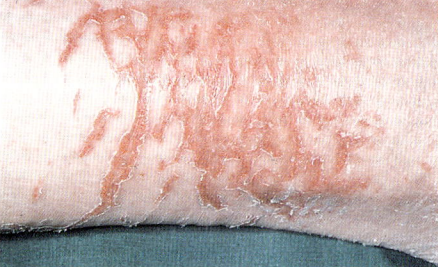

**Plate 13.14.** Eczema craquelé. Linear cracks of eczema

changes have been apparently successfully controlled for a considerable time. The primary pathology lies in the orbital muscles, which become infiltrated with lymphocytes, mucopolysaccharides and oedema so that they become hypertrophied to many times their normal size. Lid lag and retraction are usually consistent signs, and the proptosis is due to the increased orbital volume from muscle hypertrophy. Patients require estimations of T3 and T4 and a search for thyroid autoantibodies. A high-resolution orbital CT scan with axial and coronal views is the definitive investigation (Plate 12.12). The orbital involvement may be highly asymmetrical. The inferior and medial recti are the earliest muscles to be involved; subclinical changes may be seen in other muscles or the other orbit.

Patients with thyroid eye disease may suffer from cosmetic problems from the lid retraction and proptosis and as they tend to be young and female this can be serious and should not be neglected. In many patients the appearance can be considerably improved by simple eyelid surgery. Corneal exposure is especially common in patients with acute orbital disease. Minor cases can be controlled by ointment and artificial tear drops. More severe cases require lid surgery to increase corneal cover, or orbital decompression. In view

of the primary pathology in the orbital muscles it is not surprising that diplopia is common. This is often both vertical and horizontal and requires specialized ophthalmic care. Whilst the orbital changes are unstable the diplopia must be controlled by patching one eye or using temporary prisms in spectacles; once the situation has stabilized, corrective surgery to the ocular muscles can be planned.

The most serious complication of thyroid eye disease is compression of the optic nerve. This occurs in about 5 per cent of cases and is caused by the hypertrophic muscle bellies in the tight confines of the orbital apex. It is particularly common in patients who have relatively little proptosis; those that have proptosis tend to decompress their own orbits. It is essential that all patients with orbital disease are asked at each outpatient visit whether or not their vision has changed as compression of the optic nerve is frequently overlooked. Other clinical signs, apart from a fall in visual acuity, are a relative afferent pupillary defect, poor colour vision and a central scotoma in the visual field. The optic disc may be swollen, normal or atrophic. Treatment lies initially in high-dose steroids; surgical decompression or orbital radiotherapy are useful in cases that fail to respond to steroids.

# 13

# DERMATOLOGY

Irene Leigh

## INTRODUCTION

Skin diseases are very common: 15 per cent of consultations in general practice concern skin problems. One in 10 of the Western population will experience eczema at some stage of their life; psoriasis affects another 1 to 2 million in the UK; 5 per cent of the population will experience the common physical urticarias—cholinergic and dermatographic; and, of course, >95 per cent of the population will meet the common skin viruses—wart virus (human papillomavirus) and herpes simplex virus.

The skin subserves many functions other than simply providing a barrier and protection, particularly in regard of sexual and social interaction. Damage to the skin by disease may cause problems of temperature control and fluid and electrolyte balance. The individual may also have systemic effects, such as fever, toxicity and malaise, and abraded skin can be penetrated by infection. Conversely, the skin can provide important and often disregarded clues in the diagnosis of systemic disease, which could allow invasive investigations to be bypassed—better surely a skin biopsy than a mediastinoscopy in the diagnosis of sarcoidosis. Unfortunately, doctors often fail to appreciate the significance of skin signs and simply do not see gross changes visible to the trained eye. Very fine discrimination of the enormous complexity of skin signs is undoubtedly an acquired skill but do not be misled by the apparent ease of diagnosis by the dermatologist. Pattern recognition is not the mainstay of diagnosis for the inexperienced. Patients don't match the pictures in the book, especially once they have received treatment. It is crucial to analyse the type and distribution of the skin lesions and follow a diagnostic pathway.

## TAKING A SKIN HISTORY

### Essential facts

(1) *Time course of the eruption*. The first essential is to develop a clear picture of the time course of the skin eruption. Did it evolve slowly or rapidly? Is it recurrent or persistent? In what order did the skin signs appear?

Patterning is often characteristic of a skin disease. Pityriasis rosea can often be diagnosed in retrospect given the history of a solitary lesion (herald patch) appearing in a pale-pink oval patch with a circle of scale, usually treated as ringworm, one week before the generalized eruption of similar small lesions, which last six weeks and then fade spontaneously.

The time course of the individual lesion may differ from the time course of the overall eruption—in urticaria, individual weals last for less than 24 h although urticaria may recur nightly for many weeks and the eruption appear continuous to the patient. It may be necessary to draw a ring around a lesion to establish the accurate time of disappearance.

Changes in the appearance of the skin lesions with time should also be noted—did the rash look different at the start? Are there any marks left when the rash fades?

(2) *Skin symptoms.*

  (a) Itching (pruritus): itching like pain has a widely variable individual threshold of tolerance so some rashes that are not supposed to cause itching, such as psoriasis, do so in some people. Itching is not a very useful differential diagnostic feature but is of tremendous importance to the patient—chronic itch is as miserable as chronic pain and may become unbearable so it needs to be acknowledged and treated even if only symptomatically. The patients, as well as those living and sleeping with them, may be kept awake by the constant rubbing and scratching. Severe itching will both stop the patient going to sleep and repeatedly wake them in the night, especially as the skin warms up in bed. Disturbed nights are common.

Atopic children particularly scratch at night and the repeated waking of the household may cause parental exhaustion and desperation.

(b) Burn, pain, tingling: ischaemic ulceration and infection can cause severe pain in leg ulcers. Some acute eczemas present with tingling or pricking discomfort rather like pins and needles.

(c) Systemic features: is there any fever, shivering, rigors or malaise referable to the skin disease?

(3) *Triggers*. Are there any triggers that can predictably reproduce the eruption? Physical triggers such as heat, cold, sweating, bathing, light touch and deep pressure are particularly important in urticarias. Food allergy can cause swelling of the tongue on eating the food or swelling of the hands on food handling, particularly in the atopic person.

## Personal past history

Previous skin diseases should be described or diagnosed as far as possible. Public knowledge of skin disease is low and that 'nervous rash' usually wasn't! A personal history of infantile eczema, asthma or hay fever is usually relevant in eczema patients. Atopics have an increased risk of hand dermatitis or industrial or domestic exposure to irritants. Many skin diseases are recurrent and patients often learn to manage them better than many doctors, so listen to their past response to therapy. The effects of pregnancy may be to aggravate psoriasis and eczema in addition to causing specific skin problems such as toxic erythema of pregnancy (near term) and herpes gestationis. A recent baby may be relevant in diffuse hair loss due to postpartum shifts in the hair-growing cycle. Past treatment of malignant or benign disease may be relevant to skin tumorigenesis. Skin diseases treated with X rays in the distant past include scalp ringworm, acne, pruritus and chronic eczema.

## Drug history

A drug history should detail every item of topical treatment such as over-the-counter creams and potions, including herbal and homeopathic medications. Previous applications may alter the appearance of a typical rash or may cause a supervening contact dermatitis. Inappropriate therapies are widely used—Dettol, TCP, etc. A drug history of ingested or inhaled agents is also relevant given the variety of drug eruptions that may mimic naturally occurring skin diseases. All drugs taken up to two weeks before the eruption should be noted. Patients often mistakenly think that only new drugs cause drug eruptions although in fact allergy can develop after any period of exposure. Patients should also be directly questioned about reagents they do not consider drugs—phenolpthalein-containing laxatives can cause a fixed drug eruption; quinine in tonic water can cause lichenoid eruptions. Contraceptives may alter the severity of acne and can cause pigmentary problems.

## Family history

Many skin diseases are genetically determined—psoriasis, eczema, icthyoses—and should be asked for by name in all the first-degree relatives. Other atopic features, such as hay fever and asthma in first-degree relatives, are also relevant. A family history of itching of recent onset strongly suggests scabies as does an itchy boyfriend or girlfriend—eczema isn't catching!

## Occupational history

Occupational history is very important in skin disease; industrial dermatitis is the major cause of claims for industrial disease benefit. It is not enough to know the patient's job title—a full job description is required particularly about industrial exposure to irritants and allergens, such as solvents, soaps, detergents, dyes, metals, oils, epoxy resins and contact adhesives.

## Recreational history

Hobbies can cause skin disease—woods and adhesives in woodwork and plaster and cement in do-it-yourself construction, for example. Frequent swimming may aggravate eczema. Sport may aggravate sweat-induced dermatoses. Recreational sun exposure is a major contribution to skin carcinogenesis: cumulative exposure in epitheliomas and sunburn in melanomas. Has the patient lived abroad? Does the patient sun worship or even work outdoors? Use of a sunbed is also likely to be carcinogenic.

### Personal habits

Elderly skin cannot tolerate soap and detergent so bathing with bubble bath or use of a soap-filled flannel for a daily wash down may be contributing to elderly pruritus. Cleansing of dentures may be inadequate, contributing to chronic oral candidiasis. Patients may be aggravating skin problems by the use of strong irritants (TCP, Dettol) on the flexural skin in particular.

Cosmetics, perfumes and over-the-counter creams contain multiple allergens and many cause cross-sensitivity due to a common ingredient. Again allergy can develop on chronic use—it is not necessary to have changed to the preparation recently. Patients often say 'it can't be allergy because it hasn't caused trouble before'. In fact, previous exposure for at least 5 to 21 days is essential to become allergic. Herbal remedies and 'natural' creams do not contain preservatives so may spread infection in addition to the risk of sensitization to the potent plant allergens.

### Social history

This should include the social consequences of skin disease for the patient. People react thoughtlessly to skin diseases and not every skin patient can shrug off the inevitable comments about appearance. Some shun relationships, particularly sexual, and some refuse to go out at all, especially in the teenage years. Job prospects are altered, especially in uniformed services, which may add to depression. Teenage atopics often rebel against parentally directed treatment and the eczema gets worse. Sexual preference should be determined as skin manifestations of acquired immune deficiency syndrome (AIDS) and secondary syphilis are more common in homosexual men at present.

### SKIN SIGNS

The analysis of skin signs depends on two components:
(a) the morphology of the individual skin lesion;
(b) the distribution of the skin lesions.

Plates 13.1 to 13.8 show some typical types of lesion.

### Morphology of the individual skin lesion
(Table 13.1)

The terminology used to describe skin lesions is rather cumbersome to learn but it is a language that helps diagnosis once you have acquired it. It is important to assess whether all skin lesions are the same or whether there is evolution with time or space—for example, steroid-induced acne is characterized by monomorphic lesions, usually papulopustules, all at the same stage of evolution, whereas in acne vulgaris, lesions are polymorphic with comedones, papules, pustules and scars occurring together. The colour of skin lesions varies enormously and also has implications for diagnosis (Table 13.2).

### Distribution of skin lesions

Most skin diseases produce well-defined, often symmetrical patterns (Table 13.3). If the patterning doesn't fit a particular disease, then it is worth considering exogenous factors such as drugs, which often mimic the natural disease. Other exogenous factors that have to be considered are ultraviolet radiation (photosensitivity), heat, plants and exposure to allergens on the skin (contact dermatitis, contact urticaria). In contact dermatitis the main clue to diagnosis lies in the distribution of skin lesions because the lesions only develop where the skin has actually been in contact with the allergen.

### *Photosensitivity*

Photosensitivity eruptions affect the areas maximally exposed to light—even where the whole body has been exposed the lesions will be denser in those areas exposed to light in everyday life. On the face, the bridge of the nose, over the cheekbones, the forehead and chin are affected but around the eyes and under the nose and chin are spared. The 'V' of the neck, the side and back of the neck in the short haired, and the back of the hands are prime targets. Chronic actinic dermatitis is an eczematous eruption of the photoexposed sites, varying from an exudative eczema to pebbly lichenification of juicy, infiltrated areas. Other photosensitive eruptions include the very common papular eruptions—polymorphic light eruption

**Table 13.1 Morphological types of skin lesion**

| Name | Description | Example |
|------|-------------|---------|
| Macule | Colour change only—no substance palpable | Freckle |
| Papule | Palpable, small | Lichen planus |
| Nodule | Palpable, spherical | Erythema nodosum |
| Plaque | Palpable, large | Psoriasis |
| Pustule | Pus-filled | Acne |
| Vesicle | Fluid-filled, small | Herpes simplex |
| Bulla | Large, fluid-filled sac with intact roof | Bullous pemphigoid |
| Erosion | Partial-thickness loss of epidermis | Impetigo |
| Ulcer | Full-thickness loss of epidermis | Venous ulcer |
| Telangiectasia | Visible, dilated venules | Spider naevi |
| Scale and hyperkeratosis | Loose skin surface (stratum corneum) often silver or yellow | Psoriasis |
| Crust | Dried serum/tissue fluid | Eczema |
| Atrophy | Loss of skin thickness giving paper-thin, wrinkled, featureless skin | Lichen sclerosis et atrophicus |
| Hypertrophy | Increase in skin thickness | Hypertrophic lichen planus |
| Excoriation | Removal by scratching | Prurigo |
| Lichenification | Increase in skin thickness but preservation of markings giving deep clefts | Atopic eczema |

**Table 13.2 Colour of skin lesions**

| Colour | Name (if any) | Implications |
|--------|---------------|--------------|
| Red | Erythema | Acute inflammation, e.g. cellulitis |
| Magenta | | Dermatomyositis |
| Purple | Violaceous | Lichen planus |
| Brown/black | Pigmentation | Iron or melanin deposition |
| Yellow | | Lipid-xanthomas/drug, e.g. mepacrine |
| Orange | | Carotenaemia |
| Green | | Pigment-producing bacteria e.g. *Pseudomonas* in leg ulcers/nails |

**Table 13.3 Distribution of skin lesions**

| Distribution | Example |
|--------------|---------|
| Flexor | Atopic eczema |
| Extensor | Psoriasis |
| Flexural | Intertrigo |
| Acral (centrifugal) | Erythema multiforme |
| Central (centripetal) | Chickenpox |
| Palmoplantar | Palmoplantar pustulosis |

and solar urticaria. Photosensitive drug eruptions also occur.

## Contact allergens (Table 13.4)

Contact urticaria is shown by wealing of the skin within minutes of contact with the allergen—usually food and on the hands. Contact dermatitis is a delayed hypersensitivity reaction: the patterning is the distinctive diagnostic feature, which varies with the allergen as the lesions appear mainly at sites of allergen contact. Nickel dermatitis affects 10 per cent of women, especially those with pierced ears. The dermatitis thus appears under jewellery, jean studs, watches, coin/key-containing pockets and hands that handle metal objects.

### Heat

Thermal injury causes burns of varying depth—full thickness being through the dermis, partial thickness with remaining dermal elements, and superficial just epidermal erosions. However, chronic low-grade heat will cause fixed, reticulate erythema and pigmentation—erythema ab igne.

### Plants

Allergic contact dermatitis to plants tends to affect the hands and face due to airborne exposure to the plant allergens or handling of plants. Classical examples of this are allergies to chrysanthemum and primula. Many plant reactions are urticarial (cf. nettle rash) but these occur within minutes and are usually obvious. Poison ivy dermatitis is a common cause of a severe contact dermatitis: because its onset is delayed the initiating contact may not be so obvious to the patient, and the rash

**Table 13.4 Common contact allergens**

| Allergen | Source | Site of dermatitis |
| --- | --- | --- |
| Nickel | Jewellery, coins, keys, jean studs | Wrists, ears, thighs, hands, discs on trunk |
| Dichromate | Cement, matches | Hands—widespread |
| Cobalt | Metal | As nickel plus paint, china |
| Rubber | Gloves | Back of hands/wrists |
| | Shoes | Contact areas of soles |
| Lanolin (wool alcohols) | Medicaments, cosmetics | Face, hands, treatment sites, e.g. leg ulcers |
| Neomycin | Eyedrops, eardrops, skin creams | Site of application |
| Paraphenylene diamine | Hair dye | Ears, eyes, neck |
| Formaldehyde resins | Clothing | Armpits, chest, neck |
| Azo dyes | Clothing + stockings | Dorsa of feet, thighs |
| Parabens | Preservatives in creams | Site of application |
| Chlorocresol | Preservatives in creams | Site of application |
| Dowicil 200 | Preservatives in creams | Site of application |
| Epoxy resin | Industrial exposure | Hands, face |

can even appear after departure from the country in which it was acquired. Phytophotodermatitis is a phototoxic response to the release by plants of bergapten, which is activated by light and causes streaky pigmented erythema, often blistering. Commonest causes are umbelliferous plants, such as cow parsley, and the distribution depends on what the patient was specifically doing in that field of hay. Usually only arms and legs are affected.

## Key additional signs

### Nail involvement

Nail involvement is characteristic of some skin diseases, particularly psoriasis, lichen planus and fungus infection. In psoriasis, the nails show fine pitting of the plate and separation of the plate from the nail bed (onycholysis); the combination of these changes is diagnostic. In fungus infections, onycholysis with destruction of the nail plate to give thick and crumbly nails (nail dystrophy) which affects individual nails asymmetrically. In lichen planus, there is destruction of the nail-growing area by inflammatory infiltration, often leaving a central triangle of residual nail—the wing or pterygium.

### Scalp/hair involvement

Psoriasis and seborrhoeic dermatitis commonly affect the scalp. The lesions in psoriasis are well-defined, hyperkeratotic plaques of erythema, but in seborrhoeic dermatitis, diffuse fine scaling and poorly defined erythema are more typical. Alope-

cia (hair loss) is unlikely in psoriasis or eczema. Much alopecia occurs without skin disease. Alopecia areata shows completely smooth, bald, growing circles due to autoimmune attack on the hair follicles. Other causes of alopecia tend to reduce the number of hairs rather than producing complete baldness; commonly these follow childbirth or illness, especially anaemia or thyroid disease. Male-pattern baldness in men and women (constitutional alopecia) shows a pattern of temporal recession and vertex thinning.

### Mucous membrane involvement

Aphthous ulceration of the mouth is very common, with sharply marginated, punched-out ulcers appearing for no apparent reason. Mucous membrane involvement occurs in a disparate group of skin diseases. In acute eruptions, such as erythema multiforme, painful aphthous-type ulceration usually heals within a few weeks. In pemphigus, mucosal ulceration is indolent, irregularly progressive and fails to heal. Mucous membrane involvement in lichen planus seldom ulcerates but forms a lacy pattern of white, coalescent papules on the buccal mucosa and tongue.

### Nail-fold changes

Nail-fold telangiectasia with secondary cuticle involvement giving a ragged appearance is a subtle and often early sign of connective tissue disease, much beloved of dermatologists. It does not distinguish between lupus erythematosus, scleroderma or dermatomyositis but other, equally subtle clues should be able to support the diagnosis. Nail-fold inflammation occurs in candidal paronychia, with separation of the nail fold from the nail allowing further maceration and invasion on exposure to water. This is the commonest form of paronychia, which may cause nail-plate infection and discoloured dystrophic nails with time. Nail-fold lesions occur in lichen planus: these purplish infiltrations presage nail damage so need to be treated aggressively otherwise the nail will be permanently destroyed (see above).

## MANAGEMENT AND THERAPY OF SKIN DISEASE

### Topical therapy—general principles

The basis of skin therapy is that drugs affecting the skin should be delivered to that organ in a way that spares systemic side-effects. As much therapy as possible should be applied to the surface of the skin—topical rather than systemic. Remember, though, that the skin can absorb many drugs, depending on their physical formulation, the area treated and the total dosage applied. This property is now being exploited in transdermal administration of drugs such as glyceryl trinitrate and scopolamine through adhesive patches. Systemic side-effects can therefore be obtained from topical therapy—for example, adrenal suppression from high-potency topical steroids.

### *Formulation*

The formulation of the topical reagent must be appropriate for the skin problem or the active ingredient will not reach the skin cells. The same drug, e.g., hydrocortisone, can be delivered in a variety of formulations—ointment, cream, lotion or paste.

(1) *Ointments* (unguentum). Ointments are mixtures of waxes, often paraffin-based, which are thick, greasy and sticky. They are immiscible with water and so should not be applied to wet or exudative skin—the effect will be the same as putting a lump of lard in a bucket of cold water: it will float off the surface. Ointments are very good greasing agents and so help to protect the skin surface and offer some insulation.

(2) *Creams*. These are emulsions of oil in water or water in oil. They have a high water content and may act inadvertently as sensitizers because they must contain a preservative to prevent bacterial contamination. They are miscible with water so can be used on exudative skin.

(3) *Lotions*. These may be (a) solutions of soluble reagent, e.g., potassium permanganate, or (b) suspensions of insoluble agents, e.g., calamine lotion. They cool the skin by evaporation and tend to have an astringent or drying effect.

(4) *Pastes*. Dermatological pastes are usually insoluble powders in an ointment base so they are very thick and sticky and cosmetically unacceptable. They deliver insoluble reagents to the skin (e.g., dithranol in Lassar's paste). Bandages impregnated with paste are very useful to occlude the skin surface of arms and legs (unfortunately not of head and neck!) in atopic children, and in exudative eczemas of the lower legs in stasis eczema, or where rubbing and excoriation is a problem, as in lichen simplex chronicus or self-induced injury (dermatitis artefacta).

### Topical therapy—active ingredients

### *Topical steroids*

Topical steroids are potent anti-inflammatory re-agents that provide the mainstay of treatment in a wide range of skin problems, particularly eczemas. They suppress appropriate inflammation due to infection as well as less appropriate inflammation in skin disease so they tend to encourage the spread of bacterial and fungal infections. They should not, therefore, be used unless a firm diagnosis has been made—'blunderbuss' therapy 'just in case' should be avoided: a dermatological opinion should be sought in diagnostic difficulties. Topical steroids vary in potency, related to the steroid molecule itself and also to the absorption and penetration of the steroid. A range of potency from weak to very strong is available, and progression up or down the potency scale is logical. The lowest possible potency of steroid should always be used and movement towards lower potency is always the aim. However, the potency selected depends on the natural history of the disease: it may be good therapy to treat a severe acute eczema with a potent steroid but not a chronic lichenified eczema. In addition, some diseases are only steroid responsive at higher potency, e.g., lupus erythematosus, lichen planus.

Side-effects of steroids are predictable: application of high-potency steroids over a large area will cause adrenal suppression and, in children, growth retardation. Thus children should only receive low-potency steroids. Cutaneous side-effects centre on the atrophic action on subcutaneous tissue—wrinkled, cigarette-paper skin with telangiectasia—or on the spread of infection, which is the reason for including antibacterial agents and antibiotics in many steroids. Potent topical steroids on the face can cause an acneiform eruption (perioral dermatitis/rosacea) so only weak steroids should be used there. Flexural skin absorbs steroids well due to skin occlusion so lower potency steroids should be used there.

### Emollients

Dry skin needs grease, partly to prevent water loss and partly to increase the cohesion of the surface scale. This is particularly important in atopic children and elderly patients. The emollients range from simple oils, such as liquid paraffin, arachis oil and waxes, and including the emulsifying ointments and Vaseline (white soft paraffin, yellow soft paraffin), to more complex formulations. The grease from sheep wool can be extracted by alcohol, and these wool alcohols are good emollients (called lanolin rather than sheep grease) that provide the base of many dermatological medicaments and cosmetics. However, wool alcohols are allergens (see below) and care is needed in their use. Atopic children have reduced contact hypersensitivity so can often use lanolin-based emollients.

### Other active ingredients

(1) *Coal tar* is antimitotic and anti-inflammatory, the first-line treatment of psoriasis. Crude coal tar is very effective (1–10 per cent) but black and messy so the alcoholic extracts of coal tar (liquor picis carbonis; LPC) are more commonly used (e.g., 6 per cent liquor picis carbonis in yellow soft paraffin).

(2) *Dithranol* is a highly concentrated tar product containing antimitotic activity. It is very insoluble and as a paste is usually used for in-patient treatment. Cream forms are available and are better tolerated in outpatients. Dithranol is irritant and burns normal skin so must

be accurately applied in low concentrations (0.05–2 per cent). Short contact (half an hour) therapy can be used for outpatients and is effective.

(3) *Keratolytics*. Salicylic acid, benzoic acid and lactic acid desquamate the skin and help peel off hyperkeratoses such as warts, corns, psoriatic scale and icthyotic skin. They also peel off fungus-infected squames and are widely used over the counter for athlete's foot. They enhance penetration of other drugs.

(4) *Antifungal agents*. Potent fungicidal agents now exist, such as clotrimazole, miconazole and econazole. They are non-toxic but cannot penetrate hair roots or nails so ringworm of the scalp and nails must be treated systemically with griseofulvin or terbinafine. Imidazoles are also effective against candida and other skin organisms.

(5) *Antibiotics*. Many antibiotic preparations are allergenic so antiseptic agents are preferable. Topical antibiotics are now in use for acne—clindamycin, erythromycin and tetracycline in lotion form.

(6) *Antibacterial agents*. Antiseptics are less of a problem as potential sensitizing agents although they can be irritant and cytotoxic to newly forming epithelia. Most release iodine (povidone iodine), chlorine (sodium hypochlorite) or oxygen (hydrogen peroxide). Chlorhexidine is also useful especially against Gram-positive organisms. Most antiseptics are inactivated by tissue exudate.

(7) *Sulphur* is a traditional remedy having anti-scabies, antiyeast, antibacterial and anti-inflammatory effects. It is helpful in seborrhoeic dermatitis and other infectious eczematides.

(8) *Gamma benzene hexachloride lotion*. This insecticide is used in the treatment of scabies by whole-body applications (except face) of three treatments. All people in contact with the patient must be treated at the same time. Itching continues for 7 to 10 days because of the dead mites.

### Topical therapy—side-effects

Apart from the side-effects of the active ingredients, a major risk in skin therapy is the development of allergic contact dermatitis to a topical reagent—'dermatitis medicamentosa'—or irritancy of the ingredients.

## Allergic contact dermatitis

The development of an allergic reaction through the skin is common and a well-known reason for a worsening of the skin rash or a failure to heal. If in doubt the medication should always be stopped as the reaction will subside in 7 to 10 days. The ingredients that cause allergic contact dermatitis in medicaments are:

(1) *Bases*, e.g., lanolin.
(2) *Preservatives* in creams and cosmetics—parabens, chlorocresol, formaldehyde, dowicil 200.
(3) *Active ingredients*, e.g., antibiotics especially neomycin, gentamicin: once a patient has been sensitized through the skin, a population of sensitized T cells circulates and systemic drug administration will trigger a generalized allergic response, so antibiotics that are essential for systemic administration, e.g., gentamicin, should not be given topically.

Primary sensitization is a classical delayed hypersensitivity response and takes 10 to 21 days to develop. Subsequent re-exposure to the allergen will cause a reaction in 48 to 96 h, which is the basis for patch testing.

*Rules*:

Use ointments not creams.

Consider ingredients and if a reaction is suspected, use an unrelated drug and remove preservative in the base.

No antibiotics.

No systemic drugs.

Listen to the patient.

## Irritancy

Acids, alkalis and solvents are all irritants and can cause erythema and maceration of the skin but the effect of irritancy can be removed by resting, dilution or less frequent application. Irritancy is a particular problem in leg ulcers as it tends to cause pain in the ulcer and maceration around the ulcer edge.

## Intralesional steroids

Depot preparations of triamcinolone can be used intralesionally for lesions that are potentially steroid responsive but too thick to allow penetration of topical steroids. They are used for keloids, lupus erythematosus, alopecia areata and hypertrophic lichen planus/lichen simplex. As

they are difficult to inject through a syringe or needle, a high-pressure jet (Dermojet) is used.

## Systemic drug therapy

Some of the skin diseases mentioned here are described in the next section and some above.

## Antihistamines

Antihistamines are the treatment of choice in urticarias but the response is dose-dependent so the dosage needs to be increased steadily until the weals are controlled. Adequate dosage is often limited by the sedative effect so the new, peripherally acting antihistamines, such as terfenadine and astemizole, are useful. In pruritus a centrally acting drug is often helpful for anxiolysis and nocturnal sedation as the itch is often worse at night. Useful drugs are trimeprazine, hydroxyzine, promethazine, chlorpheniramine and brompheniramine. Atopic children with severe pruritus have an amazing tolerance of antihistamines and during exacerbations need very high dosage (although not more than 60 mg of trimeprazine, four times a day).

## Systemic steroids

These should only be used for skin disease by dermatologists. They are usually necessary to manage pemphigus and pemphigoid, pyoderma gangrenosum and sometimes erythrodermic eczema. They should be avoided if possible in atopic eczema because it may be difficult to wean the patient off them. They are not indicated in urticarias and toxic erythemas just because the acute eruption alarms the doctor. They may increase mortality in toxic epidermal necrolysis and Stevens–Johnson syndrome.

## Immunosuppression

Azathioprine is a useful adjunct to therapy in pemphigus and pemphigoid. It is also helpful in other immunological diseases such as chronic actinic dermatitis, lupus erythematosus and dermatomyositis. Side-effects are uncommon but the long term risk of lymphoma/leukaemia may be increased.

### Aromatic retinoids

An exciting group of drugs has been developed from retinoic acid and provides a new type of therapeutic weapon. Retinoids alter the keratinization and proliferation of the skin and have effects on intercellular adhesion and the sebaceous gland. Isotretinoin (1 mg/kg body weight) has revolutionized treatment of cystic acne and the aromatic retinoids (etretinate) are used in psoriasis and other keratinizing disorders. They have proved useful in the previously untreatable genodermatoses: icthyosiform erythrodermas, Darier's disease, palmoplantar keratoderma. The side-effects include cheilitis and mucous membrane fragility, hyperlipidaemia, hepatotoxicity and skeletal problems. They are only prescribable by dermatologists.

### Antimitotic drugs

Methotrexate has been used for severe psoriasis, pustular psoriasis and erythrodermic psoriasis since 1951 and is very useful systemic therapy. Haematological complications are uncommon in the regimens used (0.2–0.5 mg/kg body weight once per week orally) but hepatic fibrosis is a risk. Patients therefore have liver biopsies before this treatment and regularly after it (at 1.5 g accumulative dosage).

### Dapsone

Dapsone is the treatment of choice in dermatitis herpetiformis and linear IgA disease where the eruption can be dramatically switched on and off. Dosage ranges from 50 to 200 (up to 600) mg/day and problems are common, with dosage-dependent haemolytic anaemia being the most frequent. Dapsone is also helpful in other neutrophil-mediated skin disorders, such as pyoderma gangrenosum and leukocytoclastic vasculitis.

### Griseofulvin

Griseofulvin is systemically active against the dermatophytes that cause ringworm but not against candida or tinea versicolor. Dosage of 500 mg to 1 g/day can give idiosyncratic reactions with severe headache and nausea, but is usually well tolerated. Treatment needs to be given for six weeks to clear skin, 2 to 3 months for hair, 9 to 12 months to clear finger nails and 18 to 24 months to clear toe nails. Chronic nail carriers usually re-

infect themselves due to an immune defect to trichophyton so should not be treated unless there is a compelling reason. Ketoconazole is only indicated in chronic mucocutaneous candidiasis and systemic mycoses. It should not be used as an alternative to griseofulvin because of its hepatotoxicity. Terbinafine is an alternative for griseofulvin intolerant patients.

## Surgical treatment

### Cold-point cautery/Hyfrecator

A fine-point cautery needle can be used to diathermy and obliterate spider naevi, telangiectasis and small papular lesions. A tiny pinpoint scar will result.

### Cryotherapy

Cryotherapy is a useful tool but must not be used without a definite diagnosis. Cold injury from the liquid nitrogen causes separation of the skin through the dermo-epidermal junction so epidermal lesions tend to separate off with the blister roof. A cryotherapy gun is used: this directs a fine spray of liquid nitrogen at the lesion, which gradually turns white, and a spread of cold around the lesion in a ring is necessary to show cold penetration. Two freeze/thaw cycles are usually applied. Cryotherapy is useful in the treatment of warts and keratoses but should only be used for tumour therapy in the hands of a dermatologist. Epidermal cysts can also be treated by liquid nitrogen.

### Laser therapy

Lasers can be used to treat vascular lesions but there is always some scarring. Treating a substantial cavernous haemangioma is a very time-consuming business. Lasers cannot prevent skin ageing in spite of claims to the contrary in the lay press.

### Electrolysis

Electrolysis consists of passing a fine electrical probe down the shaft of a hair and passing a small current across the hair-growing area. Three treatments will permanently destroy hair and a skilled electrologist will treat about 100 hairs in a single session. To treat a hirsute face will take one to two years.

## Skin grafts (may need general anaesthetic)

If a defect after primary excision of a skin lesion is too large for primary closure, a number of procedures can be used to close the defect as healing from the edge tends to cicatrize (contracted scarring):

(1) *Split skin grafts.* A sheet of epidermis and upper dermis is shaved off in a continuous sheet using a keratotome—usually the donor site is on the thigh. The graft is sutured over the primary defect. The donor site heals over time from the edge and hair follicle and healing may be a problem in the elderly. The area of skin can be meshed using an instrument to punch holes regularly and then increasing the area.

(2) *Full thickness graft.* This procedure is used in reconstructive surgery and as it involves full thickness skin including fat, a blood supply must be taken with the graft.

(3) *Pinch grafts.* Small pieces of skin (1–2 mm) are taken from the donor site, often the thigh, under local anaesthetic and seeded as islands across the epidermal defect to provide foci of healing that migrate outwards and join together.

(4) *Culture grafting.* Skin grown in the laboratory by a variety of techniques provides a new technological advance in grafting that is very exciting but at an early stage of development.

## COMMON SKIN DISEASES

Various of these are shown in Plates 13.9 to 13.14.

## Eczemas

Eczema is a clinicopathological entity spanning a spectrum from acute to chronic. Acute eczemas are characterized by erythema, oedema and vesiculation with rapid formation of serous crusts, whereas in chronic eczema the skin is greatly thickened as a response to rubbing, with an increased depth of skin markings—lichenification. At the microscopic level, spongiosis (intercellular oedema) is often found, with spongiotic vesicles in the acute phase, and blunt acanthosis or thickening of the prickle cell layer in the chronic phase. Thus eczema is a well-defined entity.

There are many different patterns of eczema falling into two groups—endogenous and exoge-

**Table 13.5 The two groups of eczemas**

| Endogenous | Exogenous |
|---|---|
| Atopic eczema | Irritant dermatitis |
| Discoid eczema | Allergic contact |
| Vesicular hand/foot eczema | dermatitis |
| (pompholyx) | Photodermatitis |
| Seborrhoeic eczema | Phytodermatitis |
| Lichen simplex | Phytophotodermatitis |

nous (Table 13.5)—and they have typical time courses and patterns of skin involvement.

Atopic eczema is a most important endogenous eczema being inherited with a predisposition to asthma and hay fever. Any combination of the three features may be found in the patient or their first-degree relatives. The child usually develops widespread itchy patches of acute eczema within the first six months of life but by the age of 1 to 2 years the pattern changes to become predominantly flexural with marked lichenification. The pruritus makes the child and family miserable and is the major symptom to treat with antihistamines and frequent emollients. Weak topical steroids are very helpful.

Children with atopic eczema have impaired cell-mediated immunity and are vulnerable to disseminated herpes simplex (and previously vaccinia) infections, which should be treated as a potentially fatal dermatological emergency. They also suffer repeated staphylococcal infections due to widespread carriage of staphylococci on moist, eroded skin. Infections, food allergy, mite allergy and emotional upheaval all make eczema worse but there is no magic cure—95 per cent of children with atopic eczema are clear by the age of 15 years. A positive and consistent relationship with an experienced physician is essential through the ups and downs for severely affected families; unfortunately, these are the most vulnerable to the often misguided theories written of in the lay press and/or promoted by other therapists.

Chronic eczema of the hand is a common form of exogenous eczema and it is a major domestic and industrial problem. Chronic exposure to detergents, washing-up dishes, solvents, oils, soaps, etc. degreases the skin, which then becomes chronically inflamed with a dry, powdery surface and painful fissures. This is an irritant problem usually rather than allergy and simply due to cumulative insult. It is the major cause of industrial dermatitis in this country. Given adequate protection with avoidance of irritants, heavy plastic protective gloves and lashings of emollients and barrier creams, the skin will slowly recover but this is difficult and the problem may continue in the domestic worker until children are grown up and housework lessens. Workers in some occupations, such as hairdressers and nurses, often accept it as an occupational hazard. The individual threshold to irritant dermatitis varies greatly so workers in industry may have recurrent problems even after moving jobs.

### Psoriasis

Psoriasis is characterized by epidermal hyperproliferation and neutrophil-mediated inflammation. Although a genetically determined disease it usually manifests between the ages of 15 and 25 years but any age can be affected. The rapid cell turnover causes thick scaly well-defined erythematous plaques on the extensor aspects of elbows and knees, on the scalp, and also scattered truncal lesions. The surface is made of loosely attached silvery scales because of immature differentiation of keratinocytes. Nail and joint involvement occur in a substantial percentage of patients (15–20 per cent) and there are many clinical variants. Classical plaque psoriasis tends to improve in summer with ultraviolet radiation but also fluctuates with time. Most patients can be managed by coal tar, dithranol and ultraviolet radiation but patients who are erythrodermic or who have pustular or disabling psoriasis, may need systemic treatment with methotrexate, etretinate or PUVA (photochemotherapy with long-wave (A) ultraviolet irradiation).

### Acne vulgaris

Acne is normal. It is impossible to find someone who has never had a spot. Occlusion of the hair follicle by keratinous debris causes the blackhead or comedone. Inflammatory breakdown of lipid by *Proprionobacteria acnei* is associated with erythematous papules and pustules that rupture and may leave scars. Deep-seated inflammatory lesions may give cystic acne. Usually lesions are found at all stages of evolution in the acne areas—face, chest, back. As acne is androgen-dependent, women often have other androgenic features such as hirsutism and greasy skin. The social effects of acne should not be underestimated. Topical treatment with benzyl peroxide or retinoic acid or long-

term, low-dose antibiotics (oxytetracycline, 500 mg twice a day) will help most patients. Few patients with severe cystic acne will need isotretinoin orally.

### Skin cancer

Cancer of epidermal cells—basal cell carcinoma and squamous cell carcinoma—is usually caused by excessive, cumulative ultraviolet radiation, particularly from life in the subtropics in patients who have poor protective tanning ability. They are usually therefore on the sun-exposed sites, being maximal on the head and neck. Basal cell carcinomas are pearly nodular lesions, slow growing and sometimes ulcerating (rodent ulcer) but only locally invasive. Squamous cell carcinomas are more keratotic and may metastasize. A good prognosis usually follows radiotherapy, surgical excision, cryotherapy or local antimitotic agents.

Melanomas are different. For reasons that are incompletely understood, melanomas are greatly increasing in frequency and the incidence is doubling every ten years. Melanomas have several growth patterns: they can spread as nests of malignant melanocytes along the dermo-epidermal junction (junctional activity), or they can spread vertically into the dermis (nodular melanoma). Prognosis depends very much on the level of invasion and the thickness of the tumour so early diagnosis is crucial, especially as the tumours are poorly radiosensitive and not chemosensitive. Early excision is the rule. The critical clinical features suggesting the diagnosis are in Table 13.6; any pigmented lesion showing these features should be examined histologically. It is wise to err on the side of caution.

**Table 13.6 Signs of melanoma**

Increase in size
Increase in pigmentation
Variation in colour
Variation in pigmentation
Irregular edge
Irregular surface
Spontaneous bleeding
Crusting
Itching
Satellite pigmentation
Halo of erythema/pigment

## Lichen planus

Lichen planus is characterized by flat-topped, shiny, purple, polygonal papules, especially on the inner wrist and thighs but also disseminated. Pruritus is a typical symptom. Oral lesions form a lacy network on the buccal mucosa. Lichen planus occurs in graft versus host disease so it appears that the dense dermal infiltration of lymphocytes is pathogenic and causes the characteristic destruction of basal cells. Lichen planus-like (lichenoid) eruptions are seen with many drugs, especially gold, antimalarials and thiazide, but most cases are idiopathic and 87 per cent are likely to be cleared spontaneously by 18 months. Potent topical steroids or a short course of systemic steroids may be necessary in severe cases.

## Urticaria

Urticaria is common, in particular the physical urticarias—cholinergic urticaria and dermato-graphism—an exaggerated triple response after light touch. It often becomes symptomatic after some other minor dermatological complaint. Cholinergic urticaria consists of tiny, transient weals or papules, especially triggered by heat, bathing, sweating and exercise. True urticaria has large weals, each lasting less than 24 h but often recurring, especially in the evening and early morning. Gross facial oedema is sometimes associated. Although drugs (especially penicillin) and foods may be triggers, often a cause is not found. Increasing doses of antihistamines will at some stage control urticaria, though often well above the normal dose range. Patients may benefit from diets free of azo dyes, benzoates and salicy-lates.

## Lupus erythematosus

The classical lupus lesion—fixed erythema, atrophy, telangiectasia, follicular plugging and scarring—is identical in both discoid and systemic lupus erythematosus. It is usually light-induced and -exacerbated, and so occurs in a photosensitive eruption. Patients need immunological classification and a search for organ involvement, especially of the brain, joints, kidneys and blood before definitive diagnosis. All patients with lupus should avoid sun exposure and wear a sun-blocking preparation (with a sun protection factor [SPF] of 15 or over); potent topical steroids or intra-lesional steroids are very helpful but antimalarials, such as hydroxychloroquine and mepacrine, may be necessary. Dermatomyositis can be distinguished from lupus as its magenta-coloured lesions are particularly periocular and on the knuckles.

## Warts

Warts are caused by human papillomaviruses. They incubate for three to six months, then the hyperkeratotic papilliferous lesions develop particularly at sites of trauma. On the feet they are compressed into the sole by pressure and become hyperkeratotic and uncomfortable to walk on. The patient slowly develops immunity, on average taking two to three years, and then the warts vanish. They can be treated by any physically destructive method—cryotherapy, curettage—but these do not kill the virus or improve host immunity. Keratolytic agents can be used on the feet if pain is a problem.

## Fungus infection

### Ringworm

Ringworm on the body (tinea corporis) and in the groin (tinea cruris) shows as a migratory erythema with a superficial scale, slowly spreading outwards. Scalp involvement (tinea capitis) usually destroys hair and shows a moth-eaten scaly erythema, which may be grossly inflammatory and form a soggy purulent mass (kerion) as in some animal ringworm. Nail involvement (tinea unguum) is asymmetrical and destructive of nail architecture, so thickened discoloured powdery nails (dystrophy) result. Usually nail ringworm is associated with chronic infection of the fourth and fifth interdigital spaces (tinea pedis). Systemic therapy with griseofulvin is necessary for hair and nail involvement but topical therapy will suffice with most other forms.

### Candidiasis

Candida flourishes in flexural sites, which are warm and moist. Candida may complicate underlying flexural seborrhoeic dermatitis, and dermatitis of infancy or age, and shows the classical sign of satellite pustules around a glazed erythema. Candidal paronychia are a problem of wet hands, and chronic inflammation of the nail fold with a gaping nail cuticle junction is nearly always candidal. Candida is common in the patient on antibiotics, immunosuppressives and steroids, and in diabetics. Treatment may need to eradicate multiple sites of oral, genital, and gastrointestinal infection. Angular cheilitis is also a sign of candida, particularly in denture wearers.

## DERMATOLOGICAL EMERGENCIES REQUIRING INTENSIVE TREATMENT IN HOSPITAL

### Erythroderma

In erythroderma the skin becomes uniformly and universally inflamed, red and oedematous with a fine brawny scale, and no normal skin can be seen anywhere. The patients often lose their hair and sometimes their nails. The four major causes are psoriasis, eczema, drug reactions (see Table 13.7) and lymphoma/leukaemia, although many other causes infrequently occur. Once the patient has become erythrodermic, features of the underlying skin problem have been obliterated and unless there is a history of a preceding skin disease, diagnosis may be very difficult. Skin biopsies are often not diagnostic when the clinical picture is not clear. The primary problem of the erythrodermic patient is temperature control: the inflamed skin can radiate so much heat to the environment that the patient becomes hypothermic and starts shivering to maintain core temperature. Unfortunately, thermometer readings through a hyperaemic mucosa may be falsely high and the problem is compounded by well-meaning attempts to cool the patient by fans, tepid sponges and open windows. The patient must be warmed by raising the environmental temperature to high levels so they stop shivering. They will feel a lot better when warm. Other patients with widespread erythemas (and not erythrodermas) often feel cold and uncomfortable as well and can be helped by warmth. Other problems from erythroderma include difficulties with fluid and electrolyte balance due to an increase in insensible water loss. Sweating may be impaired by duct occlusion. Pooling of fluid in oedematous skin can aggravate hypotension. Patients may become hypoproteinaemic, which often aggravates the inflammatory oedema. Elderly patients run the risks of high-output heart failure.

### Toxic epidermal necrolysis (TEN)

This is caused either by a toxin-producing staphylococcus (uncommon in the adult) or a drug reaction (see Table 13.7). The skin dies and falls off (necrolysis) leaving extensive areas of superficial ulceration with little erythema. Mucous membrane involvement occurs in drug-induced TEN. The patients are toxic and febrile and the mortality is high—10 per cent in drug-induced TEN. Patients are particularly vulnerable to the entry of bacteria through the eroded skin causing septicaemia, but also there are problems of fluid and electrolyte balance like the erythrodermic or burns patient.

### Stevens–Johnson syndrome

This is the severe end of the spectrum of drug-induced erythema multiforme (Table 13.7) with severe mucous membrane involvement. It is similar to TEN in the problems caused. The lesions start as erythematous papules, which develop concentric rings like typical erythema multiforme but then become widespread, confluent and often erosive.

**Table 13.7 Drug causes of acute skin reactions**

| Erythroderma | Toxic epidermal necrolysis/ Stevens–Johnson syndrome |
|---|---|
| Sulphonamides | Sulphonamides |
| Hydantoins | Hydantoins |
| Allopurinol | Penicillin |
| Gold | Barbiturates |
| Carbamazepine | |

### Generalized pustular psoriasis

Generalized pustular psoriasis may develop as a rapidly migrating acute exanthematic form (von Zumbusch). The lesions are fine, monomorphic pustules (sterile, inflammatory, non-infective lesions) migrating with erythema, oedema and little evidence of classical psoriasis. Patients are toxic, with fever, leucocytosis and hypocalcaemia. They may mistakenly be treated for infection because of the toxicity but treating with antibiotics may cause fatal delay—the correct treatment is systemic antipsoriatic therapy.

## Pemphigus and bullous pemphigoid

Patients with pemphigus have an autoimmune loss of cell to cell cohesion in the epidermis caused by binding of an autoantibody to the intercellular glycoprotein pemphigus antigen. The skin cells part company and the skin and mucous membranes develop shallow blisters that rapidly disintegrate to form indolent erosions, which fail to heal and spread inexorably. Once body lesions have developed the patient is at risk of septicaemia and all the problems of skin loss (see 'TEN' above).

Bullous pemphigoid lesions are subepidermal blisters, which form due to an autoantibody to the basement membrane. The roof is the full thickness of epidermis and so the blisters remain intact, although haemhorragic and on an erythematous base. The problems of infection do occur but the patients are less toxic. Active management and hospitalization are required. Treatment of both pemphigoid and pemphiguis with high-dose steroids and immunosuppression.

## Eczema herpeticum

Atopic children have poor cell-mediated immunity and are particularly vulnerable to disseminated herpes simplex infection (eczema herpeticum) and, previously, eczema vaccinatum with vaccinia. The child develops disseminated herpetic vesicles on primary exposure to the virus. The small, punched-out lesions particularly affect the skin around the eyes and face so herpes keratitis is a common complication. The child is usually toxic with a fever and the complication is potentially fatal so early hospitalization is indicated. Early management with intravenous acyclovir may prevent spread but a major problem is postviral septicaemia (often Gram-negative bacteria) so erosions should be treated with topical antiseptics such as vioform or povidone iodine, or with a topical silver sulphadiazine cream, which is particularly effective against Gram-negative organisms.

## SPECIAL INVESTIGATION OF SKIN DISEASE

Systemic investigations of skin diseases are aimed at detecting underlying disease or other organ involvement in classical multisystem diseases such as lupus erythematosus. Immunological investigations are particularly important in many skin diseases because their immunopathogenesis is becoming clearer. However, there are some skin-specific investigations of which biopsy is fundamental; indeed, some feel that this is the major role of a skin doctor.

## Skin biopsies

Skin biopsies are usually taken for histopathological or immunofluorescent examination. Interpretation of both is a considerable skill given the immense diversity of skin diseases and adequate clinical information must be given to the pathologist so that appropriate special stains can be used. Skin biopsies may be:
(a) elliptical, either incisonal or excisional;
(b) punch biopsies;
(c) shave biopsies.

Other procedures providing histological material include curettage and cautery and cutting diathermy but here the architecture is distorted and so the techniques are only applicable to certain types of lesions.

### Elliptical skin biopsies

Biopsies must be taken along the skin lines and not across them or the resulting scar will be obtrusive. If in doubt about the lines, pinch the skin and see in which direction the lines form. Biopsies should not be cut on the face or any other visible area if a covered site can be used. Children form active, noticeable scars so cosmetic excisions should be delayed until adult life. Incisional biopsies should be taken across the edge of the lesion to include some normal skin. The biopsies are taken under local anaesthetic and a straight-sided ellipse confidently cut down to fat. The edge may need to be undermined to permit primary closure as a straight scar. Excisional biopsies are preferable for solitary lesions if at all possible although shave biopsy can be used in a clearly benign pedunculated lesion for cosmetic reasons. Excisional biopsy should be performed for malignant melanomas wherever possible in view of the debate about whether incisional biopsies enhance the risk of metastasis. A clearance of 1 cm/mm thickness of melanoma is the rule.

### Punch biopsies

Punch biopsies are cut with a sharp punch that looks like a mini apple corer of diameter 1 to 6 mm. The punch needs to be twisted down to fat or there will be problems in extracting the biopsy and obtaining adequate tissue for histological assessment. Adequate architectural information is not always obtained by punch biopsy but they are useful for immunocytochemistry, experimental purposes and difficult sites. A stitch will improve the cosmetic result but is not absolutely necessary.

### Shave biopsies and cutting cautery

These consist of shaving flat with the skin a pedunculated or raised lesion. It does not provide histological clearance and is a cosmetic procedure that should only be undertaken if the diagnosis is not in doubt.

### Curettage and cautery

Many solitary lesions, such as seborrhoeic warts, viral warts and basal cell carcinomas, have a clear separation zone and so can easily be scooped out with a spoon-shaped curette with a sharp cutting edge. Bleeding points in the base can then be staunched with cautery. This provides fragments of tissue and poor architectural information but may be appropriate for benign lesions or for areas where excision is difficult, e.g., nose, nasolabial fold.

### Cytology

There are a few situations where a scraping from the surface of a skin lesion can aid in diagnosis if the cells are fixed and stained. A Tzanck smear may show degenerate balloon cells in suspected herpes simplex. Acantholytic cells may be seen in a scraping from suspected pemphigus. In expert hands, dark small basaloid cells from basal cell carcinoma can be diagnostic. However, a negative result must be followed by biopsy. Cytological examination cannot tell you the type of tumour— morphoeic, etc.—and is only suitable for situations when it is preferable to avoid a scar and when definitive treatment will follow shortly.

### Immunofluorescent studies on skin

### Direct immunofluorescence

A punch biopsy of perilesional skin or uninvolved skin may be helpful in the analysis of immunological disease because deposition of diagnostic immunoreactants can be found in bullous and connective tissue diseases (Table 13.8). The skin biopsy is examined by fluorescent microscopy after labelling with a type-specific fluorescein-tagged antibody to immunoglobulin and complement. Fluorescence provides better resolution of the sites of deposition than immunoperoxidase histochemistry.

**Table 13.8 Immunofluorescent patterns in skin disease**

| Disease | Involved skin | Uninvolved skin |
|---|---|---|
| Pemphigus | *Intercellular epidermal IgG and C3 | +ve |
| Bullous pemphigoid | *Basement membrane, linear IgG and C3 | +ve |
| Dermatitis herpetiformis | Basement membrane, granular IgA | *+ve |
| Linear IgA disease | Linear IgA in basement membrane | +ve |
| Discoid lupus erythematosus | Granular basement, membrane IgM & C3 (lupus band test) | −ve |
| Systemic lupus erythematosus | | +ve |

* The diagnostic test for this particular disease.

### Indirect immunofluorescence

This detects circulating antibody to skin antigens and, by serial dilution, the titre of such an antibody. The patient's serum is incubated with normal skin (or appropriate substrate such as rodent oesophagus) so that the circulating antibody binds to the skin antigen and this is then tagged with the fluorescein-labelled second antibody.

### Immunoblotting

This is a new technique whereby an antibody can be detected by reactivity with skin antigens transferred from an electrophoretic gel to nitrocellulose paper. These tests have shown the heterogeneity of bullous diseases and may lead to new classifications and diagnostic criteria.

### Notes on Kveim test

The Kveim antigen is prepared from pulverized sarcoidal tissue. It is injected intradermally and the site biopsied six weeks later. A punch biopsy is adequate for interpretation but must be accurately sited. Injection of Indian ink into the Kveim test site produces misleading histological appearances and, if used, markers should be injected away from the site in several places to allow accurate pinpointing of the biopsy. It is usually unnecessary to use a marker as most patients have enough skin freckles or other markings to allow an accurate map of the Kveim site to be obtained.

### Patch tests

Patch tests are used to detect contact dermatitis. A small extract of the putative allergen is placed under an aluminium disc and a hypoallergenic plaster for 48 h. A positive reaction will be shown by the development of an eczamatous disc at the application site. The European patch test battery contains an agreed set of the most common allergens encountered in Europe and patients are routinely tested to this in addition to specific preparations suggested by the history. Readings are taken at 48 and 96 h. False-positive irritant responses may occur particularly at 48 h so interpretation must be by an experienced observer.

### Mycology

Fine surface scales can be scraped off with a blunt scalpel and examined for dermatophytes and yeasts. Some of the scales can be dissolved in 5 per cent KOH to allow dissolution of the skin cells, whereby invading mycelia can be seen by microscopy. The remaining sample is plated onto Sabouraud's medium when cultures of dermatophytes can be distinguished by their colonial morphology and pigment production.

### Further reading

Baran R., Dawber R. P. R. eds. (1984). *Diseases of the Nails*. Oxford: Blackwell Scientific.

Braverman I. M. (1981). *Skin Signs of Systemic Disease*. Philadelphia: W. B. Saunders.

DuVivier A. (1987). *Atlas of Clinical Dermatology*. Edinburgh: Churchill Livingstone.

Fitzpatrick T. B., Eisen A. Z., Wolff K., Freedberg I. M., Austen K. F. (1987). *Dermatology in General Medicine*. New York: McGraw-Hill.

Harper J. (1985). *Handbook of Paediatric Dermatology*. London: Butterworths.

Levene G. M., Calnan C. D. (1974). *A Colour Atlas of Dermatology*. London: Wolfe Medical.

Lever W. F., Schaumberg-Lever G. (1983). *Histopathology of the Skin*. Philadelphia: Lippincott.

Marks R. (1987). *Skin Disease in Old Age*. London: Martin Dunitz.

Rook A., Dawber R. (1982). *Diseases of the Hair and Scalp*. Oxford: Blackwell Scientific.

Rook A. J., Wilkinson D. S., Ebling F. J. G., Champion R. H., Burton J. L., eds. (1986). *Textbook of Dermatology*. Oxford: Blackwell Scientific.

# 14

# VASCULAR DISORDERS

John Davies

## HYPERTENSION

It has always been difficult to define the 'normal' blood pressure. Probably blood pressures over 160/95 are abnormal. The significance of high systolic readings is controversial because these are a common finding, particularly amongst the elderly. A diastolic pressure over 95 and certainly over 100 is significant and it has been well established that readings in this range carry an increased risk of cerebral vascular accidents and early ischaemic heart disease. It has been estimated that about 10 per cent of the population of the UK have blood pressures over 160/95.

In 95 per cent of cases, the cause is unknown and the patient is labelled as having 'essential hypertension' or 'primary hypertension'. This should only be done when the following 'reversible' causes of hypertension have been excluded:
(1) *Endocrine diseases:*
    (a) Cushing's syndrome;
    (b) Conn's syndrome;
    (c) acromegaly;
    (d) phaeochromocytoma.
(2) *Renal disease:*
    (a) renal artery stenosis;
    (b) polycystic kidneys;
    (c) polyarteritis nodosa;
    (d) chronic glomerulonephritis;
    (e) chronic pyelonephritis.
(3) *Coarctation of the aorta.*

Hypertension may occur in pregnancy and be asociated with other symptoms and signs of pre-eclampsia. Hypertension can be drug-induced and may revert to normal on withdrawal of steroids or the contraceptive pill.

A patient should be carefully assessed and seen on several occasions before being labelled 'hypertensive'. If borderline readings are found, the patient should be allowed to relax for at least half an hour and the blood pressure recording repeated. If the patient is obese, care should be taken to use a special, commercially available, 'large' cuff that encircles at leat two thirds of the arm. Blood pressure readings should be taken in the lying and standing positions. For the assessment of adequate therapy, take the blood pressure after some exercise (climbing up and down two steps attached to the examination couch about 20 times will suffice). Surprising alterations in blood pressure may be found.

## Symptoms

Most hypertensive subjects are asymptomatic. Headache and mild visual disturbances may occur. A patient with a phaeochromocytoma usually complains of attacks of flushing, headaches and diarrhoea during which, if taken, the blood pressure will be particularly high. Symptoms of renal disease, such as nocturia or haematuria, should be enquired after.

## Signs

There may be no other abnormal signs apart from a raised blood pressure. Evidence of endocrine abnormalities such as Cushing's disease should be obvious. Patients with Conn's syndrome (this is very rare) usually look normal.

It is important to assess the patient carefully for signs of organ damage that may have resulted from longstanding hypertension. Three important areas to consider are as follows:
(1) *The kidneys.* A specimen of urine should be tested for the presence of albuminuria, which may be a sign of ongoing kidney damage. Kidney failure may be causing the hypertension.

(2) *The heart.* Signs of left ventricular hypertrophy may be present and the patient may have a sustained left ventricular apex beat as well as an aortic ejection murmur and a loud aortic component to the second heart sound.

(3) *The eyes.* Both optic fundi should be searched for signs of small-vessel damage produced by longstanding hypertension. This occurs due to fibrinoid necrosis within the arteriolar walls.

The presence and severity of ocular changes should be graded thus:

*Grade I.* Arterial narrowing, increased tortuosity and silver wiring.

*Grade II.* Arterial on venous nipping.

*Grade III.* Haemorrhages and exudates.

*Grade IV.* All the changes seen in Grade I to III with papilloedema.

(Grade IV is usually termed 'malignant hypertension.)

## Examination

A careful examination for the absence of femoral artery pulsations is essential in all hypertensive patients, particularly short men, in order to exclude coarctation, a surgically correctable cause of hypertension. Palpation of the abdomen may reveal bilateral masses due to polycystic kidneys. The dramatic physical appearances of acromegaly are usually strikingly obvious. In renal artery stenosis it may be possible to hear a systolic bruit on auscultation of the lower part of the back to one or both sides of the lumbar spine but this is unusual! In advanced and longstanding cases of hypertension there may be signs of heart failure. The presence of other findings suggestive of longstanding hypertension, such as hypertensive retinopathy, will confirm hypertensive heart failure.

## Investigations

Over the last decade the investigation of hypertensive patients has been rationalized and rather than performing a battery of screening tests in all such patients a small, selected group are now being investigated more thoroughly. Any factors pointing to a specific cause in patients with secondary hypertension will obviously require special investigations. For instance, when glycosuria occurs with hypertension, investigations for Cushing's syndrome, acromegaly and phaeochromocytoma are indicated.

Routine investigations include assessment of cardiac and renal function. A chest X-ray and an ECG should be performed to look for cardiomegaly and left ventricular hypertrophy. Two midstream specimens of urine should be examined for the presence of cells, casts, proteinuria and evidence of infection. If proteinuria is discovered, a 24-h sample of urine should be collected for estimation of creatinine clearance and total protein output. If a phaeochromocytoma is suspected, three 24-h urine samples should be analysed for the presence of vanillylmandelic acid. Blood urea, creatinine and electrolytes should be measured for kidney function and for the presence of specific electrolyte abnormalities in Conn's and Cushing's syndromes.

If there is evidence of kidney damage, an intravenous pyelogram (IVP) should be performed both to search for a renal cause of the hypertension or, in primary hypertension, to assess how much kidney damage has occurred. Most physicians would also ask for an IVP in young patients with considerably raised pressures. Radioactive renography, where available, is a simple technique that can quickly and accurately diagnose renal artery stenosis or outflow obstruction. If either of these conditions is suspected, this investigation is probably preferable to an IVP. Further investigations, such as digital angiography and selective renal arteriography, should be made if renal artery stenosis is suspected, and it may be possible to organize angioplasty immediately after arteriography if facilities are available.

## Management

There is increasing interest and some controversy over non-pharmacological methods of treating hypertension. These methods include weight loss, salt reduction, decreased alcohol intake, relaxation and stopping cigarette smoking.

### Weight reduction

Although weight reduction is always indicated on general health grounds in obese people, it will only be effective for mild hypertension.

### Salt restriction

Salt intake in the Western world is so high that it would now be difficult to reduce it to a level that might significantly affect blood pressure.

Although it has been shown that a salt-free diet can lower blood pressure, it is generally thought to be so unacceptable that compliance is a major problem. As an overall rule, it is wise to recommend that patients do not avoid salt in their cooking but that they refrain from adding more salt at the table.

### Alcohol

Chronic alcoholism raises blood pressure and cessation of drinking may be all that is required in these patients. A study of two groups in hospital, both of whom had moderate to large daily alcohol intakes, showed that it was much easier to control hypertension in the group that abstained from alcohol than in those who continued their daily intake.

### Relaxation

A relaxed patient certainly has a lower blood pressure than somebody who is rushing around. Relaxation techniques can be enjoyable and should be encouraged but their effect on blood pressure tends to be transitory.

### Cigarette smoking

Although cigarette smoking has not been shown to cause hypertension, patients who continue to smoke are more difficult to manage pharmacologically than those who stop smoking. Because cigarette smoking is an additional and important risk factor in the early development of ischaemic heart disease and in the incidence of cerebral vascular accidents, hypertensive patients should be advised to stop smoking.

### Drug therapy

Having ensured that the patient does have significant primary hypertension, and having applied the methods outlined above without significant success, most physicians would adopt the following stepwise approach to the pharmacological management of the hypertensive patient:
(a) a diuretic;
(b) a diuretic plus a β-blocker;
(c) a diuretic, plus a β-blocker, and a calcium antagonist;
(d) a diuretic, a β-blocker, a calcium antagonist plus an ACE inhibitor.

Thiazide diuretics have become less popular over recent years because there have been reports suggesting that they are associated with an increased incidence of myocardial infarction amongst men. β-blockers have been extremely popular over the last decade but physicians are increasingly aware of their side-effects. Few young, active patients enjoy being β-blocked and, in the middle-aged, symptoms such as impotence and depression are not uncommon. Calcium antagonists lower blood pressure and seem to be free of major side-effects although they are associated with frequent minor side-effects including headaches and flushing in about 20 per cent of patients. The angiotensin-converting enzyme (ACE) inhibitors are an exciting new group of drugs that at first were unfortunately used in much higher doses than needed and therefore fell into disrepute because of a high incidence of side-effects. Their correct dosage has since been rationalized so they cause few side-effects and indeed a sense of well-being. These agents are likely to become 'first-line agents' after further trials and general clinical experience.

### Other hypotensive agents

Before the arrival of ACE inhibitors, the two most commonly used groups of drugs as third-line antihypertensive agents were vasodilators (hydralazine) and centrally acting drugs such as methyldopa and clonidine. Apart from clonidine, all these drugs are effective antihypertensive agents and are preferred by some physicians to the drugs mentioned in the step-wise guide above. Clonidine is ineffective as an antihypertensive agent and may produce a dangerous rebound in severe hypertension if stopped suddenly. Ganglion-blocking agents are no longer used but the post-ganglionic blocking drugs, guanethidine and bethanadine, still have a place in the management of severe hypertension. They all tend to cause postural hypotension.

### Combined preparations

There are now a number of preparations where one tablet appears to have two and even three or four different modes of action! It is wise to use these preparations with caution. One drug can adversely affect the absorption of another and it is obviously impossible to vary the dose of one drug while leaving the dose of the other component stable. Also, the detection and monitoring of side-effects is difficult when using a combined therapy because it is impossible to identify the offending drug.

### Aim of therapy

The aim of therapy is to lower the blood pressure to acceptable levels, in particular the diastolic pressure to below 90 mmHg without causing side-effects. Starting patients on antihypertensive therapy is, in most cases, a lifelong sentence and should not be undertaken lightly. First it is essential to ensure that a patient actually is hypertensive; and if he or she is, that they understand what exactly this means, particularly in terms of the need for treatment and how long it will last. Time should be devoted to a discussion of assessment, treatment and shared follow-up between hospital and general practitioners. Many patients are now buying sphygmomanometers and taking their own blood pressure which, in some cases, can be a good idea.

A decision needs to be taken about a 'target' blood pressure and treatment instituted. Attempts at too rigorous control can produce unacceptable side-effects and may result in default from follow-up. A realistic approach therefore is necessary and although every attempt should be made to get the patient's blood pressure down to 120/80, higher levels may have to be accepted.

### Management of malignant hypertension

Accelerated or malignant hypertension is characterized by a very high blood pressure (diastolic greater than 130 mmHg) and quite severe fibronoid necrosis of smaller arterioles, often visualized by fundal examination, with evidence of haemorrhages, exudates and papilloedema. Although it is a medical emergency and such patients should be admitted to hospital and treated, there is rarely an indication for very rapid reduction of blood pressure (within minutes) and indeed this can be dangerous. There have been reports of strokes, for example, resulting from precipitous reductions in blood pressure in these patients.

It is usually found that bed rest over a 24-h period will produce quite a profound fall in even the most severe hypertension. If a short-acting agent is needed after a period of observation and bed rest, hydralazine intramuscularly (10 mg),

repeated as necessary, is safe and acceptable. An oral β-blocker such as atenolol (which starts to act after about three hours) can also be started unless there is a specific contraindication such as bronchospasm or heart failure. If further treatment is needed, diuretics or vasodilators (see above) can be used in combination with the β-blockers, topping up as necessary with intramuscular hydralazine.

Intravenous labetalol has been advocated, particularly in pregnancy, and this seems a safe drug. Rarely, if ever, are powerful drugs such as nitroprusside (a potent vasodilator) or diazoxide required unless there is a dramatic hypertensive encephalopathy when the patient may be fitting continuously.

## PULMONARY THROMBOEMBOLISM

### Acute pulmonary thromboembolism

The management of acute pulmonary embolus has already been discussed in Chapter 2.

### Chronic thromboembolic disease

This is common and should always be considered as a cause of chronic exertional dyspnoea. Predisposing conditions include prolonged immobilization, such as after recent surgery, trauma or paralysis. A recent acute myocardial infarction and any period of congestive cardiac failure also predispose. Cigarette smoking is a further risk factor.

After chronic thromboembolism, pulmonary hypertension usually occurs. This is partly due to the mechanical obstruction produced by embolic material and partly secondary to vasoactive substances, including serotonin and prostaglandins, released after multiple pulmonary emboli. Pulmonary hypertension then gives rise to right ventricular hypertrophy and consequent right ventricular failure with the usual physical signs.

### Symptoms

These may be nonspecific. The usual indicators of acute thromboembolism, such as pleuritic pain, dyspnoea and haemoptysis, are seldom found in chronic disease. Dyspnoea and particularly tachypnoea are common symptoms and may be associated with cyanosis and a tachycardia. Fatigue, breathlessness and general lethargy occur.

There may well be no signs of peripheral vascular problems because many of the emboli arise silently within the large pelvic veins.

### Signs

The signs are those of right heart failure with frequent third and fourth heart sounds. A loud pulmonary second heart sound is often present and there may be a functional tricuspid incompetent murmur.

### Investigations

The ECG often shows right ventricular enlargement, right axis deviation is common and there may be a 'P pumonale'. The chest X-ray may be normal. The most sensitive and useful investigation is a radionucleotide perfusion scan, which can be complemented by a ventilation scan if there is a suspicion of concomitant airways obstruction. Pulmonary angiography is also sensitive and specific.

### Management

Mobilization is important, stopping smoking essential, and where there is proven evidence of longstanding chronic thromboembolic disease, patients should be anticoagulated with warfarin for life.

## VENOUS THROMBOTIC DISEASE

### Acute deep venous thrombosis

The management of an acute deep vein thrombosis (DVT) has already been covered in Chapter 2.

### Chronic venous deep thrombosis

Repeated pulmonary emboli should be regarded as a complication of widespread DVTs. The larger leg and pelvic veins are the most common cause of clinically significant pulmonary emboli and these are often silent, particularly those within the pelvis. The three factors that promote chronic venous thromboses are stasis, abnormality of the vessel wall, and alterations in the blood coagulation system. Coagulation studies have been undertaken extensively, but as yet there is no reliable test for the so-called state of 'hypercoagul-

ability'. Polycythaemia, thrombocytosis and excessive cigarette smoking should of course be excluded. Other conditions associated with a high risk of chronic venous thrombosis include the postpartum period, left ventricular failure, fractures and other injuries of the lower extremities, prolonged bed rest, carcinoma and obesity.

Although the clinical diagnosis of an acute deep venous thrombosis may be obvious, clinically 'silent' thrombosis is frequently present. For example, the classical signs of pain, heat and swelling have been reported to be absent in over half of patients in whom proven DVTs were later demonstrated on thermography.

### Prophylaxis

A commonly used method of prophylaxis is small-dose, subcutaneous heparin in patients at risk, such as those with multiple fractures, severe myocardial infarction and chronic congestive heart failure. Heparin is given in a dose of 5000 u every 12 h and continued until the patient is fully ambulatory. This approach is associated with little risk of haemorrhage while maintaining a significant effect on the coagulation system.

## PERIPHERAL VASCULAR DISEASE

### Acute arterial obstruction

This is an acute and painful event associated with numbness, paraesthesiae and weakness of the affected limb. There is pallor and coldness of the limb below the obstruction, frequently followed by cyanosis. The peripheral pulses distal to the obstruction are impalpable. Ninety per cent of these obstructions occur in the legs. The cause may be local chronic thrombosis in the large arteries supplying the limb but an embolic cause should always be considered, especially in patients with mitral stenosis or atrial fibrillation.

### Management

The limb should be maintained at room temperature or below to decrease local cell metabolism; hyperbaric oxygen, if available, may be helpful. The patient should be heparinized before early assessment for surgery, which is the definitive treatment. Thrombolytic agents and vasodilators may be tried if surgery is delayed or contraindicated. Embolectomy is a relatively simple procedure (usually using a Foggarty balloon catheter) and is commonly associated with a very gratifying return of sensation, power and colour to the affected limb.

## Chronic arterial obstruction

Careful chiropody is of paramount importance in these patients, particularly in diabetics with their frequently associated chronic neuropathy. Sympathectomy may improve superficial blood supply and relieve symptoms. Endarterectomy or vascular grafting procedures are seldom of any use as the pathology is often within the small vessels. Unfortunately, amputation is frequently required and is usually done above the knee. Conservative management includes stopping smoking and giving antiplatelet drugs (aspirin) and vasodilators. However, no drug therapy is of any proven merit in this condition.

## Intermittent claudication

This usually occurs in the legs and is more common in males over the age of 50 years. It is usually a manifestation of generalized atheromatous arterial disease and is frequently associated with angina pectoris or a history of myocardial infarction. Most of the patients are heavy smokers. It may be worsened by diabetes and occasionally precipitated by anaemia.

The history is of pain in the calf on effort, which is rapidly relieved by rest. Leriche's syndrome produces claudication within the upper part of the legs and the buttocks, and is associated with impotence. Major arterial peripheral pulses are reduced or absent. There may be bruits over the femoral or carotid arteries. Arteriography should be performed if surgery is contemplated; angioplasty can be easily repeated and is less traumatic than endarterectomy and/or vascular bypass grafting. Usually angioplasty is performed at the same time as angiography if the patient has a clinically suitable lesion and facilities are available.

Associated problems such as diabetes mellitus should be treated. The patient should be emphatically told that smoking is associated with a much worse prognosis.

Medical management has not been shown to be of use in this condition, although many vasodilators and other drugs are marketed for it. If angioplasty or surgery is contraindicated, then sympathectomy often helps to relieve symptoms. Polycythaemia or indeed anaemia should be excluded.

## Raynaud's phenomenon

This is defined as intermittent attacks of pallor and cyanosis of the digits without evidence of arterial obstruction. Initially the fingers become white and painful, they then turn blue and finally there is a reactive arterial dilatation producing a dusky-red hue. It is commonly unilateral and can be exacerbated by working with vibrating tools. Otherwise, it is more common in women, where there may be a strong family history. Related collagen diseases such as scleroderma should be carefully looked for. Exacerbating factors such as β-blocking drugs should be enquired after, as stopping these medications may be the only treatment required. Long-term management is disappointing but recent reports have suggested that nifedipine produces significant relief in some patients. Otherwise the treatment is symptomatic, the hands and feet being kept warm, particularly in cold weather. Extra gloves and sometimes battery-operated, electrically heated gloves and socks may produce tremendous symptomatic relief. Patients should be advised to stop smoking.

# Section Four

## Special Clinical Subspecialities

# 15

# APPROACH TO THE PSYCHIATRIC PATIENT

## Glyn Lewis

Patients with minor psychiatric illness are commonly encountered in general hospitals and every physician needs to be able to provide adequate psychiatric care for this group. In addition, attending to the psychological aspect of a consultation should improve compliance, clarify the diagnosis and assist in many aspects of management. Occasionally a psychiatric diagnosis features in the differential diagnosis, though usually psychiatric illness occurs simultaneously with physical illness. These issues have ensured that general hospital psychiatry has become increasingly important, leading to the increased provision of psychiatric services in general hospitals and in the psychiatric education of medical students, many of whom now face a large proportion of psychiatric cases in their final exam.

This chapter will try to introduce some parts of psychiatry that are important to a general physician. For details about the various psychiatric syndromes and treatments the reader is referred to textbooks of psychiatry.

## PRINCIPLES OF PSYCHOLOGICAL MEDICINE

Psychiatrists tend to approach their patients from a slightly different point of view than that of the physician, and there are three main areas in which their assessments differ—the use of informants, the specific mental state examination and the involvement of other professionals.

### Informants

It is often valuable to interview someone apart from the patient about the presenting problem and background and this becomes especially important in elderly patients, or in seriously mental ill (e.g., schizophrenic) patients, who may have a very distorted view of their own history. Relatives or close friends can often provide important information, but perhaps the most valuable informant is the general medical practitioner (GP), whose knowledge of the patient's background may be difficult to summarize in a letter. It is always worth talking to the GP over the phone if a psychological problem is at issue.

### The mental state examination

Non-psychiatrists are often reluctant to ask about upsetting things, but this is essential if the patient is to be properly assessed and probably helps the patient's treatment, as long as the doctor listens sympathetically. Most doctors also tend to reassure automatically when someone appears upset, and though this is usually the most appropriate thing to do, it is also important to acknowledge someone's distress and talk about the distressing subject, even if it is only for a minute or two.

### Involvement of other professionals

The GP should be involved in the treatment offered for a psychiatric disorder. The GP usually has a much better idea of local circumstances, friendly and unfriendly neighbours, and other community resources. Furthermore, the GP will be involved in long-term follow-up and will have to deal with any recurrences.

It is also essential to contact any psychiatric teams that are still involved with a patient, or have been involved in the past. Always ask the patient about past psychiatric history, and if psychiatric care is necessary or relevant, contact the team that usually deals with the patient. This has become more important recently, both because hospitals tend to interpret rigidly the boundaries of their catchment area, and also because the growth of community care forces a local approach.

## DETECTION OF MINOR PSYCHIATRIC ILLNESS

Between 30 to 40 per cent of medical outpatients have a minor psychiatric condition, usually a mixture of anxiety and depression. Only a minority of these requires the help of the psychiatrist and it is important that physicians can adequately manage these patients. The high prevalence is partly because those suffering from anxiety and depression are more likely to seek help for a physical complaint and be referred to hospital but also because physical illness also increases the risk of psychiatric disorder. Minor psychiatric illness therefore usually coexists with physical illness.

Some authors have advocated routine screening of medical patients with questionnaires, but most doctors are reluctant to adopt this strategy despite failing to detect at least half of the psychiatric disorders they are presented with. Most patients do not actively volunteer psychiatric symptoms to their physician, so it is wise to include a few questions about these in the routine clerking of a patient. For instance, 'Have you been cheerful recently, or have you had spells of feeling miserable or unhappy?', 'Have you been feeling under strain?' and 'Are there times when you become anxious or nervous?'

## MANAGEMENT OF MINOR PSYCHIATRIC ILLNESS

Detection of minor psychiatric illness is important because the disorders are treatable. In general this group of patients do not require drug treatment and benzodiazepine anxiolytic drugs should be avoided whenever possible because of the risk of dependence and their lack of efficacy in cases of chronic anxiety. The drugs used in psychiatry are not that effective and the mainstay of treatment remains counselling and 'talking over problems'.

The most important rule is to tell the patient that they have depression and/or anxiety and to acknowledge their distress. It is also important to inform the GP, who may want to manage the patient him/herself. The patient needs an opportunity to discuss their concerns and worries, which

will often be focused on their physical health. This kind of support can, of course, be provided by social workers, nurses, physiotherapists and occupational therapists as well as by medical staff. 'Self help' books have also been written and may help some patients (see Further Reading).

Those that have anxiety provoked by situations or specific things can be effectively treated with behaviour therapy. 'Self help' books exist that show a patient how to devise his/her own behavioural programme, otherwise the patient can be referred to a clinical psychologist. Behavioural treatment for anxiety may seem paradoxical, as treatment initially increases anxiety by exposing the patient to the anxiety-provoked stimulus. In one sense making the patient anxious is treatment for anxiety.

Tricyclic antidepressants should only be described if there are 'biological' symptoms of depression (poor appetite with weight loss, loss of libido, disturbed sleep with early morning wakening, depression worse in the morning) and these are often difficult to assess in the physically ill. Furthermore, they have physical side-effects that can complicate management. Amitriptyline remains the drug of first choice, though it is sedative. A healthy adult of average size should be started on a dose of 50 to 75 mg daily, increasing to 150 mg daily in the course of a week, as this helps the patient tolerate the anticholinergic side-effects. Before prescribing an antidepressant it is worth observing the patient to see if nonspecific treatment will lead to improvement. Some of the newer non-tricyclic antidepressants have fewer side-effects, but there are still doubts about the efficacy of these.

Patients with minor psychiatric disorders will benefit from a psychiatric referral if they are ready to accept psychiatric help and they have persistent symptoms. The patient must be prepared for a psychiatric visit as some people become very offended if the doctor suggests they have any psychological problems. Telling the patient he or she is to see 'another doctor' without specifying the doctor is a psychiatrist is unhelpful and can alienate the patient.

## ORGANIC PSYCHOSYNDROMES

Organic psychiatric syndromes are those that result from a physical condition, either of the brain or of the rest of the body. These are very common in a general hospital. It is useful to distinguish between the acute confusional states and the chronic organic syndromes, of which the most important are the dementias. Both acute and chronic organic syndromes are characterized by a loss of intellectual functioning, and this is the clinical means of distinguishing these syndromes from the functional psychiatric disorders, where changes in intellectual functioning are much rarer. Confusional states and dementia are the commoner organic psychosyndromes.

## Acute confusional states

The diagnosis is made by a history of a relatively sudden change in intellectual functioning, provided by an informant, and a mental state that provides evidence of a cognitive deficit, in particular: disorientation, poor recall of an address, inability to draw a clock face accurately, poor digit span, or inability to do simple arithmetic. Acute confusional states are sometimes characterized by rapid fluctuations in attention, the patient appears to wander off in mid sentence, though at other times appears to understand the interviewer for a few seconds. Visual hallucinations are rarely seen in other psychiatric disorders but are relatively common in this group. In addition, they often have loosely held paranoid ideas.

There is always a physical cause for an acute confusional state, and the patient requires urgent physical investigation. It is more common in children, elderly people, and in those with pre-existing brain damage, including those with dementias. An acute confusional state is therefore a common cause for a rapid deterioration in the behaviour of a demented patient. Many drugs can also lead to acute confusional states, especially those with anticholinergic effects (e.g., tricyclic antidepressants) and sedatives.

Treatment is of the underlying cause, but disturbed behaviour can often force medical staff to sedate the patient. Promazine, and if this is not effective, haloperidol in small doses can be used, and both drugs can be given intramuscularly if necessary.

## Dementia and other chronic organic reactions

Dementia is a permanent and global loss of intellectual functioning. There are two main causes, Alzheimer's disease and multi-infarct dementia, resulting from cerebrovascular disease. Alcoholic brain damage can also present as dementia, though the classical Korsakov's psychosis, resulting from thiamine deficiency secondary to alcoholism, is a chronic specific memory deficit with other intellectual functions relatively spared.

The diagnosis is made clinically, though a CT scan if available helps to exclude some of the rarer causes. Thorough cognitive and neurological assessments are essential, and there is a suggestion that parietal lobe signs are more common in patients with Alzheimer's disease.

Management depends on the degree of disability, and this is always gleaned from informants, including the GP. The ability of the patient to manage at home requires information about the physical layout of the home, the availability of relatives and neighbours, and evidence of dangerous behaviour, for instance, of burning themselves with fires. If admitted, the ward nurses can assess whether the patient needs nursing care, or whether he/she can cope in local authority homes for the elderly (Part 3 accommodation). For very disturbed patients there are a very small number of ESMI (elderly severe mentally impaired) beds managed by a psychiatrist specializing in the elderly, but for the vast majority of patients the psychiatric services have no appropriate inpatient facilities. However, it is important to inform the GP and Old Age psychiatrists of early or suspected cases of dementia, as emergency admissions can sometimes be prevented if social services and other community supports can be arranged before any crises develop.

## PSYCHIATRIC EMERGENCIES

### Attempted suicide and assessing suicide risk

Self poisoning and other suicide attempts are one of the commonest reasons for medical admission, though the incidence has begun to fall recently. Anyone who has attempted suicide or to harm themselves, however trivial, requires a psychiatric assessment.

When taking a history of the overdose (or other attempt) the incidents surrounding the event and any precautions to prevent discovery must be elicited. Many patients have little medical knowledge, and an assessment of medical risk from the point of view of the patient is also useful. Had the attempt been planned or was it impulsive? Previous attempts must be asked after and the presence of any precipitants.

The following items appear to be associated with an increased risk of suicide: middle age or older, male sex, social isolation and lack of important close relationships, unemployment, separated or divorced, a history of alcohol dependence and previous suicide attempts. All patients with a serious psychiatric illness, including personality disorders, also have an increased suicide risk, so a past psychiatric history must be obtained.

The mental state examination must concentrate on assessing the patient's mood including 'biological' features, but more importantly asking if they are still considering suicide, and about their views of their future. If patients admit to feeling that their 'life isn't worth living' or that they 'no longer look forward to things they used to enjoy', then such hopeless views of the future indicate a more serious depression and a greater suicide risk.

It is always useful to contact the GP, particularly if the patient is discharged.

One group of patients, those with personality disorders, often cause confusion amongst non-psychiatrists. This is a rather unsatisfactory and widely criticized diagnosis, made if someone has had symptoms since adolescence, so current abnormalities are attributed to personality rather than to an illness. Though there are difficulties in making this diagnosis reliably, it is used to describe that group of patients who do not usually benefit from inpatient treatment. When the diagnosis of personality disorder is made, most psychiatrists are therefore reluctant to admit the patient. However, these patients are often severely disabled, require specialized psychiatric help, and they have a substantial risk of suicide.

## Management of acute psychotic episodes

Occasionally, someone with an acute psychosis presents in the casualty department or in other areas of medical practice. There are two situations that a physician may have to manage. Firstly, whether to admit the patient and 'section' (see below) and secondly, potential or actual violent incidents.

### Admission

It always helps to involve the local psychiatric team, or the psychiatric team that has been involved with the patient in the past. There are no rules about when to admit, but if there has been a recent change in mental state, admission should be considered after taking the outcome of previous admissions into account.

If the patient refuses voluntary admission, a 'section' (of the 1983 Mental Health Act) must be considered. There are two requirements: firstly, that the person is suffering from mental disorder, and secondly, that the patient is a danger to the health or safety of him/herself or others. The act specifically excludes people who are addicted to alcohol, heroin or other substances and do not suffer from other mental disorders, but it does include those who are severely mentally handicapped and those with organic psychiatric conditions, including dementia and acute confusional states.

A section 2 should be sought whenever possible. The application must be recommended by two doctors, one of whom must be a psychiatrist approved under the Mental Health Act, usually a senior registrar or above. In addition an approved social worker or 'nearest relative' must agree to the section. This section lasts for 28 days and the patient must be informed of his or her right of appeal against the decision. The 'nearest relative' is carefully defined in the act: the spouse, if appropriate is the first choice, and if not the eldest child then the elder of the parents, etc. In general a social worker should always be involved in a section and should attempt to contact the nearest relative. If there is an urgent need for admission and a second medical opinion would delay matters dangerously a section 4 can be applied for. This allows a single doctor and an 'approved social worker' or nearest relative to admit for 72 h. It can be converted to a section 2 if a second opinion is obtained. Ideally, the doctor applying for a section 4 should have known the patient before, for instance the GP.

This Act does not allow treatment for physical conditions against someone's will, and only a section 3 (which is similar to section 2 but admits patients for six months) specifically allows psychiatric treatment against a patient's will. All other treatment is given under common law, which allows urgent treatment to be given to avoid serious suffering, to save the patient's life or to prevent deterioration in an urgent situation. Bluglass has written a useful reference book that describes the Act (see Further Reading).

### Disturbed behaviour and violence

If a patient is violent or potentially so, a decision must be made about whether physical restraint is necessary. If physical restraint is used, enough staff to safely restrain the patient must be immediately available. Most patients with functional psychoses tend to calm down if there is a sufficient number of determined staff around them, and calling staff to a ward may be enough to control the situation. Before the patient is restrained, a suitable dose of medication to sedate the patient should be made ready. Haloperidol, 5 to 10 mg intramuscularly, repeated if there is no response, is suitable, but an anticholinergic (e.g., procyclidine, 5–10 mg intramuscularly) should be available for treatment of a dystonic reaction or severe extrapyramidal side-effects should they arise. Chlorpromazine, 100 to 200 mg intramuscularly, is also used and is more sedative than haloperidol; however, it can lead to hypotension and the blood pressure needs to be monitored. These neuroleptics cannot work on their own and good nursing, ideally by psychiatrically trained staff, is essential.

## THE ADDICTIONS

### Alcohol dependence and problem drinking

Excessive alcohol consumption is a major cause of physical ill health and leads to considerable social and psychological damage to the drinkers' personal lives. The latest Royal College of Psychiatrists' report (see Further Reading) suggested that someone should not drink more than 21 'units' per week and drinking 50 'units' a week leads to some harm. One unit is 8 g of alcohol and is equivalent to about one pub measure of spirits (30 units per bottle), half a pint of normal strength beer or a table glass of wine (7 units per bottle). Some strong lagers (e.g., Carlsberg Special and Tennants' Super) have 4 units per can. There are therefore many people who need advice to cut down.

Many people with drinking problems are not identified by physicians. The CAGE, a four-item questionnaire, has been advocated to improve detection by doctors. The four questions are 'Have you ever felt you ought to cut down on your drinking?'; 'Have people annoyed you by criticizing your drinking?'; 'Have you felt bad or guilty about your drinking?'; and 'Have you ever had a drink first thing in the morning to steady your nerves or get rid of a hangover?' If someone answers 'yes' to two or more of these questions then they have a 50 per cent chance of being a problem drinker.

Alcohol problems are more common in men, in publicans and those who work in the catering industry, in those businessmen who regularly have business lunches and in the medical profession. Tests for liver damage or macrocytosis are very unreliable ways of detecting heavy drinkers. It is much better to ask the patient how much they drink, as long as bland responses like 'social drinker' are followed with more detailed questioning.

There are two major categories of heavy drinker. The 'problem drinker' is drinking to such an extent that their personal lives or physical health are endangered. For instance, drunkenness at work may lead to dismissal, alcohol may lead to marital difficulties or be at such a level that liver damage is likely.

The second category of heavy drinker is 'dependent on alcohol' and this is characterized by the following features:

(1) Alcohol becomes an important priority compared to their relationships, job and health, etc.

(2) There is increased tolerance to the effects of alcohol.

(3) There is a subjective awareness of a compulsion to drink and difficulty in controlling the amount.

(4) There are repeated withdrawal symptoms, e.g., morning nausea, retching, 'shakes'.

(5) Withdrawal symptoms are avoided by further drinking ('relief drinking').

(6) Heavy drinking reinstates rapidly after periods of abstinence.

Almost all dependent drinkers will also have social or other problems, though it is possible for people to drink heavily and for this not to interfere with their work, for instance in the catering industry. However, many heavy drinkers, including those with physical complications of alcohol use, may not be dependent on alcohol.

The management of these two groups differs and a drinking history, often forgotten in both general medical and psychiatric practice, must elicit enough information to distinguish them as well as determining the amount drunk.

It is essential to tell a heavy drinker of the

potential problems they have had or will have with alcohol. A problem drinker must be urged to reduce their alcohol consumption unless there are medical reasons for abstinence. Simple advice can be effective treatment for problem drinkers—for instance, to alter social habits, keep a diary of alcohol intake, use non-alcoholic drinks to quench thirst and to try alcohol-free beers and wines. On occasions a period of abstinence may help.

The dependent drinker, however, must be told to stop drinking, and most authorities recommend lifelong abstinence as the only realistic goal. The patient can be recommended to attend Alcoholics Anonymous or other voluntary groups.

Dependent drinkers will suffer withdrawal symptoms if they stop drinking suddenly and medication (and parenteral thiamine) is needed to cover withdrawal. Chlordiazepoxide, 40 to 80 mg four times a day, is a suitable drug and appears to be less addictive than chlormethiazole, which is also a drug of abuse amongst dependent drinkers. The chlordiazepoxide should be tailed off within 10 days. Benzodiazepines should not be prescribed for more than short periods to anyone with a drinking problem because of the risk of dependence. If someone is being withdrawn as an outpatient the drug should be dispensed daily to avoid the possibility that alcohol and sedative drugs are taken simultaneously.

Delirium tremens is an acute confusional state caused by the withdrawal of alcohol. It is characterized by disorientation and confusion, visual hallucinations and paranoia. Medical problems, including chest infections and dehydration, commonly coexist. The treatment is the same as withdrawal, and there is usually a rapid response to chlordiazepoxide.

## Dependence on heroin and other illegal drugs

It is best to contact the local drug dependence unit and act in accordance with their protocol. The withdrawal symptoms are less severe than those of alcohol withdrawal, but are usually covered by a short course of methadone syrup. It is inadvisable to give any narcotic to an addict on an outpatient basis. The patient should be encouraged to attend voluntary groups, including Narcotics Anonymous, and be referred to a specialist unit if they are prepared to keep an appointment.

Only doctors with a special licence may prescribe diamorphine or cocaine to addicts.

## Dependence on minor tranquillizers

Some people find it extremely difficult to stop taking benzodiazepine tranquillizers and the withdrawal phenomena are now well documented. If someone is to be withdrawn the drug should be tailed off slowly, and a maximum of two weeks should be left between successive reductions in dose. Referral to a psychiatrist may be appropriate in someone who has great difficulty in stopping.

## PHYSICAL SYMPTOMS AND PSYCHOLOGICAL ILLNESS

This is a difficult area in which to make diagnoses and manage patients. It is widely accepted by both physicians and psychiatrists that some physical complaints have a psychological origin, but there is still no definite way of deciding whether a symptom is a result of psychological factors or due to a physical condition. The doctor often has to diagnose a psychological cause by exclusion, and this can be dangerous. However, accurate diagnosis is aided if there is a clear idea of the sort of psychological cause being suggested in a particular case. Minor cases of anxiety and depression are also common, and so a psychiatric disorder will usually coexist with a physical disorder.

Psychiatric disorder is still a stigmatizing label, and patients often feel that symptoms with a psychological cause are 'imaginary' or 'faked'. The terms hysteria and hypochondriasis have therefore both become rather pejorative so it is important for the doctor to convey that psychiatric disorder requires as much sympathy as physical disorder and that symptoms with a psychogenic cause can be as disabling and as 'real' as any physical symptom. The rather acrimonious and unhelpful debates about some conditions, for instance the postviral fatigue syndrome, appear to rest upon the premise that it is insulting for people to be given the label of a psychiatric disorder. Whatever the cause of this syndrome it is sad that psychiatric disorder is seen to be so stigmatizing, even within the medical profession.

## Somatic manifestations of anxiety and depression

Anxiety leads to a variety of physical symptoms that can sometimes be confused with physical conditions, particularly if the patient is concerned about their cause. Palpitations and a variety of aches and discomfort, including chest pain and epigastric discomfort, are quite common. Hyperventilation and the subjective feeling of breathlessness is also a frequent accompaniment of anxiety and can lead to paraesthesiae and even tetany and loss of consciousness.

The diagnosis of anxiety is more likely if the person becomes anxious at the times of the symptoms, and if there are definite situational precipitants of anxiety, for instance, the patient may become anxious in social circumstances or when in crowded supermarkets. Furthermore, when anxious the patient may have anxiety-provoking thoughts, for instance, of imminent death, of disease or of making a fool of themselves in public.

A depressed mood is frequently associated with anxiety, and feelings of tiredness and fatigue are commonly found in depression, usually with a loss of enjoyment for activities that the patient enjoyed in the past. On occasions, persistent pains are associated with depression, and appear to improve when the mental state improves.

It is rare for bad anxiety attacks to start in the elderly, without evidence of previous episodes of anxiety.

### Hysterical conversion symptoms

Hysteria is an old term, and unfortunately implies a particular psychogenic mechanism for the symptoms, unlike most other psychiatric diagnoses, which are purely descriptive. Freud suggested that hysterical conversion symptoms were a result of denied unconscious conflicts, which were then 'converted' into physical symptoms as a way of dealing with the conflict. Nowadays, the term is usually used for physical symptoms that can neither be explained by a physical cause nor as concomitants of anxiety or depression. Classically, hysterical paralysis, for instance, occurs in someone with no psychiatric symptoms and with neurological signs that cannot be explained by neuroanatomy. The diagnosis of hysteria must be made with extreme caution as there are few reliable clinical signs that can lead to a definite diagnosis.

More recently the term 'somatization' has been used, particularly by North American psychiatrists. It also refers to physical symptoms that arise for psychological reasons. It has been preferred because it lacks the specific connotations of hysteria.

### Hypochondriasis

Hypochondriasis is the excessive fear of physical illness or the conviction that one suffers from a physical illness. Though hypochondriasis does not lead to physical symptoms, it can make the management of patients very difficult and is sometimes associated with physical symptoms caused by psychological factors.

One of the main difficulties in managing hypochondriacs comes in deciding when to stop investigating. Often investigations are used as a way of reassuring both patient and doctor that all is well, but it is difficult to reassure those labelled as hypochondriacs, and the physician has to decide whether there are any indications for further investigation, ignoring the patient's own anxiety. This is a real challenge for the clinical skills of the doctor, as the decision must be based purely on clinical symptoms and signs.

It is important to give the patient a full explanation of the reasoning behind all investigations and when hypochondriasis coexists with psychogenic symptoms or with conditions exacerbated by psychological factors, a physiological account of the connection is useful. In general, when the clinician has finished investigation, it is unwise to reinvestigate unless new symptoms present. If the doctor changes his or her mind, it tends to increase the patient's anxiety.

'Hypochondriac' has become a rather derogatory term and it is important to give someone who is very worried about illness proper sympathetic medical care.

### Physical conditions affected by emotional state

There are some conditions that appear to be worsened by the patient's psychological state, including duodenal ulcer, irritable bowel syndrome, asthma, some skin disorders and 'brittle' diabetes. In general there is only clinical evidence to support these conclusions, but it may be useful to consider psychological issues when managing someone who responds poorly to standard management, as psychological help for dealing with stress may have a beneficial effect on their medical condition.

## Factitious disorders

Some patients either mutilate themselves or simulate medical and surgical conditions. These include the factitious skin disorders and Münchhausen's syndrome. The term factitious suggests that the patient is aware of the attempt to deceive, in contrast to those with hysteria, who are unaware of the psychological nature of their condition.

## Eating disorders

### Anorexia nervosa

This condition is characterized by a loss of weight because of inadequate food intake, cessation of menstruation and a fear of putting on weight. The highest incidence is in teenage women and the patient tends to describe themselves as fat despite an objectively emaciated condition. Medical problems can result from the malnutrition, and also from the abuse of laxatives and/or repeated vomiting, which are also used to reduce weight. Patients with anorexia nervosa tend to be very secretive about their eating habits and can present with weight loss, amenorrhoea or diarrhoea. Anorexia nervosa must be considered in any woman less than 30 years of age who presents with substantial weight loss. It is rarely found in men. Patients with anorexia nervosa need specialized psychiatric treatment.

### Bulimia nervosa

This closely related condition is commoner than anorexia and almost always occurs in women. The patient eats large quantities of food at one sitting and then has a compulsion to vomit and/or to abuse laxatives. There is also a fear of putting on weight, though the patient is usually close to their ideal weight. Other psychiatric symptoms, especially depression, are commonly found. Electrolyte disturbances can occur, and repeated vomiting also leads to dental problems (erosion of enamel by stomach acid).

## PSYCHOLOGICAL CARE OF THE DYING AND THE SERIOUSLY ILL

Minor psychiatric disorder is very common in those with serious physical illness but is not an inevitable consequence of receiving a life-threatening diagnosis. There is no advantage for a patient to have the additional disability of a psychiatric disorder as well as a physical disease. Psychiatric disorder in the terminally ill, and in those with cancer, must therefore be detected and adequately treated.

When most physicians or nurses are confronted with a dying patient, they tend to use 'distancing tactics' (see Maguire's paper in Further Reading) rather than enquire after psychiatric symptoms. Even when emotional issues are raised, doctors tend to talk exclusively about physical symptoms. Denial is an important way of coping with serious illness, but asking a few questions routinely about psychiatric symptoms does not prevent the patient from using denial as a means to cope, but does allow the doctor to detect those patients that may need help.

Present evidence shows that disorders in patients with cancer can be effectively treated by counselling, behavioural treatment or antidepressants. The former non-pharmacological methods seem preferable in the physically ill, and some authors advocate helping the patient accept physical changes, if any, but to regard psychological symptoms as reversible. The patient should be encouraged to keep busy and continue doing the things they enjoy.

## Further reading

Blackburn I. M. (1988). *Coping with Depression*. Edinburgh: Chambers.
Bluglass R. (1983). *A Guide to the Mental Health Act*. Edinburgh: Churchill Livingstone.
Burns D. (1980). *Feeling Good*. New York: New American Library.
Maguire P. (1985). Barriers to psychological care of the dying. *Brit. Med. J.*, **291**, 1711–13.
Marks I. (1977). *Living with Fear*. New York: McGraw-Hill.
Royal College of Psychiatrists (1986). *Alcohol: Our Favourite Drug*. London: Tavistock.

### Textbooks

Kendell R. E., Zealley A. K. (1988). *Companion to Psychiatric Studies* 4th edn. Edinburgh: Churchill Livingstone.
Gelder, M., Gath D., Mayon R. (1989). *Oxford Textbook of Psychiatry* 2nd edn. Oxford: Oxford University Press.

# 16

# INFANTS AND CHILDREN

## Neil McIntosh

## INTRODUCTION

The application of clinical method in adult medicine is straightforward, the patient usually being cooperative. In paediatric medicine, clinical method must be modified in accordance with the age of the child and the degree of cooperation, and it is thus more taxing to the specialist and non-specialist alike. In the UK it is usual for children to be assessed in primary care by general practitioners (GPs) not by paediatricians. Some such practitioners have had little or no specific post-graduate paediatric training. Casualty officers are frequently training for surgical careers and similarly have had little postgraduate training in pae-diatrics before their experience in casualty. The inclusion of a chapter on paediatric method within a book on practical clinical medicine can be justified on these grounds alone. The addition of sections on non-accidental injury and child sexual abuse also seems appropriate, not only because of the current interest in these subjects but because their presentation may well be to GPs or adult specialists through an emergency department.

## HISTORY TAKING

The history-taking session represents the major proportion of the paediatric examination as physical signs are comparatively uncommon in children. The session offers not only the opportunity for the patient to transfer pertinent information to the doctor but also the opportunity for the doctor to study the relationship of the child with the parents. If the child is attending for the first time it also establishes the doctor's relationship with both the parent and the child. Some areas of the history may be deferred until the end of the interview when rapport has been more firmly established. It is worth emphasizing that many questions routine and innocuous to the medical profession may be upsetting and threatening to the family. For instance, the term abortion medically relates to expulsion of a fetus before 28 weeks gestation. In lay terms, miscarriage is used for this event and abortion is reserved for more therapeutic/elective procedures, some of which may be outside the framework of the law. It is also sometimes more appropriate to ask about the child's father rather than the mother's husband.

Even when the child concerned is quite young the history should be obtained, if possible, from them first and then with confirmation of the facts from the parent. The parent may have areas to discuss that cannot or should not be revealed in front of an older child (and vice versa). It is important to consider interviewing each separately. Possibly the appropriate time is during the physical examination, when the child may be questioned apart from the parents and the parents may be questioned outside the room as the child dresses or undresses.

During the history taking one should note whether the history is estimated to be reliable or coloured by the parents' concern or their lack of information about things that are important. Biased medical comment should not be entered into the notes unless justified. Even so, the pae-diatrician frequently gets information second-hand via the parent and so must question how the history given has been acquired. Examples of this are:

(1) 'The baby has abdominal pain.' (The baby draws his or her legs up while crying.)
(2) 'The baby has pain in the ear.' (He or she has been rubbing the ear.)
(3) 'My baby doesn't like the milk.' (My baby has stopped sucking at the bottle.)

If parents use semitechnical terms, e.g., wheezy, diarrhoea, constipation, ask them to explain what they mean!

## Present complaint

The present complaint is the response to the question, 'Why are you here today?' It may or may not be related to the child's medical condition. However, it is the most significant part of the paediatric history and adequate time should be allowed to obtain a detailed account, arranging this in significant, chronological order. It is appropriate to make brief notes while the parent or child gives the history, rewriting in more detail later. Scribbling busily during the whole of the history taking makes eye-to-eye contact impossible and distances the developing relationship between doctor and parent. Be precise about dates when recording the history: remember that last Monday is useless in the notes, use '5 days before admission (21st May)'; one month ago should be dated to 'about the 25th January'. When this is attempted as the parent or child first tells the story, important details of the history can later be inserted when they are presented out of chronological order. It is important to obtain what the parent or child observed rather than the diagnosis told by the GP or a more distant relative. Show interest in the parent's observations—if the child is said to have had a fever, enquire (with tact) whether the temperature was taken. What medicines or other treatments has the child had during the illness and what has been the response to these?

When a complete story has been heard, supplement this by questions that may provide significant positive or negative information—example: in a wheezy child—how much school has been missed? Is this because he or she is kept at home or sent home from school (each may have a very different implication)?

At the end of the account of the present illness it is often useful to give a history back to the parent in chronological order. This shows that you have understood and heard all the information provided and it also allows the parent to insert any forgotten details.

## Previous medical history

(1) Enquire about: The pregnancy, gestation, delivery and condition in the neonatal period with details if appropriate, for example:

(a) *gestation*—duration, discrepancy of size of infant during pregnancy, medications and illness of mother;

(b) *delivery*—was this spontaneous, induced, instrumental or caesarian section?—elaborate reasons if abnormal;

(c) *neonatal period*—did the child require special treatment, what was this and why was it necessary—(the clinic Baby Book may be useful as a source of information)?

(2) *Development* up to the time the present complaint started. A developmental guide is useful here, e.g., the Denver development chart for a young child. Consider the development under the categories (a) physical growth (comparing with sibs and peers and considering pubertal information if relevant), and (b) mental development (again comparing with sibs and peers with details of the latest school report if appropriate).

(3) *Immunizations*—what has been given and when, and were they believed to have been successful? Have boosters been given? If any immunizations were omitted, ask why. (A charted UK immunization schedule is shown in Table 16.1.)

(4) *Response to infectious diseases*. Record details of any acute exanthemata and of coughs and colds, with their frequency and treatment.

(5) *Hospital admissions and accidents*. Details should be recorded of these as appropriate.

(6) *Allergy or atopy*. Record both the severity of these from the history and any medication that has been used.

## Family history

The purpose of a family history is to gain insight into the genetic and epidemiological background of the child and also to anticipate the setting in which the disease and the medical care of the child with the disease will take place. In recording familial disease a kinship diagram with standard symbols should be used and pursued as appropriate to each generation (Fig. 16.1). If through death or divorce both natural parents are not the acting parents this should be noted.

The age, health and occupation of the parents and siblings should be recorded and other household members and animals should be noted, with their state of health. Recent travel history may be of importance—travel to exotic parts of the world or to a new playgroup may be equally significant.

**Table 16.1 UK immunization schedule**

*General*

| | |
|---|---|
| 2 months | Diphtheria, tetanus, pertussis as triple vaccine, intramuscularly (1) |
| | Polio, oral (1) |
| 3 months | Triple vaccine, intramuscularly (2) |
| | Polio, oral (2) |
| 4 months | Triple vaccine, intramuscularly (3) |
| | Polio, oral, (3) |
| 12–18 months | Measles, mumps and rubella vaccine, intramuscularly |
| 4–5 years | Preschool booster: diphtheria and tetanus |
| | Polio, oral |
| 11–14 years | Rubella vaccine for girls |
| 15–19 years | Oral polio vaccine |
| | Tetanus toxoid |

*Additions in high-risk populations*

| | | |
|---|---|---|
| Birth | BCG | If close family history of tuberculosis or of Asian origin |
| Birth | Hepatitis B vaccine (1) with hepatitis B immunoglobulin | If mother hepatitis B-positive (particularly e antigen) |
| 1 month | Hepatitis B vaccine (2) | If mother hepatitis B-positive (particularly e antigen) |
| 6 months | Hepatitis B vaccine (3) | If mother hepatitis B-positive (particularly e antigen) |
| 11–14 years | BCG vaccine | If tuberculin negative |

*NB.* If baby born preterm, it is now thought correct to give the immunizations at their true age *not* their corrected age.

*Gentle* enquiry about miscarriages and infant deaths is appropriate as these will seldom be spontaneously mentioned.

## Social history

Much of this may have been covered in taking the family history:

(1) *Physical environment.* Are the parents living in a house or flat and what is the neighbourhood, what are the sanitary conditions, how many are there in the family and how many are there in the bedrooms of the apartment? Is there a play area for the child?

(2) *Economic factors.* The parental occupation will have been recorded during the family history but more detail may be required of income and aid, depending on the type of illness of the child. If unemployed, how long for, and was there a previous trade, training or profession?

(3) *Cultural factors.* Race (sickle cell anaemia, thalassaemia), religion (Jehovah's Witness—implications for blood transfusions; vegan), complementary medical practices (goat's milk user; homeopath).

(4) *Social adaptation.* Does the child go to nursery school or playgroup, does he or she partake in school activities, scouts, church, etc? Get details of the school.

(5) *Medical contacts.* How many doctors has the family seen and how often do they see them? It is frequently worth a phone call to the general practice to find out the details. If the child is preschool, which child health clinic is used?

## THE EXAMINATION

### Introduction

Every child must have a careful and complete physical examination. The first step is to get the confidence and cooperation of the patient but this is not always possible in paediatrics. There are some tough customers—younger children often do not like being handled by strangers.

In the very young child (age 1 to 2 years) a useful approach is to take the initial history about the child from the family, completely ignoring the child with no eye-to-eye contact. During this time, the child can play around or sit on a chair or the parent's lap as he or she wishes. The fact that you and the parents are talking relaxes the child. Toddlers are often frightened and are usually best examined on the parent's lap. Inspection of the whole child as he or she plays is often most revealing and should not be neglected in one's haste to listen to the heart or look at the eyes. What is available should be examined first. You should not insist on an orderly examination with the child lying down as this will particularly frighten children between the age of 18 months and 3 years.

The child may gain confidence during the examination if the examiner plays with him or her.

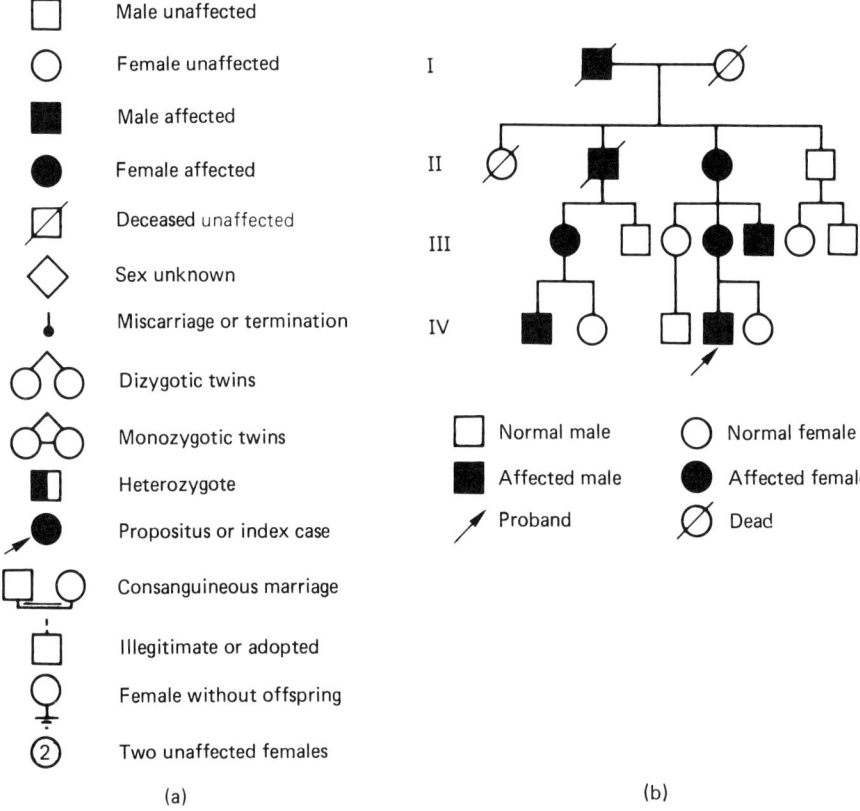

| | |
|---|---|
| □ | Male unaffected |
| ○ | Female unaffected |
| ■ | Male affected |
| ● | Female affected |
| ⊘ | Deceased unaffected |
| ◇ | Sex unknown |
| ● | Miscarriage or termination |
| ⚭ | Dizygotic twins |
| ⚭ | Monozygotic twins |
| ◧ | Heterozygote |
| ● | Propositus or index case |
| □—○ | Consanguineous marriage |
| □ | Illegitimate or adopted |
| ♀ | Female without offspring |
| ② | Two unaffected females |

(a)

Normal male   Normal female
Affected male   Affected female
Proband   Dead

(b)

*Figure 16.1*   Symbols used in a kinship diagram and family pedigree pattern of an autosomal dominant trait through four generations.

Allowing the child to handle the examining instruments may remove much of their fearful image. Use the instruments only later in the examination. The stethoscope may be used to listen to a knee or an arm before putting it on the chest; it warms it up and it shows the child it is not a painful procedure. Listening to a teddy bear occasionally pays dividends! In children old enough to understand, a clear simple description of what is going to be done, followed by strict adherence to what has been described, may build significant trust. Limits can be set but cooperation invited within these, for instance, you should not necessarily ask children if they mind having their ears examined, but you could ask which ear you can look in first. All procedures should be explained before you do them, particularly the painful ones, which should be done last. Tell the child what is expected and don't ask permission. In the young and uncooperative child, many points will be missed in the examination. If the situation is obviously non-urgent, another outpatient appointment may be made to clarify missed aspects, but if the situation is obviously urgent the child should be admitted and occasionally even sedated or given an anaesthetic to define the presence or absence of some physical signs.

The physical examination should be written up with special attention to the relevant history, and all the negative findings pertinent to the history should be recorded. For example, in the asthmatic *no wheeze* is just as relevant as *bilateral wheeze.*

### General condition

An overall comment on the child's nutrition, physical development and behaviour for the age should be noted. The height, weight and head circumference should be plotted on a centile chart and developmental progress should be assessed if appropriate.

## Vital signs

The pulse and respiration of the child should be taken, as should the blood pressure. Children as well as adults have a blood pressure! Temperature may be taken with a rectal thermometer in babies or with an oral thermometer in the older child. Remember that the respiratory rate or pulse may be exaggerated by the stress of the examination and if an odd result turns up, note down the child's state and obtain a sleeping value.

## Skin

Texture, colour, rashes, birthmarks, spots, oedema, bruises or other trauma should be noted. Are there signs of dehydration or wasting? Is the hair distribution normal?

## Lymph nodes

These should be assessed in the usual fields. Children usually have palpable cervical nodes, but fixity would be very important.

## The head

The size, shape and symmetry of the head and the size of fontanelles should be noted. The head circumference should be plotted on a centile chart. The condition of the fontanelle is particularly important (full—possibly meningitis or increased intracranial pressure; sunken in dehydration). Stiffness and swelling of the neck should be assessed.

## The eyes

Is there photophobia, conjunctivitis, cataracts? Are the pupil reactions normal? Are the sclera icteric? Is there strabismus (is the reflection of a distant light at the same position on each pupil?)? Try to get some idea of the visual activity and examine the fundi (see 'Central nervous system' below).

## Chest

Examine this as for an adult but auscultate before percussing. The most important physical sign in chest medicine applied to paediatrics is the respiratory rate. In a peaceful child a raised respiratory rate is an exceedingly good index of lung path-ology. Note recession and the presence or absence of stridor.

## The heart

Examine as for adults. The most important sign in paediatric cardiology is the quality of the pulmonary component of the second sound. Do try and listen to it and describe it. It should only be audible in the pulmonary area. Murmurs should be graded out of 6; 5 and 6 have thrills.

## The abdomen

Examine as for adults. In children a change in bowel habit does not usually indicate the necessity for a rectal examination but it should be done if one is considering appendicitis or an acute abdomen.

## Urinogenital system

Do examine the genitalia of all children, male and female, and describe the state of puberty in older children. Before telling parents that their boy is cryptorchid, get a second opinion in a warm environment!

## Musculoskeletal systems

Is there a scoliosis or kyphosis of the spine, or spina bifida occulta, or a sacral dermal pit? Comment where relevant. Test for dislocation of the hips in the newborn by Ortolani's sign.

## Central nervous system

This examination requires considerable patience and a fair amount of cooperation and play in small children. To do a fundal examination, get a parent to stand 6 ft (about 2 m) behind you, showing the child objects, and ask the child to tell you about these. When the child focuses on the parent, the disc is usually easily seen. If you are worried about raised intracranial pressure, percuss the skull—a boxy, cracked-pot sound indicates suture separation. Head circumference should be measured.

## Ears, nose and throat

It is exceedingly important that the younger child should be held properly if information is to be complete here (Figs. 16.2 and 16.3). Is there any discharge from the nose? Is the air passage bilateral? Is there a foreign body present in the nose? Is there any hearing loss or discharge from the ears? Are the drums normal? In the throat, is there pallor or cyanosis of the lips and mouth? Are there any clefts or the enanthem of measles (Koplik's spots); redness of Stensen's duct as in mumps; petechiae on the soft palate as in infectious mononucleosis? In older children, asking them to pant like a dog may permit the visualization of the pharynx without the need to use a tongue depressor, which usually causes gagging. Note the presence of a postnasal drip or pus on the tonsils. The throat should probably be examined last in the examination as this is frequently a cause of distress.

## Summary

A short summary of the history and examination with relevant positive and negative features will crystallize the case. A differential diagnosis can then be considered in order of likelihood.

## NON-ACCIDENTAL INJURY

This may take the form of:
(a) physical abuse;
(b) neglect and mental abuse;
(c) sexual abuse.
Any abnormality should be photographed.

### Physical abuse

Physical abuse may mimic natural childhood injury. If the nature of an injury is not consistent with the account of how the injury occurred, then a child should always be admitted to a paediatric unit until the circumstances are clarified. It may be impossible to be certain that a single injury is the result of abuse or accident, but one of the most helpful signs of physical abuse is the presence of injuries at different stages of resolution, indicating that injury has occurred on more than one occasion. The diagnosis of osteogenesis imperfecta when bones are fractured and of bleeding tendency, e.g., haemophilia, when there are multiple bruises should be viewed sceptically because of their individual rarity. If there is any suggestion

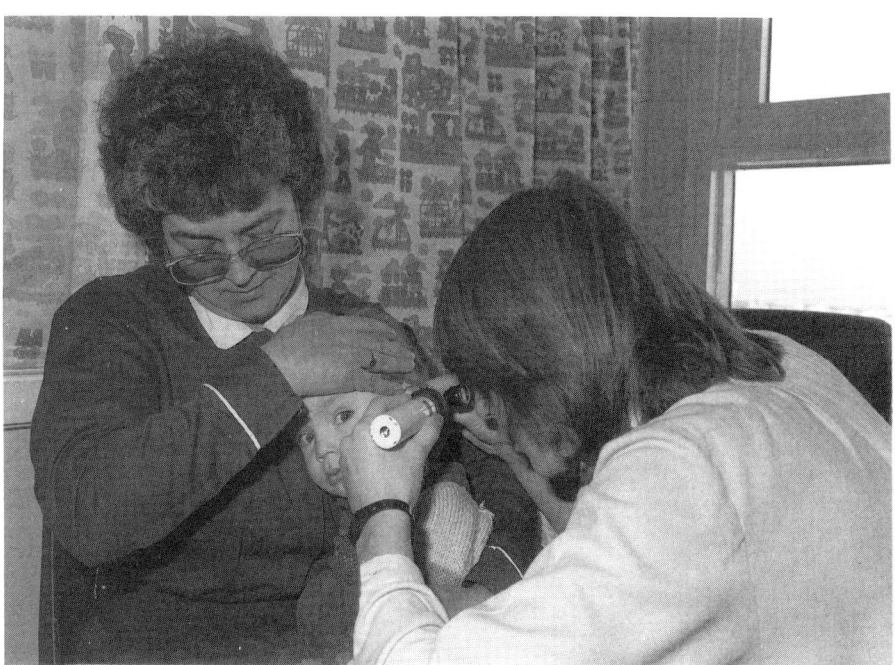

*Figure 16.2* Holding child for ear examination (the penultimate part of the general examination). Child sits sideways on the parent's lap. One of the parent's hands holds the child's head firmly onto the parent's own body. The other parent's hand holds the child's arms.

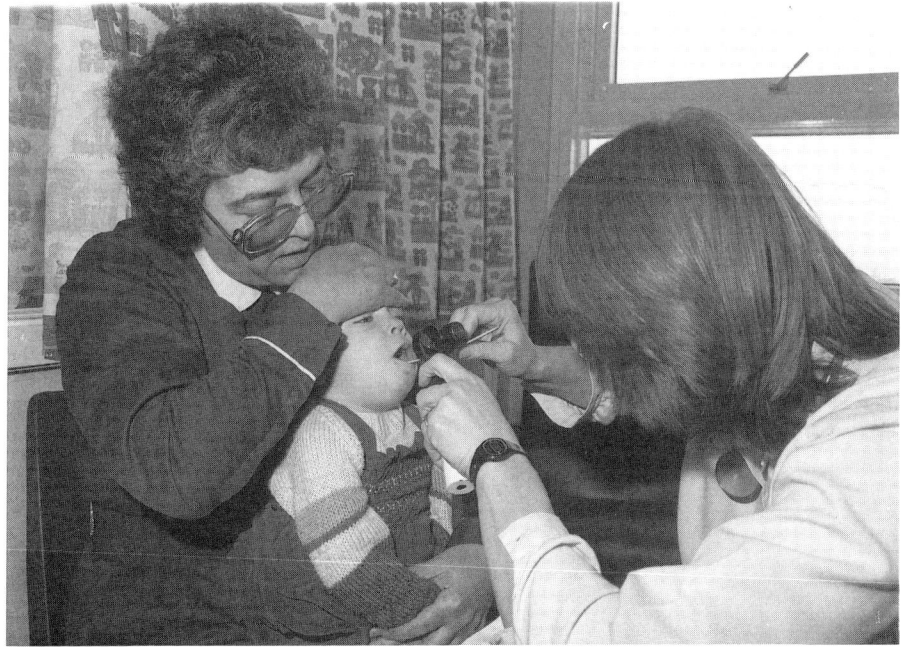

*Figure 16.3* Holding young child for throat examination (the last part of the general examination). Child sits on parent's lap facing forward. One of the parent's hands holds the child's forehead firmly tipped back, the other encompasses the child's body and arms, so that wriggling is impossible.

that a child has been wilfully injured, that child should be immediately referred for a paediatric opinion while the signs are present. The paediatrician should almost always admit the child to substantiate or disprove the diagnosis. The interests of the child are paramount. If the primary presenting problem is bruising, a full clotting screen is needed to rule out an inherited or acquired bleeding tendency. If the presentation has been a fracture, then a complete skeletal survey is required to assess bone texture and structure generally and to identify previous trauma. Physical abuse can also take the form of:

(1) *Shaking*, with the production of intracranial haemorrhage from rupture of delicate veins. This leads to subdural haematoma formation with disturbed sensorium. The fundi should always be visualized in an attempt to identify retinal haemorrhages.

(2) *Systematic burns* (often with cigarette) or scalds.

(3) *Poisoning*. Children with disturbances of sensorium or apparent encephalopathies should always have urine and blood samples stored for analysis of toxic products if natural illness cannot be confirmed.

### Neglect

Neglect may be obvious, leading acutely to cold injury or starvation, or chronically to failure of the infant to thrive. Hospital admission should always occur and, if not accepted by the parents, social services and sometimes the police should be notified. Classically the child who is neglected or failing to thrive because of emotional deprivation will rally in the hospital environment, putting on significant amounts of weight in a short period of time. However, there may be a delay period before this weight gain begins.

### Child sexual abuse

Child sexual abuse is defined as the involvement of dependent, developmentally immature children and adolescents in sexual activities that they do not truly comprehend, to which they are unable to give informed consent or that violate the social taboos of family roles. Any child below the age of consent may be deemed to have been sexually assaulted when any person by design or neglect involves the child in any activity of a nature that is intended to lead to the sexual arousal and gratification of that person or any other person. This definition stands whether or not this activity involves genital contact and whether or not this is initiated by the child.

Child sexual abuse is not new. It is, though, being increasingly recognized both because society is more ready to confront uncomfortable facts and because paediatricians are more aware of the presentations. Sustained sexual abuse of children causes not only physical injury but also has adverse effects on physical and emotional health, growth and development. This is why a complete physical examination is required for children with physical or behavioural complaints. If the possibility of child sexual abuse arises, a paediatrician should be asked to examine the child fully. The anogenital examination is important but not pre-eminent. Sexual abuse may occur without anogenital contact; conversely, physical abnormalities may have an innocent explanation. It is naive to diagnose child sexual abuse on physical evidence alone except when there has been gross assault. The painstaking inquiry that is initiated once suspicion has been raised should be performed by the expert, with the interview and examination if possible being videoed for future evidence.

### Signs and symptoms of child sexual abuse

Physical indicators on genital and anal areas:
(a) bruises, scratches and other injuries;
(b) itchiness, soreness, discharge or unexplained bleeding;
(c) foreign bodies in the urethra, bladder, vagina or anal canal;
(d) abnormal dilatation of urethra, anus or vaginal opening;
(e) pain on micturition;
(f) signs of sexually transmitted infections;
(g) semen in the vagina or anus or on external genitalia.
  Physical indicators generally:
(a) bruises, scratches, bites on body;
(b) difficulty in walking or sitting;
(c) torn, stained or bloody underclothes or evidence of clothing having been removed or replaced;
(d) semen on skin or clothes;
(e) pregnancy in teenagers;
(f) recurrent urinary tract infections;
(g) psychosomatic features such as recurrent abdominal pain or headache.

Behavioural indicators:
(1) *Sexual*:
  (a) a child who hints at sexual activity through words, play or drawings;
  (b) a child with excessive preoccupation with sexual matters and a precocious knowledge of sexual behaviour; one who repeatedly engages in inappropriate sexual play with peers; a child who is sexually provocative with adults;
  (c) an older girl who behaves in a sexually precocious way; she may be 'a vamp';
  (d) requests for information on contraception, though this is rare.
(2) *General*:
  (a) a sudden change in mood;
  (b) regressive behaviour, e.g., onset of bed-wetting;
  (c) change in eating patterns, loss of appetite, faddiness;
  (d) lack of trust in familiar adults or marked fear of men;
  (e) disobedience, attention-seeking or restless, aimless behaviour and poor concentration;
  (f) sleep disturbance with fears, vivid dreams or nightmares;
  (g) social isolation, child playing alone;
  (h) girl takes on mother role in family whether or not mother is present;
  (i) inappropriate displays of affection between fathers and daughters or mothers and sons; behave more like lovers than parent and child.
(3) *Behaviour especially noticeable at school*:
  (a) poor peer relationships and inability to make friends;
  (b) inability to concentrate; learning difficulties or a sudden drop in school performance; some may see school as a haven, they arrive early, are reluctant to leave and perform well;
  (c) marked reluctance to participate in and change clothing for PE and games;
  (d) avoidance and fear of school medical examinations.
(4) *Behaviour in older children*:
  (a) antisocial behaviour or delinquency;
  (b) hysterical attacks;
  (c) suicide attempts and self-mutilation;
  (d) dependence on alcohol and drugs.

Should child sexual abuse be suspected on grounds of history, it is more appropriate for a specialist paediatrician with an expertise in this area to carry out a full interview and examination. This is not an area for the amateur.

### Summary

If a child presents in a casualty or outpatients department and there is suspicion of actual or potential abuse, the child should be admitted. Suspicion should not be expressed to the parents at this stage and no attempt should be made to obtain an admission of guilt. Explain that admission is necessary for investigation and treatment. If the child presents to the GP and there is definite evidence of abuse of any sort, the child should be admitted to hospital. Arrangements for this should be made directly with the paediatrician or deputy, and the casualty department should be warned that the child must be admitted straight to the wards without the usual procedures of being admitted from a casualty or admissions office. If there is no evidence of injury but certain of the factors associated with child abuse have been clearly identified, the family doctor should discuss the problem with a medical colleague, the principal physician in child health, health visitor and social worker. If the child presents in clinic or school, the clinical medical officer should be informed, who should inform the principal physician in child health and the social services. If parents refuse to collaborate in the investigation of child abuse, it is appropriate to obtain a place of safety order, which will usually define the paediatric ward of the local hospital as the place of safety.

## ACUTE CRISES

### Severe wheeze

In the child with a history of previous wheezing or cough, severe wheezing is likely to be due to an exacerbation of asthma. Although classically asthma gives wheezing in expiration, if it is of any severity the wheeze will also be evident in inspiration. If the child has an extremely severe attack, then very little wheezing may be present, simply because the air entry is so poor. In this situation, the child may be cyanosed and hyperinflated with a pronounced tachycardia and tachypnoea and an easily definable pulsus paradoxus. If the child is of an age when he or she can talk, the speech may be

in monosyllables or even absent (from breathlessness). If the child is a known asthmatic, then treatment at this stage may well be more urgent than investigation with chest X-rays or blood gases; indeed arterial sampling for blood gases in the young child may result in deterioration. If there is any suggestion that the diagnosis is not asthma, a chest X-ray is indicated, but it would be more appropriate to do this investigation on the ward, than to send the child in a critical condition to the X-ray department.

The treatment of the severe attack is initially with oxygen given by nasal catheter or by a parent holding a mask (oxygen/steam tents are very frightening for young children), and with nebulized salbutamol, which if necessary can be given by mask ventilation by a physiotherapist. As soon as this therapy is underway, it is appropriate to ensure adequate hydration with a drip to which aminophylline and steroids should be added (care in theophylline dosage is needed if the child has been on this medication previously). The intravenous therapy should continue until blood gases are normal and the intermittent nebulized β-sympathomimetic should be continued until the child is wheeze free. If the child is of an age when a peak flow meter can be used, this should be measured frequently (before and after nebulized therapy) to identify the improvement in condition. The normal values are related to the child's height.

The dosages for the above regimen are:
Salbutamol nebulizer, 3- to 4-hourly, diluted in 2 ml of normal saline.
Aminophylline, 4 mg/kg intravenously over 10 min—loading dose; 20 mg/kg/24 h—infusion. (If on theophylline at home— *no loading dose*.)
Hydrocortisone, 4 mg/kg, 2-hourly, intravenously.
Oxygen—as much as the child will take to relieve cyanosis. (There is *no* danger that oxygen will cause respiratory depression as there is in an adult with chronic bronchitis.)

Rarely, severe wheeze may be due to acute obstruction caused by a foreign body or by an anaphylactic reaction to drug, food or possibly a bee sting. In these cases, the history of a very sudden onset of wheeze and the absence of a previous history is important. On examination, the child who has inhaled a foreign body may have signs predominantly on one side—hyperinflation and wheeze. If the cause is anaphylaxis there may be other signs of this. Removal of the foreign body may be urgent by laryngoscopy and bronchoscopy carried out by an experienced ENT surgeon. While this is being organized, oxygen should be given. If the obstruction is part of an anaphylactic reaction, the treatment of the anaphylaxis is urgent and again oxygen should be given while this is having its effect.

## Acute upper airway obstruction

This may be caused by croup or *Haemophilus influenzae* epiglottitis or the inhalation of a foreign body. An anaesthetist should be called urgently to assist in management if the airway is compromised and resuscitation equipment must be made available. Do not be fooled by the apparent lack of chest signs, which may be related simply to the poor entry of air caused by severe obstruction. Oxygen and a sitting, leaning forward posture may improve oxygenation. It is crucial in the acutely ill child to avoid delays, (e.g., in the accident and emergency department or particularly in the X-ray department) and to arrange assessment of the child urgently in the operating theatre before radiographs, 'drugs and bloods' are done. A paediatrician, anaesthetist and ENT surgeon with experience would be the optimal team.

If the diagnosis of epiglottitis is confirmed, orotracheal intubation is carried out. This tube may be changed for a nasotracheal tube as these are easier to secure. Chloramphenicol (50–100 mg/kg/day—divided into 6-hourly doses) should be given intravenously; it is much more effective than ampicillin (and recently about 15 per cent of *Haemophilus* isolates have been resistant to ampicillin).

If the diagnosis of epiglottitis is not confirmed, laryngoscopy and bronchoscopy by the ENT surgeon may assist diagnosis of an aspirated foreign body or viral laryngotracheobronchitis (croup). Clinically, viral croup may have been suspected from the absence of toxicity in the child, even if he or she is very tired. Endotracheal intubation may be required on clinical grounds, e.g., with subglottic oedema or exhaustion.

There is no proven place for steroids in viral croup. Most children get treated with antibiotics (ampicillin) because of the clinical anxiety of a bacterial cause.

Continued management by a multidisciplinary team is crucial until there is no longer a danger of airway obstruction and senior staff should be alerted rapidly if there is any deterioration.

## Severe dehydration

In the UK, severe dehydration is usually due to gastroenteritis with diarrhoea and vomiting and the situation may have been exaggerated by a poor fluid intake. Before beginning fluid therapy, four aspects of the patient should be evaluated:
(a) fluid volume deficit;
(b) body fluid osmolality;
(c) acid–base status;
(d) extracellular electrolytes.

### Fluid deficit

Accurate assessment of the fluid deficit is important as fluid replacement is based on this estimation. Classically there are three levels of dehydration:

*Less than 5 per cent*, with dryness of the skin and mucous membranes, oliguria and slight depression of the fontanelle if the child still has one.

*5 to 10 per cent*, where the dehydration is leading to a circulatory disturbance, manifested by tachycardia, mottled skin, cool extremities and severe oliguria. Usually there is associated loss of elasticity or turgor of the abdominal skin and depression of the eyeballs and, if present, the fontanelle, though this may not be so evident if there is significant hypernatraemia (see below). The child is usually lethargic and uninterested in its surroundings.

*10 to 15 per cent*, where the signs are as above doses but the patient is in a moribund condition (the previous record of body weight may be helpful in assessment).

An infant estimated to be 10 per cent dehydrated and weighing 10 kg has a fluid deficit of 1 l, which will need replacement in addition to (a) the ongoing losses after the initial assessment, and (b) the maintenance requirements.

### Osmolality

When a child is dehydrated the remaining body fluids may remain isotonic (because of parallel loss of electrolytes) or they may become hypotonic, or if free water loss predominates, the body fluids may become hypertonic and hypernatraemic. The latter is particularly likely if the parents have attempted to rectify the fluid loss with too concentrated a feed or solids. In this situation, the abdominal skin may have a thickened or doughy feel and the infant may develop neurological disturbances.

### Acid–base

The acid–base status of the child should be assessed by a blood gas, the acidosis being representative of the inadequate tissue and, in particular, renal perfusion. Kussmaul's breathing may be clinical evidence of this. Only in the more severe cases should correction be made as the repletion of body fluids and the correction of electrolyte disturbance will usually allow the kidney to rectify the situation.

### Electrolytes

Finally, fluid replacement should be done in parallel with electrolyte replacement and the early measurement of serum electrolytes is mandatory.

If the child is in actual or impending shock, the rapid expansion of the vascular space with 20 ml/kg of plasma in 30 min will allow better oxygen transport to the periphery and ensure that the kidneys remain perfused. If plasma is not available, 10 per cent dextrose in normal saline will support the plasma volume for a few hours. The remaining treatment depends on whether the dehydration is hypotonic or isotonic or hypernatraemic. The first two are treated similarly; half the deficit is replaced in 6 h and the other half over the subsequent 12 to 18 h. In addition, provision must be made for ongoing losses and the maintenance requirements. This is all best done with a glucose and multiple electrolyte solution (e.g., 5 per cent dextrose and 50–60 mmol Na/l, 30–40 mmol K/l).

If the child is significantly hypernatraemic (serum sodium greater than 150 mmol/l), having supported the extravascular compartment with plasma or normal saline, very slow fluid replacement is undertaken with 10 per cent glucose in half-normal saline with 30 mmol potassium/l of solution at a rate no greater than 150 ml/kg/24 h. Faster correction leads to rapid osmolar shifts across the blood–brain barrier with the possibility of fitting. The high sodium content of the replacement solution makes rapid sodium shifts less likely. (Despite being hypernatraemic, these children have a total body deficit of sodium and the kidneys will sort things out satisfactorily if renal plasma flow is adequate.)

If the child is cooperative and the dehydration is clinically less than 10 per cent, oral rehydration with a dextrose electrolyte solution is quite effective. If the child cannot cooperate, or the vomiting is excessive, or the dehydration is severe, intravenous replacement is essential. An occasional uncooperative child who is *not* vomiting will tolerate a nasogastric tube for rehydration.

### Fitting

The causes of convulsions are summarized in the list below. Not only is it essential to stop the fitting because prolonged convulsions themselves may cause significant secondary damage to the brain, but, if it is known, it is essential to treat the cause.
(1) *Central nervous system disorders*:
    (a) prenatal or perinatal malformations, e.g., vascular (Sturge–Weber syndrome), porencephaly, etc.;
    (b) tuberous sclerosis;
    (c) infections (bacterial meningitis, viral meningo-encephalitis);
    (d) intracranial space-occupying lesions (cysts, abscesses, tumours);
    (e) intracranial haemorrhage;
    (f) trauma;
    (g) acute cerebral oedema (e.g., acute glomerulonephritis);
    (h) degenerative (e.g., Tay–Sachs disease, leucodystrophies).
(2) *Toxic*—e.g., lead encephalopathy and glue inhalation.
(3) *Metabolic*—e.g., hypoxia, hypoglycaemia, hypocalcaemia, inborn errors (phenylketonuria).
(4) *Fever*.
(5) *Idiopathic epilepsy*.

If a first convulsion occurs between 6 months and 3 years of age, and it is associated with fever, it may well be a febrile convulsion. If this convulsion is generalized and lasts for no more than 15 min, and if examination shows no neurological abnormality (after the convulsion has stopped) and an obvious cause for the fever is discernible, it is reasonable to assume that it is a simple febrile convulsion with a good outlook. One in five such children (25–50 per cent depending on age, sex and family history) will have a repeat episode but only 1 to 5 per cent will go on to develop epilepsy. If the diagnosis of a febrile convulsion is not ascertained or substantiated, multiple investigations may be required to elaborate the cause.

The termination of a prolonged convulsion is

urgent. The use of rectal diazepam by the parents (in children who have had several previous convulsions) and by accident and emergency departments has greatly helped prevent secondary brain damage from intracerebral acidosis and infarction. In resistant cases intravenous infusion of diazepam (Valium), phenytoin (Epanutin) or chlormethiazole (Heminevrin) may be necessary but this should only be used when airway maintenance is ensured and ventilatory assistance can be readily provided. If diazepam does not work, many would suggest anaesthesia.

The dosages for the above regimen are:

Rectal diazepam—5 mg rectal sachet for those under 3 years of age; 10 mg rectal sachet for those older than this.

Intravenous diazepam—50 µg/kg/h or bolus of 300 µg/kg.

Intravenous phenytoin, 10 to 15 mg/kg over 30 min (not exceeding 50 mg/min).

Chlormethiazole—up to 3 mg in 5 min for those under 3 years of age; 1 to 4 mg in 3 to 5 min if older, then reduce the rate.

## Breath-holding attacks

These may be confused with convulsion. They occur between 6 and 36 months of age and are usually precipitated by pain, fright or frustration. The baby cries and at the end of expiration fails to breathe in, becoming cyanosed and then unconscious, with or without a convulsion. Though frightening, these attacks are self limiting because when unconsciousness occurs so does respiration. They are short-lived but may be quite frequent.

## Unconsciousness

Immediate supportive therapy to prevent hypoxia and prompt aetiological diagnosis to ensure proper specific treatment are both mandatory. If there is satisfactory respiratory effort and cardiac output, the airway should be cleared and the child nursed in the semiprone position. The stomach should be emptied and continuous or frequent nasogastric suction should be given. A reliable intravenous access should be ensured for administration of parenteral fluids, blood, plasma and drugs as indicated. If the child is convulsing, the fits should be controlled (see above).

The elaboration of a cause is from a consideration of the history obtained from the parents or witnesses, a meticulous physical examination and the use of special laboratory and radiological tests, which may also be used to ascertain the need for specific emergency measures. Remember that the lack of oxygen and glucose for brain metabolism can lead to permanent damage and at least until an aetiological diagnosis is clear, both oxygen and intravenous glucose can do no harm.

The level of consciousness should be determined and sequential observations started using a Coma Scale. Unconscious patients must be turned very carefully, with no differential spinal movement, until spinal injury can be discounted. Is there any evidence of external injury elsewhere? If so, is all the trauma visible likely to be of the same time of causing? If it is not, non-accidental injury must be considered. Needle punctures may indicate a history of diabetes or narcotic usage, depending on site. Angiomas about the head and face may suggest an intracranial arteriovenous malformation. Neck stiffness may suggest meningitis or intracranial bleeding with a subarachnoid component. The conjunctivae, oropharynx and skin should be carefully examined for the petechiae of meningococcal septicaemia. Erythematous eruptions may indicate both viral and severe bacterial infection. In the cardiovascular system a very rapid heart rate may suggest syncope associated with paroxysmal tachycardia. Evidence of old rheumatic or congenital heart disease may be associated with emboli (septic or non-septic). In the abdomen a large spleen may suggest a sickle cell disorder or the possibility of cerebral malaria. Hypertrophy of the penis or clitoris may suggest an Addisonian crisis associated with congenital adrenal hyperplasia or hypoglycaemia. In the examination of the central nervous system, particular attention should be paid to any localizing signs.

If the history and examination give no indication for the cause of unconsciousness, blood should be sent for a full count and stained film, sugar, gas, urea and serum electrolytes, calcium and magnesium and ammonia. Ask about medicines around at home and where there is any suspicion of drug ingestion do a toxicology screen. Vomit and urine should be saved for analysis. A skull and chest X-ray should be done and if there is any suggestion of intracranial trauma or abnormality, a CT scan of the head should be organized. Evidence of raised intracranial pressure (slow pulse, raised blood pressure—*do not* automatically expect papilloedema) is a contraindication to lumbar puncture unless this decision is made with neurosurgical facilities immediately available.

## Acute heart failure

Heart failure may be due to (a) major cardiac malformation; (b) an acquired myocardial disorder; or (c) an extracardiac cause. The predominance of these varies with the age of the child and it is usual to consider heart failure as occurring in either the neonatal period, in infancy or in childhood.

Heart failure in the neonate may be caused by lesions incompatible with postnatal life, e.g., hypoplastic left heart or right heart, transposition of the great vessels or severe coarctation of the aorta. The tachycardia may be associated with marked tachypnoea, which prevents the infant from feeding. There may be a marked weight loss or a poor weight gain, or occasionally excessive weight gain from oedema. Cyanosis may be pronounced with some causes.

Later in infancy the presentation is similar but the heart lesions are essentially those compatible with the postnatal circulation. Obstructive lesions like coarctation (femoral pulses) and infradiaphragmatic anomalous pulmonary venous drainage may present at this time as may left to right shunts (septal defects and patent ductus arteriosus) and myocardial disorders (cardiomyopathies and arrhythmias).

After infancy, cardiac failure is unusual with congenital heart disease (except ostium secondum defects and aortic stenosis) and is more likely to be related to a systemic disorder, e.g., bronchiolitis, pneumonia, anaemia or acute nephritis. Acquired heart disease, such as rheumatic fever, or viral myocarditis or pericarditis also occur in this group. The sudden onset of breathlessness with poor perfusion or a rapid increase in weight may be accompanied by the signs of right ventricular failure (raised jugular venous pressure, hepatosplenomegaly and oedema) or left ventricular failure (crepitations in the lung fields). There may well be a triple cardiac rhythm.

Diagnosis is based on the history, clinical signs and the use of special cardiac tests, such as ECG, chest X-ray, echocardiogram, and sometimes cardiac enzyme studies and invasive tests.

The use of the diuretic frusemide while diagnostic tests are being carried out is of value; with the establishment of the diagnosis, more definitive operative or supportive medical treatment may be indicated. Electrolyte monitoring is mandatory with chronic diuretic therapy. Appropriate dosages in early management are:

Frusemide—1 mg/kg intravenously.

Digoxin—10 to 15 µg/kg/day intravenously; double this dose to digitalize in the first 24 h.

## Further reading

### *General*

Athreya B. H. (1980). *Clinical Methods in Paediatric Diagnosis*. New York: Van Nostrand Reinhold.

Gill D., O'Brian N. (1988). *Paediatric Clinical Examination*. Edinburgh: Churchill Livingstone.

Illingworth R. S. (1987). *The Development of the Infant and Young Child: Normal and Abnormal*, 9th edn. Edinburgh: Churchill Livingstone.

Smith D.W. (1977). *Growth and its Disorders*. Philadelphia: W. B. Saunders.

### *Child sexual abuse*

CIBA Foundation (1984). *Child Sexual Abuse within the Family*. London: CIBA/Tavistock.

Hobbs C. J., Wynne J. M. (1987). Child sexual abuse—an increasing rate of diagnosis. *Lancet*, **ii**, 837–45.

Kempe H., Kempe R. (1978). *Child Abuse*. London: Fontana.

# 17

# THE ELDERLY

Anne Freeman and Paul Finucane

Old age is the most unexpected of things that happen to man.

(*Diary in Exile*, Trotsky 1935)

Over the last 40 years geriatric medicine has developed into one of the most important sub-specialties of general medicine. It now has to be accepted that the middle-aged and elderly are responsible for a very high proportion of all hospital admissions.

The specialty has become recognized as an essential part of undergraduate education and many junior doctors are choosing to work in a geriatric department as part of their training for either general medicine or general practice. Elderly patients are also appearing, with increasing frequency, in both final MB and postgraduate diploma examinations.

Improved living standards and advances in medical care in Britain (and the other developed countries) have resulted in an increasing pro-portion of our population now living to pension-able age (60 years for women; 65 years for men) and beyond. Figure 17.1 shows that the greatest proportional increase has been among those sur-viving into their ninth decade, most of whom are female. These demographic changes pose an immense challenge that society in general and the medical profession in particular must address.

In parts of Asia and the underdeveloped areas of Africa, the average life expectancy at birth is only about 40 years. Mortality in places like Ethiopia is high due to war and famine and these countries have no need at present for specialized services for elderly people. However, health education and preventative medicine are import-ant for these people.

Ill health is more common in old people due to both pathological and physiological changes. It is not surprising, therefore, that elderly people are making increasing demands on medical services.

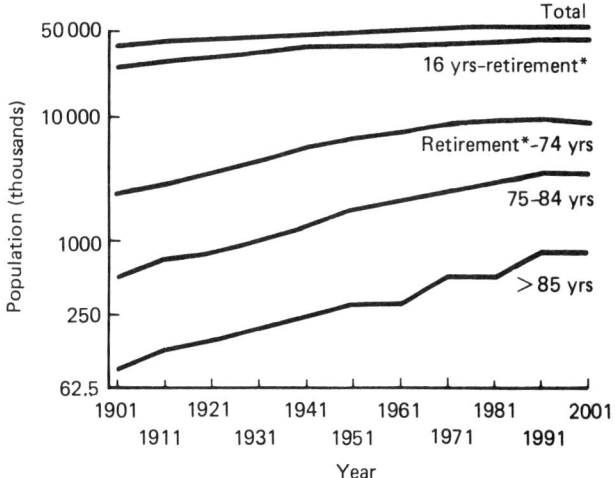

*Figure 17.1* Age structure of the population 1901–2001, United Kingdom. (OPCS 1980.) * Retirement age 65 years for men; 60 years for women.

In the 1960s, about 20 per cent of patients admitted to acute hospital beds were elderly; the figure today is just over half and is expected to reach 80 per cent by the end of this century. While approximately 16 per cent of an average general practitioner's list consists of patients aged over 65 years, this group accounts for more than 30 per cent of his or her workload.

It is, therefore, essential that all doctors, irrespective of their primary sphere of interest, understand and implement the principles of modern geriatric medicine. It is no longer traditional for elderly people to remain in hospital or long-stay wards. Instead, there must be a policy of immediate assessment and treatment of all acute illnesses and a multidisciplinary approach to active rehabilitation with the aim of returning the patient to their own home with the provision of community support services where necessary.

Earlier chapters in this book have outlined the basic approach to history taking and physical examination as well as describing the investigation and management of illnesses relating to the various systems of the body. Elderly people can present with a wide variety of problems—physical, psychological and social. The fact that the elderly do differ in many important ways from younger people is the *raison d'être* for geriatric medicine as a specialty in its own right. It is the purpose of this chapter to bring forward the special problems that may arise in the recognition and management of illness in the elderly.

## WHY THE ELDERLY PATIENT IS DIFFERENT

Many elderly patients (and sometimes their doctors) accept illness as an inevitable accompaniment of old age. Problems such as impaired mobility, joint pain, anaemia, impaired vision and hearing, incontinence and depression are particularly underreported and therefore underdetected. The aphorism 'We see only what we look for, we look for only what we know' should be borne in mind.

The clinical manifestations of illness in old age can be very different to those in younger patients. A single diagnosis can usually explain all the symptoms and signs of an illness in a young patient. However, in elderly people, clinical features are commonly attributable to a combination of coincidental diseases. Thus, dyspnoea in an old person may be due to a combination of heart failure, obstructive airways disease and anxiety. Similarly, an exacerbation of existing symptoms in a young person is most often due to a worsening of the underlying disease. In the older person, however, it may well reflect a new problem. For example, an increase in back pain in a patient with osteoarthritis of the spine may be due to a vertebral collapse secondary to coexistent osteoporosis.

When multiple diseases coexist there is a danger that clinicians may focus on the main condition that has caused the medical breakdown whilst neglecting those non-acute illnesses that affect the overall management of the patient. For this reason a problem-orientated approach is particularly appropriate in the assessment of ill-health in the elderly. Rather than just concentrating on labelling diseases the clinician must also consider the limitations caused by such conditions and attempt to reduce them. Thus he or she must not only think of arthritis but also of the immobility resulting from the arthritis. The patient's care plan may need to include physiotherapy, the modification of their home and the provision of a home help, in addition to the prescription of, say, a non-steroidal anti-inflammatory drug.

The body's response to illness alters with advancing age so that symptoms and signs of disease differ to those found in younger patients. This is particularly seen with pain and fever. For example, chest pain and dyspnoea become less frequent manifestations of an acute myocardial infarction while acute confusion and syncope become more common. Often an acute infarction is completely asymptomatic. Similarly, the examination of a patient with an acute abdomen may just reveal absent bowel sounds with no rigidity or guarding. The reason for diminished sensitivity to pain in old age is unclear. Fever is not an automatic accompaniment of an infective illness because of impairment of the thermoregulatory mechanisms. Being aware of these facts is the key to correct diagnosis.

Some malignancies are less active in elderly people and progress slowly. For example, carcinoma of the breast can remain static for many years and can often be treated conservatively.

Physical illness in the elderly commonly presents with psychiatric symptoms. These should not be accepted as due to dementia or depression until a physical cause has been considered and excluded.

While the interaction of environmental and

health problems is important in all patients it is of special relevance in the case of elderly people. Inappropriate housing and inadequate social support can often compromise the person's ability to cope at home. Management of the patient's problems may require input from other health professionals, such as physiotherapists, occupational therapists and social workers. The so-called multidisciplinary approach to the care of the elderly involves the coordinated efforts of the whole team, usually under the direction of the geriatrician.

Elderly people frequently have illnesses that are not 'socially acceptable'. Problems such as dementia and incontinence may invoke negative feelings among sufferers, their relatives and even among doctors and other health workers. So these problems are either not reported or are not further investigated. Adopting a positive approach to elderly people and their problems is the responsibility of all members of the health service.

## THE CLINICAL ASSESSMENT OF THE ELDERLY PATIENT

The clinical assessment is the key to the correct diagnosis and management of every patient. Common sense, patience and understanding are required from the clinician when dealing with an elderly person. Contact with a doctor, either in the hospital or at home, can be stressful and confusing for many elderly people. Reassurance and a careful explanation of any procedures must be given. The format of the clinical assessment does not differ from that used for young patients but there are certain aspects of the history taking and physical examination that require special consideration.

### The history

The best history is always that obtained from the patient. While ideally they should be allowed to give their history without interruption it is often necessary, by direct questioning, to steer the conversation along pertinent lines. Communication problems can arise in patients who are deaf or dysphasic. Perseverance, though time consuming, is generally the best approach. Deaf people can often lip-read so they should be faced and spoken to slowly in simple but adult language. Hearing aids should be worn and be in good

working order. Communication aids, such as pen and paper, visual aids and voice amplifiers, can be used when appropriate.

Patients with an acute or chronic confusional state may not give a reliable history, so any information obtained needs to be verified. This should usually be from whoever knows the patient best. It may be necessary to see the spouse, another relative, neighbour, friend, clergyman, etc. in order to get an accurate history. Interviewing a third party should be undertaken in person and at the time when the patient is first seen. If this is not practicable, then efforts should be made to get the information as soon as possible by any available means. A telephone conversation, though not ideal, is better than nothing. Old clinical notes giving details of the past medical history and the previous condition of the patient are often invaluable, especially if they can be obtained quickly.

As elderly patients tire easily it may be useful to combine part of the history taking with the physical examination. For example, while examining the abdomen it may be possible, by chatting to the patient, to get valuable insight into the social history. This may have the added advantage of allowing a tense patient to relax the abdominal musculature.

Several points in the history require emphasis, as are described in the next subsections.

### Presenting complaint

As already indicated, vague symptoms, such as funny turns, dizziness, feeling generally unwell or 'gone off her feet', may be due to an underlying medical condition such as a myocardial infarction. All reported symptoms must be taken seriously and the circumstances surrounding their presentation should be explored.

### Social history

In addition to recording the patient's marital status, it is important to know with whom the patient lives. If accommodation is shared or rented, who owns the dwelling? A brief description of the property is important. How many storeys are there? Does the patient have a problem getting to the front door? Where are the toilet and bathroom and are these readily accessible?

Facts about the patient's community support

services must be obtained. Are there relatives in regular contact? Are the neighbours friendly and helpful? Do voluntary or religious organizations give help? Does the patient have 'meals on wheels' or a home help and if so, how many times each week? Does the person attend a day centre or a day hospital? Does he or she have any community nursing services?

It is essential to know how the patient copes with the activities of daily living. Are there difficulties with getting about the house, dressing, washing, using the toilet, cooking, shopping or doing essential housework? How are any difficulties overcome? What hobbies or interests does the person have? Are there any household pets?

Does the patient smoke or drink? Remember that alcohol abuse is not uncommon in the elderly.

Although it will not be necessary to document all this information for every elderly person it will be found to be relevant in most cases. However, with practice, gathering this information is not time consuming and it can be postponed to a later time if the patient is extremely ill.

### Drug history

A significant proportion of ill health in the elderly is drug induced. Many old people take multiple combinations of inappropriate or unnecessary drugs. Patients must be asked about all preparations being taken, their dosage and duration of treatment. It may be useful to know the initial indication for the treatment, as people may continue to take drugs that were originally intended for only a short period of time. The use of products that are particularly liable to cause toxicity in the elderly (e.g. digoxin, diuretics and hypnotics) should be specifically asked about.

Remember to ask about topical preparations (including eye drops) and injections, as elderly people often forget to mention these. A history of a drug allergy is as relevant in the elderly as in younger patients and must always be asked for.

### Psychiatric history

Psychiatric disorders are a common cause of morbidity in the elderly and symptoms should be looked for. Depression, in particular, is often overlooked unless the patient is asked about worries, episodes of tearfulness, sleep disturbance or loss of appetite. People vary in their sleep requirements but the important point is that sleep should be restful and refreshing. Enquiry should be made regarding recent bereavements, including the loss of pets.

If the patient is confused it is essential to clarify the approximate duration of this state. As a rule of thumb, less than three months suggests an acute confusional state and a longer period suggests dementia. If confused, an assessment of the mental state must be carried out by means of a simple questionnaire. The following has come into common usage:

(a) the patient's age;
(b) time of day (to nearest hour);
(c) year;
(d) recall of address (42 West Street);
(e) name of institution;
(f) recognition of a person (e.g., doctor, nurse);
(g) date of birth;
(h) dates of First World War;
(i) name of Prime Minister;
(j) count from 20 to 1.

Four or more inaccuracies indicate significant cognitive impairment.

### Review of systems

As mentioned earlier, elderly people tend to be stoical and to regard disease symptoms as part of growing old. Reluctance to report symptoms must be anticipated and therefore the systems review has to be thorough. The basic format has already been described but certain points require emphasis.

In reviewing the *respiratory system* remember to ask for a history of cough. Elderly people may have had chronic bronchitis for so many years that they regard their cough as unimportant. In the *cardiovascular system*, peripheral oedema is a common symptom and is more often due to hypostasis and venous insufficiency rather than cardiac disease.

In reviewing the *alimentary system*, enquire whether the patient wears dentures and if they fit properly. Are there problems with chewing due to other factors such as a facial palsy? A brief dietary assessment may be valuable. How many meals does the patient have each day and how much is generally eaten? How often is a cooked meal prepared? How often are meat, fresh fruit and vegetables eaten? Ask about bowel function, as diarrhoea and especially constipation are common problems which can cause much distress.

When asking questions relating to the *urinary system* enquire about urinary frequency, nocturia and incontinence. The circumstances surrounding episodes of incontinence must be explored. Immobility rather than urinary tract dysfunction can cause incontinence when the person is unable to get to the toilet on time. Prostatism is very common in elderly males and surgical resection is indicated if the history suggests that it is causing the patient significant discomfort or disability.

Review of the *nervous system* should include an assessment of the special senses. Is vision impaired and if so to what extent? Does the patient collide with objects? Are there problems reading books or newspapers or watching the television? Can normal conversational voices be heard?

## The physical examination

The basic approach to the physical examination is the same for all age groups. Each system of the body must be examined properly using a well-practised routine so that no physical signs are missed. However, in the elderly, frailty, immobility and confusion can cause lack of cooperation. Examination of the abdomen and the nervous system is particularly difficult if the person is apprehensive and time spent reassuring the patient will be well rewarded.

The physical examination begins as the patient enters the consultation room, even before the history taking. Watch how he or she walks from the door to the chair. Is a stick or a walking frame used and how dependent on this does the patient appear? Are there any abnormalities of gait? Later, as he or she moves from the chair to the examination couch, note any difficulties encountered in rising from the chair. Such difficulties may be due to arthritis of the hips or knees, polymyalgia rheumatica, proximal myopathy or wasting of the quadriceps muscles. Note the ease with which the patient gets onto the examination couch and any difficulties with undressing. At least initially he or she should undress unaided. Are there problems with raising the arms above the head? Can buttons be unfastened easily? Are there difficulties with removing shoes or stockings? In this way a functional assessment is also made as part of the physical examination.

Some parts of the physical examination require special emphasis in the case of the elderly patient; these are detailed in the next subsections.

## General appearance

Look at the general appearance and at the state of dress. Many debilitating disorders prevent people from washing and grooming themselves. If the patient is unkempt does he or she appear to be aware of this? Lack of concern may indicate dementia or depression. Is the male patient clean-shaven or is the facial hair well groomed? Is there any evidence of infestations? Are the finger nails and toe nails short and clean? Is there a smell of urine, which suggests a problem with continence? Generalized hair loss is common and does not necessarily signify an endocrine disorder.

## Nutritional status

All patients should have their weight recorded. This is a good indicator of nutritional status, especially when interpreted with the height. Furthermore, serial weights taken over a period of time give valuable information regarding the person's general health. A progressive and significant loss of weight usually indicates an underlying disease. Inspection of the patient even when dressed can reveal evidence of weight loss as the clothing and rings may be loose. When undressed, inspection may reveal evidence of protein and calorie malnutrition. In addition to looking thin there may be lax skin folds, particularly on the abdominal wall, due to the loss of subcutaneous fat, and this can cause difficulty when assessing the degree of hydration.

If the patient is obviously undernourished look for evidence of deficiency syndromes. A scorbutic rash is occasionally seen, usually over the buttocks and calves. Soft gums that bleed easily are further evidence of vitamin C deficiency. A magenta-coloured tongue is classically seen in riboflavin deficiency while an atrophic glossitis together with a lemon-yellow skin discoloration characterizes vitamin $B_{12}$ deficiency. Iron deficiency is the commonest deficiency syndrome found in the elderly and it clinically manifests as angular stomatitis, a depapillated tongue and occasionally koilonychia. Obesity is another nutritional disorder that should be recorded and, when present, conditions such as hypothyroidism must be considered.

## The cardiovascular system

As people age certain physiological changes occur in the heart and vascular tree that result in impaired cardiovascular performance. This is particularly seen when the elderly person is 'stressed'. In addition, compensatory mechanisms that should maintain cardiovascular function can be impaired. Ventricular compliance is reduced due to deposition of collagen and fibrous tissue in the cardiac muscle. This, together with a decreased diastolic phase of ventricular contraction, results in a diminished cardiac output and can cause cyanosis and cold extremities. The conducting system is impaired due to the deposition of fibrous tissue and results in a decreased maximal heart rate. Heart valves become progressively thickened and more rigid and the arterial tree loses some of its compliance. The net result on blood pressure is an elevation in the systolic component. However, diastolic pressure does not alter significantly with age.

Postural hypotension is common in the elderly, resulting from impaired baroreceptor function. An acute drop in venous return to the heart fails to trigger the compensatory increase in heart rate found in younger people and blood pressure falls. It is therefore important to measure blood pressure both in the supine and standing positions. A postural drop in blood pressure may be asymptomatic but become suddenly symptomatic if exacerbated by diuretic therapy.

As a result of these physiological changes some findings that are abnormal in younger subjects may have no pathological significance in the elderly patient. Thus, on auscultation of the heart, an S4 gallop rhythm in the absence of other features of cardiac failure can be attributed to a physiological reduction in ventricular compliance. Similarly, an apical systolic bruit is more often due to physiological thickening of the valve than to true mitral valve disease. An aortic ejection systolic bruit is more likely to be due to aortic sclerosis than to stenosis, especially if the other manifestations of aortic stenosis are absent. Other physical signs are so frequently found in the elderly that their presence can be accepted as normal. One such example is arcus senilis, which seldom indicates hyperlipidaemia.

Examination of the cardiovascular system must be systematic and thorough. Examination of the pulses should include an assessment of the degree of atherosclerosis in the vessel wall. This is best appreciated by performing Osler's manoeuvre. The radial artery is compressed proximally to obliterate the pulsation. If the vessel wall is palpable by rolling the finger over it, then this indicates arteriosclerosis. This manoeuvre can help to differentiate between genuine and spuriously high readings of systolic BP. All the peripheral pulses, including the femoral, popliteal, dorsalis pedis and posterior tibial pulses, should be examined, though in the elderly the latter may be difficult to feel. Look for arterial stenosis by auscultating for bruits over the carotids, abdominal aorta, renal and femoral vessels. The apex beat may be hard to feel and if displaced can be due either to kyphosis of the thoracic spine or true cardiac enlargement. Remember to palpate the abdominal aorta for aneurysmal dilatation.

### The respiratory system

Physiological changes in the ageing respiratory system involve both the lung and the chest wall. The elastic recoil of the lung diminishes, resulting in a decreased vital capacity and peak expiratory flow rate. This is exacerbated by increasing stiffness of the chest wall and a tendency to kyphoscoliosis. In addition, morphological changes in the alveoli together with a reduction in the capillary bed result in decreased oxygen transfer to the blood. However, this may not be noted in a relatively healthy older person until they are 'stressed'. Furthermore, a reduction in the number and function of cilia lining the bronchial tree impairs the ability of the lung to remove inhaled particles. Again, these physiological changes may lead to physical signs of no pathological significance. For example, scattered basal crackles found on auscultation are unlikely to be of importance in the absence of other signs of chest or cardiac disease.

Physical examination of the chest does not differ from that of younger patients though the thoracic spine should be examined for curvatures and the extent to which this appears to compromise chest expansion should be assessed. An increase in the respiratory rate suggests active lung disease. Many older patients have been habitual cigarette smokers and evidence of chronic obstructive airway disease is commonly seen.

### The alimentary system

Inspection of the mouth is of particular relevance in the elderly. Does the person have natural teeth and what are their condition? If dentures are worn do they occlude properly? Is there any gingival or mucosal ulceration? The absence of bowel sounds suggests an acute abdomen even without the other signs of tenderness and guarding. The hernial orifices should be examined and a rectal examination must *always* be performed. Unless this is done, pelvic, prostatic and rectal pathology, including faecal impaction, will frequently be missed.

### The genito-urinary system

Diseases of this system are particularly prevalent in the older patient and may be asymptomatic. Chronic urinary retention is often painless and it is surprising how frequently a palpable bladder is found on routine examination. The kidneys should be palpated and the external genitalia inspected.

The testes usually become harder and smaller with age. In the female patient a vaginal examination may be necessary as both a uterine prolapse and atrophic vaginitis can cause urinary incontinence. A bimanual examination, if indicated, may reveal a pelvic tumour.

### The nervous system

Lack of cooperation on the patient's part may make the evaluation of muscle tone, power, reflexes, sensation and coordination extremely difficult. Some physical signs that would be considered abnormal in younger patients can be accepted in the elderly so long as any possible underlying causes have been considered and excluded. Thus diminished sensation in the lower limbs, particularly involving the modalities of proprioception and vibration, is commonly seen. Abdominal reflexes and ankle jerks are often absent though the latter, as in younger patients, should prompt a search for conditions causing peripheral neuropathy. Constricted and irregular pupils that have lost their ability to constrict further with convergence may be seen and upward, conjugate deviation of the eyes can be impaired. Cataracts are common and lead to difficulty when examining the fundi. Wasting of the small muscles of the hands is much more likely to be due to osteoarthritis than to motor neurone disease.

Evidence of diseases that are particularly common in the elderly should be looked for. Signs of Parkinson's disease are often missed, especially if they are unilateral or predominantly characterized by bradykinesia. In most of these patients a careful clinical assessment will usually show evidence of tremor and dystonia, though sometimes these are absent. Assessment of the gait should never be neglected. The patient should be asked to walk in a straight line and to turn around. In addition to giving diagnostic information it allows for a further functional assessment of the patient. An elderly person who has significantly impaired mobility is likely, sooner or later, to become dependent on others. Romberg's test is used to assess balance.

If there are features in the history to suggest a dementing process then the signs of re-emergence of the primitive reflexes may be present. These include:

(1) *The palmomental reflex.* By stroking the palm an ipsilateral contraction of the facial muscles is elicited.
(2) *The snout* or *snarl reflex.* Lightly tapping the skin over the angle of the mouth causes contraction of the ipsilateral facial muscles.
(3) *The sucking reflex.* Continuous stimulation of the skin over the angle of the mouth results in a sucking or pouting action of the mouth.
(4) *The grasp reflex.* Firm pressure across the palm from the ulnar to the radial side causes the fingers to clasp. This is particularly found with involvement of the frontal lobes.

### The musculoskeletal system

Muscle strength declines with age due to muscle atrophy and an increase in fibrous tissue. Bone disorders such as osteoporosis and osteomalacia are found almost exclusively in the elderly population. In addition, about 80 per cent of people reaching retirement age have a rheumatological complaint and this emphasizes the importance of a careful examination of the musculoskeletal system in the older patient.

In assessing muscle strength it is important to compare each muscle group with that on the opposite side of the body. Asymmetrical muscle weakness points to either local disease, a neurological disorder or a localized myopathic disorder. Each joint should be put through its full range of movement, both actively and passively. Again, it is important to make a functional assessment. In a patient with rheumatoid arthritis of the hand it is as important to know how he or she writes with a pen or raises a cup to the lips as it is to note the physical manifestations of the disease.

### The special senses

Eye disorders are particularly common in the elderly and visual impairment is one of the important causes of loss of independence. Inspection of the eye and of the optic fundus is essential, though the latter is sometimes difficult to see clearly. Visual acuity and visual fields should also be tested. In addition to yielding information on local eye disease, such as cataract, macular degeneration or glaucoma, evidence of systemic disease may also be found—examples being diabetic retinopathy or ischaemic optic neuropathy due to temporal arteritis.

The majority of elderly people have some degree of hearing loss. Auditory acuity should be assessed and the auditory canal inspected. Often deafness is due to easily treated conditions, such as occlusion of the auditory canal by wax.

## DIFFERENTIAL DIAGNOSIS IN THE ELDERLY

Many medical conditions occur in both the young and the old. However, in general, the genetic and autoimmune disorders become less prevalent with advancing age while the degenerative and neoplastic diseases become more prevalent. Multiple pathology is much more common in the elderly than a single diagnosis. Table 17.1 lists some of the conditions that are more common in the elderly.

Accidental hypothermia (core temperature below 35°C) is particularly common during the winter months and can be precipitated by alcohol,

**Table 17.1 Conditions that are more common in the elderly**

Ischaemic heart disease
Peripheral vascular disease
Cerebrovascular disease
Bronchopneumonia
Malignant disease
Constipation
Incontinence
Immobility
Parkinson's disease
Osteoarthrosis
Diabetes mellitus
Anaemia
Osteoporosis
Hypothermia
Polymyalgia rheumatica
Confusion (acute, chronic)

drugs (hypnotics and phenothiazines), myxoedema and, most importantly, by a cold environment. Many old people are unable to afford adequate heating and clothing.

## INVESTIGATION AND TREATMENT OF THE ELDERLY PATIENT

Work pioneered by Dr Marjorie Warren in the late 1940s confirmed that illnesses in the elderly should be properly investigated because accurate diagnosis made possible effective treatment and management. Since that time the advances in diagnostic and therapeutic technology have benefited the elderly as they have all age groups.

It is essential to remember that age itself is no barrier to performing diagnostic and therapeutic procedures. Biological age does not always reflect chronological age and many people remain fit and active into their ninth decade and well beyond, while others have prematurely aged before reaching retirement.

### Investigation

The practice of performing a range of 'screening' investigations in the elderly hospitalized patient has now gained widespread acceptance. This reflects the frequency with which unexpected but treatable abnormalities are found. Table 17.2 shows the 'routine' investigations that are commonly performed on admission to hospital. Other haematological, biochemical, bacteriological and radiological investigations should be requested as indicated (see Chapters 4 and 5).

The normal ranges quoted by laboratories are usually compiled from information gathered from

**Table 17.2 'Screening' investigations recommended for elderly patients**

Full blood count
Erythrocyte sedimentation rate
Plasma urea and electrolytes
Blood glucose
Serum calcium, phosphate and alkaline phosphate
Serum protein and liver function tests
Thyroid function tests
Chest X-ray
Electrocardiograph

younger people and therefore may not apply to the elderly. Thus a mildly elevated plasma urea in a well-hydrated patient usually reflects an age-related deterioration in renal function rather than active renal disease. Table 17.3 shows the laboratory values that are altered in the elderly.

Specialized investigations, such as ultrasonography, bone marrow aspiration, tissue biopsy, bronchoscopy, gastroscopy, colonoscopy, barium examinations of the upper and lower gastrointestinal tract and other radiological procedures, are generally well tolerated by the elderly. In fact, if any investigation is likely to supply information that will benefit the patient in either their short-term or long-term management then it is warranted. However, the hazards of any invasive test should always be considered and the nature and indication for any proposed investigation must always be discussed with the patient and informed consent obtained. Should the patient be incapable of giving consent, the wishes of the next of kin should be taken into account provided one is happy that they are acting in the patient's best interest.

Sometimes an investigation is appropriate, even if curable disease is unlikely to be found. An example is a patient who presents with a slowly progressive hemiplegia that could be due to a stroke or to a cerebral neoplasm. A CT brain scan, if it clarifies the cause, can help plan the further management of the patient and in counselling the family.

Basic investigations should be arranged from the general practitioner's surgery, hospital outpatient department or day hospital wherever possible because admission to hospital is not only expensive but stressful for many elderly people. Obviously, admission is essential for acutely ill patients or those requiring more extensive and sophisticated investigation.

**Treatment**

Treatment should be aimed first at the most serious conditions affecting the patient's health. However, remember that every drug is potentially harmful and multiple drug therapy carries unique hazards for the elderly patient. Iatrogenic illness is a major problem, often attributable to the over-prescribing of combinations of inappropriate drugs. The elderly patient commonly requires smaller doses of drugs than the younger one because of decreased renal excretion. Failure to realize this can lead to the accumulation of the drug and toxicity. Digoxin, diuretics, hypnotics and anticoagulants are examples of drugs that commonly cause adverse reactions. As complex drug regimens are confusing to the patient and can lead to accidental self-poisoning it is important that as few drugs as possible are prescribed. Time spent counselling the patient about the drugs, the use of simple written instructions and ensuring supervision of the medication wherever possible are efforts that will be well rewarded. All drug regimens must be reviewed regularly and routine 'repeat prescriptions' should never be allowed. The management of disability and the attainment of optimum domestic function is the role of the rehabilitation team.

With advances in anaesthetic and, to a lesser extent, in surgical skills the results of surgery in the elderly continue to improve. The quality of life has been dramatically improved for many following ophthalmic, orthopaedic, urological and other surgical procedures. However, considerable skill is often required in deciding when surgical intervention will benefit the individual patient. Postoperatively, adequate analgesia and early mobilization are important. Increasingly the surgeon and the geriatrician are combining their expertise and sharing postoperative care.

So far, this chapter has emphasized the importance of a positive approach to elderly people. This does not mean that all elderly people require extensive investigation and treatment. A complete cure is not always a realistic goal but most can be helped to live as normal a life as possible. When some degree of disability is inevitable, the aim of treatment is then to relieve symptoms and to ensure adequate rehabilitation.

Not surprisingly, the care of the terminally ill

**Table 17.3 'Normal ranges' in the elderly compared with standard ranges**

| Normal range increased | Normal range unchanged | Normal range decreased |
| --- | --- | --- |
| ESR | Haemoglobin | White cell count |
| Urea, creatinine | Platelet count | Iron, TIBC |
| Prothrombin time | Sodium | Serum T3 |
| Uric acid | Potassium | |
| Calcium | Chloride | |
| Alkaline | Bicarbonate | |
|   phosphatase | Bilirubin, AST | |
| | Thyroxine | |

patient is frequently the responsibility of those caring for the elderly. It is important to recognize when someone is unlikely to benefit from further diagnostic and therapeutic intervention. Death should be regarded as a natural process and not an incurable disease. So, irrespective of the age of the patient, it is important to know when to move from a 'cure' to a 'care' approach. A full discussion of this important topic is outside the scope of this chapter.

## THE 'GERIATRIC GIANTS'

Certain problems present themselves with such regularity in sick elderly people that they have assumed special significance. Isaacs has highlighted the importance of intellectual impairment, incontinence, instability and immobility and has termed these the 'Geriatric Giants'.

Almost any condition that can cause an elderly person to be ill can result in an acute confusional state (delirium). The long litany of possible causes includes disorders such as pneumonia, urinary tract infection, myocardial infarction, a malignancy, electrolyte disturbances (hyponatraemia, uraemia, etc.,) and faecal impaction. The side-effects of drug therapy are an especially important cause. Often the acutely confused elderly person will be made worse by having to adjust to a strange, hospital environment. Some patients will already have a degree of underlying chronic intellectual impairment (dementia), which is then exacerbated by the intercurrent disease. Other important predisposing factors are impaired hearing and vision, together with increasing age.

Dementia is usually due to Alzheimer's disease but multiple small cerebral infarcts also have a cumulative effect on intellectual function and are another important cause of dementia. It is usually possible to separate the two conditions on clinical grounds. With senile dementia of the Alzheimer's type (SDAT), a progressive deterioration in intellectual ability occurs whereas with multi-infarct dementia (MID) the deterioration is step-wise, each sudden deterioration coinciding with a small stroke. A CT brain scan can also help to differentiate these two conditions. With SDAT, cortical atrophy is apparent, whereas with MID, discrete infarcts within the brain parenchyma may be seen. In addition the two conditions can coexist. Unfortunately, once established, both of these conditions are irreversible.

Dementia can occasionally be a result of a treatable disease, such as vitamin $B_{12}$ deficiency, hypothyroidism, a chronic subdural brain haemorrhage or normal pressure hydrocephalus. If these conditions are suspected on clinical grounds, then the appropriate investigation and treatment is mandatory and the results of treatment can sometimes be gratifying.

Urinary incontinence of recent onset is often another nonspecific indicator of an underlying condition. Local disorders should be looked for, such as an acute urinary tract infection. Bladder outflow obstruction resulting from prostatic hyperplasia or carcinoma can result in urinary retention with overflow incontinence.

Alternatively the incontinence can reflect a systemic disease. Any condition that impairs cerebral function can cause the loss of the cerebral control of reflex bladder emptying. Thus urinary incontinence can accompany acute confusional states and resolve as the confusion improves. Drugs are again an important cause of incontinence, particularly diuretics. Other causes of urinary incontinence are uterine prolapse and atrophic vaginitis.

Faecal incontinence can be due to either faecal impaction or to cerebral impairment. Faecal impaction causes chronic faecal soiling and is managed by disimpaction and by keeping the stools soft. When due to brain failure a regular toileting regimen can be established with the help of suppositories.

A history of recurring falls in old people often heralds severe medical breakdown. They can result in serious morbidity, such as fractures, and can cause an elderly person to lose confidence and to become progressively less mobile. While increasing instability occurs with increasing age, falls are usually attributable to acquired disorders. Environmental hazards both inside (loose rugs) and outside (uneven pavements) the home can cause the elderly to trip over. Endogenous factors are of even greater importance and these include those disorders that impair mobility and vision.

Again, the aetiological role of drug therapy needs emphasis. The sedative agents and alcohol are particularly important. Some 20 per cent of falls are associated with a syncopal episode. Syncope can be due to cardiovascular disorders, such as arrhythmias and postural hypotension, or to neurological disorders, such as cerebral ischaemia and fits.

The causes of impaired mobility include a variety of neurological and locomotor lesions. Joint disease is a particular problem among old people with osteoarthritis affecting the weight-bearing joints in the legs and spine. Neurological causes include strokes, Parkinson's disease, motor neurone disease, multiple sclerosis and cerebellar disorders. Locomotor and neurological dysfunction often coexist and the cause of impaired mobility in any old person can seldom be attributed to a single disorder.

## THE PROVISION OF SERVICES FOR THE ELDERLY

At any given time about 94 per cent of the elderly population in this country is living in the community (in their own homes or in sheltered housing), either with a spouse, alone, with their children or with others. The remainder are either in hospital (1–2 per cent in long-stay geriatric or psychogeriatric wards) or in other institutions in the community (4–5 per cent in local authority residential homes, private residential or private nursing homes).

For patients of all ages the function of a hospital is to diagnose disease, to cure when possible and to minimize residual disability in non-reversible conditions. Modern departments of geriatric medicine have radically altered the medical care of the elderly. They have developed expertise in the management of older people, who usually present with multiple problems that involve a combination of acute and chronic conditions.

Most geriatric departments now have beds in the district general hospital for acute assessment and rehabilitation. There are usually additional beds in peripheral hospitals for 'slow-stream' rehabilitation and continuing care. Most departments run an age-related service, accepting as many acutely ill elderly patients as possible (the lower age limit varies from 65 to 75 years in different departments). It would be ideal for all elderly patients to be admitted directly to acute geriatric beds but the vast numbers now make this impossible and it is inevitable that general medical intakes will include elderly people.

The geriatric assessment wards have easy access to all the diagnostic facilities and the other specialist departments within the hospital. The average length of stay is about 18 days. These wards also benefit from the services provided by the paramedical professions. Any acute illness or period of enforced bedrest in an elderly person may considerably impair their mobility. This can usually be minimized by a policy of early mobilization. However, for some patients a longer period of rehabilitation will often be required to enable them to return to their previous level of independence. It is then usual to transfer them to a rehabilitation ward, where all the members of the multidisciplinary team (Fig. 17.2) work together under the direction of the geriatrician. They help to restore impaired function and to teach the patient how to adapt to any residual disability. The progress of the patients and the plans for their future management are discussed at regular weekly meetings. Particular attention is paid to the social requirements (home help, 'meals on wheels', day-centre care, etc.) following discharge as well as to the patient's home environment and the need for aids or adaptations.

The patient's discharge plan should be formulated as soon after admission as possible to prevent unnecessary delay at the time of discharge. The community liaison nurse and the social worker coordinate the efforts of the hospital staff and the primary health care teams to ensure a smooth discharge. A home assessment by the occupational therapist (occasionally accompanied by the social worker or the physiotherapist) is usually arranged before discharge where there is concern as to whether the patient will be able to manage at home. The support available from the family, friends and neighbours is assessed and often the voluntary organizations are asked to provide support in addition to the community services available from the statutory bodies (Fig. 17.3). The majority of elderly patients admitted to hospital are discharged back to their homes. Attendance at the day hospital is often arranged in order to continue the rehabilitation programme. Every geriatric department has a few beds set aside for respite care so that relatives of very dependent patients can have a 'holiday'. Only a very small number of patients are considered for longer term care either in Part 3 accommodation, a nursing home or a continuing care hospital.

The same principles of care apply to elderly patients admitted to the general medical wards. Early mobilization, the use of the multidisciplinary team and, when necessary, referral to the department of geriatric medicine will ensure a speedy and successful return home.

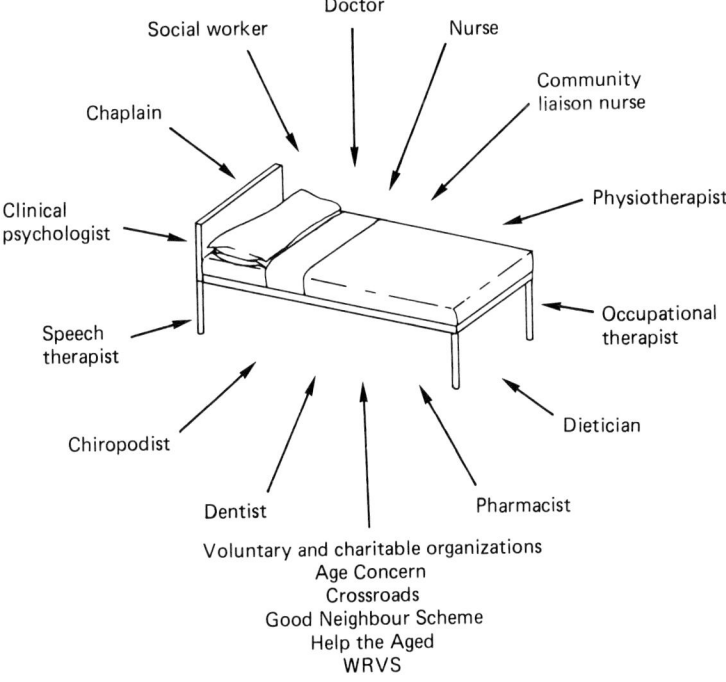

Figure 17.2   Care team for the elderly patient in hospital.

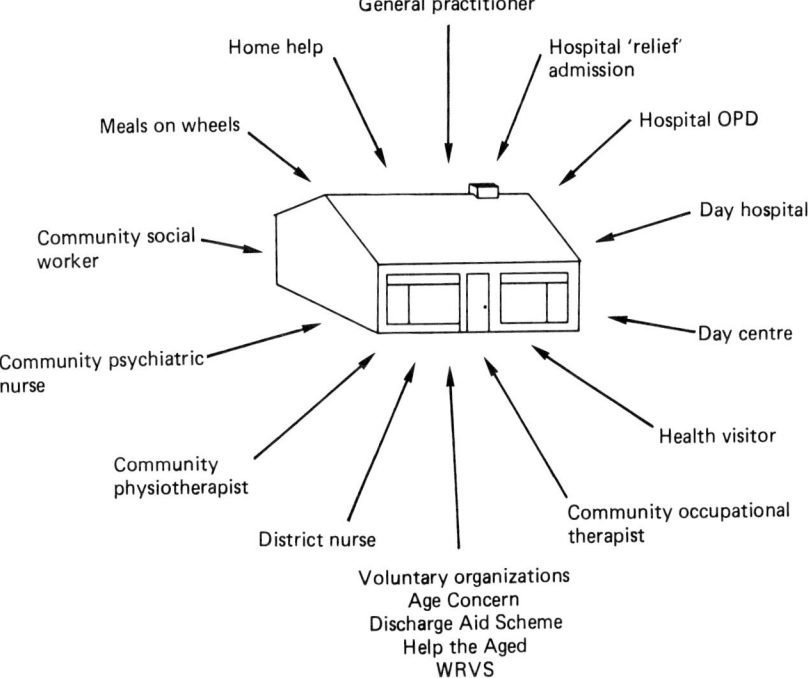

Figure 17.3   Support for the elderly disabled and their carers at home.

Whatever commitment there may be to exclusive specialties in the future, whatever prompts divorce and reconciliation between geriatricians and 'special interest physicians', the fact will remain that all doctors of the future will need education early in their careers if they are to provide a better and more positive approach to old people.

(M. Keith Thompson, 1984)

## Further reading

Arie T. (1981). *Health Care of the Elderly*. London: Croom Helm.

Coni N., Davison W., Webster S. (1977). *Lecture Notes on Geriatrics*. Oxford: Blackwell Scientific.

Hall M. R. P., MacLennan W. J., Lye M. D. W. (1978). *Medical Care of the Elderly*. Chichester: John Wiley.

Kafetz K. M. (1986). *Clinical Tests in Geriatric Medicine*. London: Wolfe Medical.

Pathy M. S. J., Finucane P., eds. (1989). *Geriatric Medicine—Problems and Practice*. Heidelberg: Springer-Verlag.

Thompson M. K. (1984). *Care of the Elderly in General Practice*. Edinburgh: Churchill Livingstone.

# APPENDIX

Normal values

*Serum or plasma*

| | |
|---|---|
| Acid phosphatase: | |
| total | 1–5 iu/lit |
| prostatic | 0–1 iu/lit |
| ACTH | <10–80 mg/l |
| Alkaline phosphatase | 30–115 iu/l |
| Alanine aminotransferase | 5–35 iu/l |
| Amylase | 70–300 iu/l |
| Aspartate aminotransferase | 5–45 iu/l |
| Bicarbonate | 22–30 mmol/l |
| Bilirubin | <17 fmol/l |
| Calcium | 2.26–2.60 mmol/l |
| Chloride | 95–105 mmol/l |
| Cholesterol | <5.7 mmol/l |
| Complement: | |
| C3 | 0.69–1.5 mg/l |
| C4 | 0.12–0.27 mg/l |
| Cortisol: | |
| midnight | 80–320 nmol/l |
| 9.00 a.m. | 280–700 nmol/l |
| Creatinine | 70–150 fmol/l |
| Creatine phosphokinase | <200 iu/l |
| α-fetoprotein | <10 ku/l |
| γ-glutamyl transferase: | |
| men | 11–51 iu/lit |
| women | 7–33 iu/lit |
| Glucose (fasting) | 4.5–6.0 mmol/l |
| Growth hormone | <20 mu/l |
| Immunoglobulins: | |
| IgG | 6–13 g/l |
| IgM | 0.5–2.0 g/l |
| IgA | 1.0–4.0 g/l |
| Lactate dehydrogenase | 240–525 iu/l |
| Magnesium | 0.7–1.0 mmol/l |
| Osmolality | 275–300 mosmol/kg |
| Phosphate (inorganic) | 0.8–1.4 mmol/l |
| Potassium | 3.4–5.2 mmol/l |
| Prolactin | male 450 |
| | female 600 |

Protein:
   total                                      60–80 g/l
   albumin                            33–50 g/l
Sodium                                    133–145/l

Thyroxine:
   total                                      70–140 nmol/l
   free $T_4$                            9–20 pmol/l
Tri-iodothyronine                1.2–3.0 nmol/l
TSH                                       <6 mu/l
Triglycerides                     <0.55–1.90 mmol/l
Urea                                     2.5–7.5 mmol/l
Uric acid:
   men                                     0.15–0.42 mmol/l
   women                            0.10–0.36 mmol/l

*Arterial blood gases*
pH                                        7.35–7.45
$P_{CO_2}$                                35–45 mmHg (4.6–6.0 k$Pa$)
$P_{O_2}$                                95–105 mmHg (10.6–14.0 k$Pa$)
Base excess                       +2.0 mmol/l
*Urine*
Cortisol                                  <280 nmol/24h
Creatinine clearance:
   men                                     90–140 ml/m
   women                            80–125 ml/m
5-hydroxyindole acetic acid       16–73 fmol/24 h
Hydroxymethylmandelic acid      16–48 fmol/24 h
$\beta_2$-microglobulin                4–370 µg/l
Osmolality                         30–370 fg/24 h
                                         350–1000 mosmol/kg
Oxalate                                  <450 fmol/24 h
24 h protein                         <150 mg
   (pregnancy)                  <300 mg
*Cerebrospinal fluid*
Pressure                               80–180 mm $H_2O$
Protein                                  <0.4 g/l
Glucose                               2.2–3.8 mmol/l (1.5–2.0 mmol/l <blood)
*Haematology*
Haemoglobin:
   men                                      13.5–18.0 g/100 ml
   women                            11.5–16.5 g/100 ml
Red cell count:
   men                                     $4.5–6.5 \times 10^{12}$/l
   women                            $3.8–5.8 \times 10^{12}$/l
Packed cell volume:
   men                                     0.4–0.54
   women                            0.37–0.47
Mean corpuscular haemoglobin     27–32 pg
Mean corpuscular volume         77–93 fl
Mean corpuscular haemoglobin concentration     31–35 g/100 ml
Reticulocyte count                  0.2–2.0%
White cell count:
   Total                                     $4.0–11.0 \times 10^9$/l
   Neutrophils                     $2.0–7.5 \times 10^9$/l

| | |
|---|---|
| Lymphocytes | $1.5–4.0 \times 10^9/l$ |
| Monocytes | $0.2–0.8 \times 10^9/l$ |
| Eosinophils | $0.04–0.4 \times 10^9/l$ |
| Basophils | $<0.1 \times 10^9/l$ |
| Platelets | $150–400 \times 10^9/l$ |
| Serum $B_{12}$ | 160–925 ng/l |
| Folate: | |
|   serum | 3–20 µg/l |
|   red cell | 160–640 µg/l |
| Serum iron: | |
|   men | 14–32 µmol/l |
|   women | 10–30 µmol/l |
| Total iron binding capacity | 50–80 µmol/l |
| Ferritin | 12–250 ng/ml |
| Fibrinogen | 2.0–4.0 g/l |
| Bleeding time | <6 min |
| Fibrinogen degradation products | <0.8 fg/l |
| Thrombin time | 10–15 s |
| Prothrombin time | 10–14 s |
| Activated partial thromboplastin time | 35–40 s |
| Erythrocyte sedimentation rate | 0–10 mm (Higher values in healthy old people) |

# INDEX